The Routledge International Handbook of Psychosocial Resilience

Psychological resilience has emerged as a highly significant area of research and practice in recent years, finding applications with a broad range of different groups in many settings. Contemporary discourse is not limited to ways of effective coping with adversity but also introduces mechanisms that can lead to enhanced capacity after dealing with difficult circumstances and recognizes the importance of enriching the field with varied perspectives. *The Routledge International Handbook of Psychosocial Resilience* is a comprehensive compendium of writings of international contributors that takes stock of the state-of-the-art in resilience theory, research and practice.

The Routledge International Handbook of Psychosocial Resilience covers the many different trajectories that resilience research has taken in four parts. Section I delineates the **'Conceptual Arena'** by providing an overview of the current state of theory and research, exploring biological, psychological and socio-ecological perspectives and discussing various theoretical models of personal and social resilience. The **'Psychosocial Correlates'** of resilience are discussed further in Section II, from personal and personality correlates, socio-environmental factors and the contextual and cultural conditions conducive to resilient behaviour. In Section III, **'Applied Evidence'** is introduced in order to build upon the theoretical foundations in the form of several case studies drawn from varied contexts. Examples of resilient behaviour range from post-disaster scenarios to special operation groups, orphaned children and violent extremism. Finally, Section IV, **'Proposed Implications and Resilience Building'**, sums up the issues involved in discussing post-traumatic growth, well-being and positive adaptation in the varied contexts of personal, familial, organizational and societal resilience.

The volume provides a comprehensive overview of resilience theory, practice and research across disciplines and cultures, from varied perspectives and different populations. It will be a key reference for psychiatrists, psychologists, psychotherapists and psychiatric social workers in practice and in training as well as researchers and students of psychology, sociology, human development, family studies and disaster management.

Updesh Kumar, Ph.D., is Scientist 'G' and Head of the Mental Health Division at Defense Institute of Psychological Research (DIPR), R&D Organization (DRDO), Ministry of Defense, Delhi, India. His previous books include *Suicidal Behaviour: Underlying Dynamics* (Routledge, 2015), and he is the recipient of the DRDO's *Scientist of the Year Award,* granted by the Indian Government.

The Routledge
International Handbook
of Psychosocial Resilience

Edited by Updesh Kumar

Routledge
Taylor & Francis Group

LONDON AND NEW YORK

First published 2017
by Routledge
2 Park Square, Milton Park, Abingdon, Oxon OX14 4RN

and by Routledge
711 Third Avenue, New York, NY 10017

Routledge is an imprint of the Taylor & Francis Group, an informa business

British Library Cataloguing in Publication Data
A catalogue record for this book is available from the British Library
Library of Congress Cataloging-in-Publication Data
Names: Kumar, Updesh, editor.
Title: The Routledge international handbook of psychosocial resilience / edited by Updesh Kumar.
Description: 1 Edition. | New York : Routledge, 2016. | Includes bibliographical references and index.
Identifiers: LCCN 2016002741 (print) | LCCN 2016005946 (ebook) | ISBN 9781138954878 (hardback) | ISBN 9781315666716 (ebk) | ISBN 9781315666716 (ebook)Subjects: LCSH: Resilience (Personality trait) | Psychology.
Classification: LCC BF698.35.R47 .R68 2016 (print) | LCC BF698.35. R47 (ebook) | DDC 155.2/4—dc23
LC record available at http://lccn.loc.gov/2016002741

ISBN: 978-1-138-95487-8 (hbk)
ISBN: 978-1-315-66671-6 (ebk)

Typeset in Bembo
by Apex CoVantage, LLC

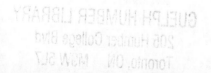

My wife Anju, son Kushal, and daughter Dakshi for their unconditional support and encouragement.

Contents

Contents

Contents

Figures

Tables

Chart

About the editor and contributors

The editor

Updesh Kumar, Ph.D., is Scientist 'G' and in the chair of the Head, Mental Health Division at Defense Institute of Psychological Research (DIPR), R&D Organization (DRDO), Ministry of Defense, Delhi. After obtaining his doctorate degree in the area of suicidal behaviour from Panjab University, Chandigarh, India, he has more than twenty-five years of experience as a Scientist in an R&D organization. He specializes in the area of personality assessment, suicidal behaviour and test development (Personality and Intelligence). Dr Kumar has been involved in the selection of officers and other ranks as well as responsible for monitoring the selection system of the Indian Armed Forces for the last twenty-four years. Dr Kumar has edited eight quality volumes including *Suicidal Behaviour: Assessment of People-at-Risk* (SAGE, 2010); *Countering Terrorism: Psychosocial Strategies* (SAGE, 2012); *Understanding Suicide Terrorism: Psychosocial Dynamics* (SAGE, 2014); *Suicidal Behaviour: Underlying Dynamics* (Routledge, 2015); *Positive Psychology: Applications in Work, Health and Well-being* (Pearson Education, 2015) and most recently *The Wiley Handbook of Personality Assessment* (John Wiley & Sons, 2016). Dr Kumar has also authored field manuals on *Suicide and Fratricide: Dynamics and Management* for defense personnel, *Managing Emotions in Daily Life & at Work Place* for general populations, *Overcoming Obsolescence & Becoming Creative in R&D Environment for R&D Organizations* and *Self-Help Techniques in Military Settings*. He has authored more than fifty other academic publications in the form of research papers, journal articles and book chapters and has represented his institute at the national and international levels. Dr Kumar has been a psychological assessor (Psychologist) in various Services Selection Boards for eight years for the selection of officers in the Indian Armed Forces and also on the selection panel with the prestigious Union Public Service Commission (UPSC), Government of India. He is a certified psychologist by The British Psychological Society with level 'A' and level 'B' Certificates of Competence in Occupational Testing. He has to his credit many important research projects including the project directorship of a mega project titled "Comprehensive Soldier Fitness Program: Resilience Building" for the Indian Armed Forces. He was conferred with the DRDO's Best Popular Science Communication Award–2009 by Hon'ble Defense Minister of India. He has also been the recipient of DRDO Technology Group Award in 2001, 2009 and 2015; the Professor Manju Thakur Memorial Award–2009 and 2012 by Indian Academy of Applied Psychology (IAAP); and the Professor N. N. Sen Best Paper Award for 2010 by the Indian Association of Clinical Psychologist (IACP). Recently, he has been conferred with Laboratory Scientist of the Year Award–2012–2013 and prestigious DRDO's Scientist of the Year Award–2013 by the Government of India.

The contributors

Gary A. Ackerman, Ph.D., is the Director of the Special Projects Division of the National Consortium for the Study of Terrorism and Responses to Terrorism (START) and is responsible for integrating and incubating innovative research programs. He is also the acting director of START's Unconventional Weapons and Technology Research Program, where he manages large research projects, explores new avenues for research and establishes collaborative research relationships. Prior to taking up his current positions, Ackerman held the post of Research Director at START and of Director of the Center for Terrorism and Intelligence Studies, a private research and analysis institute. He has also served as the Director of the Weapons of Mass Destruction Terrorism Research Program at the Center for Nonproliferation Studies in Monterey, Calif., and chief of operations of the South Africa-based African-Asian Society. Originally hailing from South Africa, Ackerman possesses an eclectic academic background, including past studies in the fields of mathematics, history, law and international relations. His research encompasses various areas relating to terrorism and counterterrorism, including terrorist threat assessment; motivations for using chemical, biological, radiological and nuclear (CBRN) weapons; radicalization; the relationship between terrorism and technology, and the modeling and simulation of terrorist behaviour. He is the co-editor of and contributing author to *Jihadists and Weapons of Mass Destruction* (CRC Press, 2009), is the author of several articles on terrorism-related subjects and has testified on terrorist motivations for using nuclear weapons before the Senate Committee on Homeland Security.

J. C. Ajawani, Ph.D., D. Lit., is the Head of Department of Psychology, Govt. Art's and Commerce Girls' College, Raipur (C.G.), India. He has been engaged in the teaching of psychology since 1975. His wide research interests include personality and applied psychology, and he is an expert in emotional and spiritual intelligence. He has seventy-three research papers published in international and national journals to his credit. He has presented 112 research papers in international and national seminars. So far, twenty-five Ph.D. degrees have been awarded to scholars, and five scholars are continuing their Ph.D. research under his guidance. He has completed three research projects sponsored by University Grants Commission, New Delhi, India, and presently is working on the "Identification of emotional intelligence correlates of stress resistance: Development of an intervention programme for adolescents" project, sponsored by the Chhattisgarh Council of Science and Technology. He has contributed chapters to three books. He is life member of various academic organizations and an International Affiliate of the American Psychological Association (APA). He constructed various psychological tests including emotional intelligence, spiritual intelligence etc. He also has developed emotional intelligence and spiritual intelligence training programmes. He is the editor of the *Journal of Psychology Applied to Life and Work*, published by the Chhattisgarh Academy of Applied Psychology, of whom he is the vice-president.

Lyle M. Allen III, M.A., has an A.B. Duke Scholarship, from Duke University and an M.A. in Clinical Psychology from Appalachian State University (ASU) in Boone, NC. In his early career he was engaged in outcome research at Duke University Medical Center and later became an entrepreneur and now pursues academic interests in retirement. Mr Allen holds three patents related to remotely administered dosage adjustment and was Principal Investigator or a key consultant on several National Institute of Health (NIH) and National Institute of Mental Health (NIMH) grants related to weight loss in diabetes, computer-assisted depression management, computer-assisted head injury self-management and physician-assisted remote semi-automated adjustment of medication for chronic diseases for diabetes and warfarin therapy. This later technology was acquired by Roche Diagnostics (RHHBY) and Alere (ALR). Mr Allen is the principal author of the Computerized Assessment of Response Bias and co-author of the Pain Assessment Battery (Eimer & Allen), Resourcefulness for Recovery Inventory (Celinski & Allen, rehabilitation psychology), Word Memory Test (Green, Allen & Astner), Psycho Assistant (Celinski & Allen) and other less well-known instruments. He is a co-recipient of the 2002 Nelson Butters Award from National Academy of Neuropsychology for best empirical paper of 2002 for work describing the relationship between depression, neuropsychological test performance and symptom validity (malingering) test results.

Shaima Y. Almahmoud is a Doctoral Researcher in the Clinical Psychology program at Kent State University. She holds a B.A. and an M.A. in general psychology from Kuwait University. She previously worked as a teaching assistant at Kuwait University and as a school counselor in public schools in the State of Kuwait. Currently, she has a graduate scholarship from Kuwait University for her doctoral program. For her master's research topic, she examined "Psychological Resilience in Adult Patients with Transfusion Dependent Thalassemia". Her research interests include emotion, health behaviour and chronic illnesses.

Archana, Ph.D., is Scientist 'E' at Defence Institute of Psychological Research and is associated with R&D activities in the areas of organizational behaviour, mental health and well-being of soldiers in the peace as well as field locations. She has to her credit a number of papers in the national journals of repute. She has authored two field manuals on *Stress Management* and *Psychological Well-Being of Soldiers at High Altitude*. In addition, she has made valuable contributions by organizing many workshops and seminars for the soldiers in the area of military psychology. She has been the course coordinator in organizing training programs for service officers in the area of counselling. She has also been actively involved in delivering lectures on stress management and other related areas in active field environments.

Reuven Bar-On has worked as a clinical and organizational psychologist for both public and private organizations since 1972. One of his primary areas of scholarly involvement has been in emotional and social intelligence, and he is acknowledged as one of the leading theorists, researchers and practitioners in this field today. The "Bar-On model of emotional intelligence" is described in the *Encyclopedia of Applied Psychology* as one of the three main approaches to this concept, and the term "EQ" was coined by him in 1985 to describe his approach to assessing it. He began developing the precursor to the *Emotional Quotient Inventory (EQ-i)* in 1980, which is the first measure of this concept to be published by a psychological test publisher. He developed or co-developed twelve additional psychometric instruments since 1978. The most recent psychological test that Dr Bar-On has developed is the *Multifactor Measure of Performance*, which measures the various aspects of his conceptual model of human behaviour, performance and well-being. Dr Bar-On has contributed over 50 publications to the professional literature, which have been cited nearly 8,000 times in articles, books, encyclopaedias and doctoral dissertations.

Paul T. Bartone, Ph.D., is Professor and Senior Research Fellow at the Center for Technology & National Security Policy, Institute for National Strategic Studies, National Defense University. Dr Bartone's research focuses on understanding and measuring resilient responding to stress and applying this knowledge to improve selection, training and leader development programs.

During his twenty-five years with the US Army, Bartone served as Commander of the US Army Medical Research Unit in Heidelberg, Research Psychology Consultant to the Surgeon General of the Army, and Medical Service Corps Assistant Corps Chief for Medical Allied Sciences. He taught leadership at the US Military Academy, West Point and at the National Defense University, Washington DC. A Fulbright scholar (Norway, 1996), Bartone is former President of the American Psychological Association's Society for Military Psychology, a Fellow of the American Psychological Association, a Fellow of the Inter-University Seminar on Armed Forces and Society and a charter member of the Association for Psychological Science. Dr Bartone holds an M.A. and Ph.D. in Psychology and Human Development from the University of Chicago.

Cara L. Blevins, is a Senior Doctoral Researcher in Clinical Health Psychology at The University of North Carolina, Charlotte (USA). She received her B.A. in Psychology from George Mason University in Fairfax, VA, and has held positions working for the US Army STRONG Bonds program and conducting military suicide prevention research at the Uniformed Services University of the Health Sciences in Bethesda, MD. She currently works under the mentorship of Dr Richard G. Tedeschi and the Posttraumatic Growth Research Group at UNCC and her research interests include biological outcomes and determinants of stress-reactivity and PTG in civilian and military populations, mindfulness and compassion. She is also interested in the biopsychosocial benefits of physical exercise and meditation, is a certified yoga instructor and enjoys teaching yoga and meditation to members of the community in Charlotte, NC.

Bruce Bongar, Ph.D., is the Calvin Distinguished Professor of Psychology, Palo Alto University, Consulting Professor of Psychiatry and the Behavioral Sciences, Stanford University School of Medicine. Dr Bongar received his Ph.D. from the University of Southern California and served his internship in clinical community psychology with the Los Angeles County Department of Mental Health. Past clinical appointments include service as a senior clinical psychologist with the Division of Psychiatry, Children's Hospital of Los Angeles and work as a clinical/community mental health psychologist on the psychiatric emergency team of the Los Angeles County Department of Mental Health. For over twenty-five years, he maintained a small practice specializing in psychotherapy, consultation and supervision in working with the difficult and life-threatening patient. He is past president of the Section on Clinical Crises and Emergencies of the Division of Clinical Psychology of the American Psychological Association, a diplomate of the American Board of Professional Psychology, a fellow of the Divisions of Clinical Psychology (12), Psychology and the Law (41), and Psychotherapy (29) of the American Psychological Association, a fellow of the American Psychological Society and of the Academy of Psychosomatic Medicine and a chartered psychologist of the British Psychological Society. Dr Bongar is also a winner of the Edwin Shneidman Award from the American Association of Suicidology for outstanding early career contributions to suicide research and the Louis I. Dublin award for lifetime achievement in research on suicidology. In 2008, he was awarded the Florence Halpern award by the Division of Clinical Psychology of the American Psychological Association for distinguished contributions to the practice of clinical psychology. His research and published work reflect his long-standing interest in the wide-ranging complexities of therapeutic interventions with difficult patients in general and in suicide and life-threatening behaviours in particular.

David J. Brooks, Ph.D., is the Security Science Course Coordinator at Edith Cowan University, Australia. David commenced his career in Military Air Defence, moving into the Electronic Security sector and later into Security Consultancy prior to his current academic role. He has broad industrial security experience within Defence, Critical Infrastructure, Resources and Corrections. Research interests include security science education, psychometric risk, entropic security decay and the role of resilience in vetting. David has published widely, with books, chapters, and academic journals. David's books include *Security Science: The Theory and Practice of Security* with Elsevier, *Corporate Security in the Asia Pacific Region: Crisis, Crime, Fraud and Misconduct* with Taylor & Francis, and *Engineering Principles in the Protection of Assets in the Handbook of Security* with Palgrave Macmillan.

Julia V. Bykhovets, Ph.D., is a Researcher in the Laboratory of Psychology of Posttraumatic Stress, Institute of Psychology at Russian Academy of Sciences. His areas of expertise are post-traumatic stress disorder, sensitivity to a terroristic threat, personality psychology and family psychology. Dr Bykhovets is an author of thirty-four papers in Russian and international journals. In his doctoral dissertation, he has investigated the impact of terrorist threat on indirect victims. He was a fellow of the President of the Russian Federation Grant for young scientists with the topic "Experiencing of the terrorists' threat as a factor of decreasing psychological well-being".

Marek J. Celinski, Ph.D., a registered psychologist in the Province of Ontario (Registration Number 1276) and affiliated with the Ontario, Canadian and American Psychological Associations; with the Canadian Register of Health Services Providers in Psychology; and with the Canadian Academy of Psychologists in Disability Assessment. Dr Celinski is also a member of the National Academy of Neuropsychology and International Neuropsychological Society and has been working as a rehabilitation psychologist and a provider of neuropsychological services since 1977 both in private practice focusing on rehabilitation and assessment of head injury and as a Consultant to the Head Injury Programme and the Psycho Traumatic and Pain Programme at the Downs View Rehabilitation Centre (WCB) until its closure. He remained a part-time head-injury/rehabilitation consultant with the Workplace Safety and Insurance Board until the end of October 2009. In the years preceding his early retirement (which began in February 1998 to focus on private practice), he occupied the position of a senior psychologist, presented at national and international conferences and published more than fifty papers and book chapters on the subjects of clinical psychology, rehabilitation, neuropsychology and hypnosis. Currently, a number of clinical and rehabilitation tests that he co-authored or developed alone are being prepared for publication. At this time, five of his tests have already been published: Rehabilitation Survey of Problems and Coping (Multi-Health System of Toronto); Resourcefulness for Recovery Inventory – Research Edition; Resilience to Trauma Scale – Research Edition; Psychoassistant/ Concentration and Remote Memory Test – Research Edition; and Social Intelligence Test – R (all published by Cognisyst of Durham, N.C.). Furthermore, he is the co-editor of a four-book series on *Resilience and Resourcefulness*, which has already been published by internationally reputed publishers.

Captain Thomas Chaby is an active duty Naval Officer (SEAL) currently serving as the Director for the Preservation of the Force and Family Task Force (POTFF-TF) in Tampa, FL. In his present position, Tom focuses on programs that will holistically build resiliency for the 67,000 men and women of United States Special Operations Command and their families. He has been in the Navy for twenty-five years during which time he has worked and lived in Central America, South America, Guam and various locations throughout the US. His deployments have taken him throughout the Middle East, the Pacific, Africa and South America. He is a graduate of the University of Delaware and has a Master's Degree from National University where he attended night school.

Chris Cocking, Ph.D., is a Senior Lecturer in the School of Health Sciences at the University of Brighton, UK, and has research interests in the psychology of crowd behaviour (particularly during mass emergencies such as fires and terrorist attacks) and collective resilience. His work has been disseminated to a wide audience in both the theoretical and applied field, including in peer-reviewed publications, end-user reports, public consultation documents and in both the printed and broadcast global media. He has worked in the crowd management sector, advising on crowd behaviour at large events in London and the South East. Other consultations he has provided have been for the London Resilience Team and the Greater London Assembly (where he contributed to their report into the 7/7 terrorist bombings). He has also been a qualified Psychiatric Nurse since 2002, with experience of working in Child and Adolescent Mental Health Services (CAMHS).

Lynne Cohen, Ph.D., is a Professor of Psychology and Community Psychologist and brings approximately thirteen years of experience in resiliency research with children and university students. She has successfully developed transition programs that empower students and positively impact on their experience and outcomes. Professor Cohen has led a number of interdisciplinary research teams and is committed to a collaborative model involving community organizations. She teaches in both the undergraduate and post-graduate psychology programs and has been awarded a National Teaching Award by the Australian University Teaching Committee. She also has extensive experience in working with children with learning difficulties.

Karin G. Coifman, Ph.D., is an Assistant Professor of Psychology in the Department of Psychological Sciences, Kent State University. Her research is focused on developing a more thorough understanding of how basic emotional processes contribute to psychological health. Dr Coifman's research is currently focused on explicating the link between executive cognitive deficits and problematic patterns of emotional responding. She conducts her research on both clinical and community samples using a broad range of experimental and experience-sampling assessments. Dr Coifman attended Yale University where she completed an undergraduate degree in English. From there, she worked for several years for a community health and education agency in New York, NY, where she first began to work within the field of psychology. In 2001, Dr Coifman commenced graduate studies at Columbia University, working under the mentorship of Dr George Bonanno, completing a Ph.D. in Clinical Psychology in 2008. Dr Coifman then completed a post-doctoral fellowship in personality and emotion also at Columbia University, under the mentorship of Drs Geraldine Downey and Eshkol Rafaeli. She has been an Assistant Professor of Clinical Psychology at Kent State University since 2010.

Jeff Corkill served in the Australian Army for twenty years. A graduate of the Royal Military College he served as an officer in the Australian Intelligence Corps specializing in the areas of counter-intelligence and security. His post-military career has included an appointment as the Ashton Mining Security Manager followed by a period as the Security Intelligence Specialist at Argyle Diamonds. He has provided specialized strategic security and intelligence consultancy and training to corporate and government clients both in Australia and overseas. In 2007, Jeff joined ECU as a lecturer in Intelligence and Security and Ph.D. scholar.

Mark Dechesne, Ph.D., is an Associate Professor at Leiden University-Campus The Hague, Netherlands. He obtained his Ph.D. in 2001 on the effects of fear on social behaviour. His subsequent research activities have increasingly focused on the motivation of terrorists, the workings of terrorist organizations and reactions to terrorism. From early 2006 until September 2008, he worked at the DHS Center of Excellence NC-START (National Consortium for the Study of Terrorism and Responses to Terrorism) of the University of Maryland in the United States. Since 2008, he has been connected to Leiden University Campus The Hague, first as a senior researcher at the Centre for Terrorism and Counterterrorism, and since September 2011, he has been working for the Dual Ph.D. Centre. He is responsible for the quality control and advancement of the current dual Ph.D. tracks. Next to this he is working on research projects concerning psychological themes such as knowledge, human motivation, fear, radicalization and large-scale violence.

Nora Didkowsky is a Doctoral Candidate in the Interdisciplinary Ph.D. Program at Dalhousie University, Canada. She has coordinated programs with an emphasis on youth-engagement, youth-adult partnerships, and participatory-action research with Genuine Progress Index Atlantic since 2007. This work is centered in Nova Scotia and Bhutan. Her previous position was as coordinator of the Negotiation Resilience Project, at the Resilience Research Centre, Dalhousie University. That international research used an innovative combination of photo-elicitation, videotaping a *day in the life*, observation and interviews to understand the processes associated with positive development among youth in transition between two (and possibly more) culturally distinct worlds. Nora is on the Board of Directors for the Atlantic Council for International Cooperation.

Chandra Bhal Dwivedi, Ph.D., is presently Emeritus Professor at Banaras Hindu University (BHU), Varanasi, India. Professor Dwivedi completed several research projects among which are two major international research projects with Professor Bruce M. Ross, USA, and Professor Gerald Matthews, UK. He has just completed an ICSSR research project entitled "The Mundane and Incorporeal Aspects of the Psychology of Yoga." He has been a Co-Principal Investigator of two major projects from the University Grant Commission (UGC) and DRDO. He has been conferred with several awards by various organizations. As a recipient of the Fulbright Fellowship, he joined the Catholic University of America, Washington, DC, as a Visiting Professor in 1993. He was also offered a one-year visiting professorship at the Brown University, Providence, RI, USA. He has published more than 125 research papers in reputed national and international journals and authored six books besides contributing more than a score of chapters in edited books. His areas of current research interest are indigenous Indian psychology, spiritual psychology and counseling psychology.

Cath Ferguson is a Postdoctoral Researcher and Lecturer in the School of Law and Justice at Edith Cowan University in Perth, Western Australia, having previously worked as an integral member of the Lifespan Resilience Research Group on a number of projects. Catherine currently applies her knowledge of resilience in her research on re-integration of offenders into the community and as a protective factor within families who support a member with criminal behaviour.

Logan A. Favia, Ed.S., is a Senior Researcher in school psychology at the University of Washington. Logan received a Specialist in Education (Ed.S.) degree in school psychology from the University of Washington. As part of her graduate training, she evaluated students and provided evidence-based interventions to students with academic, social, emotional and behaviour issues in the clinical and public school setting. She completed her School Psychology Internship in the Federal Way Public Schools. Ms Favia's work focuses on the implementation and evaluation of universal, social-emotional learning programs in order to foster children's social and emotional development in the school setting.

Brooke M. Fowler, M.A., is a doctoral student with a focus on public relations and communication technology at the University of Maryland, US. She also has a strong interest in crisis management and relationship building, particularly across cultures. Her research utilizes primarily qualitative research methods. Brooke received her B.S. in Business Communication from Stevenson University in 2010 and her M.A. in Integrated Marketing Communication from Duquesne University in 2012. Prior to beginning the doctoral program, Brooke taught public speaking, intercultural communication, interpersonal communication and speech at Stevenson University and Carroll Community College.

Karen J. Friday is currently a Clinical Professor of Medicine (affiliate) at Stanford University and a staff cardiologist at the Palo Alto Veteran Affairs Medical Center. She graduated from Case Western Reserve University with a bachelor of science as well as a Master's degree in chemistry and eventually her medical degree. Dr Friday did her residency in internal medicine at Johns Hopkins Hospital followed by a fellowship in clinical pharmacology/critical care at University Hospital of Cleveland. She received her cardiology training at St. Louis University Hospital and did her fellowship in cardiac electrophysiology at Jewish Hospital in St. Louis. Dr Friday was a part of the cardiology faculty at the University of Oklahoma and subsequently was a Director of Medical Research and Clinical Pharmacology at Syntex Laboratories, which later became Roche Bioscience.

Abigail Gewirtz, Ph.D., is an Associate Professor in the Department of Family Social Science and Institute of Child Development at the University of Minnesota, Director of the University's Institute for Translational Research in Children's Mental Health, and the Director of Graduate Studies for the Prevention Science Minor at the University of Minnesota. Dr Gewirtz's research focuses on the development, testing and widespread implementation of evidence-based practices focused on parenting in highly stressed families. Her research projects have included diverse populations of families exposed to adversity, including projects with families exposed to homelessness, intimate partner violence and war.

Lokesh Gupta, Ph.D., from Department of Psychology, Maharishi Dayanand University, Rohtak, India. He has been a Research Investigator in Defence Institute of Psychological Research, Delhi, and Project Assistant at Department of Humanities and Social Sciences, Indian Institute of Technology, Delhi. His areas of interest are psychometrics and positive psychology. He has presented papers in conferences and published research papers in refereed national journals.

Kathryn M. Gow, Ph.D., is a University Professor, Psychologist and Researcher at School of Psychology and Counselling, Queensland University of Technology, Australia, who also currently practices in medical clinics, and undertakes disaster interventions in rural communities. The majority of her publications (over a hundred) are in quality journals and are published in peer reviewed journals and books. Her research projects include competencies, education and training, hypnosis, coping, trauma, emergency services, natural disasters, climate change and other social psychology topics. She has presented papers in seminars and conferences and has delivered keynote addresses at state, national and international levels.

Captain Gordon Hanson is a retired USCG Captain, he spent much of his life in the Coast Guard, as a deck officer, engineering officer and pilot. He rounded the "Horn" on a polar icebreaker en route to Antarctica, crossed all the "lines" and sailed six of the seven seas. He flew hundreds of rescue missions as a USCG helicopter and C-130 pilot, including four years in San Francisco. Captain Hanson holds a 50-Ton USCG Near Coastal license and is a USSA- and ASA-certified sailing instructor, teaching courses from basic keelboat through advanced cruising and coastal navigation. He has taught and run charters in San Francisco since 2000. Captain Hanson has skippered sailboats up and down the West Coast, Mexico, New England, Florida and throughout the Caribbean.

Meena Hariharan, Ph.D., is Professor in Health Psychology in University of Hyderabad. She is the Founder Director of the Centre for Health Psychology, University of Hyderabad. She has been working as faculty in this University since the year 1992. Prior to this, she worked in National Institute of Nutrition, Hyderabad. She has three books and about sixty articles to her credit. Her research areas are coping with stress, ICU trauma, psychosocial factors in non-communicable diseases. She has completed thirty research projects funded by national and international agencies.

Craig Harms works as a lecturer and researcher in the School of Psychology and Social Science at Edith Cowan University as well as a Clinical Psychologist in private practice in Wembley, Australia. He worked as a Psychologist at the Western Australian Institute of Sport between 2011 and 2014. His research and practice interests include factors impacting on and the psychological consequences of personal achievement (in sporting and academic settings); psychological aspects of health and exercise; resilience; and emotional regulation as well as the treatment of psychological distress.

Kira Harris, Ph.D., is an Associate of the School of Arts and Humanities at Edith Cowan University. Kira completed her Ph.D. on the psychology of exiting from marginalized and extreme groups. Kira has taught in the domains of psychology, criminology and terrorism studies. Her research interests include social psychology, one percent motorcycle clubs, extremism and de-radicalization and resilience.

Todd I. Herrenkohl, Ph.D., is Professor in the School of Social Work, University of Washington and Co-Director of the 3DL Partnership, an interdisciplinary center at the University of Washington focused on social, emotional and academic learning in children and youth. Dr Herrenkohl's work focuses on the study and promotion of positive youth development and the amelioration of risk factors related to interpersonal violence. His funded projects and numerous publications examine various health-risk behaviours in children exposed to violence, resilience and protective factors that buffer against early risk exposure in children and methods and approaches to promoting wellness by investing in the whole child.

Lori Holleran is a Doctoral Researcher in the Clinical Psychology at Palo Alto University with an emphasis in forensic psychology. She received her undergraduate degree in Psychology and Sociology from Arizona State University, and a Master's degree in Psychology from Pepperdine University. Lori's previous research experience at the University of California, Los Angeles's Alzheimer's Disease Research Center focused on the impact of white matter breakdown on depressive symptoms and cognitive impairment among individuals with Alzheimer's disease. In addition, Lori assisted in research at the Palo Alto VA's National Center for Posttraumatic Stress Disorder, where she was involved in research examining factors that predict an individual's likelihood of experiencing chronic PTSD. Currently she assists in research at the Substance

Abuse and Anxiety Program at the Palo Alto VA. Here she conducts neuropsychological and psychiatric assessments as part of a study examining the impact of a mobile, neuroscience-based cognitive remediation intervention for veterans with PTSD and alcohol use disorder. Clinically, Lori has focused on working with individuals diagnosed with borderline personality disorder and substance use disorders, as both of these conditions are highly prevalent among traumatized and incarcerated populations. She is currently serving the veteran population as an extern at the Neuropsychological Assessment and Intervention Clinic at the Palo Alto VA. Her research interests include examination of trauma-related behavioural outcomes, including subsequent risk for suicide and antisocial acts, and specifically violent acts towards others. In addition, Lori is focused on research initiatives that integrate technology with mental health treatment in order to offer more comprehensive and accessible care to a broader group of individuals.

Irina Illes, is pursuing her Ph.D. with an emphasis in Persuasion and Social Influence. She is interested in culture-centered approaches to health communication, mainly in the adaptation of health messages according to cultural values and beliefs and the motivation of behaviour change by using culture and core values as a medium.

Jasleen Kaur did her doctorate in Psychology from Panjab University, Chandigarh. Her areas of interest include developmental psychology, positive psychology and psychometrics. She has worked in the Department of Humanities and Social Sciences, Indian Institute of Technology (IIT), Delhi, from 2010–2013, in the capacity of research assistant, where she was closely involved in the field of positive psychology and has several published papers on the same. She is a member of National Positive Psychology Association (NPPA).

Kateryna V. Keefer, Ph.D., is an adjunct research professor at the University of Western Ontario, Canada. Her research interests concern personality structure and assessment; social-emotional competencies; and resiliency, coping and wellness.

Brooke Fisher Liu, Ph.D., serves as the Director of START'S Risk Communication & Resilience Program and an Associate Professor of Communication at the University of Maryland, US. Her research investigates how effective risk and crisis communication can optimally prepare the public to respond to and recover from disasters. In recent years, her research has focused on the unique roles that governments' social/news media can play in building community resilience. Liu serves as a member of the Food and Drug Administration's (FDA) Risk Communication Advisory Committee and on the editorial boards for *Communication Yearbook, Communication Quarterly, Public Relations Review, Journal of Applied Communication Research* and the *Journal of Public Relations Research.* Her research has been published in outlets such as *Communication Research, Communication Theory,* the *Handbook of Crisis Communication,* the *Journal of Applied Communication Research,* the *Journal of Communication Management,* the *Journal of Public Relations Research* and *Public Relations Review.*

Salvatore R. Maddi, received his Ph.D. in Clinical Psychology with honors from Harvard University in 1960. While at the University of Chicago, from 1960 to 1986, he went up through the academic ranks to full professor. From 1986 to the present, he has been a Professor at the University of California, Irvine. Throughout his career, he has developed the hardiness approach, which is the existential courage and motivation people need in order to turn stressful circumstances from potential disasters into growth opportunities instead, thereby enhancing their performance, leadership, morale, stamina and health. By now, there are well-accepted procedures for assessing and training hardiness. In demand for speaking and consulting engagements, Dr Maddi has achieved an international reputation and continues to receive many awards for his work. The latest award (in 2012) was the American Psychological Foundation Gold Medal for lifetime achievements in Psychology in the Public Interest.

Alexander V. Makhnach, Ph.D., is a Senior Researcher at the Institute of Psychology Russian Academy of Sciences, Moscow. In 1994–1995, Dr Makhnach worked on the development of the international program "The Challenge of Foster Care" under the auspices of the Russian Ministry of Education that designed a system of foster care in Russia. From 1993 until the present, Dr Makhnach has been working as a rector at the NGO Institute of Psychology and Psychotherapy, Moscow. In 2000–2005, he was on the board of experts and then as deputy director for methodology at the Assistance to Russian Orphans Program. In 2003–2005, he was in a team of the International Resilience project, headed by Dr Michael Ungar (Halifax, Canada). In 2008–2012, Dr Makhnach was a principal researcher of the program of psychological evaluation of adoptive parents' applicants under the patronage of the Russian Ministry of Education and Science. His areas of expertise are orphanhood, social adaptation, adoptive family, family stress factors and resources and family resilience.

Kate Maslowski, a doctorate scholar, graduated with a Bachelor of Science Degree in oceanography. After graduation, she was commissioned into the United States Navy as a Surface Warfare Officer. During her nearly eight years on active duty, Kate was stationed in Sasebo, Japan; San Diego, CA; and Annapolis, MD and served in Operations Enduring Freedom and Iraqi Freedom. It was during her eight years on active duty that Kate realized a bigger calling and left active duty to pursue a career as a clinical psychologist. Although Kate left active duty, she is still serving her country as a Lieutenant Commander in the United States Navy Reserve. She has a master of arts in clinical psychology from Pepperdine University and is currently a first-year Ph.D. student at Palo Alto University (PAU). At PAU, Kate is currently assisting in the construction of academic articles and books related to dangerousness.

Jonathan Matusitz, Ph.D., earned his doctorate in communication from the University of Oklahoma in 2006. He is currently an Associate Professor in the Nicholson School of Communication at the University of Central Florida (UCF). He studies terrorism, globalization, culture and health communication. One of his particular emphases is the Islamist threat to America and the world. His research methodologies include qualitative interviewing, content analysis, semiotics and theoretical analysis. On top of having more than a hundred academic publications and over a hundred conference presentations, Dr Matusitz taught at a NATO-affiliated military base in Belgium in 2010. Originally from Belgium himself, he migrated to the United States in 2000. His first book on terrorism, entitled *Terrorism & Communication: A Critical Introduction*, was published by SAGE. His most recent book, *Symbolism in Terrorism*, was published in 2014 by Rowman & Littlefield. In 2012, he was honored with a prestigious teaching award by the College of Sciences at UCF. A few years later, he received another teaching award by the Nicholson School of Communication: the "Excellence in Teaching Award for 2013–2014".

Harry L. McCleary is a California-certified Marriage and Family Therapist intern and six-year United States Navy veteran. While serving under the operational umbrellas of Operation Enduring Freedom and Operation Iraqi Freedom, Harry was deployed to support missions involving antiterrorism, anti-pirating and humanitarian efforts. Harry holds a bachelor's degree in psychology from Ashford University and a master of arts in clinical psychology with an emphasis in Marriage and Family Therapy from Pepperdine University. He is currently a first-year Ph.D. student at Palo Alto University. Prior to attending Palo Alto University, Harry worked as a clinician at an inpatient dual-diagnosis treatment facility for veterans. Further, he has worked as a therapist in private practice and in inpatient and outpatient mental health programs at Brotman Hospital in Los Angeles, California. Harry's research interests include psychopathy within the military, suicide prevention among veterans and how exercise can influence the prognosis and development of post-traumatic stress disorder.

Seema Mehrotra, Ph.D., is Professor of Clinical Psychology at the National Institute of Mental Health and Neuro Sciences (NIMHANS), Bangalore. She served at faculty positions at the Kasturba Medical College (KMC) Manipal, before joining NIMHANS in 2002. She completed her M.Phil. training in Clinical Psychology from NIMHANS and subsequently completed her Ph.D. in the field of Psycho-oncology in 1996. She has eighteen years of clinical, teaching and research experience. Her areas of research and practice include positive psychology, mental health promotion, process of adaptation to major life events and emotional regulation. She has supervised several research dissertations and Ph.D. theses in these areas, published articles in peer-reviewed indexed journals and contributed book chapters on themes such as positive psychology, resilience and flourishing at work. She has also undertaken major research projects in the broad field of mental health promotion funded by the Indian Council of Medical Research (ICMR), the Indian Council of Social Science Research (ICSSR) and the Council of Scientific and Industrial Research (CSIR), which have resulted in development of promotive intervention programs.

Swati Mukherjee is Scientist 'D' at Defence Institute of Psychological Research (DIPR), Delhi. She is involved in many major research projects of the Institute including research on suicide in the Armed Forces. She has to her credit a few publications in the form of journal articles and chapters in books published by reputed publishers including Taylor & Francis and Sage Publications. She has been the associate editor of a volume on 'Recent Developments in Psychology' and has co-authored a manual on 'Suicide and Fratricide: Dynamics and Management' for the Armed Forces personnel and a manual on 'Overcoming Obsolescence & Becoming Creative in R&D Environment' for R&D Organizations. Her areas of interest are social psychology, positive mental health practices and suicidal behaviour. She has been a recipient of Defence Research & Development Organization (DRDO) Best Performance Award in the year 2008.

Laura Supkoff Nerenberg, Ph.D., is a Postdoctoral Fellow at the University of Michigan Medical School, Department of Psychiatry. She is a child clinical psychologist and received her Ph.D. from the University of Minnesota's Institute of Child Development, and her B.A. from Brown University. Her research interests include mindfulness, parenting, and children's resilience.

Crystal L. Park, Ph.D., is Professor of Clinical Psychology at the University of Connecticut, Storrs, and affiliate of the University of Connecticut Center for Health, Intervention and Prevention. Her research focuses on multiple aspects of coping with stressful events, including the roles of religious beliefs and religious coping, the phenomenon of stress-related growth, and the making of meaning in the context of traumatic events and life-threatening illnesses. She is currently Principal Investigator of NIH and foundation-funded studies of yoga interventions, breast cancer survivors' health behaviours, and college student self-regulation and success. She is co-author of *Empathic Counseling: Meaning, Context, Ethics, and skill* and co-editor of *The Handbook of the*

Psychology of Religion and Spirituality (first and second editions) and *Medical Illness and Positive Life Change: Can Crisis Lead to Personal Transformation?*

Vijay Parkash, Ph.D., is Scientist 'D' at Defence Institute of Psychological Research, Defence R&D Organization, Delhi. After completing his post-graduation as Gold Medallist in the entire social sciences faculty of Kurukshetra University, Kurukshetra he was awarded DRDO Research Fellowship and he completed his Doctorate degree in Psychology from Kurukshetra University, Kurukshetra. Health psychology, personality and psychometrics are the areas of his interest and he has ten years of research experience. He has also served as a Psychologist at Air Force Selection Board, Dehradun for around two years. He has been involved in many major research projects related to suicidal behaviour and test constructions for personnel selection in the armed forces and paramilitary forces. He has been one of the editors of two edited volumes – *Recent Developments in Psychology* and *Counseling: A Practical Approach,* and he has to his credit more than fifteen other academic publications in the form of journal articles and book chapters. The Defence Institute of Psychological Research conferred upon him the Scientist of the Year Award – 2011 for his outstanding contributions.

Elizabeth L. Petrun, Ph.D., is the Associate Director of START's Risk Communication and Resilience Program. She works to grow the risk communication and resilience portfolio and contributes to ongoing research and education. Petrun holds a Ph.D. in communication from the University of Kentucky. Her areas of expertise include public relations, social media, organizational risk and crisis communication. In addition to START, Petrun has worked with the National Center for Food Protection and Defense, the Center for Risk and Economic Analysis of Terrorism Events and the Centers for Disease Control and Prevention. She also served as a consultant and/or author for the World Health Organization and the Food and Agriculture Association. She frequently presents at national and international communication conferences and teaches undergraduate and graduate courses in communication. She has also published in scholarly journals, including *Corporate Reputation Review, Management Communication Quarterly,* and the *International Journal of Neuroscience and Behavioral Science* among others.

Julie Ann Pooley, Ph.D., is currently the Associate Professor and Associate Dean of Teaching and Learning at Edith Cowan University. Julie Ann has been involved in teaching in both the undergraduate and post-graduate psychology programs and has been a recipient of a National Teaching Award and Citation by the Australian University Teaching Committee (2003, 2011). Her research focuses on resilience at the individual and community levels. Julie Ann has been involved in and directed many community-based research consultancies, projects and workshops and has been involved in the generation of fifteen different community-oriented reports for various cities and districts.

Rabindra Kumar Pradhan, Ph.D., is Associate Professor of Psychology at Department of Humanities and Social Sciences, Indian Institute of Technology, Kharagpur, India. He has earlier been a Scientist in Defence Institute of Psychological Research, Defence Research and Development Organization, Ministry of Defence, India. His areas of specialization include social and organizational psychology, industrial psychology, managerial psychology, organizational behaviour and human resource development and management. He has more than fifteen years of experience in the field of training, teaching and research in these fields. Dr Pradhan is a member of various professional bodies including International Association of Applied Psychology,

International Association of Cross-cultural psychology, Indian Society for Training and Development, National Academy of Psychology, India, Indian Academy of Applied Psychology, and Indian Science Congress Association. He has to his credit four books and more than thirty other publications in refereed journals, newspapers, magazines and books.

Francine M. Pritchard is a qualified Statistician with over eighteen years' experience in providing high-level statistical, information management and financial analysis services to a range of state and federal government departments in Australia. She has worked in quantitative analysis, compiling statistical data from a wide variety of appropriate sources, including the design and coordination of collection instruments from Local Government Authorities in Australia. She applies her knowledge of statistical analysis, analysis of economic and financial statistics, survey methodology (including Sampling Methodologies and Estimation Techniques) to her research in disasters and emergency management. Her publications relevant to this field include many research papers and book chapters in reputed journals and books.

Sandra Prince-Embury, Ph.D., is a Clinical Psychologist and Family Therapist and current Director of the Resiliency Institute of Allenhurst. Dr Prince-Embury is author of the *Resiliency Scales for Children and Adolescents* published by Pearson Assessments. Dr Prince-Embury has co-edited two volumes on Resilience, and authored several chapters and numerous articles. While Senior Research Director at Pearson Assessments, Dr Prince-Embury assisted in the development of many clinical assessments and manual-based therapy guides. In addition to the study of resilience, Dr Prince-Embury has studied and written on psychological response in the aftermath of man-made disaster. Her work on the Three Mile Island nuclear accident is documented in chapters, articles and archives at Dickenson College and Pennsylvania State University.

Suvashisa Rana, Ph.D., is an Assistant Professor at the Centre for Health Psychology, University of Hyderabad, India. He has been the recipient of the University Gold Medal (First Rank in First Class in M.A. in Psychology) from Utkal University and the coveted Doctoral Fellowship of Government of India by the Bureau of Police Research & Development, Ministry of Home Affairs, Government of India, to pursue his Ph.D. research on Police-Public Partnership for Peace. He has served as Psychologist under the Government of India after being selected by the Union Public Service Commission for a substantial period of time. His current area of research is positive psychology, health psychology and psychometrics.

Glenn E. Richardson, Ph.D., is a Full Professor of Psychology and Director of the Center for Personalized Health Education, Research and Technology (CIPHER) in the Department of Health Promotion and Education in the College of Health at the University of Utah. He had previous appointments at the University of Kentucky and at Texas A&M University. He has presented extensively nationally and internationally on resilience and resiliency. He is the author of the seminal article "The Metatheory of Resilience and Resiliency" that was published in the *Journal of Clinical Psychology*. He is the author of six books and over fifty articles related to positive and optimal health. He teaches resilience and resiliency classes both at the graduate and undergraduate levels.

Holly A. Roberts, is a Program Manager and Researcher in START's Risk Communication and Resilience program. With a B.A. from the University of Oklahoma and an M.A. from the University of Kentucky, Roberts specializes in Public Relations and Risk and Crisis Communication. Her research interests include organizational communication, risk and crisis communication, social media, natural disasters, reputation management and health crises. Roberts has experience teaching college-level courses and has presented at a myriad of national conferences. She formerly worked with the National Center for Food Protection and Defense and is published in *Corporate Reputation Review*.

Donald H. Saklofske, Ph.D., is a Professor in the Department of Psychology, University of Western Ontario. He is a fellow of the Association for Psychological Science and the Canadian Psychological Association. An editor of two psychology journals, an associate editor of a third and a book series editor, Dr Saklofske has published more than 140 journal articles, 70 book chapters and 30 books. He serves on the boards of various professional associations including the Canadian Psychological Association and the International Society for the Study of Individual Differences.

Katrina Sims is a Clinical Psychologist currently working for the Department for Child Protection and Family Support in Western Australia. Katrina provides psychological assessment and therapeutic treatment to children in care who have often been exposed to trauma, maltreatment or neglect. Katrina offers consultation, psycho-education and support to staff, carers and parents in areas related to the impact of trauma and neglect on children.

Kamlesh Singh, Ph.D., is an Associate Professor in the Department of Humanities and Social Sciences, IIT Delhi, and has contributed greatly to the field of positive psychology. She is a board member of International Positive Psychology Association (IPPA) and secretary of National Positive Psychology Association (NPPA). Her areas of interest include positive psychology and psychometrics, and she has to her credit several national and international paper publications (sixty-five papers) and conferences.

Rajbir Singh, Ph.D., is Senior Professor at the Department of Psychology and currently the Dean of Students' Welfare at Maharishi Dayanand University, Rohtak. He has earlier served as Dean, Faculty of Social Sciences, and Head, Department of Psychology at Maharishi Dayanand University, Rohtak, and Chairperson, Department of Psychology, Kurukshetra University, Kurukshetra. He specializes in the areas of positive psychology, psychobiology and neuro-psychology. He has been the founder president of Haryana Psychological Association and is affiliated to many national and international academic bodies as a life member. He is the Coordinator of UGC-SAP-II project on Health Psychology, subject matter expert for UGC examinations, invited expert for Union Public Service Commission and a member of academic bodies of many universities. He has supervised more than twenty Ph.D. theses. He is the founder editor of the *Journal of Indian Health Psychology* and Member of Editorial Boards of numerous journals. He has authored six books and has to his credit more than fifty research papers published in national and international refereed journals.

Alena Slezackova, Ph.D., is an Associate Professor of Psychology at the Department of Psychology, Faculty of Arts, Masaryk University in Brno, Czech Republic. She specializes in positive psychology and the psychology of mental health. Her research activities are focused mainly on character strengths, well-being, life values and social capital. She has been involved in many international research projects on happiness and well-being. She teaches in both the undergraduate and post-graduate psychology programs. Beyond her research and teaching, she serves as member of the editorial boards of five academic journals. She is a founder and director of the Czech Positive Psychology Centre (CPPC), which organizes conferences, workshops and special lectures on positive psychology. Alena is a member of the board of directors of the International Positive Psychology Association (IPPA) and a country representative of the Czech Republic in the European Network for Positive Psychology (ENPP). She is also an author of the first comprehensive monograph on *Positive Psychology in the Czech Language* (Grada Publishing, 2012).

Irena Sobotkova, Ph.D., is an Associate Professor at the Department of Psychology, Philosophical Faculty, Palacký University in Olomouc, Czech Republic. She specializes in family psychology, life-span development and substitute family care. Her research activities are focused on various aspects of family life, especially family resilience, family functioning, work–family balance, personal experiences from foster families, children exposed to domestic violence, and the relationship and communication between mothers and daughters. Dr Sobotková published the first *Family Psychology in the Czech Republic* (2012 – the 3rd edition). She is Editor-in-Chief of *E-psychology* (the electronic scientific journal of the Czech-Slovak Psychological Society) and representative of the Czech Republic in the International Academy of Family Psychology (IAFP).

Nadezhda V. Tarabrina, Ph.D., is Professor at the Laboratory of Psychology of Posttraumatic Stress, Institute of Psychology of the Russian Academy of Sciences. Professor Tarabrina was a Member of Advisory Committee "RUSSIA-NATO on Social and Psychological Consequences of Terrorism" (2002–2009). He is also a member of International Society for Traumatic Stress Studies and member of the editorial boards of the journal *Counseling Psychology and Psychotherapy* and the scientific online journal *Medical Psychology in Russia*, the editorial board of *Psychology for All* and a member of the Dissertation Council of the Institute of Psychology. Dr Tarabrina is a fellow of the State scientific grant "Leading Russian Scientists". In collaboration with internationally acclaimed researchers and academicians, he has come up with the chapters in NATO security through Springer's Science Series, *Human and Societal Dynamics* (Ed. Jeff Victorov) (IOS Press: Oxford, 2006), and in the proceedings of the *NATO Advanced Research Workshop on Social and Psychological Consequences of Chemical and Biological Terrorism* (IOS Press: Oxford, 2005). His areas of expertise are the psychology of post-traumatic stress, sensitivity to terroristic threat, negative affectivity, psychological well-being, the impact of the media, traumatization and personality.

Richard G. Tedeschi, Ph.D., is a licensed psychologist and Professor of Psychology at University of North Carolina Charlotte (USA) where he is core faculty for the Health Psychology Doctoral Program. He developed the concept of post-traumatic growth and has published numerous articles and books on the subject. He serves as media consultant on trauma for the American Psychological Association and is a Fellow of the Division of Trauma Psychology. He served as a subject matter expert for the US Army's Comprehensive Soldier Fitness Program. He has provided presentations and training on trauma for the US Army, the US Navy, the CIA, the American Enterprise Institute, the Center for New American Security and many professional organizations, clinics and educational institutions.

Linda C. Theron, D.Ed., is Professor of Educational Psychology in the Faculty of Humanities, North-West University, South Africa. Her research explores why, and how, some South African youth adjust well to poverty, orphanhood and/or learning difficulties and how socio-cultural contexts shape these processes of resilience. Her regular publications, international conference presentations/lectures, post-graduate supervision, post-doctoral mentorships and research grants all relate to the aforementioned. In 2013, she received the Education Association of South Africa's research medal for her rich contributions to understanding, and promoting, resilience processes that support the positive adjustment of South African youth.

Ravikesh Tripathi completed his M.Phil. training program in Clinical Psychology as well as his Ph.D. from the Department of Clinical Psychology at NIMHANS, Bangalore. He served as a clinical psychologist in the same institute for a period of three years before joining Narayana Health City as a consultant. In his current position, he works intensively with clients dealing with major medical adversities while also contributing to teaching and carrying out research. He has authored/co-authored research papers in peer-reviewed, indexed journals and has contributed to papers presented in national and international conferences. His areas of interest include neuro-psychology, psychometrics and positive psychology.

Michael Ungar, Ph.D., is both a family therapist and a Killam Professor of Social Work at Dalhousie University where he founded and co-directs the Resilience Research Centre that coordinates more than $5 million in funded research in over a dozen countries. He has published over 125 peer-reviewed articles and book chapters and is the author of 14 books for mental health professionals, researchers and parents. Among his most recent works are *Working with Children and Youth with Complex Needs: 20 Skills to Build Resilience,* a book for counselors, and *I Still Love You: Nine Things Troubled Kids Need from Their Parents.* In 2012, Michael was the recipient of the Canadian Association of Social Workers National Distinguished Service Award. Among his many contributions to his community has been his role as Co-Chair of the Nova Scotia Mental Health and Addictions Strategy Advisory Committee, executive board member of the American Family Therapy Academy, and Scientific Director of the Children and Youth in Challenging Contexts Network. His blog, Nurturing Resilience, can be read on *Psychology Today*'s website.

Stevan Weine, M.D., is Professor of Psychiatry at the University of Illinois at Chicago College of Medicine, where he is also the Director of the International Center on Responses to Catastrophes and the Director of Global Health Research Training at the Center for Global Health. For over twenty years, he has been conducting research both with refugees and migrants in the US and in post-conflict countries, focused on mental health, health and countering violent extremism. He is currently Principal Investigator of a DHS-funded study on "Community Policing to Prevent Violent Extremism" and an NIJ-funded study on "Transnational Crimes among Somali-Americans: Convergences of Radicalization and Trafficking". He is also currently the Principal Investigator of four NIH-funded studies: 1) "Migrancy, Masculinity, and Preventing HIV in Tajik Male Migrant Workers" (R01); 2) "Labor Migration and Multilevel HIV Prevention" (K24); 3) A Case Control and Mixed Methods Study of HIV Risk and Protection among Labor Migrants" (R21); and 4) "Addressing Mental Illness and Physical Co-Morbidities in Migrants and Their Families" (D43). Weine is author of two books – *When History Is a Nightmare: Lives and Memories of Ethnic Cleansing in Bosnia-Herzegovina* (Rutgers, 1999) and *Testimony and Catastrophe: Narrating the Traumas of Political Violence* (Northwestern, 2006) – and more than eighty peer-reviewed articles and chapters.

Zvi Zemishlany, M.D., M.H.A., is currently a Professor of Psychiatry, Sackler Faculty of Medicine, Tel Aviv University, Israel. He is the author of over ninety original articles and book chapters in the journals of repute and also involved in active research in Israel and the USA (Mt. Sinai and Columbia University). Professor Zemishlany is associated with various national and international journals like the *Israel Journal of Psychiatry, PsychiatriaPolska, Harefuah* (The Israeli Medical Journal) and is a peer reviewer for national and international journals in psychiatry. He has been the President of the Israeli Psychiatric Association (2003–2006), Member of the National Council of Mental Health, Israel (2003–2013) and Board member of the European Psychiatric Association (EPA) (2011–2014) and is currently President of the Israeli-Polish Mental Health Association and Zonal Representative and board member of the World Psychiatric Association (WPA).

Foreword

It is an honour to be asked to write this Foreword to *The Routledge International Handbook of Psychosocial Resilience*. I could have used this book more than forty years ago.

I started my career as a psychologist interviewing combat veterans about what turned out to be trauma resilience. Rapport with combat vets was easy for me at that time, just as the Vietnam War was ending. Like them, I fought in that war as a US Marine and had experienced similar things.

As I reviewed this handbook, I began to recall that my expectations for these men during my early research years (1973–1983) were inconsistent with what I found. The aim of my research was to document the toll the war has taken on those who fought it that would justify a new branch of the US Veterans Administration to focus explicitly on the younger war veterans.

Those I interviewed during this time were remarkably candid. They asked me questions too. I was viewed as an expert on what they experienced that scared or depressed them. There were many stories of fear and sadness, but there were also stories of overcoming challenges and bravery. They were remarkably resilient for what they had gone through. This research resulted in my first book (*Stress Disorders among Vietnam Veterans*, 1978, Brunner/Mazel), which led to my second book with Seymour Leventman (*Strangers at Home: Vietnam Veterans since the War*, 1980, Plenum).

But I was not prepared for dealing with my own traumatic stress reactions (later called compassion fatigue) and had overestimated my capacity to spring back from such a high concentration of sadness, horror and fright I absorbed as an interviewer. The interactions with these combat veterans awakened memories of my own experiences in Vietnam, but most importantly, I learned to become more resilient in the process of my struggle. I experienced what my interviewees experienced, secondhand.

Looking back, had the concept and methods of measuring psychosocial resilience been available then I may have changed the name and focus of project. We now know that resilience is a spectrum spanning all levels of resilience. Those I interviewed were more often part of the highly resilient group of those who had been exposed to horror and experienced post-traumatic stress reactions. Viewing the traumatized through a resilience lens enables the viewer to notice more often the achievements and strengths that balance the negative symptoms found in trauma scales. For me, I was shocked to find so many who had gone through so much but were well-functioning and happy, for the most part. I marvel at how so few were damaged psychologically. Based on forty years of research, we know that war veterans appear to be especially resilient compared to others exposed to extended trauma as part of your job. Many are permanently scarred from their war and post-war experiences. Many more are not.

As you read this massive handbook, consider how resilience is connected to nearly everything that lives. Even the focus on psychosocial resilience has broad relevance. Australia's think tank on resilience provided the best explanation for the origin of resilience:

> The term resilience was introduced into the English language in the early 17th Century from the Latin verb *resilire,* meaning to rebound or recoil. There is no evidence of resilience being used in any scholarly work until Thomas Tredgold introduced the term in 1818 to describe a property of timber, and to explain why some types of wood were able to accommodate sudden and severe loads without breaking.
>
> *(Torrens Resilience Institute, 2009)*[1]

It took more than a hundred years to expand the scope of resilience beyond materials science to the ecology and environmental studies and to our current published environment. Yet, today there is no single, general theory of resilience that applies to both the origin and the current application. This handbook, edited by Dr Updesh Kumar, Indian defense psychologist and senior scientist, provides a useful step towards understanding a universal mechanism of resilience by the sheer magnitude of areas of research covered and documented.

Each of the thirty-seven chapters in this handbook provides pieces for completing the jigsaw puzzle of resilience, especially those that involved people and their interpersonal and social relationships. Like completing a jigsaw puzzle, this handbook's chapters provide the pieces linked to the current perspective of the ways resilience works, the mechanism that accounts for how resilience works and is affected by interventions. Understanding the mechanism of resilience enables us to predict who is more likely to spring back from trauma and who will not. To understand the resilience of systems, societies, organizations and families is more complicated, but we are making great progress. This handbook provides the useful pieces to this jigsaw puzzle of psychosocial resilience.

Charles R. Figley, Ph.D.
Paul Henry Kruzweg Chair in Disaster Mental
Health; Professor Traumatology Institute Chair
Tulane University in New Orleans, USA

Notes

1 Torrens Resilience Institute. (2009). *Resilience origins and utility.* Retrieved from Torrensresilience.org.

Preface

Over the past fifteen years, the field of positive psychology has gained immense momentum. Psychological resilience has emerged as a potent construct, drawing massive attention of researchers in the area. This construct has found applications across varied domains in the field of human wellness and flourishing in the face of adversity. Professionals across the globe are persistently exploring the construct from all perspectives for extracting the maximum out of it in order to prepare individuals and communities to face any kind of adversities. There is abundance of literature existing on the concept; however, the review reveals a paucity of comprehensive works in the area. Though there are many books available on resilience, there is seldom any one that brings the variance in the field under one umbrella; hence, the field remains undersupplied to some extent to provide the reader with a comprehensive perspective. There is a relative paucity of comprehensive literature that encompasses together different theoretical perspectives with varied applied wings spread through almost every field. *The Routledge International Handbook of Psychosocial Resilience* endeavours to fill this gap and brings together theoretically grounded articles from myriads of contexts and cultures. Bringing together the state of the art in the domain of resilience, the handbook attempts to be a common treasured platform for everything that one may wish to refer to.

This *International Handbook of Psychosocial Resilience* provides comprehensive coverage to the subject matter by means of systematically orchestrating it in four separate sections. The first section presents the *conceptual arena* and explains the concept of resilience from inclusive theoretical perspective. The second section tenders delineations about the *psychosocial correlates* of resilience including personality aspects, emotional processes, social support and other factors like social networks and spirituality. The third section of the handbook puts forth a comprehensive discourse on the applications of resilience in different fields and cites suitable *applied evidence* based on research carried out on diverse samples across the globe. The fourth and last section of the handbook is a systematic amalgamation of *proposed implications and resilience building*–related elaborative discussions. The section takes the volume beyond indicating the applied areas and emphasizes the extended utilities of resilience and the strategies that can be effective in fostering resiliency among individuals.

Opening up the handbook with an introductory note in the first chapter, Mukherjee and I attempt to provide *a conceptual review of theory and research* on *psychological resilience*. We attempt to trace the roots of the concept of resilience along with a discourse on various meanings associated with the term and follow through the different paths it has traversed. We try to provide an overview of the varied operationalizations and connotations acquired by the concept across various fields of research and practice. An attempt has also been made to critically analyze some current theories and their implications. Our discussion is taken forward by Singh and Kaur who present *an overall view of resilience in the Indian scenario*. Herein, the authors' endeavour is about presenting a generous review of existing research and programs pertaining to resilience especially in the Indian scenario so as to make the readers further better acquainted with the conceptualizations of the target construct. *Conceptual complexity of resilience* has been addressed by Hariharan and Rana in the third chapter by rationally advocating the use of a *synergy approach to its measurement*. The authors cite the limitations of existing approaches to measure resilience and posit the use of a multi-method approach as the need of the hour. Adding to the theoretical base on the construct, they propound a 'synergy model' to explain the basic principles of resilience and to simplify the rigidity and complexity in conceptualization and operationalization of resilience.

Following the elaborations focusing on simplifying the conceptual complexities of resilience, a *three-factor model of personal resiliency* is presented and deliberated upon by Prince-Embury, Saklofske and Keefer. Delineating a sense of mastery, a sense of relatedness and emotional reactivity as the three aspects of personal resiliency, highlights from resilience theory are briefly described along with associated assessment complexity and examples of interventions at different levels. *A social ecological approach to understanding resilience among rural youth* has been analyzed and discussed concisely by Didkowsky and Ungar in the fifth chapter wherein they use the social ecological model of resilience to examine the processes that make young people living in rural contexts more likely to experience resilience when exposed to stressors that are unique to their communities. Implications for contextually relevant understanding and applications of resilience are discussed. The first section further moves to the deliberations on *resourcefulness model* of resilience against *universalities of challenges*. The authors, Celinski and Allen III, review traditional understanding of resilience and cite the empirical findings of their study on two factors – resilience vis-à-vis resourcefulness. Explaining the interactions between the two, they discuss the ways in which the interactions between resilience and resourcefulness promote good outcomes. In the next chapter, Parkash, Archana and I discuss the *role of genetics and temperament in resilience*. Associations of hereditary genetics and temperament as determinants of resilience are analyzed and discussed with the help of a review of supportive empirical evidence.

Further, in an attempt to explore the *psychosocial correlates of resilience,* Archana, Parkash and I open the second section of the handbook with the eighth chapter about deliberations on *resilient personality*, taking it as *an amalgamation of protective factors*. Protective personality factors relating to explicit assets and resources essential for the process of resilience have been comprehended with relevant research illustrations. Going from general to specific, Maddi elaborates upon *hardiness as a pathway to resilience under stress.* Citing important scholastically drawn evidence, the author advocates the hardiness approach to resilience and discusses assessment and training of hardiness to learn from and endure to stress. *Evidence from social psychology* has been presented by Cocking in the tenth chapter to highlight the role of *collective resilience and social support in the face of adversity.* The author infers resilience as developable through a common identity among people facing adversity and draws upon a Social Identity Model of Collective Resilience (SIMCR). He provides adequate theoretical and empirical evidence for the existence and benefits of mutual social support and discusses the implications for emergency planning for disaster preparedness along with practical suggestions for encouraging collective resilience.

Applied metatheory of resilience and resiliency is discussed by Richardson in the next chapter. The author attempts to diminish the confusions regarding his metatheory of resilience and resiliency (MRR)[1] by clearly distinguishing between the discovery pathway and the applied pathway of resiliency inquiry. For elucidating the applied aspects of MRR, he elaborates five waves of applied resiliency inquiry and discusses in detail the postulates that need to be assumed. Extending these illuminations and providing *a contextualized perspective,* Theron illustrates *the resilience processes of*

Black South African young people in the next chapter. Putting emphasis on the role of contexts and cultures in resilience, she puts forth a comprehensive synthesis of many empirical studies delineating the resilience processes of Black South African adolescents who resisted varied negative developmental outcomes. She advocates for a contextualized understanding of the psychosocial mechanisms contributing to the process of resilience and the need for valuing social ecologies to leverage the contextualized processes that young people prioritize.

Coifman and Almahmoud extend the discourse further by discussing *emotion flexibility, psychological risk and resilience.* They review contemporary models of emotion along with current evidence that suggests role of emotions in fuelling resilient outcomes and propounds a model of emotion flexibility. The positive contributions of emotion flexibility, the psychological risks associated with lack of emotion flexibility, evidence demonstrating role of hereditary and environmental factors in emotional flexibility and methodological issues relevant to the study of emotion flexibility are discussed. Moving further in this series on the psychosocial correlates of resilience, Park elucidates the association between *meaning making and resilience.* The author thoroughly explains the significance of meaning making in fostering resilience by adequately elucidating all kinds of functions of meaning making and reviews the evidence addressing meaning-making processes in the context of resilience and their implications. *Spiritual intelligence as a core ability behind psychosocial resilience* has been assertively posited by Ajawani in the fifteenth chapter of the handbook. Concrete operationalizations of spiritual intelligence specifying its resilience-related characteristics and its specific linking associations with resilience have been well elaborated.

After ample and thorough deliberations on resilience conceptualization and the psychosocial correlates of resilience, in the third section, the handbook aims to inspire readers by presenting *applied evidence* of resilience in different contexts and varied scenarios. The section opens with the sixteenth chapter on *resilience and countering violent extremism* authored by Stevan Weine. The chapter discusses the ways in which the concept of resilience has become central in the efforts at countering violent extremism in the United States. It highlights the emphasis by the White House on building resilience for the purpose of countering violent terrorism and examines the research findings regarding some real incidents in light of the ongoing project of building effective and sustainable resilience-focused strategies to counter violent extremism in the United States. Bringing in picture a different context and culture in the next chapter, Makhnach talks about *medical and social models of orphanhood* and discusses the *resilience of adopted children and adoptive families* in Russia. The author cites the limitations of the medical model and the increasing acceptability of the social model. Medical and social models of orphanhood in their historical perspective in Russia have been elaborated. In light of disadvantageous groups of orphans, he gives a mention to the likelihood of certain disorders and emphasizes the need of positive socialization, which, as an interplay of inner and outer factors, makes each orphan more resilient, which in turn leads to their positive development.

Mehrotra and Tripathi delineate the *explored pathways and unexplored territories* between *spirituality and resilience.* Illuminating the inexplicit associations between spirituality and resilience, the chapter attempts to synthesize the global literature on the explored pathways between the two to highlight the emerging trends. In the plethora of Western literature on conceptualizations, the authors elaborate on a few concepts in Indian philosophical thought for an Indian culture-specific understanding of the linkages between spirituality and resilience. Future directions are provided for research using these concepts. Taking into consideration a very significant but diverse portion of population in the form of refugees who experience a lot of trauma, Sims and Pooley put forth their deliberations on *post-traumatic growth amongst refugee populations* and provide a systematic review of empirical research published during the last three and half decades that has studied post-traumatic growth amongst refugee populations around different parts of the world to be able to inform clinical interventions aimed at assisting refugees. In line with post-traumatic growth, Prince-Embury highlights the *importance of information for community-level resiliency intervention in a post-disaster environment* by presenting a very systematic case illustration. The case of the Three Mile Island (TMI) nuclear power facility has been described with specific emphasis on the intervention – the TMI Public Health and Environmental Information Series – a community course providing information pertaining to unanswered questions in the TMI community. The role of information in building community resilience has been given an impetus.

After a discussion of community resilience in post-disaster environment, the discourse on applications of resilience in military has been amplified by Holleran and associates by providing an explicit narrative about initiatives taken by the *United States Special Operations Command (SOCOM) for reducing risk by fostering resiliency* among the United States Special Forces operators. The chapter puts forth a detailed and clear picture of resilience-building measures taken by SOCOM to focus on physical, psychological, social and spiritual domains of well-being among the operators. The authors examine the ways in which this four-domain model is improving readiness and is building resilience in an attempt to decrease the suicide prevalence witnessed within SOCOM operators. Further on building resilience among Special Forces in the United States, Tarabrina and Bykhovets delineate *post-traumatic stress disorder (PTSD) and resilience* by putting across empirical evidence of the *experience of terrorist threats among urban populations in Russia*. The authors, on the basis of data gathered from around 500 participants, conclude that experience of terrorist threat contributes to the development of PTSD. They differentiate between two groups – vulnerable and resilient to PTSD – and discuss the characteristics of resilient people who do not develop PTSD despite terrorist threat perception.

Taking the debate on applied evidence of resilience in a diverse direction, Matusitz alludes to a *case of Palestinian suicide terrorists* and paints their *martyrdom as a result of psychosocial resilience*. Considering the social milieu a strong correlate of the psychological development of Palestinian martyrs, the author propounds certain theoretical foundations by highlighting some adaptational systems that are strongly correlated to competence, determination and resilience among the suicide terrorists. In the next chapter, Bar-On discusses *the impact of resilience on our ability to survive, adapt and thrive* and presents a comprehensive *review of research findings that empirically demonstrate the importance of resilience* in human existence, survival and adaptation. The author presents and discusses key findings that shed light on the important role played by resilience and other closely associated contributors to performance, such as flexibility, adaptability and hardiness, which impact the ability to not only *survive* but *thrive*. He focuses primarily on the impact of resilience on (1) cognitive functioning; (2) academic performance; (3) performance at work, leadership and organizational profitability; (4) physical health; and (5) emotional health and well-being. The chapter concludes with a brief summary of the major findings that emerged, their importance for better understanding resilience and what needs to be done in future research in order to gain greater insight into how it develops, what it impacts and how.

The fourth section of the volume proposes certain implications of the works carried out in the area and focuses on aspects of fostering resilience. In the opening chapter of this section, Zemishlany draws on certain implicative inferences about *resilience and vulnerability in coping with stress and terrorism*. The author asserts that identification of factors contributing to vulnerability and resilience in individuals has an important implication on mental health. The associated contributing factors and the approaches that may be adopted for identifying and preventing vulnerabilities among terror-exposed communities and resilience-enhancing probabilities have been discussed. In the next chapter, Tedeschi and Blevins establish *post-traumatic growth as a pathway to resilience* on the basis of scrupulous review of the origins and principles of the theory of post-traumatic growth (PTG) following a major loss or trauma. They distinguish PTG from resilience and discuss how PTG defines a pathway to the development of resilience with the help of a hypothesized model. Moving ahead, Dwivedi makes certain interpretive revelations about the interactive and integrative framework involving *spirituality, culture and resilience* and forming *a virtue-informed approach to well-being*. The author adequately reviews the research and focuses on the intermingling influence of spirituality, culture and resilience on developing virtuous well-being. This treatise is followed by a systematic discourse on *building resilience by teaching and supporting the development of social emotional skills and wellness in vulnerable children* by Herrenkohl and Favia. They attempt to explore and delineate the intersection between children's socio-emotional learning programs, school environments and later resilience. The authors attempt to provide certain insights about the utility of socio-emotional learning programs in positioning vulnerable children to succeed in life.

Widening the scope from individuals to organizations, Bartone attempts to explore and enumerate *leader influences on resilience and adaptability in organizations*. Highlighting the need for the workers to be highly adaptable and resilient to stress, the author explores the role of psychological hardiness as a stress–resilience resource and discusses the ways in which leaders in organizations can affect workers' hardiness. Strategies are presented for building psychological hardiness in organizations through influence of leaders. In the next chapter, Nerenberg and Gewirtz propose a *parent management training model for promoting children's resilience by strengthening parenting practices in families under extreme stress*. The authors review the literature on prevention interventions targeting parenting practices in families affected by traumatic and highly stressful events. They propose a novel agenda on the basis of a thorough review of data from parenting prevention studies around the world and across a variety of stressors. Going from parenting to families, Slezackova and Sobotkova explicate about *family resilience as a positive psychology approach to healthy family functioning*. In the form of thorough deliberations on the family resilience framework, the authors elucidate key processes of family resilience and present a research-informed overview of various approaches for understanding and strengthening family resilience. Positive psychology-based practice applications, strategies and interventions have been illustrated.

Enumerating the implications in the realm of *building resilient organizations*, Pradhan gives impetus on *introspection through the lens of psychological resiliency*. Advocating the reciprocative positive impacts of individual and organization resilience, the author assigns equal weight to the development of both, elucidates their prospects in organizational contexts and discusses practical implications for organizational behaviour and human resource professionals. Gow and Pritchard raise an imperative question – *can authorities empower individuals and communities by building resilience through self-reliance in the face of impending seasonal natural disasters?* They further try to propose an answer and call for becoming *architects of our own survival* by means of learning from the resilience of others and ascertaining how the strategies of those who are better prepared or sufficiently resourced can be inculcated into sufficient individuals, communities and organizations to create self-sufficiency and self-reliance to face catastrophic disasters. The implications of *the concept of resilience in the context of counterterrorism* have been deliberated upon by Dechesne to take the handbook towards a summing up. He reflects upon the nature of resilience in the context of terrorism and, with the help of supportive literary evidence, discusses the specific components of different kinds of resilience, which are crucial for countering terrorism, with having a collective sense of identity as the most common factor.

In the next chapter, Fowler and colleagues discuss *diffusing portable radiation detectors among first responders* and focus their deliberations on *device acceptance and implications for community resilience.* Forming a basis on challenges facing the police personnel in nations like the United States, they synthesize current knowledge and the gaps surrounding police and first responders' risk and crisis communication, with a particular emphasis on the diffusion of new, controversial security technologies. Providing empirical support to their concerns through an ethnographic field test, they highlight the ways in which a police department's first responders reacted to adopting portable radiation detectors. To take the handbook towards a summing up, in the penultimate chapter, Corkill and associates put an emphasis on *the use of resilience indicators to assist in the selection of personnel for employment in classified and covert environments* related to national security concerns. They propose vetting personnel on resilience markers with additional tools for proactive aftercare and, if necessary, interventions that will serve as an aid to security. The applicability of the 'Lifespan Resilience Scale' as a suitable tool is discussed, and an overview of the scale's construction, along with detailed information of the scale attributes, is provided.

To sum up the volume with the last chapter, Singh and Gupta expound on *psychological preparedness, combat performance and resilience* in military contexts. Basing their work on sound research evidence, the authors propose a model pointing out the significance of the soldier's individualistic strengths in combat preparedness and combat performance. Considering individual strengths as initial aspects of combat preparedness, significant interventions for improving them are suggested. The model elucidates various types of integrating combat experiences into resilience and signifies the ways in which consequential aspects of combat and combat preparedness serve as feedback to resilience building.

The conceptual deliberations on resilience put forth in the first section of the handbook by eminent scholars from varied perspectives have attempted to further expand the horizon of the reader's understanding on the much talked about concept of resilience. Going beyond existing knowledge, a comprehensive account of conceptual elucidations has been presented to the reader. The second section, devoted to revealing the psychosocial correlates of resilience, leaves no stone unturned to unearth the empirically validated, theoretically proposed and instinctually hypothesized associations of the construct with numerous relevant variables. Applications of resilience in a vast range of domains ranging from parenting, schooling and youth to family, community resilience, spirituality and resilience, to terrorism and much more are enumerated to the reader along with varied research with paradigmatically established evidence in different cultures and contexts. Probable positive extractions from the extended implications of resilience are concretely discussed in the last section of the handbook and the approaches of building resilience find significant, relevant spaces to draw the appropriate interest and attention of the reader. Having the sound notions of eminent scholars, scientists and professionals from across the globe who have dedicated enormous efforts in exploring the concept of resilience, this handbook intends to satisfy the academic curiosity of the researchers and will serve individuals, academicians, health care professionals, security agencies, policy makers and entire communities to foster resilience and develop resilient individuals and communities.

It is indubitably an arduous task and requires relentless working to edit a handbook on such a specific area with gigantic applications but relatively lesser research endeavours. Having put in the colossal efforts in the shape of this handbook, I feel indebted to one and all who offered their helping hands in this titanic venture. I express my deep sense of gratitude to all the distinguished authors for the time and effort they have devoted for this enterprise. Their exemplary inscriptions have contributed immensely to the quality of this handbook. Finally, I offer my heartiest thankful acknowledgement to Susannah Frearson and Joanne Forshaw at Routledge, UK, for their support and enormous and systematic efforts for publishing it in an appreciable constitution.

I hope it will prove to be a vital reference for lay individuals as well as eminent professionals across each and every field and will ignite the minds of budding scholars to endeavour new research, the applications of which will help build resilient individuals and resilient communities.

Updesh Kumar

Notes

1 Richardson, G. E. (2002). The metatheory of resilience and resiliency. *Journal of Clinical Psychology, 58*(3), 307–321.

Section I
Conceptual arena

Psychological resilience

A conceptual review of theory and research

Swati Mukherjee and Updesh Kumar

Originating from the physical sciences, the concept of resilience has gained significance in the psychological and social sciences in recent decades, especially in the wake of the shift in emphasis from a deficiency model of human functioning to a more positive framework delving into efficiency and well-being. Psychological resilience denotes the ability of an individual or a system to recover from a setback, adapt well in the face of trauma, and survive and thrive despite significant adversity and stress. Etymologically the word resilience has its origins in the Latin verb 'salire' meaning 'to jump' and a term derived from it – 're-salire', which means 'to jump back'. Being resilient does not merely imply dealing effectively with stress or adversity but denotes a 'springing back' into action as a more effective entity adapting to the negative incidence and construing it as a stepping stone towards positive behaviours, adaptation, and growth. Bonanno (2004) emphasises that resilience is not only about bouncing back into action but is also about being able to sustain the adaptive behaviour. The concept of resilience is used across disciplines and in varied contexts; however, the core components of defining resilience are evident in each instance, i.e. exposure to significant adversity and positive adaptation, even growth in response to the stress (Luthar, 2006). Luthar's definition that posits resilience as a two–part construct has been accepted by other scholars too (Masten, 2001; Yates, Egeland, & Sroufe, 2003). In this perspective, resilience is inferred by the coping behaviour demonstrated by an individual or a system in the face of substantial risk or adversity, and this differentiates resilient coping from normative coping. A related perspective defines resilience as normal development under adverse circumstances (Fonagy, Steele, Steele, Higgit, & Target, 1994; Masten, 2001). Another recent definition is given by Rutter who defines resilience as the relative resistance to psychosocial risk experiences (Rutter, 1999, 2000). Drawing from a variety of definitions, resilience can be conceptualised as good psychological functioning and behavioural outcomes despite facing adverse circumstances that are expected to jeopardise the normative growth and adaptation of the individual or system (Bonanno, 2004; Masten, 2001; Rutter, 2006). This conceptualisation of resilience has found applications in a variety of contexts and fields, beginning with psychopathology, developmental psychology, and disaster management to newer areas like intervention and rehabilitation programmes for war-affected communities, and people affected by ethno-political conflicts. Within the psychological literature, three general uses of the term resilience have been recognised (Werner, 1995) – good developmental outcomes despite high-risk status, sustained competence under stress, and recovery from trauma. These uses also denote the contexts of recognising resilient behaviour and indicate the path that resilience as a psychological construct has traversed.

Initial explorations aiming to understand the variability in human reactions to adversity placed the causality within the individual, labelling those with positive coping as 'hardy' or 'invincible'. Subsequent research, however, recognised the wider realm of factors implicated in positive coping and conceptualised resilience as a process rather than a trait inherent in an individual. Rutter (1990) argued that risk or protective factors in themselves are not enough in facilitating or hindering positive outcomes; rather, it is the interaction of these factors with the individual that initiates certain processes that lead to positive outcomes. He identified three such processes as building a positive self-image, reducing the effect of the risk factors, and breaking a negative cycle so as to open up new opportunities for the individual. Further, researchers conceptualising resilience as a process also argued for context and temporal specificity of resilient outcomes. Specificity of resilience as a dynamic process has also been emphasised in another context; as Luthar (2006, p. 741) puts it, resilience "is never an across-the-board phenomenon". An individual displaying resilient outcome in a particular domain may be facing negative outcomes in other areas of behavioural or emotional coping.

Origins of the resilience construct

The origins of the construct of resilience lie in developmental research, especially in developmental psychopathology, with its concern for ensuring normative development for the children facing significant adversity. The findings from this area of research have gradually been extended to populations who face extreme adversity and challenges or who have suffered traumatic experiences.

Masten (2006) refers to four waves of resilience research in the field of developmental psychology, which also have a general implication. The first wave of resilience research she refers to began in the 1970s when the question as to why certain young individuals exhibit high adaptability and growth when the opposite is expected because of their vulnerabilities and adverse environmental factors began to intrigue the psychologists. This led the pioneering researchers (e.g. Norman Garmezy, Lois Murphy, Michael Rutter, Alan Sroufe, Arnold Sameroff, and Emmy Werner) to explore the factors that provided protection to these young individuals and not only prevented them from breaking down but helped in optimising behavioural outcomes. Identification of correlates and markers of adaptive behaviours among such individuals led to developing a 'short list' of potential assets or protective factors that could be used to explain the positive behavioural outcomes despite adverse environmental circumstances. Exploration and corroboration of these factors continues to form a large portion of resilience research to date (Masten, 2004, 2006).

While the first wave of resilience research focused on description, the second wave of research built upon the 'short list' of protective factors by attempting to uncover the processes and pathways through which these protective factors operated in order to lead to positive and adaptive outcomes even under adversity. Such research sought to answer the question how the risk and protective factors disrupt or maintain adaptive functioning. Studies are still continuing with the agenda of unearthing the specific mechanisms (Luthar, 2006; Masten, 2006), with a focus on multiple levels of analysis and neurobiological processes (Cicchetti & Curtis, 2007).

Moving beyond basic research elucidating the construct, the third wave of resilience research is marked by an emphasis to extend the research insights gained through the initial explorations for the benefit of populations at risk. The third wave of research focused on applied aspects of resilience by running experimental studies regarding providing interventions and by evaluating the impact of introducing protective factors upon behavioural and mental health outcomes. This research also envisaged making an impact on policy implications for the vulnerable children and other populations facing adversity. This research runs parallel while the conceptual exploration for elucidating resilience as a construct continues. This research also gained impetus from the rise of prevention science, which focused on developing competence for preventing the occurrence of behavioural problems (Masten, Burt, & Coatsworth, 2006; Masten & Coatsworth, 1998; Weissberg, Kumpfer, & Seligman, 2003).

The initial three waves of research have amply elucidated upon the construct of resilience and have provided with a conglomerate of factors contributing to resilient outcomes. The fourth wave of resilience research currently gaining momentum focuses on integrating the research insights from concomitant fields like genetics, neurobiology, and statistics and utilises these for an enhanced understanding of the complex processes through which resilience works. Also, current research in the field focuses on integrating the insights gained from the initial research across different levels of analysis including biological, psychological and environmental systems. Integrative trans-disciplinary research in the field is paving the way for incorporating advances in research design and technological advancements in related field and thus is developing the potential to make an impact on the policy decisions that affect the quality of life of larger populations. Also, moving beyond individual resilience, researchers have begun exploring entire communities and organisations for indicators of resilience. On the other hand, with the rapid proliferation of research on resilience, concerns have also been raised regarding the rigor of methods used (Cicchetti & Garmezy, 1993; Glantz & Johnson, 1999; Luthar, 1993; Rutter, 2000) and about the conceptual definition of resilience, components of resilience construct, and the criteria used for labelling people as resilient or non-resilient. Rest of the paper reflects upon such concerns.

Theorising resilience

Integrating research insights and various conceptualisations in a given domain, a theory provides a framework for explaining the causal relationships and makes prediction possible. Given the varied approaches to the study of resilience and its usage in multiple applied domains, multiple theoretical conceptualisations emerged in the last few decades. Most of the theoretical frameworks are based on specific contexts and are thus more or less limited in their applicability. Fletcher and Sarkar (2013) have provided an exhaustive summary of these theories. Despite the varied nature of contexts in which these different theories emerged, there are certain common themes that can be identified throughout – for example most theories conceptualise resilience as a dynamic process that changes in the context of the environment with time; further, it is a multi-dimensional construct that emerges as a result of interaction of many underlying factors within the individual and in the environment; also resilience has conceptual overlap with other constructs denoting positive outcomes.

There is a vacuum for the want of a generic theory of resilience with potential applicability across domains. Fletcher and Sarkar (2013) critically analyse one such theory – the metatheory of resilience and resiliency (Richardson, 2002; Richardson, Neiger, Jensen, & Kumpfer, 1990), which has potential for generic application, as it incorporates different stressors, protective factors, and multiple levels of analysis. Richardson et al. (1990) conceptualise resilience as a striving inherent in every organism or living system for returning to a state of biopsychospiritual homeostasis, that is the original state of an organism. An adverse event causes disequilibrium in this state of balance if the organism or living system does not have sufficient resources or protective factors to buffer against the stressors. The process of reintegration begins when the individual or the system tries to adapt and overcome the adversity. There are four possible outcomes – resilient reintegration (with new protective factors and higher levels of homeo-stasis), homeostatic reintegration (maintaining the previous comfort level), reintegration with loss (with loss of protective factors and lowered homeostasis), and dysfunctional reintegration (with destructive behaviour patterns). The theory has been criticised for apparent lacunae of being uni-dimensional and of not having the potential to explain multi-dimensional interaction effects of variables on resilient outcomes; for failing to explain how meta-cognition and emo-tion affect the reintegration process; and for conceptualizing resilience as synonymous to coping (Fletcher & Sarkar, 2013). As with the conceptual issues related to the construct of resilience, theoretical concerns also indicate a need for newer theoretical approaches grounded in real-life empirical data and rigour of method.

Operationalising resilience

Resilience is an inferential construct that cannot be observed or measured directly but rather needs to be inferred from the behavioural outcomes after an individual or a living system under-goes major adversity. Naming a system as resilient thus has two prerequisites – adaptive function-ing of the system and an antecedence of adverse circumstances that had the potential to break the functioning of the system. Thus, resilience is best conceptualised as an umbrella term covering markers of adaptive functioning under adverse circumstances. Three types of indicators can be identified across resilience literature. Masten (1994) names these as (1) at-risk individuals show better-than-expected outcomes, (2) positive adaptation is maintained despite the occurrence of stressful experiences, and (3) there is good recovery from trauma.

Hence, the initial issue in identifying resilience depends on identifying what constitutes adap-tive behaviour. Murphy (1962) describes two aspects of adaptive coping – adapting to the envi-ronment (coping I) and maintaining internal integration (coping II). Initial researchers in the area of resilience focused on adaptive coping among children and markers of positive adaptive behaviour were based on the meeting of expected landmarks of development and competencies in multiple domains of achievement. The expected developmental tasks were defined in con-sonance with the developmental stage and in context of cultural and historical context (Masten & Powell, 2003). The significant issue in the approach is that it defines adaptation in behav-iourally measurable developmental landmarks and, though incorporating emotional or subjective well-being as a part of developmental tasks, does not rely on these internal criteria for defining positive adaptation. Second, the approach recognises that the criteria for adaptation need to be defined in context and in a dynamic manner so as to account for variations in populations and circumstances. Though originating in developmental research, the developmental task approach to resilience has the potential to be applied for varied populations.

The approach has generated a large body of research and has highlighted certain important issues regarding positive adaptation. Masten and Obradovic (2006) have enlisted these issues that have helped the resilience researchers in clarifying the nature of adaptation, specifically in developmental context, and extendable to generalised applications too. They conceptualise adap-tation as multi-dimensional and developmental in nature, with success in one domain positively affecting adaptation in other domains and in forthcoming tasks. Further, they posit that success or failure in multiple domains has a cumulative impact in other internal and external domains of adaptation and that interventions designed to promote success in developmental tasks helps pre-vent behavioural and emotional problems. A different perspective is provided by Luthar (2006) who contends that resilience may be demonstrated by an individual in a particular domain, while another domain of functioning remains dysfunctional. She provides the example of children who face adversity and yet remain competent in academic domains, some of whom show a variety of symptoms of emotional distress and breakdown. Resilience in one domain may not necessarily translate into resilience in general.

Besides the criteria of accomplishing salient developmental tasks adopted by some researchers (e.g. Elder, 1998; Masten & Coatsworth, 1995, 1998; Waters & Sroufe, 1983), another set of studies employed absence of psychopathology as the criterion of resilience (Conrad & Hammen, 1993; Tiet et al., 1998). Such studies originated in the field of substance abuse, parental psychopathology, and other such familial or environmental factors contributing to the vulnerability of the individual. Another set of research has used both internal as well as external criteria for determining resilient adaptation (Dubow, Edwards, & Ippolito, 1997; Felner et al., 1995; Greenberg, Lengua, Coie, & Pinderhughes, 1999).

A second domain that defines resilience besides adaptive coping is the presence of significant adversity. A risk factor is a measurable characteristic of an individual or his or her situation believed to impede positive functioning or outcome or to predict negative functioning or outcome (Masten & Reed, 2002). A large number of risk factors and challenges have been identified and tested in the context. Luthar (2006) discusses discrete risk factors like parental depression, exposure to community violence, and the like on one hand and a composite of multiple risk indices on the other like poverty, parental mental illness, and unrest in the community. Research that focuses on determining the role played by a discrete risk factor on adaptive coping of an individual helps pinpoint the causality, whereas research exploring multiple risk indices is more realistic in its predictions as most of these risk factors are found together in real-life circumstances too.

A related domain of the exploration of risk factors is the identification of protective factors. A protective factor is an asset or system that mediates the effect of risk factors by lessening their impact on the individual or the system under threat and that aids in positive adaptation.

Masten and Reed (2002) define a protective factor as a measurable characteristic of an individual or his or her circumstances believed to predict positive functioning in the context of adversity. Four broad categories of protective factors can generally be identified: a) intra-personal, b) intra-familial, c) inter-personal, and d) within the community. Though it appears that risk and protective factors lie at two opposite ends of a single continuum, the distinction is subjectively determined, and not with an objective criterion of bifurcation. As Masten (2001) asserts, the labelling of risk and protective factors is often arbitrarily decided, and the gradient on the continuum can be inversely tilted, turning the protective factors into risk factors, and vice versa. Fergus and Zimmerman (2005) similarly contend that what works as a protective factor in one context might itself become a risk in another. They provide the example of high intelligence working as a protective factor by aiding scholastic achievement when stress levels are low but having no impact when stress is high. A single protective or risk factor has limited potential for determining the causality of positive or maladaptive coping patterns. Moreover, apart from the interaction effect of various factors, the resilient outcome also varies from person to person, implying subjective meaning-making processes and a high probability of personality-based variables affecting the outcome.

Resilience and related constructs

The literature on risk and protective factors in resilience studies reflects considerable confusion regarding definition, measurement, and statistical findings (Luthar, 2006). An overview reveals two major approaches of deciphering the underlying processes – variable-based research and person-based research. Variable-based research uses multi-variate statistical analyses in order to understand the impact of risk factors on adaptive coping and to cull out the impact of mediating or moderating protective variables. Luthar (2006) describes one of the pioneering studies by

Garmezy, Masten, and Tellegen (1984) that examined the effect of protective factors like age, sex, and socio-economic status for their main effect on competence or positive adaptation outcomes. The study also examined the interaction effect of these protective factors with the risk factors using hierarchical multiple regression. This approach enables exploration of differential and specific linkages among variables and adaptive or non-adaptive outcomes. At the same time, due to enhanced focus on specificity, these studies tend to overlook patterns of resilient behaviour in lives of individuals.

Fergus and Zimmerman (2005) describe three general types of resilience models – compensatory, protective, and challenge – that use different pathways for explaining the process through which risk and protective factors operate for ensuring positive adaptation. Masten (2001) also discusses in detail the various models used in variable-based research and the pathways through which these help determine the intervention strategies. For example correlational studies exploring the main effect of variables suggest adding on to the assets in order to counterbalance the negative effects of high adversity. This concept of compensatory effects (Garmezy et al., 1984) helps design interventions based on asset enhancement where a protective factor counteracts a risk factor.

Similarly, the research models exploring mediating variables are helpful in designing interventions that alter the level of particular risk or protective variable in an individual's life. Such protective models describe the process by which assets moderate the effects of a risk on a negative outcome. Interaction models of resilience research suggest two pathways of moderation – one through an enduring personal characteristic that acts as a protective factor for the individual or system facing adversity and the second through risk-activated protection systems that come into action during or after the adversity occurs. Interventions based on these models focus on providing enhanced risk-activated protections in the environment or on improving individual coping strategies. Another category of resilience models is the challenge model, which posits a curvilinear relationship between risk factors and outcomes, implying negative outcomes at both low and high levels of risk and positive outcomes at moderate levels of risk. However, most applications of the challenge model require longitudinal data and hence find application in person-based approaches to studying resilience.

Variable-based models are useful in providing specific and pointed interventions, yet these are not fully equipped to deal with the transactional dynamics of individual and environmental variables or the bidirectional nature of these interactions (Masten, 1999). Also, variable-based analyses fail to account for the interaction of risk and protective factors for adaptive outcomes over a period of time (Masten et al., 1999).

Person-based approaches to resilience attempt to overcome these issues by studying naturally occurring cluster of risk and protective factors in the lives of individuals and provide insight into who is or is not at risk for determining holistic intervention strategies. Luthar (2006) mentions two major studies in the genre – one by Werner and Smith (1992) and the other by Cowen and colleagues (Cowen et al., 1996; Wyman et al., 1999) that identified and defined protective factors as those variables that made it possible to distinguish between high-risk children who did well and those who did not. Masten (2001) has described the approach in detail, citing these studies as prototypical examples of person-based research, which typically compares two sub-sets of individuals drawn from the same group that has faced significant adversity or that has been subjected to the same risk factors. The sub-set that demonstrates resilient outcomes is compared with the sub-set that resorts to maladaptive coping resulting in negative outcomes, thereby bringing out the assets or protective factors that shield against adverse effects and facilitate a resilient outcome. These studies have generally corroborated the evidence generated by variable-based research (Masten, 2001); however, most research, barring a few (e.g. Luthar, 1991; Masten et al., 1999), has not incorporated any low-risk groups for comparison and hence fails to provide cut-off criteria for good versus poor competence in high- versus low-risk conditions. Comparison of groups becomes a difficult task when there are multiple criteria involved. Recent research shows the trend of using both variable- and person-based approaches for analyzing multiple competency domains (e.g. Buckner, Mezzacappa, & Beardslee, 2003). Another useful approach in person-based research is demonstrated by Seidman and Pedersen (2003) who, besides comparing resilient and non-resilient groups, explored the conditional effect of risk and vulnerability factors. Luthar (2006) emphasises the need for long-term prospective studies for understanding critical turning points across a life span. Newer approaches are being used for designing long-term prospective studies that combine a variable approach with person-based approach, and the availability of newer statistical techniques that allow for sophisticated statistical analyses even with missing or discrepant data sets has ensured much scientific rigor enhancing the potential of such research to understand resilience pathways.

The way forward

As evident even from a cursory review of the field, resilience theory and research constitute a complex area. Beginning with different approaches in conceptualizing the construct – treating it either as a trait within the individual or a product of risk and protective factors in the environment, to attributing it to the dynamic interactions of the two, researchers have added to the complexity of the construct. Different approaches to designing of research studies further add on to the richness of the construct, though such complexity also makes it difficult to derive concrete and generalisable research insights and implementable conclusions. Also, context specificity of most research studies limits the applicability in different settings and for general populations. The construct of resilience is subject to much scrutiny, debate, and contention. Some of the contentious issues and challenges in the area merit specific attention, as resolution of these is crucial in determining the future trajectories of growth for the construct and in expanding its potential to provide implementable interventions in order to influence policy. Some of these issues are discussed in Luthar, Cicchetti & Becker, 2000.

First and foremost, the challenge is arriving at a consensus about defining the construct of resilience, as variations in definition are reflected in variations in operationalisation of the construct. As discussed previously, variations in conceptualizing the construct of resilience get translated into variations in operationalising the construct and in deciding the measurement criteria for resilient and non-resilient behaviours. Even when the core components of resilience are accepted as the presence of significant adversity and positive adaptation, variations in determining what constitute adversity and what behavioural indicators signify positive adaptation account for much variation across studies. There is so much diversity in measurement issues that some scholars have questioned if the various studies are even measuring the same construct (Kaplan, 1999). However, diversity in the field is also indicative of a thriving body of literature that explores divergent domains and progressively define the construct in a multi-dimensional manner. The only caveat is that researchers must diligently define behavioural indicators and parameters while operationalising resilience in their specific contexts and must take care to explicitly define risk and protective factors and their pathways of operation in the given environment. Also, it is essential to periodically consolidate diverse findings in order to establish identifiable patterns in research and expand and consolidate these domains through rigorous research designs.

Another issue that is of importance in determining the future directions of research is conceptualisation of resilience as a trait or as a process. Conceptualising resilience as a trait places it as a personal characteristic of the individual, reflecting general resourcefulness and sturdiness of character. This conceptualisation considers resilience akin to the concept of ego-resiliency developed by Block and Block (1980). Although a general consensus has developed in the field regarding differential use of the terms resilience and resiliency, there still exists some overlap in the usage of the two. As Luthar (1996) clarifies, the two concepts are differentiated on two major dimensions – resiliency is an enduring characteristic of an individual, while resilience is a dynamic developmental process; second, significant adversity is a prerequisite for inferences about resilience to be made, whereas resiliency does not presuppose any adversity. Maintaining the distinction of the two terms is essential as the term resiliency conveys the connotation of a personality trait and might lead to inappropriate labeling of individuals as not having the capability to overcome adversity (Masten, 1994) and hence hinder the designing of appropriate interventions.

The third and final challenge for future research, as discussed by Luthar et al. (2000) stems from undifferentiated usage of protective and vulnerability variables. Initial studies of resilience restricted the term protective variables for those factors that provided amelioration from adversity as a result of interaction effect; however, gradually, the distinction vanished, and the term protective variables began being used even for direct ameliorative effects. Luthar (1993) recommends using more differentiated terms in order to enable a finer distinction between salient processes.

A finer conceptualisation of the construct of resilience for future research is an essential requirement that would ensure rigour of measurement and would lead to corroboration of research findings across domains and across methods. The current divergence in the area might emerge as an advantage for it is through consolidation of findings in divergent domains that a scientific construct takes shape. Also, this would make possible expanding the construct beyond individual-based studies to the study of resilient systems and resilient communities, as generalizing research outcomes becomes a feasible option given consensus across the field.

References

Block, J. H., & Block, J. (1980). The role of ego-control and ego resiliency in the organization of behaviour. In W. A. Collins (Ed.), *Minnesota symposium on child psychology* (Vol. 13, pp. 39–101). Hillsdale, NJ: Erlbaum.

Bonnano, G. A. (2004). Loss, trauma and human resilience. *American Psychologist, 59*(1), 20–28.

Buckner, J. C., Mezzacappa, E., & Beardslee, W. R. (2003). Characteristics of resilient youths living in poverty: The role of self-regulatory processes. *Development and Psychopathology, 15*(1), 139–162.

Cicchetti, D., & Curtis, W. J. (2007). Special issue: A multilevel approach to resilience. *Development and Psychopathology, 19*(3), 627–955.

Cicchetti, D., & Garmezy, N. (1993). Milestones in development of resilience (Special Issue). *Development and Psychopathology, 5*(4), 497–774.

Conrad, M., & Hammen, C. (1993). Protective and resource factors in high- and low-risk children: A comparison of children with unipolar, bipolar, medically ill, and normal mothers. *Development and Psychopathology, 5*(4), 593–607.

Cowen, E. L., Hightower, A. D., Pedro-Carroll, J. L., Work, W. C., Wyman, P. A., & Haffey, W. G. (1996). *School based prevention for children at risk: The preliminary mental health project.* Washington, DC: American Psychological Association.

Dubow, E. F., Edwards, S., & Ippolito, M. F. (1997). Life stressors, neighborhood disadvantage, and resources: A focus on inner-city children's adjustment. *Journal of Clinical Child Psychology, 26*(2), 130–144.

Elder, G. H. (1998). The life course as developmental theory. *Child Development, 69*, 1–12.

Felner, R. D., Brand, S., DuBois, D. L., Adan, A. M., Mulhall, P. F., & Evans, E. G. (1995). Socioeconomic disadvantage, proximal environmental experiences, and socioemotional and academic adjustment in early adolescence: Investigation of a mediated effects model. *Child Development, 66*, 774–792.

Fergus, S., & Zimmerman, M. A. (2005). Adolescent resilience: A framework for understanding healthy development in the face of risk. *Annual Review of Public Health, 26*, 399–419.

Fletcher, D., & Sarkar, M. (2013). Psychological resilience: A review and critique of definitions, concepts, and theory. *European Psychologist, 18*(1), 12–23.

Fonagy, P., Steele, M., Steele, H., Higgit, A., & Target, M. (1994). The Emanuel Miller memorial lecture 1992: The theory and practice of resilience. *Journal of Child Psychology and Psychiatry and Allied Disciplines, 35*(2), 231–257.

Garmezy, N., Masten, A. S., & Tellegen, A. (1984). The study of stress and competence in children: A building block for developmental psychopathology. *Child Development, 55*, 97–111.

Glantz, M., & Johnson, J. (Eds.). (1999). *Resilience and development: Positive life adaptations.* New York: Plenum Press.

Greenberg, M. T., Lengua, L. J., Coie, J. D., & Pinderhughes, E. E. (1999). Predicting developmental outcomes at school entry using a multiple-risk model: Four American communities. *Developmental Psychology, 35*, 403–417.

Kaplan, H. B. (1999). Toward an understanding of resilience: A critical review of definitions and models. In M. D. Glantz & J. R. Johnson (Eds.), *Resilience and development: Positive life adaptations* (pp. 17–83). New York: Plenum.

Luthar, S. S. (1991). Vulnerability and resilience: A study of high-risk adolescents. *Child Development, 62*, 600–616.

Luthar, S. S. (1993). Annotation: Methodological and conceptual issues in the study of resilience. *Journal of Child Psychology and Psychiatry, 34*(4), 441–453.

Luthar, S. S. (1996). *Resilience: A construct of value?* Paper presented at the 104th Annual Convention of the American Psychological Association, Toronto.

Luthar, S. S. (2006). Resilience in development: A synthesis of research across five decades. In D. Cicchetti & D. J. Cohen (Eds.), *Developmental psychopathology: Risk, disorder, and adaptation* (2nd ed., pp. 739–795). New York: Wiley.

Luthar, S. S., Cicchetti, D., & Becker, B. (2000). The construct of resilience: A critical evaluation and guidelines for future work. *Child Development, 71*(3), 543–562.

Masten, A. S. (1994). Resilience in individual development: Successful adaptation despite risk and adversity. In M. C. Wang & E. W. Gordon (Eds.), *Educational resilience in inner-city America: Challenges and prospects* (pp. 3–25). Hillsdale, NJ: Erlbaum.

Masten, A. S. (1999). Resilience comes of age: Reflections on the past and outlook for the next generation of research. In M. D. Glantz, J. Johnson, & L. Huffman (Eds.), *Resilience and development: Positive life adaptations* (pp. 282–296). New York: Plenum.

Masten, A. S. (2001). Ordinary magic: Resilience processes in development. *American Psychologist, 56*(3), 227–238.

Masten, A. S. (2004). Regulatory processes, risk and resilience in adolescent development. *Annals of New York Academy of Science, 1021*, 310–319.

Masten, A. S. (2006). Developmental psychopathology: Pathways to the future. *International Journal of Behavioural Development, 31*(1), 46–53.

Masten, A. S., Burt, K., & Coatsworth, J. D. (2006). Competence and psychopathology. In D. Cicchetti & D. Cohen (Eds.), *Developmental psychopathology, Vol 3, Risk, disorder and psychopathology* (2nd ed., pp. 696–738). New York: Wiley.

Masten, A. S., & Coatsworth, J. D. (1995). Competence, resilience, and psychopathology. In D. Cicchetti & D. Cohen (Eds.), *Developmental psychopathology: Vol. 2. Risk, disorder, and adaptation* (pp. 715–752). New York: Wiley.

Masten, A. S., & Coatsworth, J. D. (1998). The development of competence in favorable and unfavorable environments: Lessons from successful children. *American Psychologist, 53*(2), 205–220.

Masten, A. S., Hubbard, J. J., Gest, S. D., Tellegen, A., Garmezy, N., & Ramirez, M. (1999). Competence in the context of adversity: Pathways to resilience and maladaptation from childhood to late adolescence. *Development and Psychopathology, 11*, 143–169.

Masten, A. S., & Obradivic, J. (2006). Competence and resilience in development. *Annals of New York Academy of Science, 1094*, 13–27.

Masten, A. S., & Powell, J. L. (2003). A resilience framework for research, policy, and practice. In S. S. Luthar (Ed.), *Resilience and vulnerability: Adaptation in the context of childhood adversities* (pp. 1–25). New York: Cambridge University Press.

Masten, A. S., & Reed, M. J. (2002). Resilience in development. In C. R. Synder, & S. J. Lopez (Eds.), *Handbook of positive psychology* (pp. 74–88). Oxford: Oxford University Press.

Murphy, L. B. (1962). *The widening world of childhood: Paths toward mastery.* New York: Basic Books.

Richardson, G. E. (2002). The metatheory of resilience and resiliency. *Journal of Clinical Psychology, 58*(3), 307–321.

Richardson, G. E., Neiger, B. L., Jensen, S., & Kumpfer, K. L. (1990). The resiliency model. *Health Education, 21*(6), 33–39.

Rutter, M. (1990). Psychosocial resilience and protective mechanisms. In J. Rolf, A. S. Masten, D. Cicchetti, K. H. Nuechterlein, & S. Weintraub (Eds.), *Risk and protective factors in the development of psychopathology* (pp. 181–214). New York: Cambridge University Press.

Rutter, M. (1999). Psychosocial adversity and child psychopathology. *British Journal of Psychiatry, 174,* 480–449.

Rutter, M. (2000). Resilience reconsidered: Conceptual considerations, empirical findings, and policy implications. In J. P. Shonkoff & S. J. Meisels (Eds.), *Handbook of early childhood intervention* (2nd ed., pp. 651–682). New York: Cambridge University Press.

Rutter, M. (2006). Implications of resilience concepts for scientific understanding. In B. M. Lester, A. S. Masten, & B. McEwen (Eds.), *Resilience in children* (pp. 1–11). Malden, MA: Blackwell Publishing.

Seidman, E., & Pedersen, S. (2003). Holistic, contextual perspectives on risk, protection, and competence among low income urban adolescents. In S. S. Luthar (Ed.), *Resistance and vulnerability: Adaptation in the context of childhood adversities* (pp. 318–342). New York: Cambridge University Press.

Tiet, Q. Q., Bird, H. R., Davies, M., Hoven, C., Cohen, P., Jensen, P. S., & Goodman, S. (1998). Adverse life events and resilience. *Journal of the American Academy of Child and Adolescent Psychiatry, 37*(11), 1191–1200.

Waters, E., & Sroufe, L. A. (1983). Social competence as a developmental construct. *Developmental Review, 3,* 79–97.

Weissberg, R. P., Kumpfer, K. L., & Seligman, M. E. P. (2003). Prevention that works for children and youth: An introduction. *American Psychologist, 58,* 425–432.

Werner, E. (1995). Resilience in development. *Current Directions in Psychological Science, 4*(3), 81–85.

Werner, E., & Smith, R. (1992). *Overcoming the odds: High risk children from birth to adulthood.* Ithaca, NY: Cornell University Press.

Wyman, P. A., Cowen, E. L., Work, W. C, Hoyt-Meyers, L., Magnus, K. B., & Fagen, D. B. (1999). Caregiving and developmental factors differentiating young at-risk urban children showing resilient versus stress-affected outcomes: A replication and extension. *Child Development, 70*(3), 645–659.

Yates, T. M., Egeland, B., & Sroufe, L. A. (2003). Rethinking resilience: A developmental process perspective. In S. S. Luthar (Ed.), *Resilience and vulnerability: Adaptation in the context of childhood adversities* (pp. 243–266). New York: Cambridge University Press.

2

Resilience

An overall view in the Indian scenario

Kamlesh Singh and Jasleen Kaur

The term "resilience" owes its origin to Latin word *resilio*, which means to restore a bent or a stretched object to its original shape. While "resilience" made its first appearance in physics in 1858 when Scottish engineer William Rankine used it in the context of mechanics to describe the strength and ductility of steel beams (Alexander, 2013), the successful transition of "resilience" from physics to psychology happened in early 1970s when Norman Garmezy studied the adaptive behaviour of children belonging to schizophrenic mothers, deemed to be at high risk due to unfavourable environment. This led to the development of Garmezy's project, "Project Competence", which studied the competence of children in high-risk and stressful environments. Project Competence proved to be influential in inspiring other researchers to gain an understanding as to what makes some children thrive despite their ill circumstances. This recognition was responsible for the concept of "resilience" gaining popularity in wider circles of psychology, and the focus of research gradually widened to study individuals who successfully transcended the life's adversities to emerge unscathed. Rutter (1987) aptly termed resilience as an interactive concept in which the presence of resilience has to be inferred from individual variations in outcome among individuals who have experienced significant major stress or adversity. Abrams (2001) defined resilience as the ability to readily recover from illness, depression, and adversity. The subject of resilience often broaches in the context of adversity, traumatic event, or any other stressful situation. In the face of such an event, what is it that makes people resilient? Explanations range from personality traits to role of genetics and to influence of environmental factors. For example Masten (2001) viewed resilience as part of the genetic makeup of humans and as the norm rather than the exception. According to her,

> What began as a quest to understand the extraordinary has revealed the power of the ordinary. Resilience does not come from rare and special qualities, but from the everyday magic of ordinary, normative human resources in the minds, brains, and bodies of children, in their families and relationships, and in their communities.

While Zolkoski and Bullock (2012) believed that everyone is born with an innate capacity for resilience, others (Antonovsky, 1979; Kobasa, 1982) viewed resilience as an attribute of an individual. The role of certain personality traits that make a person pre-disposed to resilience has also been explored. For example Luthar and Zigler (1991) identified certain qualities that resilient children possess. These children were found to be active, humourous, confident, competent, prepared to take risks, flexible, and, as a result of repeated successful coping experiences, confident in both their inner and outer resources. Sapienza and Masten (2011) highlighted the role of IQ, self-regulation, and positive self-perceptions in resilient children. The role of environmental factors cannot be ignored in the context of resilience. Positive parenting and schools play an important role in promoting resilience (Luthar, 2006; Masten, 2007), as well as nurturing interpersonal relationships and social support (Howell, Graham-Bermann, Czyz, & Lilly, 2010; Salami, 2010). In several studies of older adults, strong social networks predicted higher resilience (Hinck, 2004; Kinsel, 2005). Schofield (2001) identified a combination of individual and environmental factors as essential components of resilience – social support networks, the capacity to discover meaning and therefore motivation in life (such as religious or other spiritual belief), social skills to give control over life events, self-esteem, and even a sense of humour. Truffino (2010) enumerated various characteristics the degree of which decides the resiliency of individuals. It includes intrapersonal as well as interpersonal characteristics – control over the process of remembering traumatic experiences, integration of memory and emotions; regulation of emotions related to trauma; control of symptoms; self-esteem; internal cohesion (thoughts, emotions, and actions); establishment of secure links; understanding the impact of the trauma; and developing a positive meaning. Fiona (2011) believed that a secure base, good self-esteem, and a sense of self-efficacy made up the building blocks of resilience. Thus, it is not just individual or environmental factors but their interaction that is important while studying resilience.

It is also worthwhile to acknowledge the role of demographic variables in the context of resilience. Does an individual's age, gender, level of education, household income, and location affect resilience? Wagnild and Young (1993) reported that resilience is independent of age, education, income, and gender, while Bonanno, Galea, Bucciarelli, and Vlahov (2007) reported the role of gender, age, race/ethnicity, education, level of trauma exposure, income change, social support, frequency of chronic disease, and recent and past life stressors in predicting resilience. Several studies have reported both similar and/or contradictory findings. For example Lundman, Strandberg, Eisemann, Gustafson, and Brulin (2007) found resilience to be increasing with age, a finding fitting well with findings of Losoi et al. (2013). As for gender, inconsistent findings were reported. For example Campbell-Sills, Cohan, and Stein (2006) reported no gender difference in resilient levels, consistent with the Swedish finding of Lundman et al. (2007) and Losoi et al. (2013). However, Campbell-Sills, Forde, and Stein (2009) reported higher levels of resilience in men as compared to women, a finding reflected in a Nigerian study as well (Abiola & Udofia, 2011). Netuveli, Wiggins, Montgomery, Hildon, and Blane (2008) found women to be more resilient than men. Regarding the association of level of education with resilience, Campbell-Sills et al. (2009) associated lower levels of resilience with lower levels of education. Wagnild (2003) explored the role of income in resilience. Out of the three samples he studied, in two an association between lower incomes and lower level of resilience was reported. Similar findings on the positive relationship between income and resilience resonated in other studies as well (Campbell-Sills et al., 2009; Hardy, Concato, & Gill, 2004). Wells (2010) studied the association of resilience with several socio-demographic factors. Only income was found to be significantly correlated to resilience, with higher income associated with lower levels of resilience. The author did not report any difference in resilience levels of adults living in urban, rural, or suburban areas.

Since resilience and its factors have been adapted/borrowed from Western and European studies, it was necessary to understand universal/global perspective of resilience. In the next section, the chapter proceeds on how it is explored in Indian studies on different samples and stages.

While until now, the discussion on resilience has centered on the contributions of the West, we now shift focus to the work done on resilience in India. India is a developing country, and its population has already crossed one billion. With most of its population being rural (68.84%), India is also home to many states with skewed sex ratios. India has also suffered several setbacks in the form of natural adversities such as a tsunami in 2004 and many others. Despite all of this, it is today one of the fastest growing economies in the world. In such a scenario, it is important to review all the studies done on resilience in the general Indian population and on specific groups. Resilience studies in the wake of demographic factors and intervention programs have also been reviewed.

Resilience scales used and developed in India

Various components constitute resilience – novelty seeking, emotional regulation, hardiness, optimism, resourcefulness, social competence, family cohesion, control, commitment, challenge, and so on. Several unidimensional and multi-dimensional measures on resilience exist, such as the Dispositional Resilience Scale (DRS, Bartone, Ursano, Wright, & Ingraham, 1989); the Resilience Scale (RS, Wagnild & Young, 1993); the Adolescent Resilience Scale (ARS, Oshio, Nakaya, Kaneko, & Nagamine, 2003); the Connor–Davidson Resilience Scale (CD-RISC, Connor & Davidson, 2003); and so forth . Resilience research in India is still in its infancy stage as compared to the West. Indian researchers have generally used the resilience measures developed in the Western and European studies without measuring their psychometric properties in Indian scenario further, for example Mampane's (2005) resilience questionnaire in Deb and Arora's (2012) study; the Resilience Scale (RS, Wagnild & Young, 1987) in Sood, Bakshi, and Devi's (2013) study; the Resilience Scale for Adults (RSA, Friborg, Barlaug, Martinussen, Rosenvinge, & Hjemdal, 2005) in Annalakshmi's (2007) study; and so on. However, a few Indian studies have focused on the resilience measurement. Indian researchers (Singh, Kaur, & Junnarkar, under review) recently developed a new resilience measure for the Indian population. The study, carried out in three phases, reported a four-factor model of resilience consisting of self-efficacy, coping, resourcefulness, and goal orientation. With an overall reliability of $\alpha = .95$, the measure is a psychometrically sound instrument for assessing resilience in English and Hindi both. To increase its usability, the scale has also been translated in Hindi. Taking into account the increasing number of farmers' suicides, Lal et al. (2014) developed a scale to measure farmers' level of resilience towards their lives (RFL-Scale). The RFL-Scale is a uni-dimensional, eighteen-item measure of resilience with nine positive and nine negative items. Psychometrically sound, the scale has good reliability ($\alpha = .87$). Annalakshmi (2009a) developed a thirty-item resilience scale – the Bharathiar University Resilience Scale (BURS). With an overall acceptable reliability ($\alpha = .82$), BURS measures seven domains of resilience – duration for getting back to normalcy, reaction to negative events, response to risk factors (specifically disadvantaged environment) in life, perception of effect of past negative events, defining problems, hope/confidence in coping with future and openness to experience, and flexibility. Existing Western measures of resilience have also been validated on Indian population. While all these measures are standardized and psychometrically sound measures, the most popular and most validated is the Connor–Davidson Resilience Scale (CD-RISC, Connor & Davidson 2003). The original CD-RISC is a twenty-five-item measure with a five-factors solution (competence and tenacity, tolerance of negative effect, positive acceptance of change, secure relationships, and spiritual influences) with overall good reliability ($\alpha = .89$). Singh and Yu (2010) validated CD-RISC on Indian college-going students. In contrast to the original factor structure, the authors reported a four-factor solution for resilience – hardiness, optimism, resourcefulness, and purpose. With an overall reliability ($\alpha = .89$), it explained 47.38% of variance.

Resilience in different age groups in India

Children and adolescents: Resilience in children and adolescents has been studied across India by several researchers. Annalakshmi (2009b) measured resilience in adolescent girls and boys with regard to certain cognitive variables – metacognition and complexity. Adolescents scoring high on the resiliency measure were found to use more complex explanations and more metacognitions while explaining behaviour in comparison to the adolescents with lower resilient scores. The effect of religious personality on resilience was explored in a sample of 200 Muslim adolescents (Annalakshmi & Abeer, 2010). The authors reported that just the knowledge of one's religion and its rituals is not adequate for resilience until it becomes part of one's behaviour. Predictors of resilience emerging from components of spirituality were examined (Annalakshmi & Jose, 2011) in a sample of adolescents in Kerala, using BURS (Annalakshmi, 2009a). Five components emerged as strong predictors of resilience – truth, joy, discernment, synthesis, and equanimity. Deb and Arora (2012) looked into the academic achievement of high-resilience and low-resilience adolescents, using the resilience scale developed by Mampane (2005). The scale constitutes seven dimensions of resilience – commitment, future aspirations, problem solving, role models, self-awareness, sense of control, and support. Not only did high-resilience adolescents score better academically, the authors also reported a 120% greater chance for these adolescents of being successful in competitive examinations in comparison to the low-resilience group. The link between resilience and mental health was examined by Sood et al. (2013) who studied resilience in adolescents (13–18 years old) living in border areas in Jammu and Kashmir. Using the Resilience Scale (Wagnild & Young, 1987), comparisons were made on two groups of adolescents identified as having low resilience and high resilience. Poorer mental health was observed for adolescents having lower resilience levels as compared to those with higher resilience. The lower-resilience group also showed significantly greater loss of emotional control and low scores on overall positive affect. Findings also revealed resilience as being significantly positively related to overall mental health, general positive affect, emotional ties, and psychological well-being, while a significantly negative correlation was observed with loss of emotional control. A similar finding was reported by Suresh, Jayachander, and Joshi (2013), wherein the authors reported resilience as one of the predictors of psychological well-being among adolescents. Commenting on resilience in adolescents belonging to single-parent families, the authors (Manhas, Sharma, & Riya, 2013) reported a low sense of mastery and a low sense of relatedness for majority of the sample, which are considered as important components of resilience. Herbert, Manjula, and Philip (2013) studied resilience levels in children living with a schizophrenic parent. While the majority (60%) of the children reported medium resilience, 24% reported high resilience while only 15% reported low levels of resilience. For those with high and medium levels of resilience, social support was the main factor that helped them deal with life's difficulties. In a study on university students, Sharma, Bali, and Kumari (2014), examined the role of well-being in the context of resiliency to stress. Based on their scores, students were categorized in high well-being and low well-being groups. Higher resiliency to stress was observed for the high well-being group in comparison to the low well-being group. Significant positive correlation between resilience and life satisfaction was reported by Rani, Midha, and Rekha (2014) in their study of teenagers.

Adults: Annalakshmi (2007) looked at the effect of probabilistic orientation on resilience among graduate student and scientists, using the Resilience Scale for Adults (RSA, Friborg et al., 2005). Quoting Annalakshmi (2007), the probabilistic orientation refers to a typical phenomenological perspective ordaining the individual personality and is construed by seven factors: unbounded expectancy, sensing unlimited possibilities, insight into bias, healthy skepticism, unconditional acceptance, appreciation of chance, and awareness of probability. While graduate students displayed higher scores on resilience than scientists, no significant findings emerged with regard to the effect of probabilistic orientation on resilience. In a comparison of personality traits of high- and low-resilience individuals (assessed using RSA, Friborg et al., 2005), Annalakshmi (2008), in her study of more than 100 individuals aged 20 to 25 years, reported that participants with higher scores on resilience showed more dominance and a greater need for understanding, affiliation, nurturance, and exhibition in comparison to those scoring low on resilience. In a study of the well-being of managers in work organizations (Srivastava, 2009), resilience was one of the many individual factors responsible for the psychological well-being at the workplace. Resilience was also hailed as the building block of Indian identity along with connection with others, such as being hard working and so on, in a study of identity among Indian youth (Kapur & Misra, 2009). In a study of youth of Delhi and Bangalore, Kalyani, Varghese, and Velayudham (2009) reported that children's views about their parents directly correlated with their resilience levels. Resilience levels were also examined in two groups of rural women (self-help group and non-self-help group) of Telangana along with self-efficacy and psychological empowerment (Rani & Radhika, 2014). Significantly higher scores on resilience and other two dimensions were reported for women who were part of a self-help group as compared to the other group. Resilience was also found as one of the main predictors of marital satisfaction among Indian couples (Ganth, Thiyagarajan, & Nigesh, 2013). In rural Indian women, Singh, Kaur, Singh, and Suri (2014) explored the correlation between well-being with several interpersonal and intrapersonal variables. Resilience was found to be positively significantly correlated to psychological well-being, life satisfaction, social well-being, and altruism, while a significant negative correlation was seen with negative affect. In a sample of seventy female hostel wardens, who oversee school/college dormitories, Meena and Kumar (2014) examined the effect of resilience on coping strategies, perceived stress, and emotional control. Emotional control was found to be significantly affected by resilience, with emotional control varying in high- and low-resilience groups. Psychological resilience was found to be significantly impacted by spiritual as well as emotional intelligence in corporate executives across India (Ravikumar & Dhamodharan, 2014), like humour, which too was found to play an important role in impacting resilience in individuals (Pande, 2014). The role of resilience, hope, and perceived stress was examined in healthy, functioning adults (Jadhav, Dagaria, Dhavale, & Shanker, 2014). While a significant relationship between hope and resilience was found, the same did not hold true for resilience and perceived stress.

Elderly adults: In a study of 150 older adults (60–70 years), Mamta and Sharma (2013) reported significant positive correlations amongst resilience, self-efficacy, and well-being measures.

Resilience in different population groups in India

Athletes: Mehmi (2014) measured amongst other things, resilience in individual players and team game players. A total of sixty players (19–22 years), thirty for each group, were studied. No significant difference on any of the measures, including that of resilience was reported for individual or team game players. In Philip and Mathai's 2014 study pertaining to sports persons, the authors reported significantly higher levels of resilience in individuals involved in sports as compared to non-sports individuals.

Individuals with disabilities: Role of perceived environment and emotional intelligence as a function of resilience in individuals with physical disability was examined by Hariharan, Karimi, and Kishore (2014). Two groups of physically disabled persons were formed – fifty resilient and fifty vulnerable individuals. The authors reported that, not only were the resilient individuals more emotionally intelligent, but they also had more positive perceptions of their environment than the vulnerable group.

Diabetic patients: Concerned with the growing epidemic of diabetes mellitus in India, Tayal and Singh (2010) studied the predictors of healthiness in sixty-one diabetic and sixty-one non-diabetic individuals. Relationships among the measures of healthiness, self-efficacy, health locus of control, resilience, and body mass index (BMI) were also examined. A significant positive correlation of healthiness with resilience was reported as well as with internal locus of control and self-efficacy. Regression analysis further revealed resilience, chance (a component of the health locus of control), and self-efficacy as significant predictors explaining 39.1% variance in healthiness.

Natural disaster survivors: In recent years, India has witnessed large-scale devastation and loss of human lives due to natural disasters like floods, earthquakes, and so on. While the government provided all possible assistance and rehabilitated the affected people, their mental health still remains the topmost concern. The way people cope up with such traumatic events depends on their level of resilience. In a qualitative study of four coastal villages in Tamil Nadu affected by December 2004 tsunami, Rajkumar, Premkumar, and Tharyan (2008) evaluated resilience in different groups of people. Broadly, coping strategies at the individual and community level, along with spiritual coping were reported by the survivors. Authors observed that collectivizing personal trauma, a problem-focused coping style, extended social support, and one's spiritual beliefs helped the individuals and families cope with the adversity. In a comparative study of two communities of Chennai having similar exposure to natural disasters (cyclones and floods), Joerin, Shaw, Takeuchi, and Krishnamurthy (2012) examined their physical, social, and economic resilience with the help of the Climate-related Disaster Community Resilience Framework (CDCRF). The authors reported insufficient adaptive capacity for those whose houses had suffered damage due to climate hazards. These people due to limited adaptive capacity did not show more preparedness for future climate hazards and were found to be less resilient than others. In drought-prone regions of South India, Ranjan, Pradhan, Reddy, and Syme (2015) examined the roles of human, physical, social, financial, and natural capital in determining the resilience of farmers. More than health, higher skill, level of education, and number of earning members were perceived as important for future drought survival. Higher drought resilience was also seen more in farmers residing in watershed-treated areas.

Demographic variables

A glance at all the definitions of resilience gives the idea that resilience is a construct that is built upon one's personal attributes and internal and external resources, that it may be inherent or may develop over time, and that it may also fluctuate with life's changing circumstances. With resilience being such a multi-dimensional construct, it becomes all the more important to examine it more closely in the light of demographic variables. Connor and Davidson (2003) viewed resilience as a fluctuating construct that varies with age; gender; individual circumstances; and developmental, historical, and cultural contexts. However, there is a paucity of research in India focusing on the interplay of resilience and demographic factors. The studies that we came across during the review of literature mostly focus on gender differences in resilience. For example Deb and Arora (2009) explored gender differences in perception of academic adversity and resilience among 560 adolescents. Gender differences in the use of resilience resources were also probed. While females reported higher stress and lower resilience in academics than males, significant gender differences for use of internal resilience strategies (personal attributes) with males using it more than females were found. Similar findings of females being less resilient than males have echoed in other studies as well (Deb & Arora, 2011, 2012; Manhas et al., 2013). Barmola (2013) studied gender differences in adolescents across four domains of psychological capital – hope, self-efficacy, optimism, and resilience. Except for hope, no gender differences were reported in any other dimension. However, significant interaction between gender and resilience was reported by Pande (2014). Aligning to Wagnild and Young's (1993) findings, in an Indian study of well-functioning adults, Jadhav et al. (2014) found no significant correlation of resilience with any of the socio-demographic variables of age, gender, education, and marital status.

The role of income in predicting resilience has not been specifically explored much so far. We came across only one study, wherein Srivastava (2001) had examined the predictors of resilience in low-income working couples, residing in slums. The researcher took into account the past experiences (economic stress, family hassles, relative economic deprivation, future orientation, psychological symptoms, physical symptoms, quality of family life, female autonomy and social mobility) and the present experiences. These variables predicted 49.61% of the variance in resilience in wives and 63.05% in husbands, who also scored higher on overall resilience. While some predictors were found to differ across both sexes (female autonomy was a significant predictor of resilience for wives; for husbands, it was relative economic deprivation and present quality of life), future orientation and psychological symptoms predicted resilience in both husband and wife.

Resilience-based intervention programs in India

Importance of resilience enhancement programs is now being recognized the world over. In India, their implementation has started but as of now is limited to academic settings only. For example Singh and Choubisa (2009) documented the efficacy of a multi-component intervention module on college students, leading to enhanced resilience and overall well-being. Lakshmanan and Mythili (2010) administered a psychological intervention in a sample of school-going adolescent girls. Significantly higher scores on resilience were observed for the experimental group as compared to the control group. Sankaranarayanan and Cycil (2014) examined the efficacy of the Penn Resiliency Program (PRP) on school-going urban Indian adolescents. PRP is a US-based resiliency intervention program, developed by the University of Pennsylvania, for teaching coping and problem-solving skills in school-going children with the aim of promoting resilience in them. PRP proved to be an effective tool in the Indian study, wherein the researchers reported a change in negative attribution styles in the intervention group in comparison to the control group. Pareek and Mohan (2015) designed a resilience enhancement module for school-going adolescents and tested its efficacy for the same. Improved resilience scores were observed for the experimental group whereas a decrease in resilience scores was noted for the control group.

Conclusion

The study has attempted to review the work done on resilience in India in the light of various parameters. While overall, research on resilience in India has gathered pace in the last few years, there are several areas that remain unexplored, such as exploring the role of demographic factors like age, income, marital status, and so on in affecting resilience. A gap exists in resilience research on the geriatric population, which also needs to be addressed. Future, related research can also focus more on studying resilience in special groups and on the application of resilience intervention programs in different settings. There is also a crucial need for the development, standardization, and revalidation of more resilience measures for the Indian population.

References

Abiola, T., & Udofia, O. (2011). Psychometric assessment of the Wagnild and Young's resilience scale in Kano, Nigeria. *BMC Research Notes, 4,* 509–513.

Abrams, M. S. (2001). Resilience in ambiguous loss. *American Journal of Psychotherapy, 55*(2), 283–291.

Alexander, D. E. (2013). Resilience and disaster risk reduction: An etymological journey. *Natural Hazards and Earth System Sciences, 13*(11), 2707–2716.

Annalakshmi, N. (2007). Probabilistic orientation and resilience. *Journal of the Indian Academy of Applied Psychology, 33*(2), 269–274.

Annalakshmi, N. (2008). The resilient individual – A personality analysis. *Journal of the Indian Academy of Applied Psychology, 34*(Special Issue), 110–118.

Annalakshmi, N. (2009a). Bharathiar university resilience scale. In Harish Purohit, & Ajay Wagh (Eds.), *Research methods in business and management* (pp. 105–121). New Delhi: Sri Publishers.

Annalakshmi, N. (2009b). Resilience, metacognition and complexity. *Journal of the Indian Academy of Applied Psychology, 35*(special issue), 112–118.

Annalakshmi, N., & Abeer, K. C. (2010). Effect of Islamic worldview and religious personality on resilience among Muslim adolescent students. Paper presented at Indian Science Congress held at Trivandrum, Kerala.

Annalakshmi, N., & Jose, T. P. (2011). Spiritual intelligence and resilience among Christian youth in Kerala. *Journal of the Indian Academy of Applied Psychology, 37*(2), 263–268.

Antonovsky, A. (1979). *Health, stress and coping.* San Francisco: Jossey-Bass.

Barmola, K. C. (2013). Gender and psychological capital of adolescents. *Indian Journal of Applied Research, 3*(10), 1–3.

Bartone, P. T., Ursano, R. J., Wright, K. M., & Ingraham, L. H. (1989). The impact of a military air disaster on the health of assistance workers: A prospective study. *Journal of Nervous and Mental Disease, 177*(6), 317–328.

Bonanno, G. A., Galea, S., Bucciarelli, A., & Vlahov, D. (2007). What predicts psychological resilience after disaster? The role of demographics, resources, and life stress. *Journal of Consulting and Clinical Psychology, 75*(5), 671–682.

Campbell-Sills, L., Cohan, S. L., & Stein, M. B. (2006). Relationship of resilience to personality, coping, and psychiatric symptoms in young adults. *Behaviour Research and Therapy, 44*(4), 585–599.

Campbell-Sills, L., Forde, D. R., & Stein, M. B. (2009). Demographic and childhood environmental predictors of resilience in a community sample. *Journal of Psychiatric Research, 43*(12), 1007–1012.

Connor, K. M., & Davidson, J. R. (2003). Development of a new resilience scale: The Connor-Davidson resilience scale (CD-RISC). *Depression and Anxiety, 18*(2), 76–82.

Deb, A., & Arora, M. (2009). Gender differences in the perception of academic adversity and resilience among Indian adolescents. *Indian Journal of Community Psychology, 5*(2), 158–175.

Deb, A., & Arora, M. (2011). Resilience and mental health: A study on adolescents in Varanasi. *Journal of Indian Health Psychology, 5*(2), 69–79.

Deb, A., & Arora, M. (2012). Resilience and academic achievement among adolescents. *Journal of the Indian Academy of Applied Psychology, 38*(1), 93–101.

Fiona, M. (2011, July). Resilience: Concept, factors and models for practice. Briefing prepared for the Scottish Child Care and Protection Network (SCCPN) Reviewed by Brigid Daniel, Professor of Social Work, University of Stirling.

Friborg, O., Barlaug, D., Martinussen, M., Rosenvinge, J. H., & Hjemdal, O. (2005). Resilience in relation to personality and intelligence. *International Journal of Methods in Psychiatric Research, 14*(1), 29–42.

Ganth, D. B., Thiyagarajan, S., & Nigesh (2013). Role of infertility, emotional intelligence and resilience on marital satisfaction among Indian couples. *International Journal of Applied Psychology, 3*(3), 31–37.

Hardy, S. E., Concato, J., & Gill, T. M. (2004). Resilience of community-dwelling older persons. *Journal of the American Geriatrics Society, 52*(2), 257–262.

Hariharan, M., Karimi, M., & Kishore, M. T. (2014). Resilience in persons with physical disabilities: Role of perceived environment and emotional intelligence. *Journal of the Indian Academy of Applied Psychology, 40*(1), 96–101.

Herbert, H. S., Manjula, M., & Philip, M. (2013). Growing up with a parent having schizophrenia: Experiences and resilience in the offsprings. *Indian Journal of Psychological Medicine, 35*(2), 148–153.

Hinck, S. (2004). The lived experience of oldest-old rural adults. *Qualitative Health Research, 14*(6), 779–791.

Howell, K. H., Graham-Bermann, S. A., Czyz, E., & Lilly, M. (2010). Assessing resilience in preschool children exposed to intimate partner violence. *Violence and Victims, 25*(2), 150–164.

Jadhav, B., Dagaria, A., Dhavale, H. S., & Shanker, S. (2014). Study of resilience, hope and perceived stress in healthy and normal functioning adults. *Indian Journal of Social Psychiatry, 30*(1–2), 66–71.

Joerin, J., Shaw, R., Takeuchi, Y., & Krishnamurthy, R. (2012). Assessing community resilience to climate-related disasters in Chennai, India. *International Journal of Disaster Risk Reduction, 1*, 44–54.

Kalyani, V. N., Varghese, N., & Velayudham, A. (2009). Emotional intelligence and parental views of young adults: Poster presented at National Academy of Psychology (NAOP) India. *Proceedings-Psychological Studies, 54*(4), 310–352.

Kapur, K., & Misra, G. (2009). Who are we? Representation of Indianess amongst the Indian youth: Poster presented at National Academy of Psychology (NAOP) India. *Proceedings-Psychological Studies, 54*(4), 310–352.

Kinsel, B. (2005). Resilience as adaptation in older women. *Journal of Women and Aging, 17*(3), 23–39.

Kobasa, S. C. (1982). The hardy personality: Toward a social psychology of stress and health. In G. S. Sanders & J. Suls (Eds.), *Social psychology of health and illness* (pp. 3–32). Hillsdale, NJ: Erlbaum.

Lakshmanan, K., & Mythili, T. (2010). The effect of psychological intervention on resilience among early adolescent girls in Chennai corporation school. Retrieved from http://counselingchennai.com/yahoo_site_admin/assets/docs/Full_paper_Resilience_Study.22205430.pdf

Lal, S. P., Kadian, K. S., Jha, S. K., Singh, S. R. K., Goyal, J., Kumar, R. S., & Singh, S. P. (2014). Resilience scale to measure farmers' suicidal tendencies in national calamity hit region of India. *Current World Environment, 9*(3), 1001–1007.

Losoi, H., Senni, T., Minna, W., Mika, H., Juha, O., Juhani, J., & Eija, R. O. (2013). Psychometric properties of the Finnish version of the resilience scale and short version. *Psychology, Community & Health, 2*(1), 1–10.

Lundman, B., Strandberg, G., Eisemann, M., Gustafson, Y., & Brulin, C. (2007). Psychometric properties of the Swedish version of the resilience scale. *Scandinavian Journal of Caring Sciences, 21*(2), 229–237.

Luthar, S. S. (2006). Resilience in development: A synthesis of research across five decades. In D. Cicchetti & D. J. Cohen (Eds.), *Developmental psychopathology: Risk, disorder, and adaptation* (2nd ed., Vol. 3, pp. 739–795). Hoboken, NJ: Wiley.

Luthar, S. S., & Zigler, E. (1991). Vulnerability and competence: A review of research on resilience in childhood. *American Journal of Orthopsychiatry, 61*(1), 6–22.

Mampane, R. (2005). *The identification of resilient and non-resilient middle-adolescent learners in a South African township school.* (Doctoral dissertation, University of Pretoria, 2005). Retrieved from http://upetd.up.ac.za/thesis/available/etd-0204 2005–20226/unrestricted/00dissertation.pdf

Mamta, & Sharma, N. R. (2013). Resilience and self-efficacy as correlates of well-being among the elderly persons. *Journal of the Indian Academy of Applied Psychology, 39*(2), 281–288.

Manhas, S., Sharma, A., & Riya. (2013). Assessment of the level of resilience among adolescence of single parent families. *Indian Journal of Applied Research, 6*(3), 294–297.

Masten, A. S. (2001). Ordinary magic: Resilience processes in development. *American Psychologist, 56*(3), 227–238.

Masten, A. S. (2007). Resilience in developing systems: Progress and promise as the fourth wave rises. *Development and Psychopathology, 19*(3), 921–930.

Meena, S., & Kumar, A. (2014, February 24–25). *Effect of resilience on coping strategies, perceived stress and emotional control.* Paper presented at 1st International and 3rd Indian Psychological Science Congress: Psychological Well-Being: The Looming Crisis in Humanity, Chandigarh.

Mehmi, A. (2014, February 24–25). *A comparative analysis of individual and team game players on locus of control, self esteem and resilience.* Paper presented at 1st International and 3rd Indian Psychological Science Congress: Psychological Well-Being: The Looming Crisis in Humanity, Chandigarh.

Netuveli, G., Wiggins, R. D., Montgomery, S. M., Hildon, Z., & Blane, D. (2008). Mental health and resilience at older ages: Bouncing back after adversity in the British household panel survey. *Journal of Epidemiology and Community Health, 62*(11), 987–991.

Oshio, A., Nakaya, M., Kaneko, H., & Nagamine, S. (2003). Development and validation of an adolescent resilience scale. *Japanese Journal of Counseling Science, 35*, 57–65.

Pande, N. (2014). Effect of sense of humour on positive capacities: An empirical inquiry into psychological aspects. *Global Journal of Finance and Management, 6*(4), 385–390.

Pareek, H., & Mohan, M. (2015). Evaluating the efficacy of resilience enhancement module: A workshop designed for adolescents. *Indian Journal of Psychological Science, 5*(2), 61–66.

Philip, N. E., & Mathai, S. M. (2014, February 24–25). *Resilience and optimism among sports and non-sports students*. Paper presented at 1st International and 3rd Indian Psychological Science Congress: Psychological Well-Being: The Looming Crisis in Humanity, Chandigarh.

Rajkumar, A. P., Premkumar, T. S., & Tharyan, P. (2008). Coping with the Asian tsunami: Perspectives from Tamil Nadu, India on the determinants of resilience in the face of adversity. *Social Science & Medicine, 67*(5), 844–853.

Rani, B. J., & Radhika, S. (2014). Impact of self help group on self efficacy, resilience and psychological empowerment of rural women in Telangana. *International Journal of Science and Research, 3*(11), 2030–2031.

Rani, R., Midha, P., & Rekha. (2014, February 24–25). *Resilience as a correlate of life satisfaction among teenagers: A contemporary study*. Paper presented at 1st International and 3rd Indian Psychological Science Congress: Psychological Well-Being: The Looming Crisis in Humanity, Chandigarh.

Ranjan, R., Pradhan, D., Reddy, V. D., & Syme, G. J. (2015). Evaluating the determinants of perceived drought resilience: An empirical analysis of farmers' survival capabilities in drought-prone regions of South India. In V. R. Reddy & G. J. Syme (Eds.), *Integrated assessment of scale impacts of watershed intervention: Assessing hydrogeological and bio-physical influences on livelihoods* (pp. 253–285). Amsterdam, Netherlands: Elsevier.

Ravikumar, T., & Dhamodharan, V. (2014). Relationship among emotional intelligence, spiritual intelligence and psychological resilience of corporate executives in India. *Indian Journal of Applied Research, 4*(8), 349–352.

Rutter, M. (1987). Psychosocial resilience and protective mechanisms. *American Journal of Orthopsychiatry, 57*(3), 316–331.

Salami, S. O. (2010). Moderating effects of resilience, self-esteem and social support on adolescents' reactions to violence. *Asian Social Science, 6*(12), 101–110.

Sankaranarayanan, A., & Cycil, C. (2014). Resiliency training in Indian children: A pilot investigation of the Penn resiliency program. *International Journal of Environmental Research and Public Health, 11*(4), 4125–4139.

Sapienza, J. K., & Masten, A. S. (2011). Understanding and promoting resilience in children and youth. *Current Opinion in Psychiatry, 24*(4), 267–273.

Schofield, G. (2001). Resilience in family placement: A lifespan perspective. *Adoption & Fostering, 25*(3), 6–19.

Sharma, A., Bali, D., & Kumari, K. (2014, February 24–25). *Resilience to stress: Impact of well-being*. Paper presented at 1st International and 3rd Indian Psychological Science Congress: Psychological Well-Being: The Looming Crisis in Humanity, Chandigarh.

Singh, K., & Choubisa, R. (2009). Effectiveness of self focused intervention for enhancing Students' well-being. *Journal of the Indian Academy of Applied Psychology, 35*(special issue), 23–32.

Singh, K., Kaur, J., & Junnarkar, M. (under review). The Assessment of Resilience. In Singh, K. (ed.), *Measures of Positive Psychology*. New Delhi, India: Springer.

Singh, K., Kaur, J., Singh, D., & Suri, S. (2014). Correlates of well-being: A rural women study. *Journal of Indian Health Psychology, 8*(2), 31–42.

Singh, K., & Yu, X. N. (2010). Psychometric evaluation of the Connor-Davidson resilience scale (CD-RISC) in a sample of Indian students. *Journal of Psychology, 1*(1), 23–30.

Sood, S., Bakshi, A., & Devi, P. (2013). An assessment of perceived stress, resilience and mental health of adolescents living in border areas. *International Journal of Scientific and Research Publications, 3*(1), 1–4.

Srivastava, A. (2001, October). *Resilience & its predictors for low income working couples*. Paper Presented at the National Seminar on Psychology in India: Past, Present and Future. Kollam.

Srivastava, K. B. L. (2009). Social and psychological well-being: Antecedents and consequences. Poster presented at National Academy of Psychology (NAOP) India. *Proceedings-Psychological Studies, 54*(4), 310–352.

Suresh, A., Jayachander, M., & Joshi, S. (2013). Psychological determinants of well-being among adolescents. *Asia Pacific Journal of Research, 1*(11), 120–134.

Tayal, A., & Singh, R. (2010). Predictors of healthiness among diabetics. *Journal of Indian Health Psychology, 5*(1), 9–18.

Truffino, J. C. (2010). Resilience: An approach to the concept. *Revista de Psiquiatria y Salud Mental, 3*(4), 145–151.

Wagnild, G. (2003). Resilience and successful aging: Comparison among low and high income older adults. *Journal of Gerontological Nursing, 29*(12), 42–49.

Wagnild, G. M., & Young, H. M. (1987). The resilience scale. Available at www.resilience-scale.com

Wagnild, G. M., & Young, H. M. (1993). Development and psychometric evaluation of the resilience scale. *Journal of Nursing Measurement, 1*(2), 165–178.

Wells, M. (2010). Resilience in older adults living in rural, suburban, and urban areas. *Online Journal of Rural Nursing and Health Care, 10*(2), 45–52.

Zolkoski, S. M., & Bullock, L. M. (2012). Resilience in children and youth: A review. *Children and Youth Services Review, 34*(12), 2295–2303.

3

Conceptual complexity of resilience

Synergy approach to measurement[1]

Meena Hariharan and Suvashisa Rana

Resilience is a psychological resource that enhances the positivity in human life. Though 'resilience' is simple to understand, as a psychological construct, the intricacy lies in its conceptualization and operationalization. The academic debate on resilience was initiated about four and a half decades ago by psychologists like Anthony (1974) and Garmezy (1984). It started as simple research questions as to why and how a small proportion of a population exposed to severe adversity emerges successfully in life unaffected by adverse impacts. Thus, the phenomenon was very simple, referring to high achievement despite high adversity. The focus of research was the identification of the unique characteristics of this small percentage of the population that behaved in contrast to the probable consequences of adversity. The focus of research was typically on samples like children of schizophrenic parents (Garmezy, 1984); children of alcoholic parents (Chassin, Carle, Nissim-Sabat, & Kumpfer, 2004; Walker & Lee, 1998); institutionalized children (Cordovil, Crujo, Vilariça, & Caldeira Da Silva, 2011; van IJzendoorn et al., 2011); disadvantaged children (Dash & Nayak, 1998); and children with disability (Hariharan, Karimi, & Kishore, 2014), where risk is defined on statistical probability. Thus, the concept of resilience was one of the simplest to understand, where the subject of study was 'Why did that small percentage of children whose parents were diagnosed with schizophrenia not show any symptoms?', 'Why did those few children reared in impoverished physical and psychosocial environment not fail in academic fields?', and 'Why did that minor population of children with disabilities not perish like their counterparts, but excel in life?'. In other words, the subject of research was the small group of deviants from the natural, antecedent consequence path of negativity. It is this simplicity and the outlandish nature of the construct that allured many researchers to work in the field. The construct has assumed different functionally equivalent terms like 'stress-resistance' (Masten & Garmezy, 1985), 'invincible' (Werner & Smith, 1982), and 'golden lotus' (Dash & Nayak, 1998). According to Losel, Bliesener, and Koferl (1989), 'There is a multitude of constructs that are related to invulnerability, such as resilience, hardiness, adaptation, adjustment, mastery, plasticity, person-environment fit, or social buffering'.

According to Rutter (1990), resilience refers to the fact of maintaining adaptive functioning in spite of serious risk hazards. Later on he argued, 'Resilience does not constitute an individual trait or characteristic. . . . Resilience involves a range of processes that bring together quite diverse mechanisms' (Rutter, 1999). Resilience is also considered as the indication of a process that characterizes a complex social system at a moment in time (Fonagy, Steele, Steele, Higgitt, & Target, 1994). Describing as 'ordinary magic', Masten (2001) explains resilience as 'a class of phenomena characterized by good outcomes in spite of serious threats to adaptation or development'. Research findings posit that resilience is an emergent property of a hierarchically organized set of protective systems that cumulatively buffer the effects of adversity and can therefore rarely, if ever, be regarded as an intrinsic property of individuals (Roisman, Padrón, Sroufe, & Engeland, 2002). From research findings on children in institutions, Ungar (2005) observes that resilience is adequate provision of health resources necessary to achieve good outcomes in spite of serious threats to adaptation or development.

What can be termed as the initial phase of research in the field focused on marking characteristics of the individuals identified as resilient (Rutter, 1990; Werner & Smith, 1982). Among the Indian psychologists, Dash and Nayak (1998) have popularized the concept. They have, not only identified the characteristics of the resilient persons, but also traced their existence and identified characteristics from ancient Hindu scriptures. Werner and Smith (1982), in their longitudinal study running over several decades, identified the presence of a number of individual characteristics like autonomy for girls; care and nurture for boys; competence for both; and external factors such as family support, family organization, and type of family. Hariharan (1990) in her research identified certain individual characteristics such as prioritizing needs, readiness to meet challenges in resilience among socially disadvantaged and flexible coping style (Hariharan et al., 2014) in resilience among the physically challenged population. With the progress in research, several other characteristics were identified as unique to resilient children. Kobasa (1982) argued that 'hardiness', with its components of commitment, control, and challenge, is a distinct characteristic among the resilient. The literature featured many more characteristics, such as coherence (Antonvsky, 1984), ego strength, creative abilities, increased personal and physical attractiveness (Cohler, 1987), problem-solving skills, autonomy, optimism, sense of purpose, and future orientation (Bernard, 1997). Subsequent research added a few more characteristics of the resilient such as positive emotion (Tugade & Frederickson, 2004), positive affect (Zautra, Johnson, & Davis, 2005), self-efficacy (Gu & Day, 2007), self-esteem (Kidd & Shahar, 2008), and extraversion (Campbell-sills, Cohan, & Strein, 2006). Resilience is thus conceived as a constellation of individual characteristics.

Resilience: conceptual complexity

Every new impact from research in resilience added new insight to the concept, and every new insight triggered new questions. Thus, the simple concept of resilience progressively turned complex. Kaplan (1999) observes that variability in definition may be traced to four main sources: 1) the distinction between the relationship between resiliency and outcome, 2) the variation in outcomes among those definitions that equate resilience with outcomes, 3) the variation in the defining characteristics of resilience that influence outcome, and 4) the outcomes and their putative causes being defined in terms of risk factors that are themselves highly variable.

Analyzing the characteristics of the resilient, very pertinent research questions that evolved were whether these characteristics are traits and whether these children have predisposition. In fact, some studies came up with results in support of the predisposition hypothesis. For example research done on the study of monozygotic and dizygotic twins exposed to socio-economic deprivation found that evidence of resilience was high among monozygotic than dizygotic twins (Kim-Cohen, Moffitt, Caspi, & Taylor, 2004). Resilience as a trait was construed as a constellation of characteristics in the individual. However, the researchers preferred to call these individual characteristics in the resilient person as 'protective factors'. Adding little complexity, researchers envisaged the protective factors, not just as individual characteristics, but also present externally at two levels – family and community (Garmezy, Masten, & Tellegen, 1984; Rutter, 1979). Thus, the protective factors were expanded to the psychosocial level. The presence of these protective factors were assumed to have a shielding effect on the individuals insulating them from the negative impact of adversities. This in fact explained how the positive characteristics function in those who are resilient. Researchers like Sameroff, Gutman, and Peck (2003) went a step further and argued that, while the protective factors are helpful in insulating one from the negative impact, certain positive experiences like success and achievements that have intrinsic value assume the role of promoting resilience. Thus, while the protective factors are construed as the buffer, the promoting factors may be identified as the driving force. Perhaps each positive experience reinforces and strengthens the motivation to achieve or excel further.

Is the presence or absence of protective factors the sufficient prerequisite of resilience? Unless these protective and promotive factors are functional, resilience is not created. Based on this logic, Rutter (1987) argued that resilience is a process. Other researchers also subsequently explained resilience as a process (Luthar, Cicchetti, & Becker, 2000; Masten, Best, & Garmezy, 1990). Whether resilience is a process, an outcome, or a trait has been the focus of debate among the researchers for a long time. Based on the way it was conceptualized, different researchers defined resilience in different ways. A number of researchers referred to resilience as a protective factor by defining it as 'behavioural tendencies' (Agaibi & Wilson, 2005), 'capacity of the individual to cope' (Lee & Cranford, 2008), or 'personal qualities' (Connor & Davidson, 2003). Explaining the role of protective factors, Rutter (1987) clarified that the protective factors function as modifiers and ameliorators of the individual's response to the adverse environment. Thus, resilience is not just a protective factor but a process involving factors that bring a productive response outcome. Rutter identified three such processes – building positive self-image, reducing the effect of risk factors, and breaking the negative cycle – which perhaps referred to the vicious circle of exposure to adversity and negative outcome in the form of failure, underperformance, and underachievement. The merit in this argument shifted the focus of research from identifying the factors to understanding the process that facilitates the individual to emerge through the adverse environment (Luthar et al., 2000). Emphasizing the need for understanding the process, Luthar et al. (2000) defined resilience as 'a dynamic process encompassing positive adaptation within the context of significant adversity'. Two factors demand special attention in this definition – 'significant adversity' and 'positive adaption'.

Adversity in life may range from daily hassles like an unfriendly or unhygienic neighbourhood to potentially highly disruptive events such as the sudden demise of a loved one or a terror attack or losing an organ in an accident. Thus, adversity is a phenomenon that can be measured on two dimensions – the seriousness attributed through the frequency of its subjective experience and the duration of its experience. Thus, subjective perception, influenced by an array of factors, determines the seriousness. The second factor is the frequency with which one encounters such adversity. Traumatic experience such as childhood sexual abuse or humiliating experience of social discrimination may repeat themselves. What is the method by which the cumulative effect of adversity is taken into account? The other dimension is the duration of exposure to adversity. Studies on the impact of prolonged deprivation and short-term deprivation showed the potential devastating effects of duration of deprivation. Thus, when the degree of adversity is determined by the frequency and duration, adversity needs to be referred by taking into account the frequency, severity, and duration. What is referred as 'significant adversity' has an element of subjectivity in terms of attribution – what is perceived – as a significant adversity by one may not be viewed so by another. For example as per the attribution theory, the sudden demise of a parent may be perceived as devastating and has a stable and global impact on one's life. On the other hand, another sibling living far away may perceive it as a serious loss impacting the specific personal dimension. Yet he may view it as unstable, from which one recovers over a period of time.

The phrase generally used in describing resilience is 'positive adaption'. The term connotes significant limitations with reference to performance or achievement. Adaption refers to the degree to which an individual adjusts to the environment. If the environment is adverse, then logically adapting to the environment is an attempt to accommodate oneself to the demands of the environment. Here the persons change themselves to suit the environment. However, resilience refers to a context where the person manipulates, explores, and exploits the adverse environment in order to emerge unscathed or with minimum adverse impact. Hence, it may not be very appropriate to describe a resilient person who 'adapts'. Rather the resilient is the one who performs and achieves in the face of significant adversity. As propounded by Rutter (2006), repeated exposure to adversity creates a resistance to further adversity, which helps the individual to insulate oneself from its negative impacts and attain high achievement levels.

Yet another question that needs to be addressed is with regard to the level of performance or achievement. Performance assessment places the individual at different levels of achievement. Performance below the average level is considered underachievement or failure, while assessment that finds the performance above the average level varies in degrees that range between 'above average' to 'excellent'. With reference to the performance and achievement, the question that is of crucial importance is what is the level of performance and achievement in the face of adversities that qualifies one to be resilient. Does average achievement despite adversities label one as resilient, or should one's achievement be significantly nearing excellence in order to be called resilient?

If we plot the adversities and achievement on the X-axis and Y-axis, respectively, and the level of achievement by the curve R–R^1, the resilient person can be found on the extreme right end of the curve represented by R^1 (see Figure 3.1).

Thus, resilient persons are positioned where adversity is high and achievement is high. The beginning of the process of resilience can be traced where OY = OX.

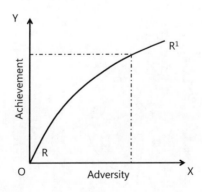

Figure 3.1 R–R^1 curve

Resilience: synergy approach to measurement

The process–product debate on resilience is converged on two essential prerequisites – the experience of adversity and achievement in the face of it. The interactive product of resilience is dynamic, varying in degree and level across situations – illness, trauma, crime, crisis, deprivation, and disadvantaged life conditions – and lifespan – childhood, adolescence, adulthood, and old age.

The availability of several psychological instruments to measure the construct of resilience is an indication of its complexity in operationalization. A critical review of the existing measures suggests that none of the measures is final in its version because of the dearth of relevant information about psychometric properties (Ahern, Kiehl, Sole, & Byers, 2006; Windle, Bennett, & Noyes, 2011). In psychological measurements, we use tests, scales, questionnaires, inventories, and checklists – each having its own advantages and disadvantages. In certain cases, we use paper-and-pencil tests whereas in other situations we depend on performance tests. In addition to these, we use projective tests to understand person's inner self. In Windle's (1999) view,

> [A]dditional efforts need to be focused on the multi-variable measurement issues surrounding the construction of risk and protective factor indexes, and the associated trade-offs in using 'clumped' summated indexes versus alternative scoring methods.
>
> *(p. 174)*

As resilience is a multi-dimensional construct and needs a multi-method approach, a battery of measures is the need of the hour in place of a single measure. Therefore, we postulate a synergy model to explain the basic principles of resilience in human life. We also propose a method to quantify resilience in more meaningful way by taking into consideration other significant constructs lying within it.

Synergy model of resilience

Our proposed 'synergy model of resilience' posits that resilience is a unique function of adversity, operating factors, and resistance across a time continuum that brings and sustains positive reflection in forms of achievement and flourishing in the person's life. Combined in a unique fashion, adversity, operating factors, and resistance – three prerequisites of resilience – interact to generate and nurture resilience. This synergy is presented in Figure 3.2 and elaborated in detail in Figure 3.3.

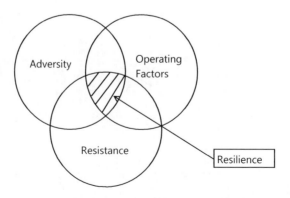

Figure 3.2 Synergy among adversity, operating factors, and resistance

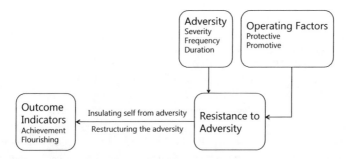

Figure 3.3 Path in synergy model of resilience

Adversity

The model (Figure 3.3) considers adversity not as a one-dimensional but rather as a multi-dimensional life condition. The adversity may be physical (e.g. disability), situational (e.g. deprivation), natural (e.g. tsunami), and parental (e.g. anti-social parents). The adversity may be congenital or accidental at any point of time after birth. There are three aspects of adversity – severity, frequency, and duration – that are to be taken into consideration while measuring resilience. How does one perceive this adversity, how often this adversity has impact on person's life, and how long the impact is felt are also the matter of high relevance in the context of resilience. Therefore, it is necessary to develop independent psychological instruments to measure these three aspects of adversity by following appropriate scaling techniques.

Operating factors

In the model, operating factors, which is intra-individual, refer to protective factors (inherent) and promotive factors (positive experiences). Like adversity, independent psychological instruments using appropriate scaling techniques are necessary to measure these two operating factors.

Resistance

We postulate that adversity and operating factors are not sufficient enough to generate and foster resilience unless there is resistance by the person. This resistance empowers the person for two actions – 1) restructuring the adverse environment and 2) insulating self from adversity. Independent psychological instruments are required to quantify these two actions of the person during adversity.

Outcome indicators

Because of the synergy among adversity, operating factors, and resistance, resilience is reflected in the form of high achievement in the face of high adversity, bringing transformation in the person's life. The major indicators of such positive growth are achievement and flourishing. Achievement and flourishing are to be measured by developing and using appropriate psychological instruments in the context of adversity, operating factors, and resistance.

Figure 3.2 depicts the presence of resilience where there is synergy between adversities, operating factors, and resistance. This indicates that any one of these factors in isolation cannot give rise to resilience. For example the positive characteristics within the individual and in the environment that are construed as protective factors by themselves are not sufficient conditions to bring resilience to those who encounter adversities. The person has to identify and endorse these strengths within and also perceive a sense of control over adversities either by using the internal resources of positive characteristics or by drawing from the external resources such as positive social support or a combination of both. This drive from within translated into action helps in the emergence of resistance to adversity. The convergence of these three brings in resilience.

As presented in Figure 3.2, operating factors contribute positively towards building and functioning the resistance to adversity. In this process, the individual either insulates from adversity (passive resistance) or restructures adversity (through active coping) to suit one's own needs towards the set goal. Either of these two options leads to high achievement and flourishing in life.

Resilience index: method of measurement

Basing on our proposed model, we suggest a method to quantify resilience in the form of the Resilience Index (RI), which determines the level of resilience of a person basing on a threshold. This method provides respective weight to each aspect of adversity, operating factors, and outcome indicators of resilience.

Step 1: Calculation of the Adversity Index (AI)

To calculate AI, we need to calculate the Adversity Severity Index (ASI), the Adversity Frequency Index (AFI), and the Adversity Duration Index (ADI). These primary indexes are to be calculated from the respective measures independently and are to be in percentages. For example

$$ASI = \frac{\text{Mean score of the participant}}{\text{Maximum score of the standard sample}} \times 100$$

The maximum score of the standard sample will be prescribed through the process of standardization by the researcher. Likewise, all other primary indexes are to be calculated depending on the obtained scores and the maximum scores of the measures concerned. After obtaining all these primary indexes, the AI is to be derived by using the following formula, where aw_1, aw_2, and aw_3 are respective weightage for the aspects of adversity.

$$AI = \frac{ASI \times aw_1 + AFI \times aw_2 + ADI \times aw_3}{aw_1 + aw_2 + aw_3}$$

Step 2: Calculation of the Operating Factors Index (OFI)

To calculate OFI, we need to calculate its primary indexes – the Protective Factor Index (PrI) and the Promotive Factor Index (PmI). These primary indexes are to be calculated from the respective measures independently and are to be in percentages by following the method mentioned under ASI, where ow_1 and ow_2 are respective weights for the two aspects of operating factors.

$$OFI = \frac{(PrI \times ow_1) + (PmI \times ow_2)}{ow_1 + ow_2}$$

Step 3: Calculation of the Resistance Index (RSI)

$$RSI = \frac{OFI}{AI} \times 100$$

Step 4: Calculation of the Outcome Indicator Index (OII)

To calculate OII, we need to calculate its primary indexes – the Achievement Index (AchI) and the Flourishing Index (FI). These primary indexes are to be calculated from the respective measures independently and are to be in percentages by following the method mentioned under ASI, where iw_1 and iw_2 are respective weights for the aspects of outcome indicators.

$$OII = \frac{(AchI \times iw_1) + (FI \times iw_2)}{iw_1 + iw_2}$$

Step 5: Calculation of the Resilience Index (RI)

$$RI = \frac{OII}{RSI} \times 100$$

The persons showing average resilience are expected to obtain RI = 100 because their RSI and OII are equal. When their RI > 100 and their OII > RSI, they are known as high resilient. When their RI < 100 and their OII < RSI, they are known as low resilient. By providing appropriate weights to all the dimensions within the construct of resilience, this method is more convenient to measure such a multi-dimensional complex construct through a multi-method approach.

The weightage given in every dimension is not equal. The weights depend upon the magnitude of such dimensions for the individual based on a standard threshold. This threshold is to be derived from extensive research. Our model helps to understand the convergence of the dimensions of resilience. Our method of calculating RI is a unique explanation to measure resilience by providing different weights basing on their importance. By using this method, one can understand the profile of resilient person. The method can be adopted for predicting resilience as well as planning intervention programmes to foster resilience among persons. The proposed hypothetical model and the method of deriving the RI, however, are the subject of further research involving various samples across the globe.

Rigorous quantitative technique, however, create a bottleneck in understanding the connotation of psychological constructs. Primarily when we try to understand resilience as a process, it is too difficult for us to understand the individual differences and its typical variation across situations. No person is resilient in absolute sense, meaning a person resilient in one situation is not found to be resilient in others. We argue that resilience as a product can be measured, whereas as a process it can be explored and understood from the qualitative research paradigm.

Note

1 We are thankful to Professor A. S. Dash for sharing his extensive experience in research in the area of invulnerability that helped us understanding issues related to resilience. We are highly indebted to Professor C. Raghavendra Rao for helping us develop a method to quantify the construct. We are also thankful to all the researchers whose findings we have cited here to build the framework of the article.

References

Agaibi, C. E., & Wilson, J. P. (2005). Trauma, PTSD, and resilience: A review of the literature. *Trauma Violence Abuse, 6*(3), 195–216.

Ahern, N. R., Kiehl, E. M., Sole, M. L., & Byers, J. (2006). A review of instruments measuring resilience. *Issues in Comprehensive Pediatric Nursing, 29*(2), 103–125.

Anthony, E. J. (1974). The syndrome of psychologically invulnerable children. In E. J. Anthony & C. Koupernick (Eds.), *The child in his family: Year book of the International Association for Child Psychiatry and Allied Professions* (Vol. 3, pp. 529–544). New York: John Wiley & Sons.

Antonvsky, A. (1984). The sense of coherence as a determinant of health. In J. D. Mastarazzo, M. W. Sharlene, J. A. Herd, N. E. Miller, & S. M. Weiss (Eds.), *Behavioural health: A hand book of health enhancement and disease prevention* (pp. 114–129). New York: John Wiley & Sons.

Bernard, B. (1997). *Turning it around for all youth: From risk to resilience.* Launceston, Tasmania: Resiliency Associates and Global Learning Communities.

Campbell-sills, L., Cohan, S. L., & Strein, M. B. (2006). Relationship of resilience to personality, coping and psychiatric symptoms in young adults. *Behaviour Research and Therapy, 44*(4), 585–599.

Chassin, L., Carle, A. C., Nissim-Sabat, D., & Kumpfer, K. L. (2004). Fostering resilience in children of alcoholic parents. In K. I. Maton, C. J. Schellenbach, B. J. Leadbeater, & A. L. Solarz (Eds.), *Investing in children, youth, families, and communities: Strengths-based research and policy* (pp. 137–155). Washington, DC, US: American Psychological Association.

Cohler, B. J. (1987). Resilience and the study of lives. In E. J. Anthony & B. Coher (Eds.), *The Invulnerable Child* (pp. 363–424). New York: Guilford.

Connor, K. M., & Davidson, J. R. T. (2003). Development of a new resilience scale: The Connor-Davidson resilience scale (CD-RISC). *Depression and Anxiety, 18*(2), 76–82.

Cordovil, C., Crujo, M., Vilariça, P., & Caldeira Da Silva, P. (2011). Resilience in institutionalized children and adolescents. *Actamédicaportuguesa, 24*(2 Suppl.), 413–418.

Dash, A. S., & Nayak, R. (1998). *When life becomes tough: The psychology of living.* Bhubaneswar: Panchajanya.

Fonagy, P., Steele, H., Steele, M., Higgitt, A., & Target, M. (1994). The theory and practice of resilience: The Emanuel Miller memorial lecture 1992. *Journal of Child Psychology and Psychiatry, 35*(2), 231–257.

Garmezy, N. (1984). Nature vs. nurture in schizophrenia: The struggle continues (Commentary). *Integrative Psychiatry, 2*(4), 141–143.

Garmezy, N., Masten, A. S., & Tellegen, A. (1984). The study of stress and competence in children: A building block for developmental psychopathology. *Child Development, 55*(1), 97–111.

Gu, Q., & Day, C. (2007). Teachers resilience: A necessary for effectiveness. *Teaching and Teachers Education, 23*(8), 1302–1316.

Hariharan, M. (1990). Invulnerable children: Some studies on disadvantaged children's competence and coping style (Unpublished doctoral thesis). Utkal University, Odisha, India.

Hariharan, M., Karimi, M., & Kishore, M. T. (2014). Resilience in persons with disabilities: Role of perceived environment and emotional intelligence. *Journal of Indian Academy of Applied Psychology, 40*(1), 97–102.

Kaplan, H. B. (1999). Toward an understanding of resilience: A critical review of definitions and models. In M. D. Glantz & J. L. Johnson (Eds.), *Resilience and development: Positive life adaptations* (pp. 17–83). New York: Kluwer Academic/Plenum Publishers.

Kidd, S., & Shahar, G. (2008). Resilience in homeless youth: The key role of self-esteem. *American Journal of Orthopsychiatry, 78*(2), 163–172.

Kim-Cohen, J., Moffitt, A., Caspi, A., & Taylor, A. (2004). Genetic and environmental processes in young children's resilience and vulnerability to socioeconomic deprivation. *Child Development, 75*(3), 651–668.

Kobasa, S. C. (1982). The hardy personality: Towards a social psychology of stress and health. In J. Suls & G. Sanders (Eds.), *The social pathology of health and illness* (pp. 3–32). Hillsdale, NJ: Lawrence Erlbaum Associates.

Lee, H. H., & Cranford, J. A. (2008). Does resilience moderate the associations between parental problem drinking and adolescents' internalizing and externalizing behaviours? A study of Korean Adolescents. *Drug and Alcohol Dependence, 96*(3), 213–221.

Losel, E., Bliesener, T., & Koferl, P. (1989). On the concept of invulnerability: Evaluation and first results of the Bielefeld project. In M. Brambring, E. Losel, & H. Skowronek (Eds.), *Children at risk: Assessment, longitudinal research, and intervention* (pp. 186–219). New York: Walter de Gruytex.

Luthar, S. S., Cicchetti, D., & Becker, B. (2000). The construct of resilience: A critical evaluation and guidelines for future work. *Child Development, 71*(3), 543–562.

Masten, A. S. (2001). Ordinary magic: Resilience processes in development. *American Psychologist, 56*(3), 227–238.

Masten, A. S., Best, K. M., & Garmezy, M. (1990). Resilience and development: Contributions from the study of children who overcome adversity. *Development and Psychopathology, 2*, 425–444.

Masten, A. S., & Garmezy, N. (1985). Risk vulnerability and protective factors in developmental psychopathology. In B. B. Labey & A. E. Kazidin (Eds.), *Advances in clinical child psychology* (Vol. 8, pp. 1–52). New York: Plenum Press.

Roisman, G. I., Padrón, E., Sroufe, L. A., & Engeland, B. (2002). Earned-secure attachment status in retrospect and prospect. *Child Development, 73*(4), 1204–1219.

Rutter, M. (1979). Protective factors in children's responses to stress and disadvantage. In M. W. Kent & J. E. Rolf (Eds.), *Primary prevention in psychopathology: Social competence in children* (pp. 49–74). Hanover, NH: University Press of New England.

Rutter, M. (1987). Psychosocial resilience and protective mechanisms. *American Journal of Orthopsychiatry, 57*(3), 316–331.

Rutter, M. (1990). Psychosocial resilience and protective mechanisms. In J. Rolf, A. S. Masten, D. Cicchetti, K. H. Nuechterlein, & S. Weintraub (Eds.), *Risk and protective factors in the development of psychopathology* (pp. 181–214). New York: Cambridge University Press.

Rutter, M. (1999). Resilience concepts and findings: Implications for family therapy. *Journal of Family Therapy, 21*(2), 119–144.

Rutter, M. (2006). Implications of resilience concepts for scientific understanding. *Annals of the New York Academy of Sciences, 1094*, 1–12.

Sameroff, A., Gutman, L. M., & Peck, S. C. (2003). Adaptation among youth facing multiple risks: Prospective research findings. In S. S. Luthar (Ed.), *Resilience and vulnerability: Adaptation in the context of childhood adversities* (pp. 364–391). New York: Cambridge University Press.

Tugade, M. M., & Frederickson, B. L. (2004). Resilience individual use positive emotions to become back from negative emotional experience. *Journal of Personality and Social Psychology, 86*(2), 320–333.

Ungar, M. (2005). Resilience among children in child welfare, corrections, mental health and educational settings: Recommendations for service. *Child and Youth Care Forum, 34*(6), 445–463.

Van IJzendoorn, M. H., Palacios, J., Sonuga-Barke, E. J. S., Gunnar, M. R., Vorria, P., McCall, R. B., . . . Juffer, F. (2011). Children in institutional care: Delayed development and resilience. *Monographs of the Society for Research in Child Development, 76*(4), 8–30.

Walker, J. P., & Lee, R. E. (1998). Uncovering strengths of children of alcoholic parents. *Contemporary Family Therapy, 20*(4), 521–538.

Werner, E. E., & Smith, R. S. (1982). *Vulnerable but invincible.* New York: McGraw-Hill Book Company.

Windle, G., Bennett, K. M., & Noyes, J. (2011). A methodological review of resilient measurement scales. *Health and Quality of Life Outcomes, 9*(8), 1–18.

Windle, M. (1999). Critical conceptual and measurement issues in the study of resilience. In M. D. Glantz & J. L. Johnson (Eds.), *Resilience and development: Positive life adaptations* (pp. 161–176). New York: Kluwer Academic/Plenum Publishers.

Zautra, A. J., Johnson, L. M., & Davis, M. C. (2005). Positive affect as a source of resilience for women in chronic pain. *Journal of Consulting and Clinical Psychology, 73*(2), 212–220.

4

Three-factor model of personal resiliency

Sandra Prince-Embury, Donald H. Saklofske and Kateryna V. Keefer

Resilience in the face of adversity has been studied extensively by psychologists for the past fifty years. This body of work has defined the common theme of resilience as the ability to weather adversity or to bounce back from a negative experience. Research on resilience suggests that psychological symptoms and disorders may be based in part on lower personal resiliency or greater vulnerability to situations and events that the person has experienced (Garmezy, 1971, 1985, 1991; Garmezy, Masten, & Tellegen, 1984; Luthar, 1991; Luthar, Cicchetti, & Becker, 2000; Luthar & Zigler, 1991, 1992; Masten, 2001; Masten & Coatsworth, 1998; Masten & Curtis, 2000; Masten & Powell, 2003; Masten et al., 2005; Prince-Embury, 2007, 2008, 2013a; Prince-Embury & Saklofske, 2013, 2014; Rutter, 1987, 1993).

More recent definitions of resilience as a product of the complex interactions of personal attributes and environmental circumstances, mediated by internal mechanisms, have presented a challenge to those interested in applying the construct to human behaviour in everyday and extreme circumstances (Luthar et al., 2000). In an effort to clarify constructs, theorists have distinguished "resilience" from "resiliency"; the former is defined as interactive and contextual, and the latter addresses personal attributes of the individual (Luthar et al., 2000; Luthar & Zelazo, 2003; Masten & Powell, 2003). Some resilience research has employed longitudinal studies, reflecting a developmental perspective, and has tried to capture contextual aspects of resilience specific to groups and sets of circumstances. Studies assessing personal resiliency, in an effort to be comprehensive, have employed extensive assessment batteries, along with various criteria of competence, achievement, or successful adaptation (Werner & Smith, 1982).

Earlier research findings on resilience were interpreted to suggest that resilient individuals are 'extraordinary' and that this quality or characteristic is not accessible to everyone. More recently, Masten described resilience as the process characteristic of normal development, an "ordinary magic", and not just applicable in adverse circumstances (Masten, 2001; Masten & Powell, 2003). Masten (2001) suggested that fundamental systems, already identified as characteristic of human functioning, have great adaptive significance across diverse stressors and threatening situations. This shift in emphasis had significant implications, and the "ordinary magic" framework suggested by Masten led to the extended application of resilience theory to a wider range of individuals in varied contexts. These systems include attachment relation-ships and social support; intelligence and problem-solving skills; self-regulation skills involved in directing or inhibiting attention, emotion, and action; agency, mastery, motivation, and self-efficacy; meaning making (constructing meaning and a sense of coherence in life); and cultural traditions.

Earlier models of personal resiliency suggested one factor: resiliency as a trait was viewed by some as present to some degree or not (Block & Block, 1980, Block & Kre-men, 1996). Other resiliency literature discussed resiliency as comprised of protective or risk factors. Variations in definitions of resiliency are reflected in the scales and mea-sures employed in research and clinical settings (see Prince-Embury, Saklofske, & Veseley, 2015). This chapter will describe a three-factor model of resiliency proposed by Prince-Embury (2007, 2014) (Prince-Embury & Courville, 2008a, 2008b) and assessed with the Resiliency Scales for Children and Adolescents (Prince-Embury, 2006, 2007). The relationship of these three factors to the psychological well-being of children and youth will be examined with an emphasis on facilitating and promoting resiliency in the school and community context.

Three-factor model of personal resiliency

One effort to simplify the construct of personal resiliency for assessment and application is the three-factor model developed by Prince-Embury (2006, 2007, 2013b, 2014). This model is based on three previously identified attributes of personal resiliency reflective of three core developmental systems: *sense of mastery*, *sense of relatedness*, and *emotional reactivity*, and the rela-tionship of these factors to one another (Prince-Embury, 2006, 2007, 2013a, 2013b, 2014). The three-factor model was based on review of the literature, based on clinical practice, and supported by factor analysis of the Resiliency Scales for Children and Adolescents (RSCA) based on this model (Prince-Embury, 2007, 2013a, 2013b; Prince-Embury & Courville, 2008a, 2008b). The three-factor model of personal resiliency focuses on the personal experi-ence of the individual and not actual ability or performance as assessed by others. Although it is recognized that actual ability and performance as assessed by others is important, the three-factor model assumes that the individual's experience mediates between external pro-tective factors and positive behavioural outcomes. The definition of resiliency according to well-researched underlying developmental systems is designed to aid in the identification of interventions that are well grounded in developmental theory and empirical research. Defini-tion and application of each of the three factors of personal resiliency are described briefly in the following sections.

Sense of mastery

One set of core mechanisms that have been consistently identified as important for resiliency in developmental and resilience research are a sense of mastery and self-efficacy. In fact, a sense of mastery and competence has been the focus of much earlier resiliency work (Masten & Coat-sworth, 1998). White (1959) proposed that children's sense of competence or efficacy provides them with the opportunity to interact with and enjoy cause-and-effect relationships in the envi-ronment. Bandura (1977, 1993) suggested that students' self-efficacy beliefs for regulating their own learning and mastering academic activities determine their aspirations, level of motivation, and academic accomplishments. Positive expectations about their future predict lower anxiety, higher school achievement, and better classroom behaviour control in students (Wyman, Cowen, Work, & Kerley, 1993). Previous research and theory suggest that children and youth who have a greater sense of competence/efficacy may be more likely to succeed in a school environment and are less likely to develop pathological symptoms.

Interventions to enhance a sense of mastery at the individual level have been described and in some cases implemented in school settings (see Prince-Embury & Saklofske, 2014). Generally, an enhanced realistic sense of mastery increases students' expectations and attempts to achieve these expectations, which in turn may enhance a sense of mastery. Rutter (1987, 1993, 2010) described pathways for increasing a sense of mastery: lessons that are matched to the ability level of students and broken into achievable steps, reducing the likelihood of negative chain reactions associated with adversity; establishing and maintaining self-esteem and self-efficacy; and creating new opportunities for success. Brooks and Goldstein (2001, 2008) have discussed the "resilient mindset" in students and have trained parents and teachers to foster a resilient mindset in students (Brooks & Goldstein, 2008); a teaching process that redefines "failure" as overcoming challenges and problem solving; and classroom environments that are responsive to the feedback of students in creating a more resilient classroom (Doll, Zucker, & Brehm, 2004, 2010).

In describing ways to foster resilient mindsets in individual children, Brooks, Goldstein, and colleagues (Brooks & Brooks, 2014; Brooks, Brooks, & Goldstein, 2012; Goldstein & Brooks, 2007; Goldstein, Brooks, & DeVries, 2013) emphasize the importance of cultivating "islands of competence", or areas of personal strength, in every child. When individuals discover that they can be successful at something, particularly in an area that is important to them and valued by significant others, they are more likely to draw on that strength for global feelings of self-efficacy and self-worth, which subsequently spread to other areas of self-concept (McConnell, 2011). Accordingly, Brooks, Goldstein, and colleagues encourage parents and teachers to make a list of their students' individual strengths and competencies and to come up with ways to reinforce those islands of competence in their everyday interactions with the students. Thus, the focus shifts from highlighting what the student cannot do to what they can do, which is essentially a strengths-based practice.

When attempting to change students' mindsets, it is important to understand the psychological mechanisms involved in the formation of self-referent cognitions. Although competence self-perceptions derive from multiple sources, personal mastery experiences exert by far the most powerful influence on self-efficacy beliefs (Bandura, 1977; Usher & Pajares, 2008). When students repeatedly achieve successful outcomes, their sense of competence is strengthened and so is their confidence in doing well in the future. In contrast, when students repeatedly fail in their attempts to achieve the desired outcomes, they begin to doubt their abilities and lose hope that things will change for the better. The resulting mindsets both contribute to, and are perpetuated by, subsequent experiences in a reciprocal fashion. Students who have developed a self-efficacious mindset are more likely to seek challenges, try harder, persevere in the face of setbacks, and ultimately fulfill their goals (Bandura, 1993). In contrast, equally able students who have come to believe that they have no control over their outcomes (i.e. helpless mindset) tend to avoid challenges, put forth less effort, give up after setbacks, and as a result are less likely to discover that they can effect positive change in their lives (Seligman, 1990).

In practice, this means that providing individuals with opportunities to experience success directly, and as a result of their own actions and sense of self, is the most effective and authentic way to build up their sense of mastery, competence, and personal control (Goldstein et al., 2013).

An important caveat to remember here is that mastery experiences are inherently subjective, for the same level of performance may be interpreted as a success by one student and as a failure by another (Usher & Pajares, 2008). These interpretations depend on a series of temporal, dimensional, and social comparisons students make in relation to their past performance, their performance in other areas, and performance of their peers (Möller, 2005). Students are more likely to experience increases in self-efficacy when their performance improves over time, when it is in the domain that is important to them, and when they are doing better than their classmates (Marsh, 2007). Students' interpretations of their performance also depend on adults' expectations for them: unrealistically high expectations set students up for failure regardless of how capable they are, whereas very low expectations trivialize students' success by implying they are not capable of doing better (Goldstein et al., 2013). Indeed, the most powerful mastery experiences occur when students successfully overcome obstacles or accomplish challenging but manageable tasks (Bandura, 1993).

Another salient source of students' self-efficacy beliefs is evaluative feedback received from significant others (Bandura, 1993; Usher & Pajares, 2008). At the very least, teachers may provide verbal encouragement to their students, communicating that they notice and value students' strengths and not just focus on their weaknesses. However, teachers also need to be aware that their verbal affirmations may not always appear welcome. Indeed, the very individuals who would benefit from encouragement the most, i.e. those with low self-esteem and little self-confidence, are often the least receptive to positive feedback, dismissing it as fundamentally incongruent with their sense of who they are (Swann, 1997). Likewise, individuals suffering from depression tend to be less accepting of others' expressions of love and support for them, which often elicits frustration and rejection by others and thereby reinforces the depressive mindset pervaded by feelings of shame and worthlessness (Joiner, Katz, & Lew, 1997). Regardless of individual circumstances, it is important to continue verbally affirming students' strengths but, at the same time, recognizing that changing such negative mindsets may require more intensive cognitive-behavioural intervention (Goldstein et al., 2013).

An important take-home message for teachers is that while mastery experiences, effort attributions, and positive feedback may not always increase students' self-efficacy, repeated experiences of failure, attributions to lack of ability, and predominantly negative feedback are almost certain to erode students' self-worth (Usher & Pajares, 2008). It is for this reason that Brooks, Goldstein, and colleagues (Brooks & Brooks, 2014; Brooks et al., 2012; Goldstein et al., 2013) encourage parents and teachers to focus their interventions, not only on the areas where students are struggling, but also on those islands of competence where students are already doing well and that matter to them a great deal. Once a foundation for mastery is established, a more resilient mindset will follow.

Similar individual-level interventions to foster sense of mastery may be applied to adults in a variety of rehabilitation settings where the task is coping with illness or injury. In such settings, the paths to recovery or improved functioning are often broken down into achievable steps that are reinforced as important steps towards recovery. Positive affirmation and recognition of small incremental steps as important are significant in maintaining a "resilient mindset" for patient recovery. For this reason, the ability of family and health care workers to recognize and acknowledge these small incremental steps as positive is crucial to patient recovery.

At a community level, enhancing sense of mastery has held many labels such as community empowerment and has taken many forms such as the provision of "a voice" or say in what happens in the community or the provision of resources to improve the functioning of the community. Community organizing has traditionally taken on the role of increasing the awareness of downtrodden or impoverished communities that there are achievable pathways for greater collective mastery, which might achieve positive outcomes at the community level. Although applied at a different level, enhancing mastery at a community level involves basic mechanisms of increasing expectations of achievable goals and providing increased awareness of pathways toward achieving these goals.

A sense of mastery is of course critical to surviving in the face of disaster and in its aftermath. Prince-Embury (in press) discusses the provision of information in the aftermath of the Three Mile Island (TMI) accident in the US in 1979, as a way of addressing unanswered questions and helping community members better process and understand what had happened in their community. Prince-Embury found that knowing a plan for emergency evacuation in the event of another crisis in the TMI vicinity was related to lower worry and psychological symptoms. We may conclude that those who have a plan on how they are going to deal with an emergency are more resilient in anticipating and dealing with such an emergency.

Sense of relatedness

Reviewing five decades of resilience research in child development, Luthar (2006, p. 780) concluded, "Resilience rests, fundamentally, on relationships." The importance of relationships for human resilience has been noted in every major review of protective factors for resilience (see Masten & Obradovic, 2006). The importance of relationships and relational ability as mediators of resilience has been supported in research by developmental psychologists. Much developmental theory has been devoted to the development of internal mechanisms of attachment and relatedness (see Prince-Embury, 2007 for discussion). Beginning in early development, the attachment figure provides a child with a secure base for reassurance under threat and, when conditions are relaxed, with the confidence to venture out to explore and learn about the world. Separation from attachment figures can cause extreme anxiety to the point of panic, particularly when a threat is perceived, and loss can induce profound grief. Sensitive attachment figures also serve a powerful regulatory function, up- or down-regulating stress and arousal or containing impulses. The presence of a secure-base attachment figure has been shown to moderate stress in threatening situations for infants and toddlers. Werner and Smith (1982) noted that resilient youth sought support from non-parental adults (especially teachers, ministers, and neighbours) more often than non-resilient youth. It must be noted, however, that previous research has indicated that perceived support, as distinguished from actual support, is the dimension of social support that is most strongly related to psychological well-being in adults and children (see Prince-Embury, 2007).

Efforts to enhance actual relatedness and perceived support in educational settings have focussed on enhancement of social skills through social emotional learning. The logic is that youth with better social skills will have better relationships and an enhanced sense of relatedness. Within the context of social emotional learning, much thought and effort has been given to enhancing social skills in children such as communication, cooperation, assertion, empathy, engagement, and self-control, which may be broken down into teachable skills such as improving eye contact, initiating and maintaining conversations, understanding others' feelings and promoting empathy, sharing, and maintaining personal space (Alvord, Zucker, & Grados, 2011; de Boo & Prins, 2007). Such programs as the Social Skills Improvement System (Gresham & Elliott, 1990) have been successfully used with children and adolescents to increase interpersonal competencies when these are lacking and are amongst the major contributors to a child's social and emotional difficulties.

Enhancing interpersonal skills in youth may enhance school engagement and performance and perhaps a more general sense of relatedness in the long run. The implication for application in the school environment is that better social skills increase the likelihood of better social relationships with peers and teachers and less conflict that interferes with learning and school attendance. In addition, research has indicated that better social engagement in school is associated with better academic performance. Students who have friends at school are more interested in academic activities and are more active participants in the classroom (Malecki & Elliott, 2002; Wentzel & Watkins, 2002). This is consistent with the assumption that learning and achievement takes place within a meaningful social context and that strength of engagement of students with teachers and other students indicates the social meaningfulness of the school environment. In summary, research suggests that a positive sense of relatedness within the school environment is essential for meaningful learning and academic achievement.

At a community level, the importance of relatedness resiliency may be viewed within the context of coping with an emergency. Disaster may present a "relatedness" threat by separating family members, disrupting contact between family members, and obscuring information about the safety among family members. In such circumstances, locator systems and means for communication among family members are critical. Disaster preparedness guidelines now recommend identifying a network of reliable adults for children to contact in the event of an emergency and reliable means for making contact.

A sense of relatedness or lack thereof can be viewed in the aftermath of a disaster as described by Prince-Embury in Chapter 20, this volume. In the vicinity of Three Mile Island, findings of loss of faith in experts (Prince-Embury & Rooney, 1987) might be interpreted within this framework, whereby officials and experts who were relied upon to safeguard the community were "lost" as credible bases of security and replaced by a sudden realization among community members that they were on their own to interpret complex risk information, which was beyond their understanding and training. Efforts at restoring sense of relatedness in this context involved identifying credible experts who were willing to educate the community in language that they could understand (Prince-Embury, 2013c).

Emotional reactivity

Research has demonstrated that children's development of pathology in the presence of adversity is related to their emotional reactivity and their inability to regulate this reactivity (Prince-Embury, 2013b). Specifically, strong emotional reactivity and related difficulty with regulation of this reactivity have been associated with behavioural maladjustment and vulnerability to pathology. Emotional reactivity is in part the individual's arousability, or the threshold of tolerance that exists prior to the occurrence of adverse events or circumstances. Rothbart and Derryberry (1981) have defined emotional reactivity as the speed and intensity of an individual's negative emotional response. Individual's reactivity varies in its intensity, sensitivity, specificity, windows of tolerance, and recovery (Siegel, 1999). Conversely, emotional regulation, or the ability to modulate emotional responses, is a significant factor in fostering resilience (Cicchetti, Ganiban, & Barnett, 1991; Cicchetti & Tucker, 1994; Eisenberg, Champion, & Ma, 2004). Regulation and redirection of emotional arousal is necessary for individuals to function adaptively in emotionally challenging situations (Cicchetti et al., 1991; Thompson, 1990).

Emotional reactivity in the school environment may impair student cognitive and behavioural functioning and thus be an impediment to learning. Importantly, academic achievement and behavioural self-control are highly interdependent. Students who are attentive, regulated, and persistent in their work often earn higher grades, whereas those who lack behavioural self-control often underachieve academically (Doll et al., 2004). Some studies have found disciplined classroom behaviour to be a better predictor of students' grades than intellectual ability (McDermott,

Mordell, & Stoltzfus, 2001). Existing programs to address Emotional reactivity in school environments may involve relaxation exercises; learning how to accurately identify, label, and verbalize emotions; and regular opportunities to discharge excess energy.

The significance of emotional reactivity and emotion regulation for resiliency in the school environment may be viewed on many levels. First, individual differences in students' physiologically based emotional reactivity may make adaptation to a structured, "sedentary" school environment difficult for those with higher emotional reactivity. Interventions for such children may involve behaviour management and relaxation techniques to lower base emotional reactivity. On the level of the school environment itself, we may examine potential triggers of emotional reactivity for children in general. Triggers may include novelty such as starting a new school or transitioning from elementary to middle, or middle to high school; presentation of material at a level too difficult for the student; punitive consequences for difficulties in learning; and difficulties in peer relationships including but not limited to bullying. Interventions in these instances would involve identifying triggers of emotional reactivity, preparation for these triggers, and efforts to modify these triggers to more emotionally neutral events. In summary, enhancing school resilience through addressing emotional reactivity might involve the following: identifying youth with higher emotional reactivity, teaching students to recognize early signs of emotional reactivity, and teaching them techniques to self-regulate and mange emotions, reducing the potential of environmental triggers to increase emotional reactivity in the school environment.

It is generally agreed that emotional reactivity is elevated by emergency, disaster, and conditions of uncertainty (Baum, Gatchel, & Schaeffer, 1983). Abundant literature exists on the importance of maintaining calm in the face of emergency conditions. The importance of access to accurate and timely information about ongoing circumstances and faith in those in charge of managing these circumstances is discussed by Prince-Embury in Chapter 20 in this volume.

Need for resiliency assessment

Assessment is the cornerstone of effective intervention. Studies of resilience have been both cross-sectional and longitudinal, have employed a developmental-psychopathology perspective, and have tried to capture contextual aspects of resilience specific to the group and sets of circumstances. Researchers of both resilience and resiliency have used different measures across studies and across populations, making it difficult to compare across studies and across groups. The resiliency measures employed in research have often been impractical for widespread use in the school or community because they are too labour intensive or expensive. On the other hand, some measures are restricted in their definition of resiliency or may not be linked with current or identifiable models of resiliency. From a psychometric perspective, some measures vary in the adequacy of their psychometric properties including both reliability and validity and may or may not have gone through the kind of standardization that would provide normative data that aid in the interpretation of an individual's scores relative to peers or clinical groups (see Prince-Embury, Saklofske, & Veseley, 2015). The lack of common metrics across different studies of resilience/resiliency constructs and across research and practice results in difficulty assessing the effectiveness of intervention strategies in a way that allows comparison across methods and populations (Prince-Embury, 2011).

On a practical level, there is work to be done to make resiliency assessment tools more field-friendly (Masten, 2001; Masten & Powell, 2003). Hence, there is a need for measures and benchmarks describing resiliency that are brief, easily administered, and simple to score and interpret.

In addition, measures used with diverse populations must be bias free with respect to gender and ethnicity and worded so that they might be used with a broad range of reading levels. In order to be acceptable to parents, students, and teachers in school settings, a measure assessing resiliency needs to be strength-based and informative while at the same time not stigmatizing or "pathologizing" of groups or individuals (Prince-Embury, 2011).

Resiliency scales for children and adolescents

Prince-Embury developed the Resiliency Scales for Children and Adolescents (RSCA; Prince-Embury, 2006, 2007) for use in preventive universal screening to identify areas of strength and vulnerability at the aggregate and individual level, for planning resiliency-enhancing interventions in the schools (Prince-Embury, 2010). The RSCA consists of three global scales based on the three-factor model of personal resiliency discussed earlier: sense of mastery, sense of relatedness, and emotional reactivity. Each of the global scales is further composed of several subscales: sense of mastery includes Optimism, Self-Efficacy, and Adaptability; sense of relatedness encompasses Trust, Comfort with Others, Support, and Tolerance; emotional reactivity comprises Sensitivity, Recovery, and Impairment. The RSCA is completed by the child (self-report), written at a third grade reading level and takes ten minutes to complete.

The three global scaled scores (mastery, relatedness, and emotional reactivity) may be used to plot each child's Personal Resiliency Profile, which highlights the individual child's relative strengths (mastery and/or relatedness) and vulnerability (emotional reactivity). At an individual level, the Personal Resiliency Profile may be used to guide the selection of an intervention or treatment plan. For example youth who are low in sense of mastery may be presented with gradually achievable tasks toward specific educational goals. Youth with a low sense of relatedness may be offered social skill training. Youth with high emotional reactivity may be presented with relaxation exercises and self-regulation skill training.

Examination of individual and aggregate Personal Resiliency Profiles indicated that, although there was considerable individual variability, the two protective factors, mastery and relatedness, were often correlated with each other and negatively correlated with emotional reactivity (Prince-Embury, 2007, 2013a, 2013b). For this reason, it is possible to condense the three factor scores into two index scores for screening. The two protective scores, mastery and relatedness, may be combined to form a Resource Index Score (see Prince-Embury, 2007, for details). Vulnerability then may be represented as the discrepancy between the Emotional Reactivity Score and the Resource Index score (see Prince-Embury, 2007, for details). These two RSCA Index scores, Resource and Vulnerability, may then be used for preventive, non-pathologizing screening in school systems.

The RSCA was standardized for three age groups (9–11, 12–14, and 15–18 years) and stratified by ethnicity and parent education level within age group and gender. The RSCA scores demonstrate good to excellent reliability at the index, global scale, and subscale levels. Also, convergent and divergent validity evidence has been demonstrated (Prince-Embury, 2006, 2007, 2008, 2010).

More recently the Resiliency Scale for Young Adults (RSYA; Prince-Embury, Saklofske, & Nordstokke, 2016) has been developed as an upward extension of the RSCA. The RSYA has been adapted for young adults and has been found to maintain the three-factor structure of the original RSCA although it is shorter (50 items) and some of the scales have been modified to fit with an older group. Future research will involve standardizing these scales for use in resiliency screening in special populations and circumstances. The RSYA will make it possible for longitudinal follow-up for youth going from adolescence to early adulthood on three major factors of personal resiliency.

Summary and conclusions

Resiliency has become a key factor in what is now termed positive psychology. The emphasis on promoting and enhancing psychological wellness has embraced a strengths-based perspective that goes beyond inoculating or "toughening-up" children to withstand life's stresses. The goal is to encourage psychologically healthy children who not only have the capacity to "bounce back" during challenging times but who are flourishing. The three-factor model of personal resiliency does not claim to be all inclusive. It is not a new theory but a model that simplifies and integrates existing theory in a way that is user friendly for practical application. The model proposed by Prince-Embury to describe and assess personal resiliency with its focus on mastery, relatedness, and emotional reactivity has implications for linking an extensive psychological research literature to the promotion of well-being in children and their journey into adulthood.

References

Alvord, M. K., Zucker, B., & Grados, J. J. (2011). *Resilience builder program for children and adolescents: Enhancing social competence and self-regulation*. Champaign, IL: Research Press.

Bandura, A. (1977). *Self-efficacy: The exercise of control*. New York, NY: Freeman.

Bandura, A. (1993). Perceived self-efficacy in cognitive development and functioning. *Educational Psychologist, 28*(2), 117–148.

Baum, A., Gatchel, R., & Schaeffer, N. (1983). Emotion, behavior and physiological effects of chronic stress at Three Mile Island. *Journal of Consulting and Clinical Psychology, 51*(4), 656–672.

Block, J. H., & Block, J. (1980). The role of ego-control and ego-resiliency in the organization of behavior. In W. A. Collins (Ed.), *Development of cognition, affect, and social relations: The Minnesota symposia on child psychology* (Vol. 13, pp. 39–101). Hillsdale, NJ: Lawrence Erlbaum.

Block, J., & Kremen, A. M. (1996). IQ and ego-resiliency: Conceptual and empirical connections and separateness. *Journal of Personality and Social Psychology, 70*, 349–361.

Brooks, R., & Brooks, S. (2014). Creating resilient mindsets in children and adolescents: A strength-based approach for clinical and nonclinical populations. In S. Prince-Embury & D. H. Saklofske (Eds.), *Resilience interventions for youth in diverse populations* (pp. 59–82). New York, NY: Springer.

Brooks, R., Brooks, S., & Goldstein, S. (2012). The power of mindsets: Nurturing engagement, motivation, and resilience in students. In S. Christenson, A. L. Reschly, & C. Wylie (Eds.), *Handbook of research on student engagement* (pp. 541–562). New York, NY: Springer.

Brooks, R., & Goldstein, S. (2001). *Raising resilient children*. New York, NY: McGraw-Hill.

Brooks, R., & Goldstein, S. (2008). The mindset of teachers capable of fostering resilience in students. *Canadian Journal of School Psychology, 23*(1), 114–126.

Cicchetti, D., Ganiban, J., & Barnett, D. (1991). Contributions from the study of high-risk populations to understanding the development of emotion regulation. In J. Garber & K. Dodge (Eds.), *The development of emotion regulation and dysregulation* (pp. 15–48). New York, NY: Cambridge University Press.

Cicchetti, D., & Tucker, D. (1994). Development and self-regulatory structures of the mind. *Development and Psychopathology, 6*(4), 533–549.

de Boo, G. M., & Prins, P. J. M. (2007). Social incompetence in children with ADHD: Possible moderators and mediators in social-skills training. *Clinical Psychology Review, 27*(1), 78–97.

Doll, B., Spies, R. A., Champion, A., Guerrero, C., Dooley, K., & Turner, A. (2010). The Class Maps Survey: A measure of students' perceptions of classroom resilience. *Journal of Psychoeducational Assessment, 28*, 338–348.

Doll, B., Zucker, S., & Brehm, K. (2004). *Resilient classrooms: Creating healthier environments for learning*. New York, NY: Guilford Press.

Eisenberg, N., Champion, C., & Ma, Y. (2004). Emotion-related regulation: An emerging construct. *Merrill-Palmer Quarterly, 50*(3), 236–259.

Garmezy, N. (1971). Vulnerability research and the issue of primary prevention. *American Journal of Orthopsychiatry, 41*(1), 101–116.

Garmezy, N. (1985). Stress-resistant children: The search for protective factors. In J. E. Stevenson (Ed.), *Recent research in developmental psychopathology (Journal of Child Psychology and Psychiatry Book Suppl. 4*, pp. 213–233). Oxford: Pergamon.

Garmezy, N. (1991). Resilience and vulnerability to adverse developmental outcomes associated with poverty. *American Behavioral Scientist, 34*(4), 416–430.

Garmezy, N., Masten, A. S., & Tellegen, A. (1984). The study of stress and competence in children: A building block for developmental psychopathology. *Child Development, 55*(1), 97–111.

Goldstein, S., & Brooks, R. (2007). *Understanding and managing classroom behavior: Creating resilient, sustainable classrooms.* New York, NY: Wiley.

Goldstein, S., Brooks, R., & DeVries, M. (2013). Translating resilience theory for application with children and adolescents by parents, teachers, and mental health professionals. In S. Prince-Embury & D. H. Saklofske (Eds.), *Resilience in children, adolescents, and adults: Translating research into practice* (pp. 73–90). New York, NY: Springer.

Gresham, F. M., & Elliot, S. N. (1990). *Social skills rating system manual.* Circle Pines, MN: American Guidance Service.

Joiner Jr., T. E., Katz, J., & Lew, A. S. (1997). Self-verification and depression among youth psychiatric inpatients. *Journal of Abnormal Psychology, 106*(4), 608–618.

Luthar, S. S. (1991). Vulnerability and resilience: A study of high-risk adolescents. *Child Development, 62*(3), 600–616.

Luthar, S. S. (2006). Resilience in development: A synthesis of research across five decades. In D. Cicchetti & D. J. Cohen (Eds.), *Developmental psychopathology: Risk, disorder, and adaptation* (Vol. 3, 2nd ed., pp. 739–795). Hoboken, NJ: Wiley.

Luthar, S. S., Cicchetti, D. C., & Becker, B. (2000). The construct of resilience: A critical evaluation and guidelines for future work. *Child Development, 71*(3), 543–562.

Luthar, S. S., & Zelazo, L. B. (2003). Research on resilience: An integrative review. In S. S. Luthar (Ed.), *Resilience and vulnerability: Adaptation in the context of childhood adversities* (pp. 510–549). New York, NY: Cambridge University Press.

Luthar, S. S., & Zigler, E. (1991). Vulnerability and competence: A review of research on resilience in childhood. *American Journal of Orthopsychiatry, 61*(1), 6–22.

Luthar, S. S., & Zigler, E. (1992). Intelligence and social competence among high-risk adolescents. *Development and Psychopathology, 4*(2), 287–299.

Malecki, C. K., & Elliott, S. N. (2002). Children's social behaviors as predictors of academic achievement: A longitudinal analysis. *School Psychology Quarterly, 17*(1), 1–23.

Marsh, H. W. (2007). *Self-concept theory, measurement and research into practice: The role of self concept in educational psychology.* Leicester: British Psychological Society.

Masten, A. S. (2001). Ordinary magic: Resilience processes in development. *American Psychologist, 56*(3), 227–238.

Masten, A. S., & Coatsworth, J. D. (1998). The development of competence in favorable and unfavorable environments: Lessons from research on successful children. *American Psychologist, 53*(2), 205–220.

Masten, A. S., & Curtis, W. J. (2000). Integrating competence and psychopathology: Pathways toward a comprehensive science of adaptation in development. *Development & Psychopathology, 12*(3), 529–550.

Masten, A. S., & Obradovic, J. (2006). Competence and resilience in development. *Annals of the New York Academy of Sciences, 1094*, 13–27.

Masten, A. S., & Powell, J. L. (2003). A resilience framework for research, policy, and practice. In S. S. Luthar (Ed.), *Resilience and vulnerability: Adaptation in the context of childhood adversities* (pp. 1–25). New York, NY: Cambridge University Press.

Masten, A. S., Roisman, G. I., Long, J. D., Burt, K. B., Obradovic, J., Riley, J. R., Boelcke-Stennes, K., & Tellegen, A. (2005). Developmental cascades: Linking academic achievement and externalizing and internalizing symptoms over 20 years. *Developmental Psychology, 41*(5), 733–746.

McConnell, A. R. (2011). The multiple self-aspects framework: Self-concept representation and its implications. *Personality and Social Psychology Review, 15*(1), 3–27.

McDermott, P. A., Mordell, M., & Stoltzfus, J. (2001). The organization of student performance in American schools: Discipline, motivation, verbal learning, and nonverbal learning. *Journal of Educational Psychology, 93*(1), 65–76.

Möller, J. (2005). Paradoxical effects of praise and criticism: Social, dimensional and temporal comparisons. *British Journal of Educational Psychology, 75*(2), 275–295.

Prince-Embury, S. (2006). *Resiliency scales for adolescents: Profiles of personal strengths.* San Antonio, TX: Harcourt Assessments, Inc.

Prince-Embury, S. (2007). *Resiliency scales for children and adolescents: Profiles of personal strengths.* San Antonio, TX: Harcourt Assessments, Inc.

Prince-Embury, S. (2008). The Resiliency Scales for Children and Adolescents, psychological symptoms and clinical status of adolescents. *Canadian Journal of School Psychology, 23*(1), 41–56.

Prince-Embury, S. (2010). Assessment for integrated screening and prevention using the resiliency scales for children and adolescents. In B. Doll, W. Pfohl, & J. Yoon (Eds.), *Handbook of youth prevention science* (pp. 141–162). New York, NY: Routledge.

Prince-Embury, S. (2011). Assessing personal resiliency in the context of school settings: Using the resiliency scales for children and adolescents. *Psychology in the Schools, 48*(7), 672–685.

Prince-Embury, S. (2013a). Translating resilience theory for assessment and application with children, adolescents, and adults: Conceptual issues. In S. Prince-Embury & D. H. Saklofske (Eds.), *Resilience in children, adolescents, and adults: Translating research into practice* (pp. 9–16). New York, NY: Springer.

Prince-Embury, S. (2013b). Resiliency scales for children and adolescents: Theory, research, and clinical application. In S. Prince-Embury & D. H. Saklofske (Eds.), *Resilience in children, adolescents, and adults: Translating research into practice* (pp. 19–44). New York, NY: Springer.

Prince-Embury, S. (2013c). The Three Mile Island health and environmental information series. In S. Prince-Embury & D. H. Saklofske (Eds.), *Resilience in children, adolescents, and adults: Translating research into practice* (pp. 227–242). New York, NY: Springer.

Prince-Embury, S. (2014). Three factor model of personal resiliency and related interventions. In S. Prince-Embury & D. H. Saklofske (Eds.), *Resilience interventions for youth in diverse populations* (pp. 25–57). New York, NY: Springer.

Prince-Embury, S., & Courville, T. (2008a). Comparison of one, two and three factor models of personal resiliency using the resiliency scales for children and adolescents. *Canadian Journal of School Psychology, 23*(1), 11–25.

Prince-Embury, S., & Courville, T. (2008b). Measurement invariance of the resiliency scales for children and adolescents with respect to sex and age cohorts. *Canadian Journal of School Psychology, 23*(1), 26–40.

Prince-Embury, S., & Rooney, R. (1987). Perception of control and faith in experts among residents in the vicinity of Three Mile Island. *Journal of Applied Social Psychology, 17*(11), 953–968.

Prince-Embury, S., & Saklofske, D. H. (2013). Translating resilience theory for application: Introduction. In S. Prince-Embury & D. H. Saklofske (Eds.), *Resilience in children, adolescents, and adults: Translating research into practice* (pp. 3–7). New York, NY: Springer.

Prince-Embury, S., & Saklofske, D. H. (2014). Building a science of resilience intervention for youth. In S. Prince-Embury & D. H. Saklofske (Eds.), *Resilience interventions for youth in diverse populations* (pp. 3–12). New York, NY: Springer.

Prince-Embury, S., Saklofske, D. & Nordstokke, D. (2016). Resiliency scale for young adults (RSYA). *Journal of Psychoeducational Assessment,* published online April 19, 2016, 1–15.

Prince-Embury, S., Saklofske, D. H., & Veseley, A. (2015). Measures of resiliency. In G. Boyle, D., Saklofske, & G. Matthews (Eds.), *Measures of personality and social psychological constructs* (pp. 290–321). New York: Academic Press.

Rothbart, M. K., & Derryberry, D. (1981). Development of individual differences in temperament. In M. E. Lamb & A. L. Brown (Eds.), *Advances in developmental psychology* (Vol. 1, pp. 37–86). Hillsdale, NJ: Erlbaum.

Rutter, M. (1987). Psychosocial resilience and protective mechanisms. *American Journal of Orthopsychiatry, 57*(3), 316–331.

Rutter, M. (1993). Resilience: Some conceptual considerations. *Journal of Adolescent Health, 14*(8), 626–631.

Rutter, M. (2010). Child and adolescent psychiatry: Past scientific achievements and challenges for the future. *European Child and Adolescent Psychiatry, 19*(9), 689–703.

Seligman, M. E. P. (1990). *Learned optimism: How to change your mind and your life.* New York, NY: Pocket Books.

Siegel, D. J. (1999). *The developing mind: How relationships and the brain interact to shape who we are.* New York, NY: Guilford Press.

Swann, W. B. (1997). The trouble with change: Self-verification and allegiance to the self. *Psychological Science, 8*(3), 177–180.

Thompson, R. A. (1990). Emotion and self-regulation. In R. Dienstbier (Series Ed.) & R. A. Thompson (Vol. Ed.), *Nebraska symposium on motivation: Socioemotional development* (pp. 367–467). Lincoln: University of Nebraska Press.

Usher, E. L., & Pajares, F. (2008). Sources of self-efficacy in school: Critical review of the literature and future directions. *Review of Educational Research, 78*(4), 751–796.

Wentzel, K. R., & Watkins, D. E. (2002). Peer relationships and collaborative learning as contexts for academic enablers. *School Psychology Review, 31*(3), 366–377.

Werner, E. E., & Smith, R. S. (1982). *Vulnerable but invincible: A longitudinal study of resilient children and youth.* New York, NY: McGraw-Hill.

White, R. W. (1959). Motivation reconsidered: The concept of competence. *Psychological Review, 66*(5), 297–333.

Wyman, P. A., Cowen, E. L., Work, W. C., & Kerley, J. H. (1993). The role of children's future expectations in self-system functioning and adjustment to life stress: A prospective study of urban at-risk children (Special issue). *Development and Psychopathology, 5*(4), 649–661.

5

A social ecological approach to understanding resilience among rural youth

Nora Didkowsky and Michael Ungar

Global economic forces and urban–centric policies, among other issues, have produced significant social, environmental, and economic transformations in rural areas (Fairbairn, 1998; Markey, Halseth, & Manson, 2008). Among the consequences of these changes has been increased out-migration by young people (Dupuy, Mayer, & Morissette, 2000). Those that remain face degraded resources such as weakened health and social services, a lack of public transportation (Halseth & Ryser, 2006), limited post-secondary educational facilities, and fewer employment opportunities (Corbett, 2005). Yet, despite the many obstacles that young people experience in rural areas, there are many who show resilience, demonstrating psychological and social well-being as they negotiate for the resources they need to cope well with adversity.

Ungar's (2012) social ecological model of resilience emphasizes the promotive and protective processes beyond individuals that enhance their capacity, and that of their communities, to navigate to the resources they need to nurture and sustain well-being, while negotiating for those resources to be provided in ways that are contextually and culturally meaningful. Both principles of a social ecological model of resilience, navigation and negotiation, appear in numerous studies of youth, adults, and families (Hart, Blincow, & Thomas, 2007; Masten, 2014) though there is a tendency to focus on one factor or process when attributing resilience to a particular population. For example, young offenders who receive social support are known to have lower rates of recidivism, though the source of that support, its impact, and its sustainability are dimensions of the resource that influence its availability and viability as a promotive factor (Hamilton, Sullivan, Veysey, & Gillo, 2007). A social ecological understanding of resilience suggests a more complex, interdependent set of multi-systemic, nested processes.

In this chapter, we use this model to examine the complex patterns of interaction young people living in rural contexts use to experience resilience. Specifically, we want to understand how the relationship between young people and their socially and physically isolated environments (in this case, natural and built environments) can successfully nurture and sustain a sense of individual and collective well-being. We begin by discussing the risks confronting young people in rural areas then explore the processes that occur at the interface of person–environment interactions related to resilience in rural contexts. We conclude with a discussion of the strengths of a social ecological model of resilience to understanding the psychological and social processes associated with successful adjustment among rural youth.

A review of the risks for youth in rural communities

Globalization, economic collapse, modernization, the erosion of public-sector support, shifts in domestic rural policies, and urban-centric development have dramatically affected rural communities (Fairbairn, 1998; Markey et al., 2008). The economic consequences of these global forces have changed the quality and quantity of employment opportunities in rural areas and have resulted in the disintegration of primary sector industries such as agriculture, fisheries, and forestry (Fairbairn, 1998); increasing out-migration of young people (Dupuy et al., 2000); growing educational and occupational mobility (Stockdale, 2006); changing demographic patterns, such as an aging and shrinking rural population (Ryser, Manson, & Halseth, 2013); and dramatic shifts, both positive and negative, to transportation, technology, and communications (Green & Meyer, 1997; Laegran, 2002).

Given these challenges, the geographic divide between rural and urban areas has resulted in higher levels of poverty, stress, and health-related problems in rural communities when compared to urban settings (Senate Standing Committee Report, 2006). Youth are particularly vulnerable to these challenges, which leave them at risk for externalizing problems like substance abuse (Senate Standing Committee Report, 2006), as well as internalizing problems such as depression and anxiety (Looker & Naylor, 2009).

Despite these patterns of risk, the extent of the problems experienced by rural youth has not been well studied. Among the exceptions is research by Matthews and his colleagues (Matthews, Taylor, Sherwood, Tucker, & Limb, 2000). They surveyed 372 children aged 9 to 16 from 28 villages in rural Northamptonshire, England, and conducted in-depth interviews with youth aged 13–16. Respondents described their childhoods as far more dangerous and far less idyllic than might be expected. Young people reported feeling a lack of power and a sense of isolation in their rural communities and noted that conflict existed between groups of young people, as well as between youth and adults, over the use of social spaces. These problems seem to persist into later adolescence and early adulthood. A study by McGrath (2001) showed that older rural youth feel dissatisfied with their work experiences due to low pay, challenging work conditions, seasonal shifts in the opportunities available, and the exploitive practices of employers. They may perceive themselves as having fewer options (McGrath, 2001), see their desires for educational attainment as unrealistic, and blame themselves for not obtaining higher education credentials despite the many structural barriers they face (Looker & Naylor, 2009). According to research conducted by Bjarnason and Thorlindsson (2006) in Iceland, youth perceptions of the occupational opportunities available to them are the strongest predictors of whether they will out-migrate, even when they prefer to reside in a rural community.

According to Corbett (2005), the educational systems currently in place in rural areas "continue to serve their traditional role of sorting and selecting for out-migration" (Corbett, 2005, p. 67). There is, he argues, a "migration imperative" (p. 62). Rural youth are taught by their educators that they must leave their rural homes if they want to be successful. Youth consequently understand leaving to be a moral responsibility. Indeed, the decision whether to stay or leave their rural homes is a personal conflict that overshadows many aspects of life for rural youth (Bjarnason & Thorlindsson, 2006; Hektner, 1995). Research conducted by Hektner (1995) showed that rural adolescents frequently feel conflicted between their aspirations for upward socio-economic and occupational mobility and their desire to remain in their rural communities, primarily because of attachments to supportive adults. Findings from a survey of 918 students in grades 8, 10, and

12 showed that males who identified as feeling conflicted about where they wanted to live were also likely to experience feelings of anger and emptiness about their futures. When confronted with choosing between two seemingly incompatible paths, some of the participants in Hektner's study indicated they would lower their educational and career aspirations in order to remain close to home.

Perhaps one of the most significant psychological threats to youth well-being in rural areas is the *perception* of rural decline. Investigators like Corbett (2007), Looker and Naylor (2009), and Stenbacka (2011) argue that the dominant discourse in Western societies that values risk-taking among youth (Beck, 1992) places value on modernity, consumption, individualistic lifestyles, and choice. These discourses endorse a mobile, rootless, and individualized workforce. Individuals' connections to place or home are considered temporary, as successful young people "disembed" (Giddens, 1991) themselves from their attachments to place and move into more robust job markets (Corbett, 2007). Against this backdrop, youth who chose to, or have limited choice but to, stay living rurally are consequently seen as backward, stagnant, or unsuccessful (Bye, 2009; Corbett, 2005, 2007; Looker & Naylor, 2009; Stenbacka, 2011).

These negative discourses of the rural are propagated by images that are produced and played out in the media (Bye, 2009; Stenbacka, 2011). Both Stenbacka (2011) and Bye (2009) dissect popular reality television shows in Sweden and Norway, respectively, to demonstrate how discourses of urban versus rural (or right versus wrong/modern versus traditional) are perpetuated and then reproduced within rural and urban identities. Bye (2009), for example shows how the rural Norwegian man is often depicted as marginal:

> Whereas "to be something in life" is often synonymous with "moving away" or "leaving", it is generally the case that youths who remain in the countryside are associated with those who make little out of life and who are backward in relation to what is happening "out there." Hence, implicit in the expression "to stay behind" is a modernist discourse of rurality which opposes traditional backward rurality to modern and progressive urbanism.
>
> *(Bye, 2009, p. 279)*

Looker and Naylor (2009) argue that these discourses are internalized by rural youth who come to perceive their decision to stay in their home communities as personal failings. Rurality is embodied as a deficit. The authors conducted an analysis of a longitudinal study that used surveys and interviews in rural and urban Canada with participants from the same cohort over the course of 11 years. The initial survey was taken with 17-year-old youth ($N = 1,209$, with approximately 400 respondents at each of 3 sites). The final survey was conducted 11 years later when participants were 29 years old, with two shorter surveys and one interview occurring in between. In-depth interviews were also conducted with 28 of the participants in year 11. The authors compared youths' satisfaction with various dimensions of their lives, their educational attainments, and their occupational situations over time across four migration patterns (rural to rural, rural to urban, urban to rural, and urban to urban). Study participants who remained living rurally were much less likely to have a full-time job in the week preceding the survey than were those in any other group. They reported lower satisfaction with their educational and occupational attainments than the youth who had moved to a city. They found that even though rural youth expressed satisfaction in their personal and family lives, and despite seeing family as very important, many interpreted their socio-economic problems as their own fault.

The perception of rural decline and stagnation also detrimentally affects the policies developed and implemented *on* rural areas (Fairbairn, 1998; Stenbacka, 2011). Fairbairn argues that, as more people leave their rural areas and the size of rural communities plummets, so too do the number of voters who that can influence vital (and contextually appropriate) rural services and policies. He states, "The *perception* of rural decline has quite likely led many urban people, and many government officials, to regard rural problems as marginal: questions of adjustment, that will go away in time" (p. 2, emphasis in the original).

Change, however, is not just happening *to* rural communities. Youth are also important actors who collectively shape the social dynamics occurring within their communities (Ryser et al., 2013). The economic and social conditions in rural communities can open up opportunities for personal and collective agency to "construct new narratives, break moulds, and reconstruct ways of understanding and relating to each other and the broader world" (Parkins & Reed, 2013, p. 6).

A social ecological approach to the study of rural youth resilience

How, then, do young people cope in rural environments? Can they adapt to changing environments in ways that make it likely they will succeed and remain in rural communities? To understand the factors that protect young people from the potentially negative impact of rural living, we can view their lives through the lens of a social ecological model of resilience (Ungar, 2012). The construct of resilience refers to the relationship between risk and positive adaptation, wherein adaptive developmental trajectories are pursued despite exposure to remarkable adversity (Luthar, Cicchetti, & Becker, 2000; Rutter, 2006). Recently, researchers have argued for a more comprehensive understanding of resilience that moves beyond subject-centered approaches to explore the interrelationship between people and their social contexts. A social ecological understanding of resilience emphasizes the role social and physical ecologies play in positive developmental outcomes (Bronfenbrenner, 1979; Sameroff, 2009; Ungar, 2011).

Bronfenbrenner (1979), and those that built on his work (see Bronfenbrenner & Ceci, 1994; Sameroff, 2009), have suggested a development-in-context approach to conceptualize the interactive and bi-directional transactions between genetic, biological, psychological, and socio-cultural processes. Accordingly, transactional processes occur within nested micro-, meso-, exo-, and macro-systems including the individual, family, community, and socio-political ecologies of the child (Dawes & Donald, 2000). More distal systems (such as broader socio-cultural values) are mediated by the closer (or proximal) systems (such as the family). The meso-system connects the different micro-systems within which the child operates. For example, a child experiencing dysfunction within her family or community context may receive support from a neighbour, who helps protect the child from further exposure to violence or neglect (Elder & Conger, 2000). Exo-systems are those in which the child is not directly involved but which can still impact the child's well-being. The child's parent's employment status, for example may result in a more or less stressful home environment (Conger, Rueter, & Conger, 2000).

Ungar's (2012) social ecological model of resilience emphasizes the opportunity structure of youths' environments that enable them and their communities to effectively use culturally meaningful resources and strategies to cope under harsh conditions. Ungars' (2011, 2013a) work across cultures has shown that the variability between what constitutes resilience-promoting or resilience-impeding processes depends upon the "fit" between persons and their social and physical ecologies. Given this need for sensitivity to a child's context, Ungar (2011) argues that resilience can be accounted for by attending to four key principles: decentrality, complexity, atypicality, and cultural relativity. He suggests that we need to place greater emphasis on the ecologies within which the child develops, and how well those ecologies facilitate resilience, rather than focusing primarily on individual characteristics (the principle of decentrality). Likewise, with regard to complexity, Ungar writes, "Resilience-promoting processes only *seem* to produce predictable outcomes. In fact, the likelihood of good outcomes depends on the degree of threat posed by a changing environment" (2011, p. 7, emphasis in the original). In Ungar's model, the principle of atypicality refers to the way children respond to risky environments and whether those around them condemn the child's behaviour as culturally inappropriate or condone it because it meets social expectations. Finally, Ungar demonstrates that resilience is a complex construct with varied outcomes that depend on culturally meaningful strategies, resources, and social structures (the principle of cultural relativity). What constitutes effective protective and promotive factors depends upon both the quality of the risk factors a young person experiences and the cultural context in which the youth lives (Kağitçibaşi, 2006; Trommsdorf, 2000).

Structural and historical constraints on young people's resilience in rural environments

Opportunities and barriers to successful adjustment in an increasingly globalized world are not equally distributed across age, social religion, ethnicity, gender (Kraack & Kenway, 2002; Wyn & Woodman, 2007), or location (Corbett, 2007). Patterns of inequality may carry forward even into new regimes, influencing who may take control of adaptive resources and consequently reinforcing the likelihood of further risks posed to certain young people (Mortimer & Larson, 2002; Wyn & Woodman, 2007). Mortimer and Larson state that

> What remains to be emphasized is the ways in which differences in family wealth, and other inequalities affecting access to resources, influence the paths young people take. Shaped within the competitive ethos of post-industrial capitalism, the new adolescence is a period of high stakes in which access to resources is critical in shaping both options and constraints.
>
> *(p. 12)*

Thus, as Looker and Naylor's (2009) work suggests, "many rural youth remain embedded in their home or similar communities, struggling with the challenges of being rural: seasonal work, little access to public transportation, limited formal support structures, and restricted educational and training opportunities" (p. 43). The age at which they experience these challenges will determine to some extent their capacity to navigate their way towards solutions. For example, are they old enough to drive, and if so, does this allow them to compensate for a lack of public transit? (Trommsdorff, 2000).

Historical forces also shape the possibilities for young people to experience resilience. Elder (1998) argues that, as historical forces shape lives, they also alter social trajectories. Decisions regarding family, education, and work are sensitive to historical events like economic downturns or changes in government policies (Dawes & Donald, 2000). Children born in different cohorts, even as little as ten years apart (or 100 miles apart) may experience disruptions and social dislocations differently (Elder, 1998; Wyn & Woodman, 2007). For example when Corbett (2005) investigated the link between formal education and out-migration in an Atlantic Canadian coastal community, he included an analysis of the spaces people identified as important. Corbett demonstrated that when compared with older generations, young people's life choices and expectations for how social institutions will provide for them depended upon the social and economic history of their communities and the values these histories helped shape. His work showed how changes in fishery policies in Canada in the 1980s left some families holding fishing licenses, which better positioned them for coastal work opportunities. Today, young people (especially young women) whose families do not hold fishing licenses face a more limited set of options and opportunities. Returning to the concept of resilience, we would argue that these young people's resilience has been compromised by historical events and that the individual decisions they can make today are limited by past events that were beyond their control.

Youth, however, are not just acted upon by social and economic forces. As youth develop new capacities, they are increasingly able to make decisions that shape their environments, their experiences within those environments, and the course of their personal development (Boyden, 2003). As interdependent actors (Punch, 2002), youth formulate goals and mold their interpersonal relationships, though may choose to circumscribe their thoughts and behaviours to fall in line with kinship obligations (Punch, 2002; Theron et al., 2011), broader systems of power, and cultural norms (Didkowsky & Ungar, 2010) that influence young people's experiences of resilience (Ungar, 2008, 2011). Empowerment (a component of resilience) can be understood as the union of internal capacities and external conditions that allow young people to take control of their lives (Boyden, 2003).

Protective and promotive factors associated with rural youth resilience

There are protective factors and processes that have been discussed in studies of social change and rural resilience. Both bodies of literature show how young people living in strained or restructuring communities can cope successfully. The protective factors that have been identified can be grouped into four mutually interdependent, ecological systems (Bronfenbrenner, 1979): the individual, the family, the community, and the socio-political context.

Protective factors at the individual level

Children's and youths' individual characteristics are inextricably linked to environmental influences on transactional developmental processes. Resilience should, therefore, not be understood as a person-centered construct but rather as the complex interaction between young people and their social and physical environments (Ungar, 2011). These processes, though, are still influenced by individual factors as it is these aspects of individuals to which environments must respond. Specifically, there are a number of individual attributes that have been found to be associated with the positive development of rural youth during periods of social and economic volatility.

Maintaining a positive attitude

Research suggests that youths' attitudes toward their transitional experiences play a role in how they make meaning from their experiences and how well they acculturate or adjust to their new environments. Maintaining a sense of hope (Marshall, 2002) and having the determination to succeed (Stockdale, 2006) are facets of a positive attitude identified in the rural literature. Youths' positive attitudes toward their rural places may be in part related to their ability to nurture and maintain social connections. Elder and Conger (2000) showed that rural youths' positive adaptations to rural restructuring were not solely determined by their economic advantage or disadvantage. Instead, they found a strong correlation between family ties, high social capital (that is having access to strong community social support networks), and youths' positive development.

Self-efficacy

The belief that one has the personal capacity, within supportive conditions, to take control of one's life as well as a strong sense of self and self-confidence have been shown to be related to the youth's ability to adjust positively when dealing with different types of challenges in rural contexts (Elder & Conger, 2000; Marshall, 2002). In the contexts of rural economic and social restructuring, strong links exist between positive self-concept, self-esteem, and group identification (Elder & Conger, 2000; Trell, van Hoven, & Huigen, 2012).

Subjective beliefs and goals

The formulation of personal goals for education and work despite significant community disruptions have been linked to the positive development of rural youth (Elder & Russell, 2000). According to Marshall (2002), it is important for youth to be future oriented but realistic about the opportunities and challenges that accompany significant dislocations.

Strong work-ethic

Being practically minded (Bye, 2009), feeling competent, having a strong work-ethic, and showing a sense of responsibility toward others (Elder & Conger, 2000; Marshall, 2002) are all factors that have been found to foster the adjustment of youth in rural settings.

Family systems

The impacts of geographical, political, and ideological transformations are often mediated by the proximal environment of the family (Trommsdorff, 2000). Family and kinship relations have been shown to mold young people's experiences of lifestyles, school, peer relationships, future plans, and work (Punch, 2002). In strained economic contexts, the concept of family is often fluid and may include networks of extended family and community relations (Theron et al., 2011). Families can themselves be sources of stress during times of change, and family economic strain has been shown to increase youth stress during times of restructuring (Conger et al., 2000). But families can also offer emotional support, connection, a sense of belonging, and exposure to positive role models (Elder & Conger, 2000). Through extended family ties, youth are provided access to work opportunities and social networks, as well as entrepreneurial pathways supported by parental and extended kinship experience and knowledge (Corbett, 2005). A number of aspects of family are known to influence whether families function as protective factors or as compound risk factors encountered elsewhere in a child's life. Given the dearth of studies in this area, we cannot assert whether these factors affect rural youth more than urban youth, though they appear thematically in studies of both populations.

Family climate

Family trust, emotional closeness, and cohesion play a protective role for youth experiencing transitions. Conger and her colleagues (Conger et al., 2000) found that families who were experiencing economic strain due to rural restructuring and were still able to resolve family conflicts constructively were more likely to sustain supportive interactions, resulting in fewer disagreements over time. They found that the support of the husband to the wife resulted in parenting that showed better communication and effective problem-solving skills. These parents were more likely to have children with better adaptive capacities.

Filial responsibility and contributions

Youths' contributions to family during times of stress can help foster better psychosocial adjust-ment (Punch, 2002; Ungar, Theron & Didkowsky, 2011). Elder and Conger (2000), for example suggest that children's contributions on family farms during economic downturns can promote a sense of self-worth. Their research with children and families in Iowa found that children who grew up on farms felt a deep sense of responsibility toward their families, were likely to spend time in communal activities, and felt strong feelings of connection and fewer feelings of isola-tion. Importantly, youth believed that their parents viewed them as important members of the household.

Community systems and collective identities

Youths' relationships with their caregivers profoundly influence their ability to interact with their broader environments and take advantage of the protective resources available to them (Cameron, Ungar, & Liebenberg, 2007). Likewise, community contexts directly influ-ence the mental health of those who care for children (Dawes & Donald, 2000), thereby indirectly affecting children's adaptive capacities. There are a number of positive commu-nity forces associated with rural youths' adaptive development during times of change and adversity.

Social cohesion and community support

Healthy communities exhibit high social cohesion, engagement, reciprocity, and extended support systems between neighbours and provide communities with the sense of shared belonging (Trell et al., 2012). In a study of well-being in rural communities experienc-ing socio-economic shifts, Jacob, Bourke, and Luloff (1997) found that stress levels were slightly lower in communities whose members perceived their neighbourhoods as inter-active. Interactional communities were those where members felt other residents were as interested in community issues as they were and where people felt at home and satisfied with their network of relationships. Likewise, McManus and his colleagues (McManus et al., 2012) interviewed 115 farmers in two rural regions in Australia and found that, despite inadequate health care services and the decline of employment opportunities, the farmers perceived their communities as strong and resilient. They attributed this resilience to the close connection between neighbours, friends, and family and a shared sense of belonging. It also appears that youth with strong emotional ties to their communities are less likely to want to out-migrate (Bjarnason & Thorlindsson, 2006).

Collective agency

The expression of rules, power, and competition shape the ways in which youth and other com-munity members access opportunities and resources for psychosocial growth, participate mean-ingfully in mainstream economies, and gain mastery over their lives. Community contexts that support youths' opportunities to experience power and control are those that allow collective decision making and foster a collective sense of power among community members (Ryser et al., 2013). Communities that demonstrate collective agency provide young people opportunities to be socialized into positive subcultures and organizations and encourage youth civic engagement (Ryser et al., 2013) and resilience.

Services and instrumental supports

Institutions, human services, and other collective resources help shape the way a community functions. Resilience-promoting communities not only offer good neighbourhood connections and access to services such as hospitals, mental health resources, and social supports but also equitable access to those structures that allow youth to successfully adjust to their changing conditions (Jacob et al., 1997; Mortimer & Larson, 2002). The structural design of community spaces – including housing density; the quality and number of social, physical, and mental-health supports in the area; the quality of housing; the kinds and costs of transportation systems; and the quality of recreational facilities and schools, along with the demographics of the community (including the community's ethnic mix, age, and gender distributions) – impact upon the opportunities young people have for positive psychosocial development (Dawes & Donald, 2000; Halseth & Ryser, 2006; Mortimer & Larson, 2002). Resilience-promoting communities provide education systems that make sense given the local context (Corbett, 2005; Ungar, Russell, & Connelly, 2014), account for students' cultural differences in programming and encourage teachers who actively engage and advocate for their students (Theron, Liebenberg, & Malindi, 2013; Ungar et al., 2014). Strong communities also offer youth access to age-appropriate work and employment opportunities (Mortimer & Larson, 2002; Ryser et al., 2013), conditions that increase the capacity of young people to show resilience in contexts where they may be marginalized.

Youth–adult partnerships, community supports, and mentors

Exposure to at least some well-functioning caregivers, role models, peers, or supportive community members can protect youth against risks in their environments (Cameron et al., 2007). While all youth benefit from adult and community support, youth from impoverished and marginalized backgrounds enjoy the differential positive impact of quality youth–adult engagement (Ungar, 2013b). Ryser et al. (2013) provide evidence that the active engagement of youth in stressful rural climates can help decrease youths' feelings of isolation and consequently encourage them to improve their behaviours. Through mentoring, experiential learning, and deliberate efforts to increase youth participation in the community, youth receive practical work experience and are exposed to previously inaccessible institutional procedures that can increase youths' personal, social, and cultural capitals.

Peers

For young people in strained rural contexts, peer relations can provide a robust support network, sources of information regarding career decisions and a sense of belonging (Marshall, 2002). Positive peer relationships and the development of healthy social identities are more likely in communities that create spaces for young people to interact in prosocial ways.

Space, place, and collective identities

The spaces within which young people interact with peers and adults shape how young people experience themselves and the individual and collective identities that follow (Jones, 1999). Community cohesion, for example and a sense of belonging to a powerful socially desirable group, both aspects of resilience, are more easily fostered in a community that provides its members access to sporting activities and recreation facilities (Oncescu & Robertson, 2010; Walia & Liepert, 2012), safe streets with street lamps, and public transportation (Walia & Liepert, 2012).

Place identity, or seeing one's sense of self as inseparable to particular geographical locations, speaks to the shared histories, socially valued practices, and ethno-cultural traditions connected with these geographic spaces (Panelli et al., 2008). To illustrate, in rural Australia, Kraack and Kenway (2002) found that economic restructuring produced changes in local attitudes regarding behaviours that were considered positive among young people. The loss of working-class modes of employment, paired with a shift toward tourism-focused work opportunities, transformed the community's expectations and perceptions of youth. New community residents actively prevented the "loitering" of young people in former youth-friendly social spaces, like the beach; places that were once locations for the production and performance of youth identities.

Socio-political systems

Studying youth development within rural contexts highlights the ways in which socio-political systems precipitate significant cultural, social, and environmental transformations and influence the relationships between young people, their families, and communities. Not only can the policies of nations *cause* significant cultural and contextual alterations for youth, they can also *moderate* the impact of socio-political forces like migration and rural restructuring on young people. For example Kerckhoff (2002) found variation in the way economic restructuring has affected young people in different countries. In America, high school dropouts have significantly fewer opportunities than college graduates; yet, regardless of their educational credentials, young people's first jobs will most likely be part-time, temporary, and on-call employment, promising few benefits or security. In contrast, European countries like Australia, Switzerland, and Germany promote a system of apprenticeship that helps young people enter into the workforce earlier and with higher wages. Resilience is, therefore, as dependent on exosystemic factors like education policies and the minimum wage as it is individual qualities, peer and family relationships, and the quality of the community in which a young person lives and forms an identity. In rural contexts, each of these processes is exacerbated (or enhanced) by the very nature of the rurality the young person experiences.

Conclusion

The investigation of resilience in rural contexts has implications for how resilience can be understood as contextually relevant in different social and geographic settings. Using rural youth as an example of a population under stress, we have shown that resilience is best understood when a person's social ecology is included in the analysis of the factors and processes that influence positive developmental outcomes. Specifically, this chapter has reviewed the factors helping to explain successful adjustment for youth experiencing transitions and strain in rural contexts, but may also inform the social change literature more broadly. We must keep in mind however, as Trommsdorff (2000) has argued, that "When looking for ways in which contextual factors transmit social change to the individual, one has to be aware of the ecological complexity of contextual variables and their different meaning in different cultural contexts" (p. 60). Though the research on the factors that influence young people's resilience in rural contexts is only just emerging, there is evidence to suggest that a social ecological model of resilience can help to explain the person-in-context and the nature of the protective and promotive processes that make it more likely rural youth succeed.

Discussion of risk and resilience shows that rural young people's coping strategies reflect their ability, and the ability of their social supports, service providers, and governments, to facilitate their navigation to, and negotiation for, the resources that are meaningful to them. By attending to the multiple and integrated aspects of young people's psychological, social, and political contexts, we are better able to show how resilience is constructed and enabled. As we have seen, the interactions engaged by youth within their social and physical ecologies are grounded in historical, geographical, temporal, and socio-cultural contexts and understood through mechanisms that are socially mediated (Boyden, 2003; Sameroff, 2009). This process-focused, contextualized stance shifts our attention from the individual, to the multi-fold, interconnected influences that shape rural communities and, by extension, the processes that impact on youths' capacity to draw upon resilience-promoting resources. This has significant implications for rural policy and community development. Rather than continuing to emphasize the need to retain youth in rural communities, we should be working toward building resilience-enabling environments that ensure young people have access to the resources (including reinforcement for their identity as a rural person) that can sustain them, thereby pre-empting out-migration and facilitating the return of young people to rural areas.

References

Beck, U. (1992). *Risk society: Towards a new modernity.* Newbury Park, CA: Sage.

Bjarnason, T., & Thorlindsson, T. (2006). Should I stay or should I go? Migration expectations among youth in Icelandic fishing and farming communities. *Journal of Rural Studies, 22*(3), 290–300.

Boyden, J. (2003). Children under fire: Challenging assumptions about children's resilience. *Children, Youth and Environments, 13*(1), 1–29.

Bronfenbrenner, U. (1979). *The ecology of human development: Experiments by nature and design.* Cambridge, MA: Harvard University Press.

Bronfenbrenner, U., & Ceci, S. J. (1994). Nature–nurture reconceptualised in developmental perspective: A bioecological model. *Psychological Review, 101*(4), 568–586.

Bye, L. M. (2009). 'How to be a rural man': Young men's performances and negotiations of rural masculinities. *Journal of Rural Studies, 25*(3), 278–288.

Cameron, C. A., Ungar, M., & Liebenberg, L. (2007). Cultural understandings of resilience: Roots for wings in the development of affective resources for resilience. *Child and Adolescent Psychiatric Clinics of North America, 16*(2), 285–301.

Conger, K. J., Rueter, M. A., & Conger, R. D. (2000). The role of economic pressure in the lives of parents and their adolescents: The family stress model. In L. J. Crockett & R. K. Silbereisen (Eds.), *Negotiating adolescence in times of social change* (pp. 201–223). Cambridge, UK: Cambridge University Press.

Corbett, M. (2005). Rural education and out-migration: The case of a coastal community. *Canadian Journal of Education, 28*(1/2), 52–72.

Corbett, M. (2007). Travels in space and place: Identity and rural schooling. *Canadian Journal of Education, 30*(3), 771–792.

Dawes, A., & Donald, D. (2000). Improving children's chances: Developmental theory and effective interventions in community contexts. In D. Donald, A. Dawes, & J. Louw (Eds.), *Addressing childhood adversity* (pp. 1–25). Cape Town: David Philip.

Didkowsky, N., & Ungar, M. (2010). Using a development-in-context approach to conceptualize the impact of sociopolitical restructuring on youth resilience in Russia. *Youth and Society.* Advance online publication. doi:10.1177/0044118X10386076

Dupuy, R., Mayer, F., & Morissette, R. (2000). *Rural youth: Stayers, leavers, and return migrants.* Ottawa, ON: Business and Labour Market Analysis Division: Statistics Canada. Report submitted to the Rural Secretariat of Agriculture and Agri-Food Canada and to the Atlantic Canada Opportunities Agency.

Elder, G. H. (1998). The life course as developmental theory. *Child Development, 69*(1), 1–12.

Elder, G. H., & Conger, R. D. (2000). *Children of the land: Adversity and success in rural America.* Chicago: University of Chicago Press.

Elder, G. H., & Russell, S. T. (2000). Surmounting life's disadvantage. In L. J. Crockett & R. K. Silbereisen (Eds.), *Negotiating adolescence in times of social change* (pp. 17–36). Cambridge, UK: Cambridge University Press.

Fairbairn, B. (1998). *A preliminary history of rural development policy and programmes in Canada, 1945–1995.* Saskatoon: University of Saskatchewan. NRE Program.

Giddens, A. (1991). *Modernity and self-identity: Self and society in the late modern age.* California: Stanford University Press.

Green, M. B., & Meyer, S. P. (1997). An overview of commuting in Canada: With special emphasis on rural commuting and employment. *Journal of Rural Studies, 13*(2), 163–175.

Halseth, G., & Ryser, L. (2006). Trends in service delivery: Examples from rural and small town Canada, 1998 to 2005. *Journal of Rural and Community Development, 1*(2), 69–90.

Hamilton, Z. K., Sullivan, C. J., Veysey, B. M., & Gillo, M. (2007). Diverting multi-problem youth from juvenile justice: Investigating the importance of community influence on placement and recidivism. *Behavioral Sciences and the Law, 25*(1), 137–158.

Hart, A., Blincow, D., & Thomas, H. (2007). *Resilient therapy: Working with children and families.* London, UK: Routledge.

Hektner, J. M. (1995). When moving up implies moving out: Rural adolescent conflict in the transition to adulthood. *Journal of Research in Rural Education, 11*(1), 3–14.

Jacob, S., Bourke, L., & Luloff, A. E. (1997). Rural community stress, distress, and well-being in Pennsylvania. *Journal of Rural Studies, 13*(3), 275–288.

Jones, G. (1999). 'The same people in the same places?' Socio-spatial identities and migration in youth. *Sociology, 33*(1), 1–22.

Kağitçibaşi, C. (2006). Theoretical perspectives on family change. In J. Georgas, J. W. Berry, F. J. R. van de Vijver, C. Kağitçibasi, & Y. H. Poortinga (Eds.), *Families across cultures: A 30-nation psychological study* (pp. 72–89). New York: Cambridge University Press.

Kerckhoff, A. C. (2002). The transition from school to work. In J. Mortimer & R. Larson (Eds.), *The changing adolescent experience: Societal trends and the transition to adulthood* (pp. 52–87). Cambridge: Cambridge University Press.

Kraack, A., & Kenway, J. (2002). Place, time and stigmatised youthful identities: Bad boys in paradise. *Journal of Rural Studies, 18*(2), 145–155.

Laegran, A. S. (2002). The petrol station and the internet cafe: Rural technospaces for youth. *Journal of Rural Studies, 18*(2), 157–168.

Looker, E. D., & Naylor, T. D. (2009). 'At risk' of being rural? The experience of rural youth in a risk society. *Journal of Rural and Community Development, 4*(2), 39–64.

Luthar, S. S., Cicchetti, D., & Becker, B. (2000). The construct of resilience: A critical evaluation and guidelines for future work. *Child Development, 71*(3), 543–562.

Markey, S., Halseth, G., & Manson, D. (2008). Challenging the inevitability of rural decline: Advancing the policy of place in northern British Columbia. *Journal of Rural Studies, 24*(4), 409–421.

Marshall, A. (2002). Life-career counselling issues for youth in coastal and rural communities: The impact of economic, social and environmental restructuring. *International Journal for the Advancement of Counselling, 24*(1), 69–87.

Masten, A. S. (2014). Global perspectives on resilience in children and youth. *Child Development, 85*(1), 6–20.

Matthews, H., Taylor, M., Sherwood, K., Tucker, F., & Limb, M. (2000). Growing-up in the countryside: Children and the rural idyll. *Journal of Rural Studies, 16*(2), 141–153.

McGrath, B. (2001). "A problem of resources": Defining rural youth encounters in education, work & housing. *Journal of Rural Studies, 17*(4), 481–495.

McManus, P., Walmsley, J., Argent, N., Baum, S., Bourke, L., Martin, J., & Sorensen, T. (2012). Rural community and rural resilience: What is important to farmers in keeping their country towns alive? *Journal of Rural Studies, 28*(1), 20–29.

Mortimer, J., & Larson, R. (2002). *The changing adolescent experience: Societal trends and the transition to adulthood.* Cambridge: Cambridge University Press.

Oncescu, J., & Robertson, B. (2010). Recreation in remote communities: A case study of a Nova Scotian village. *Journal of Rural and Community Development, 5*(1/2), 221–237.

Panelli, R., Allen, D., Ellison, B., Kelly, A., John, A., & Tipa, G. (2008). Beyond bluff oysters? Place identity and ethnicity in a peripheral coastal setting. *Journal of Rural Studies, 24*(1), 41–55.

Parkins, J. R., & Reed, M. G. (2013). *Social transformation in rural Canada: Community, cultures, and collective action.* Vancouver: UBC Press.

Punch, S. (2002). Youth transitions and interdependent adult–child relations in rural Bolivia. *Journal of Rural Studies, 18*(2), 123–133.

Rutter, M. (2006). Implication of resilience concepts for scientific understanding. In B. M. Lester, A. S. Masten, & B. McEwen (Eds.), *Resilience in children* (pp. 1–12). Boston, MA: Blackwell.

Ryser, L., Manson, D., & Halseth, G. (2013). Including youth in an aging rural society: Reflections from northern British Columbia's resource frontier communities. In J. R. Parkins & M. G. Reed (Eds.), *Social transformation in rural Canada: Community, cultures, and collective action* (pp. 189–207). Vancouver, BC: UBC Press.

Sameroff, A. J. (2009). *The transactional model of development: How children and contexts shape each other.* Washington, DC: American Psychological Association.

Senate Standing Committee Report. (December 2006). *Understanding freefall: The challenge of the rural poor.* Ottawa: HRSDC.

Stenbacka, S. (2011). Othering the rural: About the construction of rural masculinities and the unspoken urban hegemonic ideal in Swedish media. *Journal of Rural Studies, 27*(3), 235–244.

Stockdale, A. (2006). Migration: Pre-requisite for rural economic regeneration? *Journal of Rural Studies, 22*(3), 354–366.

Theron, L., Cameron, C. A., Didkowsky, N., Lau, C., Liebenberg, L., & Ungar, M. (2011). "A day in the lives" of four resilient youths: Cultural roots of resilience. *Youth & Society, 43*(3), 799–818.

Theron, L. C., Liebenberg, L., & Malindi, M. J. (2013). When schooling experiences are respectful of children's rights: A pathway to resilience. *School Psychology International, 35*(3), 253–265.

Trell, E. M., van Hoven, B., & Huigen, P. (2012). 'It's good to live in Järva-Jaani but we can't stay here': Youth and belonging in rural Estonia. *Journal of Rural Studies, 28*(2), 139–148.

Trommsdorff, G. (2000). Effects of social change on individual development: The role of social and personal factors, and the timing of events. In L. J. Crockett & R. K. Silbereisen (Eds.), *Negotiating adolescence in times of social change* (pp. 1–13). Cambridge, UK: Cambridge University Press.

Ungar, M. (2008). Resilience across cultures. *British Journal of Social Work, 38*(2), 218–235.

Ungar, M. (2011). The social ecology of resilience: Addressing contextual and cultural ambiguity of a nascent construct. *American Journal of Orthopsychiatry, 81*, 1–17.

Ungar, M. (2012). *The social ecology of resilience.* New York: Springer.

Ungar, M. (2013a). Resilience, trauma, context, and culture. *Trauma, Violence, & Abuse, 14*(3), 255–266.

Ungar, M. (2013b). The impact of youth-adult relationships on resilience. *International Journal of Child, Youth and Family Studies, 4*(3), 328–336.

Ungar, M., Russell, P., & Connelly, G. (2014). School-based interventions to enhance the resilience of students. *Journal of Educational and Developmental Psychology, 4*(1), 66–83.

Ungar, M., Theron, L., & Didkowsky, N. (2011). Adolescents' precocious and developmentally appropriate contributions to their families' well-being and resilience in five countries. *Family Relations, 60*(2), 231–246.

Walia, S., & Liepert, B. (2012). Perceived facilitators and barriers to physical activity for rural youth: An exploratory study using photovoice. *The International Electronic Journal of Rural and Remote Health Research, Education Practice and Policy, 12*(1842), 1–13.

Wyn, J., & Woodman, D. (2007). Researching youth in a context of social change: A reply to Roberts. *Journal of Youth Studies, 10*(3), 373–381.

6

Universality of the challenge–resilience–resourcefulness model

Marek J. Celinski and Lyle M. Allen III

Resilience as freedom and empowerment

From the dawn of philosophical thinking, a central concern has involved physical survival in a hostile environment along with the observation that adversity often triggers latent capabilities for coping. Reich, Zautra, and Hall (2011) cite a quotation from Horace (~ 65–8 BC): "Adversity has the effect of eliciting talents, which, in prosperous circumstances, would have lain dormant."

Plato (1937, 1992) is credited with formulation (continued later by classic Greeks, Romans and Early Christian thinkers) that courage represents endurance and perseverance through difficulty. McMartin (2011) noted that courage cannot be the only virtue guiding people but needs to be combined with prudence, which subsumes wisdom and insight:

> Almost all philosophers in the Western tradition note that living beings attempt to preserve their existence; courage and resilience become crucial because they amplify this biological drive to live. Efforts to preserve life imply judgements of value; thus courage finds support in worthy causes, sound planning, keen insight, and the discovery of meaning.
>
> *(p. 156)*

This chapter began with a reference to philosophical ideas that fundamentally address intuitions and assumptions concerning humanity and concerning the nature of our relationships with other people and with the world at large. It is the thesis of this chapter that resilience is a psychological construct that extends beyond clinical issues, a prospect of success in dealing with the social environment or a need for adaptability. In our view, resilience unifies the primary characteristics attributable to humanity, and its presence manifests beyond the way in which we react to adversities of life, such as illness, unemployment, divorce or natural disasters, even though these are opportunities for making resilient decisions. From a global perspective (Celinski, 2015a), resilience is the primary reason that cultures and civilizations have developed and offers confidence that further progress is possible. Celinski (2015b) presented a hypothetical path of development of civilizations, starting with the discovery of time as the primary organizer of the physical world and ultimately of people's lives. Recognition that something invisible profoundly impacts us manifests an ability to switch attention from the visible to invisible, or beyond the tangible and apparent, and constitutes evidence of humans' primal transcendence. Time perspective splits our awareness between "now" when our being in the world requires decisions and actions and what extends beyond now to the past, future and eternity. In the present moment, we decide how to manifest our identity so that it represents continuity and allows for transformation over time. Now is the opportunity to show our humanity, which implies that what we do will not only be a habitual, routine, "conditioned" response, but a resilient answer to a life situation. Responding in a resilient manner integrates the psychological constructs that were developed throughout the history of cultures and civilizations such as a sense of identity, meaning, values, freedom and causality, which are reflected in narratives that lead to desirable outcomes. Reich et al. (2011) described three primary meanings of the term resilience in reference to successful adaptation to stressful situations: Recovery, Sustainability and Growth:

> *Recovery* refers to the ability to rebound from a negative impact of stress that manifests as a capacity to quickly regain equilibrium and to return to an initial state of health.
> *Sustainability* refers to the capacity to go forward in life; it is defined as the extent to which ongoing purposeful engagements at school, work, in family and social life are not disrupted by stressors.
> *Growth* refers to the possibility that, as a result of healthy responses to the stressful experience the person, organization and/or community developed enhanced adaptation capacity through new learning that extends beyond pre-stress levels.

Our understanding of resilience is intrinsically connected with a sense of identity, which developed in opposition to the inevitable changes experienced over time. Resilience related to biological survival is a model for resilience in the service of identity that has individual and collective meaning because of our identification with larger groups (i.e. representing organized religion, country or a corporate mentality). McMartin (2011) referred to Aristotle's (1985) *Nicomachean ethics* by saying that our comfort or even our lives may be sacrificed "for the sake of the cause outside of the individual" (p. 156), which means that we have incorporated certain intangible values in our sense of self. Identity includes a distinct time awareness as it must remain stable in resisting the passage of time but also needs to allow for changes and improvement so that we would be able to acquire new knowledge and skills.

The second important feature of resilience is also time based. Literature on this subject (Celinski, 2011) refers to resilience in the context of how the present time reactions impact on the future. One is a possibility of "bouncing back" or to recover from any type of loss after a setback caused by illness, accident or natural disaster, another one is creating new social reality through guided and purposeful efforts. With reference to the present time, resilience manifests as preparedness and readiness to face truthfully and courageously the challenge of the situation; it is different from a tendency to ignore, minimize or reframe what the situation presents in order to lessen its emotional impact (e.g. I may try to ignore my chronic cough because I do not wish to hear bad news or to be told to change my lifestyle). Knowing as accurately as possible what given situations represent (which is the core postulate of mindfulness and phenomenology) will eventually allow accepting reality as is. When an urge to react immediately and in a compulsive (often catastrophizing) manner is diminished, this enables us to decide how to engage with reality on a certain level of freedom that represents empowerment or intention about how to impact on reality. In such a frame of mind, people know that there are often options and that they have to choose wisely to achieve the best outcomes. Values are consistently part of this process, and they guide us through choosing an optimal level of engaging and help us evaluate the results of our efforts. Behind such thinking lies more than 2,300 years of tradition (going back to Aristotle) that enabled us to comprehend external reality in terms of causal relations between successive events and to find ways to achieve what was intended. Even more importantly, this tradition has established individuals and humanity as a source of causal relations that have impact on reality. Unlike in instances of biological evolution, people did not wait for nature to equip them with skills and bodily abilities to live in various climatic or adverse conditions but instead used their creativity to withstand such conditions and thrive. In essence, resilience enables individuals to discover what represents their strength, to match perceived challenges with values and skills and to create a narrative that promotes recovery and growth. This needs to be contrasted with a regressive approach to dealing with adversity that threatens our existence or our health or may cause disintegration of our identity or lifestyle. Awareness of the options should help people choose wisely. In a similar way, Reich et al. (2011) stated the following:

> Although poor adaptation to stress is not uncommon, the "resilience solutions" approach is based on a fundamental, two-factor model suggesting that awareness of both deficits and capacities is needed for a complete understanding of sustainability of well-being following adverse events. It is now a comprehensive paradigm for understanding both stress reactivity and growth motivation and adaptation processes at many levels of analysis: individual, organizational, and community.
>
> (p. 34)

At this point it, is only briefly mentioned that such a two-factor conceptualization is behind our *Resourcefulness for Recovery Inventory – Research Edition* whose application to various clinical situations will be described in the following sections. This approach was summarized by Celinski (2013) in the following way:

> Genuine resilience starts with the appreciation of reality as mysterious and unpredictable, where the meaning and purpose of life are constructed through painful efforts and in spite of seemingly overwhelming evidence to the contrary. Resilience represents tolerance and a high threshold for development of psychopathology under the pressure of circumstances. Those who succeed have acquired the dialectic understanding and integration or at least some balanced perspective on the opposite forces that represent the dynamics of life, especially between a desire for comprehensibility, order and stability on one side, and the developmental forces opening people to novelty, exploration, challenge with a sense of freedom and hope in manageability, on the other.
>
> (pp. 19–20)

Kebza and Solcova (2013) summarized research on resilience by saying the following:

> Generally, there is agreement that resilience represents [a] multi-factorial and multidimensional phenomenon, characterized by a global aptitude which enables an individual to develop and strengthen one's competences under unfavourable life conditions (Gordon, 1995; Gordon & Coscarelli, 1996). Resilience developing processes involve complex interactions of [internal and] external factors stemming primarily from an individual's personality engaging with environmental factors.
>
> (Kumpfer, 1999, p. 15)

Celinski (2011) described a multi-level model that primarily reflects the way in which we have freedom to engage with challenging issues and to impact on the outcome. This model acknowledges that, when people stop viewing themselves as agency, it has a negative impact on their perception of reality, often resulting in helplessness. In such a frame of mind, some typical scenarios are played out that require little imagination, initiative or effort. Illness, chronic pain, being imprisoned, unemployed, living in a totalitarian system or being financially deprived may lead to a conclusion that nothing can be done except to rely on the goodwill of others or to follow rules that require responding in an expected subordinate manner. Helplessness may be overwhelming and comforting at the same time as it relieves people from responsibility to take risks and put forth significant effort. Any progress in becoming resilient starts with accepting circumstances (but not one's reaction of resignation and helplessness). Celinski (2015c) argued that, whereas humans cannot relieve themselves from a behavioural paradigm of stimulus–response, they have freedom to create various meanings of a situation (which he called *receptive meaning*) that could provide stimulus or inspiration for adaptive or value- and purpose-oriented actions. Thus, people have an option either to react based on their instinctual or acquired predispositions, or they can decide what they can do *in spite of* the circumstances that dictate some routine but suboptimal responses. This may lead an individual to a *random* or *trial-and-error exploration* until some opportunity is recognized that then should be intentionally pursued. The value of *intentional activity* is illustrated by those who acted and successfully changed a negative situation for better. If we can match the level of our functioning to some successful group of people, we may have achieved a level of *optimal freedom*. Our search for freedom either ends here, or we could aim at dealing with a challenging situation in a creative manner that represents our determination to do better than what others do in similar circumstances and perhaps to provide an inspiring example. For an individual, such an approach is often associated with risk, and it requires confidence and energy to pursue novel solutions. Therefore, we need a certain amount of social support.

If we do not want to wait until a good idea will catch the imagination of others and be inspiration for their action, and if we believe in the value of our *sovereign way* of functioning and are in a position of power (i.e. being a powerful political or corporate leader), we may introduce new ways by decree and enforce them by potentially coercive methods. Such ways of transforming a country by imposing a new mentality that changed social relations and redirected people's efforts have occurred many times in history and were made possible because of the total control over legislation and its implementation. Examples include the conversion of the Roman Empire to Christianity by Emperor Constantine the Great (reigned 306–337 CE), the forceful modernization of Russia by Peter the Great (tsar of Russia between 1682 to 1725) or of Turkey by Mustafa Kamal Atatürk (founder of the Turkish Republic and first president from 1923 to 1938), and transformation of a major part of Europe into communist states after World War II.

An opportunity of this kind is less likely to exist in democratic countries, and for this reason, yet another way is available, which we identify as *ultimate freedom*. Such a state of mind is less concerned with achieving specific goals in a specific time but rather with doing "the right thing" and hoping that this will bring good results, even though we do not know exactly what kind and when. This sense of detachment from results and focus on doing what is right may be helpful in overcoming a state of helplessness when options are limited. Moreover, if an idea is kept alive long enough and considered an indispensable part of human nature, a person or nation may seize an opportunity when there are improved chances for its expression and gaining popular support. Victor Frankl (1963) was aware of this type of freedom (which was even possible inside a concentration camp) when he appealed to his fellow inmates to express value and meaning through their actions. Celinski (2015c) regarded this particular human characteristic as manifesting *expressive meaning* when people's actions are inspired both by ideas and important values. Whereas values in the service of a meaningful life are an inspiration to hope, persevere and live in spite of unfavourable circumstances (and to even die for), fundamentalism and fanaticism are also possible outgrowths of such attitudes. A positive example is how yearning for freedom and democracy (which was never extinguished in the mentality of the European people) inspired Central and Eastern European nations to quickly overthrow (beginning in Poland in 1989) the communist economic and political model and abandon its ideology at the time when the Soviet Union underwent internal reforms that weakened its grip on the satellite countries.

The latter is an example of the inspirational forward meaning of resilience: it is not only "bouncing back" to restore a previous "status quo," but it can represent a patient and consistent effort to pursue a vision, express an ideal or create more desirable living conditions. In this process, we are guided by an inner freedom that compels us to manifest values fostering internal transformations that ultimately are recognized as progressive changes in the social environment. In this respect, Celinski (2011) stated the following:

> Resilience theory postulates that what prevents interruption is not comprehensibility of the situation alone but also commitment to values (or in Antonovsky's 1987 conceptualization what people recognize as meaningful in their lives) which motivates people to continue with chosen activities in spite of adversity or interfering circumstances. Such a perspective allows people to survive even the direst conditions relatively emotionally unscathed and to lose a lot rather than to change their beliefs. Sometimes those with a "realistic orientation" become losers and morally broken when social developments vindicate the eternal values they disregarded.
>
> *(p. 109)*

Celinski (2011) proposed a freedom-based model that unites resilience with resourcefulness as a way to act on values and ideas over time, even in the circumstances when an individual or a society does not have adequate control over the process and no assurance of desirable outcomes. Figure 6.1 (Celinski, 2004, 2011, p. 23) presents personal agency in self-transformation as it unfolds over time. In this model, a horizontal dimension of resourcefulness is contrasted with a vertical image of resilience as representing levels of engagement with reality.

The nature of resources that become available with recognition of various types of freedom will be reviewed when discussing specific research related to resilience and resourcefulness.

The Self in Evolution
Mind Transformations Through Utilization of Freedom
(Horizontal Perspective)
(Modified From Eric Fromm's Model)

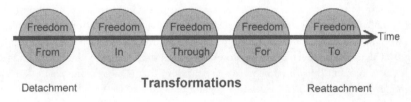

Figure 6.1 The self in evolution through various levels of personal freedom
Source: Celinski (2004).

63

Resilience may express both people's efforts to preserve the existing status quo that people consider valuable or to engage in activities leading to the personal and societal transformation when they abandon present security and accept risk, uncertainty and unpredictability with a hope that their activities can lead to a better life. In such situations, optimism and perseverance are necessary, but to succeed, they need to be combined with the availability of personal and societal resources. The primary motive behind opting for change is the recognition that the existing conditions prevent an expression of values that are an indispensable part of human identity and whose expression and realization are worthy of sacrifice. By engaging in transformation, we would need to learn new skills (and thus broaden our resourcefulness) and/or discover mental and emotional qualities needed to achieve stability or a higher level of engagement with reality, which will enhance our resilience. However, risks are involved in this process. What we aim to achieve may not be an entirely painless condition, or the assumption of new social roles may not be adaptive since both the process and its outcome may be at odds with pre-existing concepts concerning the self and reality, older values and belief systems, and may meet with social contempt or alienation. An excellent example is provided by immigration to a foreign country (Ilacqua, Celinski, & Allen, 2013). What is achieved regardless of the original goal is a broader understanding of reality and a sense of appreciation of what is important and valuable, what needs to be preserved and defended (or conversely constricted and abandoned) and what needs to be learned and expanded upon.

Bandura's (1977, 2001) description of personal agency refers to intentionality, foresight, self-regulation and self-evaluation of one's capabilities and of the meaning and purpose of one's life, which enable individuals to view themselves as a source of multiple causality. The prospect of acting in a self-efficacious manner and achieving desirable goals primarily depends on choosing an appropriate and potentially achievable level of resilience and accessing adequate resources. While we act because we are inspired by values (Frankl, 1963), it is up to individuals and humanity to create cohesive and sustainable meaning of the self and reality. We owe this insight so definitely stated to Jean Paul Sartre (2007). He postulated that for everything that exists (for example a chair) "the essence" precedes its existence; only in humans does essence follow existence as we have a potential and responsibility to create ourselves (in a psychological sense). While recognition of this concept acknowledges and inspires us to act on our freedom, we do not have an absolute freedom to manifest the "essence" of our lives because we are all subject to some physical and societal constraints and to the natural sensitivity to recognize what is "right." These limits need to be acknowledged because otherwise we risk to becoming delusional or self-destructive or causing lasting emotional, physical or moral harm to oneself and others. In this respect, social intelligence along with emotional and moral sensitivity create natural self-regulatory mechanisms (Zautra, Palucka, & Celinski, 2015).

There is no equivalent in the animal world of these uniquely human qualities. Animals have the capacity to free themselves from something that is causing discomfort or pain or prevents them from achieving what is necessary to satisfy their needs. Human freedom stemming from resilience manifests as continuity but also as disruption and violent revolutions (Satkiewicz, 2015), both of which promoted civilizations' progress in the intellectual and moral sense. We are naturally motivated, as Polish psychiatrist Dabrowski (1972) pointed out, to achieve a "higher level of psychic development [by which he means] a behaviour that is more complex, more conscious and having greater freedom of choice, hence greater opportunity for self-determination" (p. 70). There is a question as to what values are most beneficial to humanity for promoting optimal individual and societal development. History teaches us that millions of lives were lost when people struggled to introduce progressive changes or when they defended what later became obsolete, regarded as morally or intellectually wrong and which led to disastrous consequences.

The concerted efforts of historians, philosophers, theologians, social scientists, psychologists and anthropologists are needed to review the ideas that served humanity well and those that led to confusion and destruction. Alternatively, we might observe that societal change naturally occur with time – perhaps delineated by generational differences, which may be accelerated by globalization and modern communications.

In conclusion, we regard resilience as the core human ability that enables courageous engagement with life roles in a sustainable manner to express value and purpose; the construct has a definite social and developmental bias. From a social perspective, not all values are desirable, even though may be individually espoused. Developmentally, as we have a natural tendency to increase our awareness of the self and reality, it is postulated that resilience would follow broad understanding of reality rather than narrow, even though such an understanding may be sufficient. (In antiquity, a belief in a flat Earth did not prevent the Mediterranean nations from establishing colonies overseas.)

In the next section, we will present findings obtained from two measures that intend to apply the theoretical underpinnings of resilience and resourcefulness to various clinical conditions in rehabilitative psychology settings. It is our opinion that these findings may be instructive in promoting broader societal dealings with adversity (Celinski, 2015a).

Measurement of resilience

Our conceptualization of resilience is not universally shared but is nonetheless supported by other researchers. In essence, resilience is particularly needed and manifest at times of serious adversity, such as when traumatized people have to restore their life and must uncover their innate ability to "bounce back" (Bonanno, 2004; Bonanno, Papa, & O'Neill, 2001). Celinski (2013) stated that at its extreme, trauma represents destruction of heuristics, which refer to experience-based techniques for problem solving, learning and discovery. Emotionally, continuing post-traumatic self-perceptions of extreme vulnerability and expectations of further traumas or negative events manifest as a negative bias projected onto the future that frequently results in an extreme level of anxiety known as catastrophizing and a sense of helplessness; from such a perspective, the future is visualized in a fatalistic way along with an inability to change the situation for the better (p. 20).

To assess resilient behaviour in physically and psychologically traumatized individuals, Celinski, Salmon, and Allen (2005) developed the *Resilience to Trauma Scale – Research Edition (RTS-RE)* that was used to assess victims of industrial or motor vehicle accidents. (It was previously presented in detail in Celinski, Allen, & Gow, 2013, from which the scale description and test results were taken). On this scale, respondents were asked to answer questions that referred to the subjective severity of the traumatic event and their initial and long-term reactions to trauma in the context of pre-traumatic evaluation of themselves and their ability to cope. In this way, the strength of resilience represents a two-factor model of the dialectic interactions between a sense of disability and vulnerability (due to perceived multiple impacts on physical, emotional and psychosocial functioning) and a belief in manageability in the past, present and in the future. Specifically, the *RTS-RE* explores an individual's emotional experiences along with cognitive ideations pertaining to trauma or adversity and whether the event activated a sense of self-identity, the value of the self and an ability to mobilize effort and utilize specific coping styles to enable an individual to cope regardless of how disabled and vulnerable people regard themselves to be. In this respect, the *RTS-RE* addresses trauma as causing loss of meaning in life and purpose for living, and loss of one's own worth, which can profoundly affect an individual's adjustment. Another important construct measured by the *RTS-SE* is the perspective on responsibility for the event, which can result in excessive self-guilt (diminishing self-worth) or in blaming others (which may be then regarded as justification for not putting adequate effort into one's recovery). On the positive side, from the perspective of the manifestation of resilient character traits, the *RTS-RE* assesses the pre-traumatic sense of self-cohesiveness acquired through family relations and commitment to values; a sense of personal agency to shape one's life; effective or less optimal coping styles and tendencies to become frustrated, angry, overwhelmed or helpless and pessimistic about one's ability to cope in the future. The *RTS-RE* further measures the degree to which a person is prepared to sacrifice pleasure, comfort and some other values that are deemed less important for the sake of significant others, for the common good or in order to achieve higher personal goals. The scale also evaluates the level of perceived social support, which is consistently recognized as essential to prevent deterioration and to promote post-traumatic growth. The *RTS-RE* was developed and validated on a sample of 155 victims of motor vehicle and industrial accidents and refugee immigrants who escaped persecution and were sometimes tortured in their own country. The sample was 50.2% female; the average age was 43.4 years ($SD = 13.0$) and 12.8 years of education ($SD = 3.9$). They were referred for assessment of their condition and for their prospects of benefiting from rehabilitation and/or psychotherapy.

Principal components analysis (PCA) of the *RTS-RE* using varimax rotation evidenced good sampling adequacy (KMO = .75) and produced five interpretable factors that accounted for 40% of the overall variance. Factor 1 ("pre-traumatic self-cohesiveness") reflects the client's pre-traumatic perspective on their self-efficacy and self-perception of having strong, enduring personal, moral, social and religious beliefs and accounted for 13% of the total variance. The first *RTS-RE* factor could be split into two separate scales with excellent alpha reliability (alpha > .90). Sample *RTS-RE* questions related to this factor (presented as statements to be rated for their correspondence to the client's actual opinions or feelings) are presented in Table 6.1. In Factor 1, the first type of questions refers to a sense of control, while Type 2 questions exemplify strong personal beliefs.

Factor 2 ("trauma absorption") assesses the subjective severity of trauma and self-perception of pain and emotional states immediately following people's traumatic experience and accounts for 9% of the total variance. Factor 3 ("facing the challenge") accounts for an additional 6% of the variance and represents an optimistic and positive, action-oriented perspective on addressing challenges. Factor 4 ("trauma ideations") assesses the immediate impression of being a victim of a catastrophe with projection of negative consequences on the future and explains 6% of the variance, while Factor 5 ("severity of losses") assesses patient's perceptions of the severity of their

Table 6.1 Example statements and questions exemplifying the five major *RTS-RE* factors

Factor	Sample item content
1	Before the event, I was in control of my life.
	I have always had strong moral beliefs.
2	How severe was your trauma (mild, moderate, severe)?
	After the accident, I felt: pain, . . . anger, . . . sadness (3 separate questions)
3	In dealing with various life situations, I usually focus on finding solutions.
	I believe that everything will turn out well, even though I do not yet know how.
4	When I first realized that "I had just escaped death".
	I was sure that I would be disabled for life.
5	Do you feel that the event caused a great loss in your life?
	You lost your faith in yourself and/or others.

various material and personal losses from the longer life perspective and accounts for 5.8% of the variance. Remaining factors each account for less than 5% of the item variance and are not readily interpretable. However, Factor 9 ("traumatic amnesia"), which is comprised of only three questions, reliably identifies clients with either head injury-related post-traumatic amnesia or functional dissociation resulting in poor memory of the event.

In the same chapter, we documented the mediating impact of resilience on symptoms of anxiety, depression and PTSD, which supports the perspective that the impact of trauma is filtered through internal processes (overall labelled as resilience). Correlation analyses revealed a number of significant relationships between *RTS-RE* factors with tests typically used to measure psychopathology.

The *BDI-II* (Beck, 1987) was positively related to three *RTS-RE* factors: Factor 2 ($r = .21$, $p < .05$; trauma absorption); Factor 4 ($r = .31$, $p = .003$; immediate "traumatic ideations"); and Factor 5 ($r = .47$, $p < .001$; severity of losses). The *BAI* (Beck & Steer, 1993) was positively related to *RTS-RE* Factor 2 ($r = .22$, $p < .05$; trauma absorption) and Factor 5 ($r = .45$, $p < .001$; severity of losses). Regarding typical post-traumatic stress disorder symptomatology, significant correlations were observed between several *RTS-RE* factors and the *Davidson Trauma Scale* (*DTS*; Davidson, 1996). The *DTS* total score was significantly related to *RTS-RE* Factor 2 (trauma absorption; $r = .28$, $p = .005$), Factor 4 (trauma ideations; $r = .27$, $p = .006$) and Factor 5 (severity of losses; $r = .40$, $p < .001$). A number of *RTS-RE* factors were associated with each of the *DTS* subcomponents assessing intrusive thoughts, avoidance and hyper-arousal ($p < .05$ for all) with the strongest correlation observed between *RTS-RE* Factor 5 (severity of losses) and *DTS* hyper-arousal ($r = .47$, $p < .001$).

In order to establish relationships between the *RTS-RE* and the *Millon Clinical Multiaxial Inventory – III* (*MCMI-III*, Millon, 1977), which has empirically overlapping scales, a PCA with varimax rotation of *MCMI-III* scales was conducted. For the purpose of the present review, we will only refer to data that are extensions of the analyses discussed earlier. *MCMI-III* Factor 1 was comprised of scales measuring major depression, anxiety, dysthymia, PTSD and somatoform and thought disorders. This Factor 1 was positively correlated with *RTS-RE* Factor 4 ($r = .21$, $p < .05$) representing trauma ideations. The positive association of *MCMI-III* scales that represent DSM-IV, Axis 1 psychopathology (which may reflect accident-related sequela) with the potentially catastrophic self-evaluation of the trauma is consistent with an understanding that higher trauma severity results in more serious psychopathology. Furthermore, positive correlation of pre-traumatic self-appraisal (as reflected in *RTS-RE* Factor 1; $r = .24$, $p = .025$) with the psychopathological manifestations reflected in *MCMI-III* Factor 1 reflects a drastic contrast between how a person was and what he or she became after the trauma, which may potentiate a sense of loss and result in more severe psychopathology. Our overall conclusion was that resilience represents the flip side of catastrophizing. In evaluation of people's reaction to trauma, their perception of trauma-related experiences and subjective evaluation of trauma severity, ideations related to traumatic events and the perception of losses appear to play a significant role in development of psychopathology.

Another Celinski and Allen (2013) study focused on predicting therapy outcomes based on *RTS-RE* factors. The purpose of this study was to address other aspects of resilience (other than modifying psychopathology), which would include the ability to utilize resources to sustain involvement over time and promote recovery. As an outcome measure, we chose the *Rehabilitation Survey of Problems and Coping* (*R-SOPAC*; Salmon & Celinski, 2002), which was administered at the beginning and the end of treatment. The scale asks clients to self-rate on a zero (not a problem) to six (an extreme problem) their physical, cognitive and emotional impairments and their sense of overall disability and their current coping abilities. A summary score that combines self-ratings from physical, cognitive and emotional domains yields an overall index of patient impairment and coping difficulties/abilities.

The study summarizes findings from twenty-two cases involved in therapy for post-traumatic conditions. This sample comprised of 50% male and 50% female; the average age for the whole sample was 44.2 years (SD = 13.3), and average years of education was 13.5 years (SD = 4.5). Multiple regressions with backwards elimination were used to predict the R-$SOPAC$ total score using basic demographic data and RTS-RE factor scores. A significant overall model was produced that explained 41.5% of the total adjusted variance (Multiple R = .71) with the final solution including loadings from age (t = 3.47, p = .003), RTS-RE Factor 3 (t = 2.08, p = .05) and RTS-RE Factor 9 (t = 3.99, p = .001). Content for RTS-RE Factor 3 (that we call "facing the challenge") reflects positive and hopeful engagement, and using an active coping strategy for recovery (taking personal responsibility). Factor 9 of the RTS-RE relates to the ability to visualize the details surrounding the trauma. Factor 9 (labeled "traumatic amnesia") accounted for only 4% of total RTS-RE variance, but its association with head injury and post-traumatic amnesia (PTA) or dissociative amnesia is noteworthy and indicates that better outcomes are associated with the ability to remember and reprocess traumatic events. While this finding largely supports the usual practice of desensitization and exposure to traumatic events in cases with PTA or psychogenic amnesia, in instances when the accident was very psycho-traumatic, in order to avoid re-traumatization, therapists should exercise caution and informed clinical judgment while assisting patients in imagining "forgotten" details surrounding their accident.

Although RTS-RE Factor 5 was not retained as a significant predictor in the final model, interim results suggested a negative relationship to outcome (p < .07) that approached significance. This factor represents subjective appraisal of losses and acquired disability as having profound emotional and global consequences on peoples' lives (e.g. "Do you feel that the event caused a great loss in your life?" or that "You have lost faith in yourself and/or others. You have lost meaning and purpose of life," etc.).

In spite of the relatively small number of cases, these results make intuitive sense and are important with respect to recognizing that a future outcome is dependent on a client's courage and ability to consciously experience the emotional and cognitive content of the traumatic event, to make a deliberate effort to re-engage with the post-traumatic condition and psychosocial situation and to be able to minimize the cognitive and emotional impacts associated with objectively sustained losses.

Measurements of resourcefulness

The *Resourcefulness for Recovery Inventory – Research Edition* (*RRI-RE*; Celinski, Antoniazzi & Allen, 2007) was developed to comprehensively assess personal resources in dealing with adversity and recovery from traumas, injuries and setbacks. The items selected for the *RRI-RE* were extracted from reviews of rehabilitation and clinical literature and from polling both patients and rehabilitation personnel with respect to factors that inhibit or promote recovery (Antoniazzi, Celinski, & Alcock, 2002). The choice of the themes and composition of the subscale items was in part inspired by positive psychology and is consistent with Fredrickson's (2009) broaden-and-build theory. This theory emphasizes the importance of positive emotions that create a mind's attitude to utilize and acquire a broad range of resources that facilitate healthy transformation. The mediating effect of resourcefulness (as measured by *RRI-RE*) on symptomatology was described in Celinski and Allen (2011). The *RRI-RE* is a 239-item self-report questionnaire based on bipolar conceptualizations of stress reactions (i.e. positive and negative subscales). The inventory reflects the two-factor model, which addresses the presence of specific behavioural, cognitive, emotional and psycho-physiological responses; they either indicate regressive tendencies to catastrophizing and to becoming a helpless victim or manifest utilization of health-promoting personal resources that would promote efficient dealing with a difficult life situation. This instrument includes eighteen bipolar dimensions (e.g. control/controlled, positive/negative cognition, intentionality/lack of direction, broadening awareness/not informed, acceptance/non-acceptance, integration/ disintegration, etc.). On this inventory, a "victim" profile is reflected as strong endorsements on the negative side of the bipolar dimensions that may have become a person's "destiny." By contrast, a profile strongly leaning towards the "health-promoting pole" represents a person's ability to "choose" health over illness and is reflected in the person's cognitions, emotions and behaviours. The median *RRI-RE* full-scale alpha reliability is greater than or equal to .90.

The scale was standardized on 455 victims of motor vehicle and industrial accidents who suffered from pain, head and bodily injuries, anxiety, depression and phobias. In order to document the relation between psychopathology and resilience-resourcefulness, in this section, we will present findings from administration of this scale to the clients with various clinical conditions (both physical and psychological) that resulted from accidents, adverse social situations or severe medical illness.

In our conceptualization of resourcefulness (as reflected in the *RRI-RE*), recovery refers to gradually unravelling (spontaneously and/or after having been activated by specifically targeted therapeutic interventions) a sequence of delineated mental states, each encompassing different ideas, beliefs and behaviours to which certain emotional significance is attached. These mental states reflect efforts of personal agency (thus representing various freedoms) to make sense out of one's own illness and coping with their new and evolving physical and psychosocial conditions and can provide what Lazarus and Folkman (1984) have described as repeated self-evaluations in the course of recovery.

At their best, these mental states offer an alternative to projecting the misery of the past or present onto the future. Initial stages of therapy should promote acceptance of the situation that is forced on an individual and aim at achieving emotional stability that is usually undermined by catastrophizing, anger and frustration resulting from symptoms, limitations, dependency on others and "life unfairness." Progress begins with gradual cognitive and emotional "distancing" from the original impact of trauma and with lesser focusing on the past and on the entitlement to the life that is now no longer possible. An open-minded experience of both the negative and positive aspects of one's situation and condition is required to create a motivating dialectic tension between "archaic" and dysfunctional predispositions on the one hand, and the more adaptive progressive alternatives on the other. These dynamics are further described by Celinski and Allen (2013). Across the course of recovery, a person is encouraged to gradually regard his or her limitations as a challenge that should be an inspiration to develop (as needed) and utilize a broad range of personal resources that can facilitate and promote recovery. A positive perspective and hopeful engagement have to be primed through reference to positive experiences people have had in coping with past adversities and should be further developed in small steps.

Considering that the concept of "freedom" has a clear, common sense meaning, various types of freedoms manifesting in diverse mental states offer a convenient way of creating the narrative of recovery through a transformation that is framed as "liberation". Such a narrative moves an individual through stages in which certain ideas and emotions are especially emphasized (see Figure 6.2). Whereas these mental states pertaining to specific recovery stages are somewhat arbitrarily created, individuals are usually capable of recognizing their relevance to coping with

The Narrative Meaning of Recovery

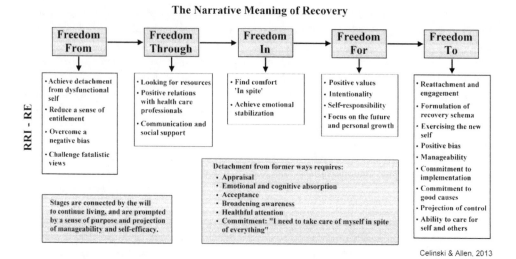

Celinski & Allen, 2013

Figure 6.2 The narrative meaning of recovery as reflected in the *RRI-RE* scales
Source: Celinski and Allen (2013).

adversity, if they are exemplified by the clients' personal history, history in general and by cultural and personal values. Such associations help integrate cognitions with emotions and with corresponding behaviours that represent an agentic manner (based on choice rather than on being compelled) of coping with the post-traumatic situations and one's own condition. By progressing through various stages, clients should become aware of the importance of "freedom in" manifesting as mindfulness and stress management, of the "freedom through", which may engage external support in learning new skills, of "freedom for", which is manifesting as mental preparation to face new challenges that would eventually enable them to act with a sense of "freedom to" that provides a mental framework for development of specific goals, along with plans for achieving better psychological adjustment and well-being.

Celinski and Allen's (2013) study attempted to predict overall *R-SOPAC* outcome with linear regression with backward elimination from *RRI-RE* factor scores. In total, fifty-nine patients were assessed with the *R-SOPAC* before and after engaging in rehabilitative efforts at the Toronto offices of three psychologists (Dr Judith Pilowsky, Dr Giorgio Ilacqua and Dr Marek J. Celinski). The sample was 54.1% male and 45.9% female; for the whole sample, the average age was 45.2 years (*SD* = 11.6) and 13.5 years of education (*SD* = 3.4). (Twenty-two clients from this sample were previously described in the study that utilized *Resilience to Trauma Scale-RE* to predict the therapy outcome.)

On average, for 4–6 months, the clients received psychological treatment "as usual" for psycho-traumatic conditions, which included cognitive behavioural approaches along with relaxation and desensitization. Variations in treatment among clients and offices cannot be reliably specified. Furthermore, the clients participated in various forms of physical therapy for bodily injuries that were provided by multiple sites using methodology as considered appropriate for their diagnosed conditions. Using *R-SOPAC*, pre- and post-comparisons, the change for the sample overall averaged a 23% reduction (range = 19–25%) in self-reported symptoms. Effect size differences ranged from moderate to large (Cohen's *g* = .50 to .80) for each of the

R-SOPAC components and for the overall total resulted in a significant model ($F = 4.05$, $df = 39$, $p = .01$). In predicting positive outcome from therapy, the first RRI-RE factor score was the only clearly significant predictor ($t = 2.38$, $p = .023$). The multiple correlation for the final model was moderate in size ($R^2 = .55$) and only accounted for 19% of the variance when adjusted for outliers. Overall improvement associated with the first RRI-RE factor reflected the absence of cognitive components of anxiety. In other words, positive outcome was dependent on a sense of self-efficacy and/or acceptance, which is a treatment-oriented conclusion drawn from the fact that it was negatively related to items concerning interference, worry, stress, feeling trapped or stuck and focusing on the past and on what has been lost. In essence, this factor is consistent with initial catastrophic reaction to trauma and indicates a need for emotional stabilization as the first step towards recovery.

A similar set of analyses to assess recovery outcome was also undertaken using RRI-RE subscales along with demographics and other variables assessing depression (*Beck Depression Inventory-II*), anxiety (*Beck Anxiety Inventory*), trauma symptoms (*Davidson Trauma Scale*) and selected scales from the *Multidimensional Pain Inventory*. Using backwards removal of variables that were found not to be significant, after their exclusion, a final regression model was highly significant ($F = 7.43$, $df = 58.10$; $p < .0001$) producing an impressive predictive fit ($R^2 = .78$) that accounted for 52.6% of total adjusted variance in outcome. Of the top nine predictors ($p < .03$ for all), in the final model, eight RRI-RE subscales were retained along with age ($p = .005$; younger patients improved more); age ranked fifth in terms of statistical significance. The *MPI Pain Interference Scale* was the only other variable retained in the final model ($p = .097$) but appeared to contribute only a small amount to the total explained variance. The top four RRI-RE subscales, associated with improvement in R-SOPAC total score were all negative in terms of face validity and, in decreasing order of importance, included Hope, Doctors, Control and Awareness. The four positive RRI-RE subscales referred to Dealing with Loss and having Fundamental Values, Hope and Control.

The fact that both negative and positive variables predict the outcome suggests that a state of high distress (characterized by hopelessness, loss of control, feeling abandoned and not being helped by professionals and not knowing how to understand one's condition), which, in the initial period of post-traumatic recovery manifest as "catastrophizing", can become a source of inspiration for proactive action in order to undo loss, better understand one's condition and regain hope and control, while also deriving strength from one's own fundamental values. This is again confirmation that the two-factor model is constantly applicable to understand the dynamics of recovery.

In the same Celinski and Allen (2013) study, we combined predictive capability of RTS-RE and RRI-RE. A limited sample of patients who engaged in rehabilitation and psychotherapy ($N = 22$) qualified for this purpose (i.e. only those who were assessed with the R-SOPAC at the beginning and end and who at the beginning of treatment were also administered both RTS-RE and RRI-RE). Nevertheless, a highly significant overall model was produced ($R^2 = .75$) that explained 49.6% of the adjusted overall variance and was associated with age, RRI-RE Intentionality and RTS-RE Factor 9 (reflecting the presence or absence of PTA or dissociative amnesia). Interim results in this backwards elimination procedure (which reduces shared variance between predictors) indicate that outcome is also significantly related to RRI-RE–assessed positive attitudes towards healthcare professionals ("Doctors", $p < .05$) and to Hope ($p = .003$), as opposed to the scales related to depression, resignation and disengagement. The other RTS-RE components predicting outcome at this step included Factor 4 ($p = .001$) reflecting a lesser degree of catastrophic appraisal of an individual's condition at the time of trauma (e.g. I had just escaped death; I was sure I would be disabled for life.) and Factor 10 ($p = .01$) that refers to subjectively assessed availability of social support; there was a negative relationship of outcome with Factor 8 ($p = .02$) whose content concerns blaming others for the accident (the more blaming, the worse the outcome) as this likely releases an individual from taking responsibility for his/her own recovery.

Conclusion

Review of the data from the administration of resilience and resourcefulness measures to clinical population revealed the results that are largely consistent with our theoretical understanding. With respect to resilience, the major point is that it manifests itself in the situation of threats, stress and adversity causing an interruption in routine functioning. Resilience is conceptualized as being on a positive end of the psychopathology-wellness/coping dimension. Resilience is about active engaging with reality rather than passivity. It represents freedom and mobilization to face adversity with a sense of identity, and recognition of the value of life and one's own efforts, and is contrasted with allowing adversity to make people think, feel and act as victims. Resilience requires courage to cognitively and emotionally absorb the truth about one's own condition and the circumstances a person has to face usually not through free choice. Attempts to forget or ignore the actual meaning of the situation prevents individuals from gradual distancing themselves from it, causes lasting vulnerability, inhibits finding adequate responses or solutions, and often results in lasting psychopathology. The resilient response depends on the severity of the trauma as being a threat to life or representing significant loss. People have a tendency to view losses in a catastrophic way. This has negative consequences, especially in terms of anxiety and depression, and may cause them to regress and feel helpless. Resilience that manifests resolve to seek solutions in an active manner precedes resourcefulness, wherein specific behaviours are selected in accordance to the type of engagement that people decide to follow to promote their recovery or efficient coping with the situation. The personal resources available to people can be identified as both strengths and weakness using of our *Resourcefulness for Recovery Inventory – Revised Edition.*

Our findings provide evidence that a two-factor model is particularly useful in understanding the dynamics of recovery from trauma or loss. Contrasting aspects of the situation can provide impetus for resilient responding. Looking forward with hope, having fundamental values and utilizing sources of support are the crucial characteristics of this process. Given the predictive significance of these psychological constructs for recovery, therapeutic efforts should initially aim at the identification and further strengthening of existing (possibly latent) resilient and resourceful characteristics so that they become the organizing principles for the new post-traumatic Gestalt. Moreover, as Ziarko and Kaczmarek's (2011) study suggests, resourcefulness has a tendency to expand. In this respect, their most important finding is that all of the *RRI-RE* resources were correlated with a measure of ego resilience. This means that people's resilient dealing with their condition or situation is associated with greater utilization of personal resources, as Casey, Gow, Crompton, Celinski & Antoniazzi's (2011) study showed with respect to PTSD. It is also very important to note that people's decisions in the present time have a strong correlation with, and significant bearing on, how they will act and cope in the future. Positive emotions play an important role as postulated by a build-and-broaden theory; they can positively affect emotional, cognitive and physical coping now and in the future, as documented by Leoniuk's (2009) research.

The reviewed findings allow us to provide clinical evidence to a long tradition of philosophical, cultural and individual intuitive views that regard courage and a sense of identity (defined in reference to values) along with commitments as the core components of dealing with life adversity and as promoting further personal and civilizational developments.

References

Antoniazzi, M., Celinski, M. J., & Alcock, J. (2002). Self responsibility and coping with pain: Disparate attitudes towards psychological issues in recovery from work place injury. *Disability and Rehabilitation, 24*(18), 948–953.

Antonovsky, A. (1987). *Unravelling the mystery of health: How people manage stress and stay well.* San Francisco: Jossey-Bass.

Aristotle. (1985). *Nicomachean ethics.* T. Irwin (trans.). Indianapolis, IN: Hackett Publishing Company.

Bandura, A. (1977). Self-efficacy: Toward a unifying theory of behavioural change. *Psychological Review, 84*(2), 191–215.

Bandura, A. (2001). Social cognitive theory: An agentic perspective. *Annual Review of Psychology, 52,* 1–26.

Beck, A. (1987). *Beck depression inventory manual.* San Antonio, TX: The Psychological Corporation.

Beck, A. T., & Steer, R. A. (1993). *Beck anxiety inventory manual.* San Antonio, TX: The Psychological Corporation.

Bonanno, G. A. (2004). Loss, trauma, and human resilience: Have we underestimated the human capacity to thrive after extremely aversive events? *American Psychologist, 59*(1), 20–28.

Bonanno, G. A., Papa, A., & O'Neill, K. (2001). Loss and human resilience. *Applied and Preventive Psychology, 10*(3), 193–206.

Casey, B., Gow, K., Crompton, D., Celinski, M. J., & Antoniazzi, M. (2011). Resourcefulness for recovery in Australian military veterans with post-traumatic stress disorder. In M. J. Celinski & K. M. Gow (Eds.), *Continuity versus creative response to challenge: The primacy of resilience and resourcefulness in life and therapy* (pp. 359–378). New York: Nova Science Publishers.

Celinski, M. J. (2004). Freedom as a mental state. *Hypnos, 31*(4), 189–200.

Celinski, M. J. (2011). Framing resilience as transcendence and resourcefulness as transformation. In M. J. Celinski & K. M. Gow (Eds.), *Continuity versus creative response to challenge: The primacy of resilience and resourcefulness in life and therapy* (pp. 11–30). New York: Nova Science Publishers.

Celinski, M. J. (2013). Challenge-resilience-resourcefulness as the essential components of recovery. In K. M. Gow & M. J. Celinski (Eds.), *Individual trauma: Recovering from deep wounds and exploring the potential for renewal* (pp. 15–34). New York: Nova Science Publishers.

Celinski, M. J. (2015a). The similarities between personal and civilizational crisis and renewal. In M. J. Celinski (Ed.), *Crisis and renewal of civilizations: The 21st century crisis of ideas and character* (pp. 3–25). New York: Nova Science Publishers.

Celinski, M. J. (2015b). The trauma of time and the development of cognition and morality. In M. J. Celinski (Ed.), *Crisis and renewal of civilizations: The 21st century crisis of ideas and character* (pp. 139–160). New York: Nova Science Publishers.

Celinski, M. J. (2015c). Introduction: Civilizations as a projection of human nature. In M. J. Celinski (Ed.), *Crisis and renewal of civilizations: The 21st century crisis of ideas and character* (pp. xi–xxxii). New York: Nova Science Publishers.

Celinski, M. J., & Allen, L. M. (2011). Resourcefulness as the art of succeeding. In M. J. Celinski & K. M. Gow (Eds.), *Continuity versus creative response to challenge: The primacy of resilience and resourcefulness in life and therapy* (pp. 343–357). New York: Nova Science Publishers.

Celinski, M. J., & Allen, L. M. (2013). Resilience and resourcefulness in predicting recovery outcome. In K. M. Gow & M. J. Celinski (Eds.), *Individual trauma: Recovering from deep wounds and exploring the potential for renewal* (pp. 139–152). New York: Nova Science Publishers.

Celinski, M. J., Allen III, L. M., & Gow, K. M. (2013). Assessing resilience in the aftermath of mass trauma. In K. M. Gow & M. J. Celinski (Eds.), *Mass trauma: Impact and recovery issue* (pp. 77–92). New York: Nova Science Publishers.

Celinski, M. J., Antoniazzi, M., & Allen III, L. M. (2007). *Resourcefulness for recovery inventory-research edition.* North Carolina: CogniSyst.

Celinski, M. J., Salmon, D., & Allen, L. (2005). *Resilience to trauma scale-research edition.* North Carolina: CogniSyst.

Dabrowski, K. (1972). *Psychoneurosis is not an illness.* London: Gryf Publications.

Davidson, J. (1996). *Davidson trauma scale.* North Tonawanda, NY: Multi-Health Systems Inc.

Frankl, V. E. (1963). *Man's search for meaning: Introduction to logotherapy.* New York, NY: Washington Square Press.

Fredrickson, B. L. (2009). *Positivity: Groundbreaking research reveals how to embrace the hidden strength of positive emotions, overcome negativity and thrive.* New York: Crown Publishing Group. A Division of Random House, Inc.

Gordon, K. (1995). Self concept and motivational patterns of resilient African American high school students. *The Journal of Black Psychology, 21*(3), 239–255.

Gordon, K., & Coscarelli, W. C. (1996). Recognizing and fostering resilience. *Performance Improvement, 35*(9), 14–17.

Ilacqua, G., Celinski, M. J., & Allen III, L. M. (2013). Resilience and resourcefulness as facilitators of adjustment in immigrants during times of adversity. In K. M. Gow & M. J. Celinski (Eds.), *Mass trauma: Impact and recovery issues* (pp. 349–364). New York: Nova Science Publishers.

Kebza, V., & Solcova, I. (2013). Trends in resilience theory and research. In K. M. Gow & M. J. Celinski (Eds.), *Wayfinding through life challenges: Coping and survival* (pp. 13–30). New York: Nova Science Publishers.

Kumpfer, K. L. (1999). Factors and processes contributing to resilience: The resilience framework. In M. D. Glantz & J. L. Johnson (Eds.), *Resilience and development: Positive life adaptations* (pp. 179–224). New York: Plenum Press.

Lazarus, R. S., & Folkman, S. (1984). *Stress, appraisal, and coping.* New York: Springer.

Leoniuk, A. (2009). *Emotions as important aspect of resilience when coping with traumatic injury.* Dissertation submitted to the faculty of The Adler School of Professional Psychology in partial fulfilment of the requirements for the degree of Doctor of Psychology. Chicago, IL.

McMartin, J. (2011). The virtue of courage in the Western philosophical tradition. In M. J. Celinski & K. M. Gow (Eds.), *Continuity versus creative response to challenge: The primacy of resilience and resourcefulness in life and therapy* (pp. 155–173). New York: Nova Science Publishers.

Millon, T. (1977). *Millon Clinical Multiaxial Inventory-III manual* (2nd ed.). Minneapolis, MN: National Computer System.

Plato. (1937). *The dialogues of Plato, Vol. 1.* B. Jowett (trans.). New York: Random House.

Plato. (1992). *Republic.* G. M. A. Grube & C. D. C. Reeve (trans.). Indianapolis, IN: Hackett Publishing Company.

Reich, J. W., Zautra, A. J., & Hall, J. S. (2011). Resilience science and practice: Current status and future directions. In M. J. Celinski & K. M. Gow (Eds.), *Continuity versus creative response to challenge: The primacy of resilience and resourcefulness in life and therapy* (pp. 33–50). New York: Nova Science Publishers.

Salmon, J. D., & Celinski, M. J. (2002). *Rehabilitation survey of problems and coping technical manual.* Toronto, ON: Multi-Health Systems Inc.

Sartre, J. P. (2007). Existentialism is humanism. C. Macomber (trans.). New Haven: Yale University Press [1946].

Satkiewicz, S. T. (2015). Revolutions: A violent encounter with eternity. In M. J. Celinski (Ed.), *Crisis and renewal of civilizations: The 21st century crisis of ideas and character* (pp. 105–115). New York: Nova Science Publishers.

Zautra, A. J., Palucka, A., & Celinski, M. J. (2015). Social connectedness and creativity: Two mutually influencing processes that promote human evolution. In M. J. Celinski (Ed.), *Crisis and renewal of civilizations: The 21st century crisis of ideas and character* (pp. 210–223). New York: Nova Science Publishers.

Ziarko, M., & Kaczmarek, L. (2011). Resources in coping with a chronic illness: The example of recovery from myocardial infarction. In M. J. Celinski & K. M. Gow (Eds.), *Continuity versus creative response to challenge: The primacy of resilience and resourcefulness in life and therapy* (pp. 379–394). New York: Nova Science Publishers.

7

Role of genetics and temperament in resilience

Vijay Parkash, Archana and Updesh Kumar

In previous times, diagnosis and treatment of mental illnesses, psychological deficits and disabilities were the focal points in psychology, and the nature versus nurture issue has loomed largely in psychological research focused since. Then, there came a paradigm shift to the field of positive psychology that emphasized enhancing personal strengths, developing and maintaining well-being and fostering and encouraging the use of positive emotions (Frederickson, 2001). Very little research so far, however, has been conducted to investigate the role of nature and nurture in psychological wellness. Resilience as an ability to bounce back to normalcy after experiencing adversities has been well deliberated upon by various scholars. There have been enormous scholarly efforts to elaborate on the conceptualizations of resilience from varied points of view. Ample evidence has been put forth by the researchers to establish resilience as a trait as well as a process. An abundance of theories and models exist to delineate the process of resilience and the way it operates.

Researchers have dedicated their scientific interests in exploring the factors associated with it and have put forth extensive descriptions of the ways in which different psychological, social, environmental and personal aspects contribute to the process of resilience. The majority of the scientific interest-holders in this concept believe that resilience is trainable and that a non-resilient or less resilient individual can become resilient. Many of these issues are being discussed in details in the other chapters of the volume. In the current chapter, we will explore whether resilience is genetically determined. Personality factors are frequently associated with the resilient behaviour but what about the biological side of personality? How does temperament relate to resiliency of an individual? Does there exist orthogonality between temperament and resilience? There is a significant paucity of literature on the issue of relationship of various genetic, biological and temperamental factors with resilience. And, similarly, the empirical evidence on these issues also remains scarce. In this chapter, we attempt to discuss the probable answers of the questions and try to make our basis on hypotetical testable assumptions and the existing few literary works.

Experience of some form of adversity is an unavoidable part of everyone's life. It is also evident that in some cases these adversities have irreversible negative impacts on the individual; however, in most other cases, people endure such adversities and reflect resilience to such effects. Different scholars have used different words to define resilience: however, the meaning more or less remains the same: that it is a person's ability to adapt effectively to stress experience, some trauma or some other forms of adversity being faced by an individual. Thus, a resilient individual is the one who has boldly faced adversity (Rutter, 2006a) and has adapted perseverely to psychological and physiological stress experiences or has demonstrated a 'psychobiological allostasis' (Charney, 2004; McEwen, 2003). Masten (2001) posits that, around five decades ago, the attention of some researchers focused on understanding of the factors that made some children capable of normal development even in the face of adversities, which gave rise to studies aimed at exploring stress resistance or 'resilience'. Initially and for many years, this research revolved around identifying the psychosocial determinants of capacity to resist stress including social competence, capacity for self-regulation and positive emotions etc. (Masten & Coatsworth, 1998; Rutter, 1985). The scope of studies later extended to understanding the factors associated with resilience among the adults exposed to adversities and trauma (e.g. Bonanno, 2004). In recent years, due to many note-worthy technological and methodical innovations, it has become possible to carry out research to comprehend the genetic underpinnings and the biological processes underlying the resilient behaviour (Charney, 2004; Cicchetti & Blender, 2006).

Resilience: an inherent trait or dynamic process?

Researchers assert that, during initial research efforts around the concept of resilience, the individuals who adaptably faced and survived adversities were regarded and labeled as 'hardy', 'invulnerable', or 'invincible' (Werner & Smith, 1982, as cited by Santos, 2011). Such individuals were considered to have a unique set of inborn qualities like a source of magical force that made them capable of bouncing back to normalcy after facing adversities and of being protected against any harm caused by them (Santos, 2011). However, many other researchers believe that rather than being inborn, trait resilience is a developmental process that builds through the experience of the individuals (Masten, 2001). There are arguments both in favour of as well as against resilience being an inborn trait. The use of terms like 'invulnerable' and 'invincible' was objected to by a few researchers by questioning the very notion of people being completely immune against the influence of adverse circumstances (Garmezy, 1993). For other researchers like Masten (2001), the resilience process is like an 'ordinary magic', given that a majority of individuals facing serious adversities remarkably manage to adapt to it and return to normal developmental process. Similarly, Bernard (1995) concludes that every individual has an innate capacity of being resilient. Resiliency building is a 'self-righting tendency' of an individual that comes into an automatic play when people face such conditions in their lives that require resilience for being faced. Bernard (1995) asserts that "we are all born with an innate capacity for resilience, by which we are able to develop social competence, problem-solving skills, a critical consciousness, autonomy, and a sense of purpose" (p. 17).

On the other hand, researchers contradicting the view of resilience as an innate capacity view it as a dynamic set of processes that can be fostered and cultivated (Masten, 2001; Padrón, Waxman, & Huang, 1999). Person–environment interactive mechanisms and various types of interplay between risk factors and protective factors have been emphasized upon by some researchers as significant underlying factors for resilience building (Santos, 2011). Some theorists like Garmezy (1991) view resilience as "a process that empowers individuals to shape their environment and to be shaped by it in turn" (Santos, 2011, p. 6). Certain models put forth by the scholars to explain resilience emphasize the interactive role of different cultural, social and situational contexts in the individual's adaptation and development of resilience.

Ecological models like that of Cicchetti and Lynch (1993) elaborate on the influences of various factors on one's development and advocate the notion of interaction between risk and protective factors as determining factor for resilience. Likewise, according to the researchers who consider resilience as a dynamic process, it is implicit that resilience can grow or decline over time depending on the roles played by different factors as mentioned earlier (Borman & Rachuba, 2001; Werner & Smith, 1992). Accordingly, rather than having a predefined inborn trait level, one may be more or less resilient at different times on the basis of the kind of circumstances and comparative strength of protective vis-à-vis risk factors (Winfield, 1991). Resilience is considered an adaptation pattern of behaviour over time in light of different kinds of risk factors and adversities (Masten, 1994). Giving impetus to external determinants of resilience, Seccombe (2002, as cited by Santos, 2011) asserted that in order to understand resilience "careful attention must be paid to structural deficiencies in our society and to social policies that families need in order to become stronger, more competent, and better functioning in adverse situations" (p. 385).

On the other hand, the researchers supporting the innate nature of resiliency posit that many of the responses to various kinds of adverse stimuli are biological kinds of responses produced by the human body, and it has been empirically established that, compared to other behavioural responses, biological responses are more influenced by an individual's genetic makeup (Hasler, Drevets, Manji, & Charney, 2004; Zhou et al., 2008). An integrative model of resilience may thus be arrived at only by analyzing individuals' stress responses at multiple phenotypic levels including psychological, behavioural, neurochemical, neuroendocrine and neural systems (Zhou et al., 2008).

Although human studies exploring the biological determinants of resilience are scarce, animal studies have been quite crucial in this direction, and they have provided many significant insights into the neural circuits and molecular pathways that influence or mediate resilient phenotypes (Krishnan & Nestler, 2008; Rutter, 2006a). In the following sections of this chapter, we attempt to trace the role of genetic and biological systems in making an individual less or more resilient. Although the early research efforts have revolved around the role of environmental and situational factors in development of resilience, Feder, Nestler, and Charney (2009) put forth that research in recent times has begun to explore the biological, neural, genetic and epigenetic mechanisms that lie beneath individual's resilience. It has been found that resilience is influenced by several adaptive changes in specific neural circuits that involve various neurotransmitter and molecular pathways. The functioning of various neural circuits is shaped by these adaptive changes, and this altered shape in turn regulates the responses of fear, stress, emotional endurance or the resilient behaviour (Feder et al., 2009). Before moving ahead to examine or infer the role of genetic factors, we will first examine the psychobiology of resilient behaviour.

Psychobiology and genetics of resilient behaviour

Literature provides us with an abundance of definitions of resilience; however, common to most of the definitions of resilience is endurance and bouncing back from stress or adversity or a relative resistance to risk (Garmezy & Masten, 1994; Masten, 2001; Rutter, 2006b). Looking at the studies conducted with the animal models to understand the psychobiological mechanisms, it has been observed that rodents show various kinds of responses to stress ranging from active or 'fight–flight' responses on one end to passive responses like freezing and submission on the other end (Korte, Koolhaas, Wingfield, & McEwen, 2005). Evidently researchers believe that, based on multiple functional endpoints, active-coping animals are often considered more resilient and that animals giving passive responses are seen as less resilient; however, depending on the specific situational context, both active as well as passive types of responses may turn out to be effective

(Feder et al., 2009). The study's efforts to understand these individual differences in the response of animals suggest that the difference in neurobiological and molecular mechanisms underlie their capability to withstand stress.

The psychobiological responses to stress involve functions of multiple numbers of bodily hormones, neurotransmitters and neuropeptides. The individual differences in the stress resilience of different individuals are the results of variations in the function, balance and interaction of these hormones, neurotransmitters and neuropeptides (Feder et al., 2009). The delineation of the role of different biological systems in the resilient responses to stress will help understand better whether resilience is merely a dynamic and cultivable capacity or whether it has to do something with the biological makeup of the individual, which has strong genetic basis. Feder et al. (2009) have opined that, in the face of stressors, the functions of various neural systems and the adaptability of various neurochemical stress response systems are determined by varied kinds of intricate interactions between an individual's genetic makeup and his specific kind of exposure to stressors or adversities. The genetic associations of these biological mechanisms may be understood by looking at the roles of specific types of genes linked with every system. Building primarily on the excellent seminal works of Feder et al. (2009) and Bowes and Jaffee (2013), the following sections of this chapter attempt to discuss the psychoneurobiological mechanisms involved in various kinds of stress responses and the genetic linkages of resilience.

Role of hypothalamus-pituitary-adrenal (HPA) axis in stress response

When an individual is faced with stress, in response to it, the hypothalamus releases corticotropin-releasing hormone (CRH); release of CRH activates the HPA axis, which in turn releases cortisol. Researchers assert that, in human and animal studies, stress experiences in early age or childhood are associated with chronically high levels of CRH (Heim & Nemeroff, 2001). In order to understand the role of biological factors in a better way, it is pertinent to mention that researchers have empirically established that, though the short-term actions of cortisol are protective against stress experiences and they help in adaptation, chronically long exposure to unusually high levels of cortisol can bring negative outcomes such as diseases like hypertension, cardiovascular disease, loss of immunity and other health problems (Karlamangla, Singer, McEwen, Rowe, & Seeman, 2002). Excessive amount of cortisol in the brain is linked with complex structural effects in the hippocampus and amygdala along with reduction in functionality of certain types of neurons (Brown, Woolston, & Frol, 2008; McEwen & Milner, 2007). Hence, controlled release of CRH and adaptive changes in CRH receptor activity may be associated with resilience promotion (Feder et al., 2009). Scientists put forth that resilience in biological terms is associated with quick launch of the stress response and its adaptive execution (de Kloet, Joels, & Holsboer, 2005).

Psychobiologists assert that resilience denotes the individual capacity to limit the increase in levels of CRH and cortisol caused due to stress experience. It encompasses optimal function and equilibrium of glucocorticoid and mineralocorticoid receptors (Charney, 2004; de Kloet, Derijk, & Meijer, 2007; de Kloet et al., 2005). In animal studies, it has been seen that animals using active responses to stress show lesser glucocorticoid responses as compared to the ones using passive responses to stress (Lu et al., 2008). The active and passive types of personalities in humans are associated with risk for different types of disorders (Korte et al., 2005). Citing Morgan and his associates (2004), Feder et al. (2009) put forth that stress also induces the release of dehydroepiandrosterone (DHEA) and has antiglucocorticoid effects in the brain. It has been observed that higher resilience is associated with higher DHEA sulphate/cortisol ratios. Military personnel performing best in the face of stress, who can be called resilient soldiers, were found having high DHEA sulphate/cortisol ratios (Morgan et al., 2004). Providing inputs in support of association of resilience with the concept of post-traumatic growth, Yehuda, Brand, Golier, and Yang (2006) empirically established that higher DHEA levels were related with regaining normalcy and psychological wellness among male veterans with post-traumatic stress disorder.

HPA axis-related genes and their association with resilience

Genetic factors play a crucial role in the functioning and regulation of the HPA axis. It has been found that the threshold regulation and control of the HPA-axis response to stress is primarily related with some functional variants of the brain mineralocorticoid and glucocorticoid receptor (GR) genes, and researchers have established that these genes have been identified in humans (de Kloet et al., 2007). Derijk and de Kloet (2008) established that, among the carriers of a specific variant of the GR gene, higher cortisol response was observed in response to certain normal stressors. Empirical testings have been performed to pinpoint the specific role of genes in resilience related outcomes and polymorphisms and haplotypes of the CRH type 1 receptor gene (CRHR1) have been found moderating the effect of abuse in childhood on development of depressive symptoms in adulthood, with the haplotypes showing exerting a shielding effect (Bradley et al., 2008).

The relationship of post-traumatic stress symptoms with the severity of childhood abuse has also been explained through the interactive association of gene FKBP5, which codes for a 'chaperone' protein regulating the GR sensitivity (Binder et al., 2008). As an example of low level of resilience and a significant risk factor for stress-related pathology by means of prolonged heightened levels of cortisol, a study on healthy adults after the Trier Social Stress Test found that inefficient recovery of HPA-axis activity has an association with genetic variation in the FKBP5 gene (Ising et al., 2008). Likewise, there has been evidence favouring genetic interconnections among various biological mechanisms associated with stressed or resilient behaviours.

Role of serotonergic, dopaminergic and noradrenergic systems in stress response

When there is a condition of acute stress, it is accompanied by increased serotonin production in many regions of brain including the prefrontal cortex, amygdala, and the nucleus accumbens (Feder et al., 2009). This serotonin function in brain is considered to have significant association with individual's mood regulation. It has both anxiety-generating and anxiety-inhibiting effects, and it controls and modulates neural responses to stress (Charney, 2004). The presence of aversive stimuli or heightened stress inhibits dopamine neurons, and the presence of positive stimuli activates them. Experiencing stress causes the release of noradrenaline from brainstem nuclei, most importantly the locus coeruleus. As a result of this, various forebrain regions involved in emotional expressions, such as hippocampus, prefrontal cortex, amygdala and the nucleus accumbens, receive noradrenergic stimulation. If the response of the locus coeruleus noradrenergic system remains continued and uncontrolled, it may lead to anxiety disorders and cardiovascular problems; however, if β-adrenergic receptors are blocked in the amygdala then aversive memories do not develop (Charney, 2003; McGaugh, 2004). Therefore, lower responsiveness of the locus coeruleus noradrenergic system may be associated with higher resilience (Feder et al., 2009).

Serotonin transporter gene and resilience

Associations have been reported between different allele of the human serotonin transporter gene (5-HTTLPR) and risk of stress-induced depression. Lesser availability of serotonin transporter gene, which results in lower uptake of serotonin from synaptic clefts, is associated with the short allele of 5-HTTLPR. Studies reveal that the individuals who carry a short allele 5-HTTLPR have been found to be at high risk for depression if exposed to stressful events in life (Caspi et al., 2003; Gillespie, Whitfield, Williams, Heath, & Martin, 2005; Kendler, Kuhn, Vittum, Prescott, & Riley, 2005). Increased susceptibility to stress can be inferred in carriers of short allele 5-HTTLPR as in these individuals the evidence of increased amygdala reactivity to environmental threat has been observed (Hariri et al., 2005). Also, variations in emotional resilience in a sample of college students have been found associated with the long allele of 5-HTTLPR (Stein, Campbell-Sills, & Gelernter, 2009).

Catechol-O-methyltransferase (COMT) as an associate gene for resilience

Resilience can be associated with another gene named catechol-O-methyltransferase (COMT), which is an enzyme with properties to degrade dopamine and noradrenaline. The level of its polymorphism allele, coded as Met158, relates to adverse psychological experience by the individual. Since it degrades dopamine and noradrenaline, a low-functioning Met158 allele leaves scope for higher levels of these neurotransmitters. Scientists infer that, due to this, such individuals with lower-functioning Met158 experience high levels of anxiety, exhibit heightened levels of plasma adrenaline in the face of stressful situations and display lesser resilience to negative affect and higher limbic reactivity to stressful events (Heinz & Smolka, 2006).

Role of brain-derived neurotrophic factor (BDNF) and neuropeptide Y (NPY)

Brain-derived neurotrophic factor (BDNF) is a vital nerve growth factor having high-level expression in the brain regions. In animal studies, it has been seen that BDNF promotes the functioning of the adult hippocampus and of newly born granule cell neurons. Research has established that in rodents BDNF expression in the hippocampus is inversely related with stress experience as it decreases with the presence of stress and its restoration to normalcy requires chronic antidepressants (Duman & Monteggia, 2006). The study of the human hippocampus post-mortem has also shown similar findings (Feder et al., 2009). In rodents, it has been observed that induction of BDNF is causally associated with the level of their resilience or stress withstanding capacity.

   BDNF expression is increased in vulnerable individuals whereas resilient ones do not show any increase in it. Similarly increased BDNF levels can also be observed in humans with depression (Krishnan et al., 2007). Neuropeptide Y is largely distributed in the regions of brain and is largely associated with an individual's capacity to endure stress. It is considered that NPY increases cognitive function in the face of stress, and thus it creates anxiolytic effects. It also resists the adverse effects of CRH in the regions of the brain, and thereby stress resilience can be a function of a balance between NPY and CRH levels (Sajdyk, Shekhar, & Gehlert, 2004). Morgan and associates (2000) have empirically established that performance of highly stress-resilient special forces soldiers has been found associated with higher NPY levels. On similar lines, higher-plasma NPY levels have been observed in combat-exposed veterans who did not develop post-traumatic stress disorder as compared to those who did (Yehuda, Brand, & Yang, 2006). On the basis of these empirical observations, it can be validly inferred that NPY levels are associated with the resilience of an individual.

Associations of brain-derived neurotrophic factor (BDNF) and neuropeptide Y (NPY) with resilience

A single nucleotide polymorphism (Val66Met) in the BDNF gene, harms the intracellular trafficking and activity-dependent release of BDNF (Chen et al., 2006). This polymorphism is also linked with reduced volume of the hippocampus (Egan et al., 2003). Looking at their associations with behaviour during adversity, animal studies have shown that rodents having the Met66 allele of BDNF exhibit higher levels of anxiety-like behaviour and impaired hippocampus-dependent learning. However, they tend to endure more against chronic stress displaying thereby a higher level of resilience (Chen et al., 2006; Krishnan, 2007). Looking at the associations of NPY gene with resilient behaviour, studies have revealed that a low-expression diplotype of the gene NPY has been found related to greater amygdala reactivity to stress-induced negative facial expressions. The echelon of NPY mRNA displayed a negative correlation with trait anxiety and positive association with the levels of stress-induced endogenous opioid release that is related to suppression of negative responses for pain and stress (Zhou et al., 2008, as cited by Feder et al., 2009).

The evidence cited earlier assertively suggests the significance of the role of various biological mechanisms in regulating emotions, mood and behaviour of the individual in the face of adversities. Varied kinds of associations have been cited, and empirical evidence has been presented in support thereof. It can be also be said that the biological nature of these mechanisms and systems would suggest that they are more influenced by the biological makeup of the individual than by the environmental interactions. Eventually, the role of genetic underpinnings becomes evident in an individual being more or less resilient.

Temperament and resilience

Just as there are numerous personality models and theories, many researchers have put forth quite comprehensive models explaining temperament. Although temperament and personality are many times used interchangeably by researchers, temperament models in particular put an emphasis on the biologically based or inborn nature of personality makeup. These models attempt to delineate the personality structure during early age and to understand individual differences in behaviour during early stages of development (Mervielde & Asendorpf, 2000; Rothbart, Ahadi, & Evans, 2000). Temperamental descriptions are more specific to the experience and expression of emotions, and their regulation (Strelau, 1983). Derryberry, Reed, and Pilkenton-Taylor (2003) differentiate the approach of studying temperament from that of other personality theories with the underlying assumption that differences in temperament have a biological foundation and center around neural reactivity (as cited by Maginness, 2007).

The biological parameters of the individual, including neural structure and function, produce the neural reactivity, and this in turn determines an individual's ability to regulate arousal (Derryberry et al., 2003; Rothbart et al., 2000). Connecting temperament with the stress response, Derryberry and associates (2003) assert that temperamental regulations can also be termed as coping mechanisms in terms of shaping the stress responses in the form of fear, anger, frustration or the like. They further posit that inefficiencies in coping responses, which are generally a function of the interplay of multiple temperamental systems, may cause vulnerabilities and increased risk to health problems and disorders (Maginness, 2007). Forming a basis on the biological side of explaining temperament Derryberry et al. (2003) elaborate on three kinds of temperamental systems playing a crucial role in resilience. Common to these three systems is the involvement of both the cortical and subcortical regions of the brain. According to them, these three systems are the appetitive system, the defensive system and the attentional system (as cited by Maginness, 2007).

Citing Derryberry et al. (2003), Maginness (2007) explains that the appetitive system involves the orbitofrontal and limbic systems and that the defensive system involves the brainstem also in addition to the orbitofrontal and limbic systems. The appetitive system is associated with seeking and reaching rewards, and increased reactivity in this system makes an individual more sensitive to rewards. Accordingly, a strong appetitive system is likely to cause the beholder to display approach behaviours and experience positive emotions such as desire and hope. On the contrary, when the defensive system becomes hyperreactive, then it increases the sensitivity of an individual to punishment and fearful/anxious emotions (Derryberry et al., 2003).

The attentional system, as the name indicates, is the system that orients the attention. This orientation of attention may be either voluntary or involuntary. Rothbart et al. (2000) have labeled the voluntary system as 'effortful control' by means of which they emphasize the ability of this system to create avenues of performing a subdominant response by suppressing the dominant response (Kochanska, Murray, & Harlan, 2000). This ability of effortful control is quite crucial since it manages self-regulation by means of initiating, maintaining and/or inhibiting responses. Heightened activation of voluntary system can be associated with better resilience as it promotes greater flexibility and maintains control over dominant tendencies (Derryberry et al., 2003 as cited by Maginness, 2007).

While exploring the linkages of these temperamental systems with resilience, it can be seen that the appetitive and defensive systems are quite primal systems for coping with stress. On one side, the appetitive system keeps an individual going towards positive outcomes even in presence of obstacles, and on the other side, the defensive system keeps a person prepared to handle threats and adversities. Moreover, these systems even have the ability to access the attentional systems, and thereby these can help enhance coping efficacy. The cortex-based system that is the attentional system has higher accuracy and elasticity in controlling behaviour. The optimal functioning of these systems exhibits enhanced resilience against the odds whereas the limitations or malfunction of any of these systems may result in inefficient or maladaptive coping (Derryberry et al., 2003 as cited by Maginness, 2007).

Drawing inferences from the understanding of the functions of these temperamental systems, it can be put forth that voluntary attention or the effortful control is the most vital factor in relation to resilience and adaptation as researchers like Derryberry and Rothbart (1997) consider it to be associated with development of conscience, impulse control and overall emotional regulation. Other scholars who have devoted their research efforts to study the nature of resilience, impulsivity and effortful control have established that the voluntary attention or the effortful control involves such processes through which children can learn the ways to regulate their behaviour and can eventually develop resilience (Eisenberg et al., 2004). It has been empirically validated that children as well as adults with high attentional or effortful control display significantly low negative affectivity, which may in turn be associated with higher resilience (Rothbart et al., 2000).

This discourse on the functioning of temperamental systems and their associations with resilient behaviour implies that significant aspects of temperament have notable influence over the emotion and overall behaviour-regulation capacity of the child. Looking through the lens of simpler conceptualizations of temperament, and taking into consideration the widely recognized trait models also, it can well be studied that how various temperamental traits are associated with an individual's resilience capacity. For an example, hardiness, a temperamental trait, has been explored a lot for its linkage with resilient behaviour. Supporting the notion of strong association between resilience and temperament traits, in a recent study conducted on a large sample of 4,355 participants, Kim, Lee and Lee (2013) found positive associations of resilience with persistence, self-directedness and cooperativeness. Inverse to that harm avoidance displayed negative association with resilience. Persistence, self-directedness and harm avoidance emerged as significant predictors of resilience, and these findings were consistent among males as well females (Kim et al., 2013).

In another study utilizing Zuckerman's model (1991), it was observed that the Activity dimension of temperament showed positive correlation with resilience whereas the Aggression-Hostility and Neuroticism-Anxiety dimensions exhibited negative correlations with resilience (Hutchinson, 2009). Zuckerman (2002) had opined that temperamental traits like 'activity' include high levels of engagement, high energy and an inclination to seek out challenges. Hence, it can be hypothesized that characteristics associated with activity temperament type help foster resilience. Individuals high on activity may thrive despite stressors and difficult life situations (Hutchinson, 2009). It has been established on the basis of empirical evidence from 100 cases of major depression disorder patients and 100 healthy individuals that resilience has a strong relationship with hyperthymic temperament among depressive as well as healthy individuals. On the other hand, it was also observed that in both groups there was a negative correlation between psychological resilience and irritable and anxious temperament (Kesebir, Gundogar, Kucuksubasi, & Tatlidil Yaylaci, 2013).

Similarly, another study conducted with 479 healthy doctors revealed positive correlations of resilience with self-directedness, persistence and cooperativeness. Going with the findings of earlier study, harm avoidance was found to be negatively correlated. Self-directedness, persistence, and harm avoidance were found to be significant predictors of resilience (Eley et al., 2013) thereby again igniting the reader to explore more in the temperamental basis of resiliency.

Concluding remarks

The discussions held in this chapter are not intended to challenge and refute the varied notions floating in the minds of researchers looking at the concept of resilience from vivid kinds of analytical lenses. However, the deliberations put forth in the preceding sections are an attempt to draw the attentions of scholars and readers toward the lesser-explored dimension for comprehension of this lay-popular concept associated largely with the well-being of every individual. We are not advocating that the researchers and scientists devote all their efforts in exploring the external links of the resilience while the other inherent side of the story is remaining ignored. Of course there have been research efforts in the direction of understanding the biological basis of resilient behaviour and elaborating its temperamental, neurological and genetic correlates. However, the number of such efforts and the focus assigned on the importance of such explorations has been quite scarce.

In the era of explaining and defining every construct in multiple terminologies, the conceptualizations and descriptions of resilience so far seem to be skewed and to converge primarily on considerations of being fosterable and cultivable. Nonetheless, the discourse presented in this chapter and the dedicated efforts of a few researchers towards continuation of exploring the root basis of one's resiliency has put forth concrete evidence of the presence of its correlates in one's biological and genetic makeup. This evidence also posits certain challenging questions to the other scholars about whether fostering or cultivation of resilience can be free from the influence of one's genetic composition. A hypothetical addressal of such a challenge lies in proper understanding of the psychobiological aspects of an individual's makeup so as to make resilience building in such individuals easier, effective and irreversible. Likewise, among other correlates of resiliency, the temperamental traits find a relatively smaller place when it comes to the research focus of the scientists. Though there have been certain attempts by some researchers to look for the temperamental correlates of resiliency, these attempts have been confined to utilizing only one or two kinds of explanations of temperament, and more focus has been given on the personality correlates. Our intention here is not to generate a fresh debate on temperament vis-à-vis personality; rather, we wish to draw the attention of the reader and of scholars toward the more stable and biologically rooted side of an individual's personality makeup.

Researchers would agree that the understanding of one's temperament, biological makeup and genetic history would help inculcate better methods of fostering resilience. Therefore, our attempt is to emphasize the need for carrying out more dedicated and focused research towards exploring the relatively unexplored side of resiliency. The utilization of newly emerging methods of research and rather a use of a multi-method approach will help provide deeper insights into the understanding of resilience and will pave the way for devising and applying better and more effective ways to develop a resilient world.

References

Bernard, B. (1995). *Fostering resilience in children.* Urbana, IL: ERIC Clearinghouse on Elementary and Early Childhood Education.

Binder, E. B., Bradley, R. G., Liu, W., Epstein, M. P., Deveau, T. C., Mercer, K. B., . . . Ressler, K. J. (2008). Association of FKBP5 polymorphisms and childhood abuse with risk of posttraumatic stress disorder symptoms in adults. *The Journal of American Medical Association, 299*(11), 1291–1305.

Bonanno, G. A. (2004). Loss, trauma, and human resilience: Have we underestimated the human capacity to thrive after extremely aversive events? *American Psychologist, 59*(1), 20–28.

Borman, G. D., & Rachuba, L. T. (2001). *Academic success among poor and minority students: An analysis of competing models of school effects.* CRESPAR (Center for Research on the Education of Students Placed at Risk), Report No. 52, Johns Hopkins and Howard Universities funded by Office of Educational Research and Development.

Bowes, L., & Jaffee, S. R. (2013). Biology, genes and resilience: Towards a multidisciplinary approach. *Trauma, Violence and Abuse, 14*(3), 195–208.

Bradley, R. G., Binder, E. B., Epstein, M. P., Tang, Y., Nair, H. P., Liu, W., . . . Ressler, K. J. (2008). Influence of child abuse on adult depression: Moderation by the corticotrophin releasing hormone receptor gene. *Archives of General Psychiatry, 65*(2), 190–200.

Brown, E. S., Woolston, D. J., & Frol, A. B. (2008). Amygdala volume in patients receiving chronic corticosteroid therapy. *Biological Psychiatry, 63*(7), 705–709.

Caspi, A., Sugden, K., Moffitt, T. E., Taylor, A., Craig, I. W., Harrington, H., . . . Poulton, R. (2003). Influence of life stress on depression: Moderation by a polymorphism in the 5-HTT gene. *Science, 301*(5631), 386–389.

Charney, D. S. (2003). Neuroanatomical circuits modulating fear and anxiety behaviors. *Acta Psychiatrica Scandinavica, 108*(Suppl s417), 38–50.

Charney, D. S. (2004). Psychobiological mechanisms of resilience and vulnerability: Implications for successful adaptation to extreme stress. *American Journal of Psychiatry, 161*(2), 195–216.

Chen, Z. Y., Jing, D., Bath, K. G., Ieraci, A., Khan, T., Siao, C. J., . . . Lee, F. S. (2006). Genetic variant BDNF (Val66Met) polymorphism alters anxiety-related behavior. *Science, 314*(5796), 140–143.

Cicchetti, D., & Blender, J. A. (2006). A multiple-levels-of-analysis perspective on resilience: Implications for the developing brain, neural plasticity, and preventive interventions. *Annals of New York Academy of Sciences, 1094,* 248–258.

Cicchetti, D., & Lynch, M. (1993). An ecological-transactional analysis of children and contexts: The longitudinal interplay among child maltreatment, community violence, and children's symptomatology. *Development and Psychopathology, 10*(2), 235–257.

de Kloet, E. R., Derijk, R. H., & Meijer, O. C. (2007). Therapy insight: Is there an imbalanced response of mineralocorticoid and glucocorticoid receptors in depression? *Nature, Clinical Practice, Endocrinology and Metabolism, 3*(2), 168–179.

de Kloet, E. R., Joels, M., & Holsboer, F. (2005). Stress and the brain: From adaptation to disease. *Nature Reviews Neuroscience, 6*(6), 463–475.

Derijk, R. H., & de Kloet, E. R. (2008). Corticosteroid receptor polymorphisms: Determinants of vulnerability and resilience. *European Journal of Pharmacology, 583*(2–3), 303–311.

Derryberry, D., Reed, M. A., & Pilkenton-Taylor, C. (2003). Temperament and coping: Advantages of an individual differences perspective. *Development and Psychopathology, 15*(4), 1049–1066.

Derryberry, D., & Rothbart, M. K. (1997). Reactive and effortful processes in the organization of temperament. *Development and Psychopathology, 9*(4), 633–652.

Duman, R. S., & Monteggia, L. M. (2006). A neurotrophic model for stress-related mood disorders. *Biological Psychiatry, 59*(12), 1116–1127.

Egan, M. F., Kojima, M., Callicott, J. H., Goldberg, T. E., Kolachana, B. S., Bertolino, A., . . . Weinberger, D. R. (2003). The BDNF val66met polymorphism affects activity-dependent secretion of BDNF and human memory and hippocampal function. *Cell, 112*(2), 257–269.

Eisenberg, N., Spinrad, T. L., Fabes, R. A., Reiser, M., Cumberland, A., Shepard, S. A., . . . Thompson, M. (2004). The relation of effortful control and impulsivity to children's resiliency and adjustment. *Child Development, 75*(1), 25–47.

Eley, D. S., Cloninger, R., Walters, L., Laurence, C., Synnott, R., & Wilkinson, D. (2013). The relationship between resilience and personality traits in doctors: Implications for enhancing well being. *PeerJ, 1*, e216.

Feder, A., Nestler, E. J., & Charney, D. S. (2009). Psychobiology and molecular genetics of resilience. *Nature Reviews Neuroscience, 10*(6), 446–457.

Frederickson, B. L. (2001). The role of positive emotions in positive psychology: The broaden-and-build theory of positive emotions. *American Psychologist, 56*(3), 218–226.

Garmezy, N. (1991). Resiliency and vulnerability to adverse developmental outcomes associated with poverty. *American Behavioral Scientist, 34*(4), 416–430.

Garmezy, N. (1993). Children in poverty: Resilience despite risk. *Psychiatry, 56*(1), 127–136.

Garmezy, N., & Masten, A. S. (1994). Chronic adversities. In M. Rutter, L. Henov, & E. Taylor (Eds.), *Child and adolescent psychiatry* (pp. 191–208). Oxford, England: Blackwell.

Gillespie, N. A., Whitfield, J. B., Williams, B., Heath, A. C., & Martin, N. G. (2005). The relationship between stressful life events, the serotonin transporter (5-HTTLPR) genotype and major depression. *Psychological Medicine, 35*(1), 101–111.

Hariri, A. R., Drabant, E. M., Munoz, K. E., Kolachana, B. S., Mattay, V. S., Egan, M. F., & Weinberger, D. R. (2005). A susceptibility gene for affective disorders and the response of the human amygdala. *Archives of General Psychiatry, 62*(2), 146–152.

Hasler, G., Drevets, W. C., Manji, H. K., & Charney, D. S. (2004). Discovering endophenotypes for major depression. *Neuropsychopharmacology, 29*(10), 1765–1781.

Heim, C., & Nemeroff, C. B. (2001). The role of childhood trauma in the neurobiology of mood and anxiety disorders: Preclinical and clinical studies. *Biological Psychiatry, 49*(12), 1023–1039.

Heinz, A., & Smolka, M. N. (2006). The effects of catechol O-methyltransferase genotype on brain activation elicited by affective stimuli and cognitive tasks. *Reviews in the Neurosciences, 17*(3), 359–367.

Hutchinson, A. M. (2009). *Biological contributors to well-being: The relationships between temperament, character strengths and resilience* (Unpublished Doctoral Thesis). University of Johannesburg, Johannesburg.

Ising, M., Depping, A. M., Siebertz, A., Lucae, S., Unschuld, P. G., Kloiber, S., . . . Holsboer, F. (2008). Polymorphisms in the FKBP5 gene region modulate recovery from psychosocial stress in healthy controls. *European Journal of Neuroscience, 28*(2), 389–398.

Karlamangla, A. S., Singer, B. H., McEwen, B. S., Rowe, J. W., & Seeman, T. E. (2002). Allostatic load as a predictor of functional decline: MacArthur studies of successful aging. *Journal of Clinical Epidemiology, 55*(7), 696–710.

Kendler, K. S., Kuhn, J. W., Vittum, J., Prescott, C. A., & Riley, B. (2005). The interaction of stressful life events and a serotonin transporter polymorphism in the prediction of episodes of major depression: A replication. *Archives of General Psychiatry, 62*(5), 529–535.

Kesebir, S., Gundogar, D., Kucuksubasi, Y., & Tatlidil Yaylaci, E. (2013). The relation between affective temperament and resilience in depression: A controlled study. *Journal of Affective Disorders, 148*(2–3), 352–356.

Kim, J. W., Lee, H. K., & Lee, K. (2013). Influence of temperament and character on resilience. *Comprehensive Psychiatry, 54*(7), 1105–1110.

Kochanska, G., Murray, K. T., & Harlan, E. T. (2000). Effortful control in early childhood: Continuity and change, antecedents, and implications for social development. *Developmental Psychology, 36*(2), 220–232.

Korte, S. M., Koolhaas, J. M., Wingfield, J. C., & McEwen, B. S. (2005). The Darwinian concept of stress: Benefits of allostasis and costs of allostatic load and the trade-offs in health and disease. *Neuroscience and Biobehavioural Reviews, 29*(1), 3–38.

Krishnan, V., Han, M. H., Graham, D. L., Berton, O., Renthal, W., Russo, S. J., . . . Nestler, E. J. (2007). Molecular adaptations underlying susceptibility and resistance to social defeat in brain reward regions. *Cell, 131*(2), 391–404.

Krishnan, V., & Nestler, E. J. (2008). The molecular neurobiology of depression. *Nature, 455*(7215), 894–902.

Lu, A., Steiner, M. A., Whittle, N., Vogl, A. M., Walser, S. M., Ableitner, M., . . . Deussing, J. M. (2008). Conditional mouse mutants highlight mechanisms of corticotropin-releasing hormone effects on stress-coping behavior. *Molecular Psychiatry, 13*(11), 1028–1042.

McEwen, B. S. (2003). Mood disorders and allostatic load. *Biological Psychiatry, 54*(3), 200–207.

McEwen, B. S., & Milner, T. A. (2007). Hippocampal formation: Shedding light on the influence of sex and stress on the brain. *Brain Research Review, 55*(2), 343–355.

McGaugh, J. L. (2004). The amygdala modulates the consolidation of memories of emotionally arousing experiences. *Annual Review of Neuroscience, 27*, 1–28.

Maginness, A. (2007). *The development of resilience: A model* (Unpublished Doctoral thesis). University of Canterbury, Canterbury.

Masten, A. S. (1994). Resilience in individual development: Successful adaptation despite risk and adversity. In M. C. Wang & E. W. Gordon (Eds.), *Educational resilience in inner-city America: Challenges and prospects* (pp. 3–25). Hillsdale, NY: Lawrence Erlbaum.

Masten, A. S. (2001). Ordinary magic: Resilience processes in development. *American Psychologist, 56*(3), 227–238.

Masten, A. S., & Coatsworth, J. D. (1998). The development of competence in favorable and unfavorable environments: Lessons from research on successful children. *American Psychologist, 53*(2), 205–220.

Mervielde, I., & Asendorpf, J. B. (2000). Variable-centred and person-centred approaches to childhood personality. In S. E. Hampson (Ed.), *Advances on personality psychology* (Vol. 1, pp. 37–76). New York, NY: Psychology Press.

Morgan, C. A., 3rd, Southwick, S., Hazlett, G., Rasmusson, A., Hoyt, G., Zimolo, Z., Charney, D. S. (2004). Relationships among plasma dehydroepiandrosterone sulfate and cortisol levels, symptoms of dissociation, and objective performance in humans exposed to acute stress. *Archives of General Psychiatry, 61*(8), 819–825.

Morgan, C. A., 3rd, Wang, S., Southwick, S. M., Rasmusson, A., Hazlett, G., Hauger, R. L., & Charney, D. S. (2000). Plasma neuropeptide-Y concentrations in humans exposed to military survival training. *Biological Psychiatry, 47*(10), 902–909.

Padrón, Y. N., Waxman, H. C., & Huang, S. L. (1999). Classroom behavior and learning environment differences between resilient and nonresilient elementary school students. *Journal of Education for Student Placed at Risk, 4*(1), 63–81.

Rothbart, M. K., Ahadi, S. A., & Evans, D. E. (2000). Temperament and personality: Origins and outcomes. *Journal of Personality and Social Psychology, 78*(1), 122–135.

Rutter, M. (1985). Resilience in the face of adversity: Protective factors and resistance to psychiatric disorder. *British Journal of Psychiatry, 147*(6), 598–611.

Rutter, M. (2006a). Implications of resilience concepts for scientific understanding. *Annals of the New York Academy of Sciences, 1094*, 1–12.

Rutter, M. (2006b). The promotion of resilience in the face of adversity. In A. Clarke-Stewart & J. Dunn (Eds.), *Families count: Effects on child and adolescent development: The Jacobs foundation series on adolescence* (pp. 26–52). New York, NY: Cambridge University Press.

Sajdyk, T. J., Shekhar, A., & Gehlert, D. R. (2004). Interactions between NPY and CRF in the amygdala to regulate emotionality. *Neuropeptides, 38*(4), 225–234.

Santos, R. S. (2011). *Why resilience? A review of literature of resilience and implications for further educational research* (Unpublished qualifying paper submitted to Claremont Graduate University & San Diego State University). San Diego State University, San Diego.

Seccombe, K. (2002). "Beating the odds" versus "changing the odds": Poverty, resilience, and family policy. *Journal of Marriage and Family, 64*(2), 384–394.

Stein, M. B., Campbell-Sills, L., & Gelernter, J. (2009). Genetic variation in 5HTTLPR is associated with emotional resilience. *American Journal of Medical Genetics. Part-B: Neuropsychiatric Genetics, 150B*(7), 900–906.

Strelau, J. (1983). A regulative theory of temperament. *Australian Journal of Psychology, 35*(3), 305–317.

Werner, E. E., & Smith, R. S. (1982). *Vulnerable but not invincible: A longitudinal study of resilient children and youth.* New York, NY: R. R. Donnelley and Sons, Inc.

Werner, E. E., & Smith, R. S. (1992). *Overcoming the odds: High risk children from birth to adulthood.* Ithaca, NY: Cornell University Press.

Winfield, L. F. (1991). Resilience, schooling, and development in African-American youth: A conceptual framework. *Education and Urban Society, 24*(1), 5–14.

Yehuda, R., Brand, S. R., Golier, J. A., & Yang, R. K. (2006). Clinical correlates of DHEA associated with posttraumatic stress disorder. *Acta Psychiatrica Scandinavica, 114*(3), 187–193.

Yehuda, R., Brand, S. R., & Yang, R. K. (2006). Plasma neuropeptide Y concentrations in combat exposed veterans: Relationship to trauma exposure, recovery from PTSD, and coping. *Biological Psychiatry, 59*(7), 660–663.

Zhou, Z., Zhu, G., Hariri, A. R., Enoch, M. A., Scott, D., Sinha, R., . . . Goldman, D. (2008). Genetic variation in human NPY expression affects stress response and emotion. *Nature, 452*(7190), 997–1001.

Zuckerman, M. (1991). *Psychobiology of personality.* New York, NY: Cambridge.

Zuckerman, M. (2002). Zuckerman–Kuhlman Personality Questionnaire (ZKPQ): An alternative five factorial model. In B. De Raad & M. Perugini (Eds.), *Big five assessment* (pp. 377–396). Toronto: Hogrefe.

Section II
Psychosocial correlates

8

Resilient personalities

An amalgamation of protective factors

Archana, Vijay Parkash and Updesh Kumar

Research in the area of resilience has grown tremendously during the past few decades. Resilience is an expedition involving the growth and transformation of an individual, which are considered vital for survival. It is a process of endurance that depends on multiple factors involving one's capability to remain flexible during adversities, adapting to the ongoing changes occurring in life and recuperating at a faster pace by building on own strengths. The cumulative effect of these factors depends on an individual's resilient skills, which are dynamic in nature. Resilience is an important aspect for understanding how human beings deal with stressors and recover constructively in the face of crisis by remaining positive and compliant in nature. According to Luthar (2006), resilience refers to positive adaptation despite adversity. It relates to acknowledging change as a means towards continuous growth and prosperity that enhances strengths and deals with vulnerabilities. It is a universal ability to spring back from negative influences and convalesce from illness and the feelings of hopelessness.

A resilient individual displays a strong sense of commitment towards the task, by accepting it as a challenge and putting efforts towards accomplishing it. They have the capability to flourish, prosper and recover instinctively from hindrances by bouncing back and dealing effectively with daily hassles. It is a gradual course of action that takes place in the presence of life-threatening situations. In other words, resilience is also referred as "the capacity for successful adaptation, positive functioning, or competence despite high risk, chronic stress, or prolonged or severe trauma" (Henry, 1999, p. 521). It relates to the ability to take control of stressful events by maintaining strength, enthusiasm and good health. Resiliency signifies dynamism, flexibility, ability to thrive, resistance to change and sustained competence irrespective of facing extreme stress that threatens an individual's skill for survival. It is a vigorous revival from excessive and traumatic sufferings. There's no doubt that there are certain challenges in life that are inevitable. But these challenges are part of the developmental processes of an individual that build upon the strengths and well-being.

The concept of resilience came into existence when research carried out on children depicted it as a positive outcome irrespective of childhood adversities (Luthar, 2006). During these investigations, it was observed that children with parents suffering from mental health difficulties were still flourishing and functioning well. Also, early psychiatric studies revealed that these children were observed to be invulnerable irrespective of experiencing unpleasant life situations. Over a period of time, this invulnerability was substituted by the word 'resilience' (Earvolino-Ramirez, 2007). During adulthood, resilience was found to be positively associated with mental health and well-being despite unfavourable conditions. Bonanno (2005) has opined that resilience can be explained both in terms of pathways and end results, wherein an individual presents their explicit skills for attaining preferred outcomes. Resilience is not stagnant in nature; rather, it is a process that changes with respect to time while dealing with the hardships of life. High-rated resilient individuals are good in sustaining their psychological health by overcoming the stressful situations as compared to those who are rated low on resilience. Also high resiliency is associated positively with optimistic outlook, strong social networks and effective coping skills in dealing with the vulnerabilities of life.

Resilience is characterized by the utilization of coping skills to reinstate an internal and external process that gets affected during stress, revitalization at the time of adversities and making use of protective factors that reduces the intensity of risk factors and inculcate competence in individuals (Smith & Carlson, 1997). Resilient individuals exemplify interpersonal skills and problem-solving ability in dealing with anxiety-prone circumstances. They display inbuilt strength and have the capability to withstand stress by holding a broader perspective and keeping high expectations in life. They have often been observed to be proficient in dealing with the turmoil of life irrespective of the obstacles that occur due to the lack of resources available at their end. In a study carried out by Luthar (2006), it was observed that, despite suffering from mental disturbances in one way or the other, certain children were found to be displaying resilience. On one hand, these children exhibited some trouble on the psychological or emotional fronts whereas on the other they showed academic competence. Individuals high on resilience express greater resistance to inevitable circumstances by being more optimistic and socially equipped, upholding psychological well-being and relying more on healthy coping style. They cope with catastrophe in spite of the anticipated effects of harsh conditions and are able to excel under both chronic as well as acute circumstances. It is thus a process of change that provides a buffer against adversities by thriving and fostering the overall mental and emotional health of the individual.

Resilient people have confidence in their ability for solving problems and coping with stressors. Due to their past experiences in dealing with stressful situations, they display a strong sense of personal control that helps in facing adversities. Since resilience is not a stable personality trait, it varies from situation to situation; like, a person may show resilience at workplace but may display disturbances at interpersonal level. Resilience as one of the vital components of well-being promotes health and is found to be a strong indicator of psychological maturity that reflects higher levels of self-directedness and cooperativeness along with low harm avoidance and high persistence (Cloninger, Salloum, & Mezzich, 2012). Researchers like Reich, Zautra, and Hall (2010) assert that resilience depends upon two important dimensions: recovery and sustainability. Recovery relates to the capability of an individual to return to the original form in a systematic manner so as to conquer adversity. Susceptibility refers to the adaptive nature of the individual that helps them to flourish and maintain well-being in the face of unforeseen changes of environment. Being resilient does not lead to a desired goal; rather, it is a product of numerous approaches that result in continuous growth and development.

Personality in context of resilience

To have a thorough understanding of personality with reference to resilience, first of all, it becomes essential to follow a line of conceptualization about what personality is all about and how it develops over a period of time. Every individual holds a unique personality in terms of attitudes, beliefs and perceptions, and due to these individual differences, they respond in a special way to everyday circumstances. Since no two individuals are alike, therefore, personality cannot just be labeled as stable over time, it is, however, a dynamic process that brings out a person's unique way of behavioural regulation in dealing with complex situations. The overall personality of an individual involves certain mental processes that vary from person to person and make them unique; for example some individuals go to pieces while experiencing traumatic events in their lives while others are capable enough in handling stressors in an effective manner.

There is a wide array of factors responsible for figuring out an individual's personality. Both personality traits and environmental factors play a key role in determining resilience. The dynamic personality along with the non-static environmental factors determine the ways a person responds to and copes with the damaging effects of adversities. If an individual finds difficulty in dealing with the adversities of life, then they cannot be termed as having resilient personality. It is difficult to predict any one particular trait responsible for making an individual resilient. An individual's response to traumatic events may vary depending upon the situation, as the same person may fail to adapt to all the situations at all the times. Resilient individuals do not trim down the prevalence of stress in their day-to-day life; rather, these stressful events are generally observed as prospects for one's progress leading to enhanced mental health (O'Rourke, 2004).

A resilient personality possesses three important characteristics: the capability to generate a context of meaning, to relate oneself to others and to remain flexible (Frogge, 2000). There are certain other traits that are equally found unique to resilient people. These include dealing with dissatisfactions, adapting well at the time of setbacks, exhibiting higher levels of self-sufficiency, empathy, good interpersonal relations, inquisitiveness, and problem-solving capabilities (Jew, Green, & Kroger, 1999). During the past few decades, the Big Five Factor model of personality has emerged as one of the most prominent models that help in comprehending the role of various personality traits in different kinds of coping behaviour patterns. They are observed to affect resilience in adolescents by showing a negative association between resilience and neuroticism and a positive linking between extraversion and conscientiousness (Nakaya, Oshio, & Kaneko, 2006). On similar lines, in a study by Annalakshmi (2007), resilience was found to be positively correlated with well-regulated personality dimensions. It showed that low psychoticism, high extraversion and low neuroticism tend to display higher resilience that resulted in enhanced problem-solving skills and healthier lifestyles. Resiliency in children generally tends to increase their competence by making them more amiable and emotionally stable.

Other researchers like Hurtes and Allen (2001) put forth that the profile of a resilient individual includes seven factors – insight, independence, creativity, sense of humour, initiative, supportive relationships and value orientation. Insight is the capability to comprehend people and the circumstances around them. Independence relates to being self-sufficient and capable of dealing with others. Creativity focuses on creating innovative ideas for coping with unfavourable conditions. Sense of humour refers to laughing and remaining cheerful in oneself. Initiative signifies a proactive behaviour to explore and remain focused in one's life. Supportive relationship means maintaining good interpersonal relationships with others. Value orientation works on the principle of morality. Lerner, Dowling, and Anderson (2005) highlighted the 'Five Cs' observed in resilient individuals that add to their overall growth and development. These are Confidence (having faith in one's own abilities by remaining self-reliant), Competence (skills to meet demands by doing things efficiently), Connection (having strong social networks), Character (qualities that are measured in terms of moral values and societal norms) and Caring/Compassion (a gesture of showing concern and empathy for others).

Resilient individuals display quick reaction to threat, high level of maturity, information seeking behaviour, healthy relationships, optimistic approach towards future, altruistic behaviour and cognitive restructuring of traumatic events (Mrazek & Mrazek, 1987). Resilience involves interplay of biological, psychological and environmental factors wherein environmental factors can alter biological traits by helping an individual develop specific behaviours that can be learned over a period of time (Kim-Cohen, Moffitt, Caspi, & Taylor, 2004).

Interplay of risk and protective factors

The presence of protective factors contributes towards human growth and development. At the same time, there are certain situational factors that may put an individual at risk. These are called risk factors, which negatively affect an individual's health and well-being. According to Compas, Hinden, and Gerhardt (1995), risk factors relate to the traits of an individual along with their immediate milieu that enhance the scope of their maladaptive behaviour. An individual cannot be labeled as resilient unless and until they are exposed to risk factors. Those exposed to risk conditions generally deal with numerous stressors that serve as a barrier towards their enhancement. The stressors may be experienced either due to the prevalence of certain vulnerable attributes of an individual that are innate or may occur because of external conditions like illness, trauma, maltreatment, natural disasters and homelessness (Masten & Reed, 2002). The stressors experienced by an individual may be acute, episodic or chronic in nature (Miller, Smith, & Rothstein, 1993). Acute stress is experienced by almost all individuals on a regular basis while dealing with the various demands of life. This kind of stress is not permanent in nature as it fades away as soon as the complexities get resolved. Episodic stress occurs when people keep unrealistic expectations along with undesirable demands that hinder their ability to attain goals. Chronic stress takes place due to prolonged exposure to stressors and usually results in life-threatening behaviour that obliterates the mind and body of the individual completely. Every individual in one situation or another becomes vulnerable to stressful life events, but this vulnerability depends upon an individual's threshold level for tolerating stress. If stress in the form of risk factors increases beyond a particular threshold, then it results in the breakdown of an individual.

The interplay of both risk and protective factors is essential to lead towards a particular outcome that may either help an individual to attain the set goals or may serve as a barrier towards achieving the desired output. The balance between risk and protective factors depends upon the rate and extent of recurrence and intensity as well as the developmental phases at which they take place. Werner (2000) has asserted that till the time the balance between risk and protective factors is maintained, successful adjustment is feasible, but when risk factors outweigh the protective factors, then it may lead to adversities. Protective factors serve as a buffer against risk factors, and the sum of protective factors promotes resilience. Beyond genetic makeup, these factors include culmination of one's personal traits, the environmental surrounding in which an individual resides, their personality makeup, presence of external support system, interpersonal skills and the capability of an individual to make use of the available means for dealing with adversities. As observed by Seligman (1992), resilience generally occurs in people who remain positive in their lives, display cheerfulness, bravery, self-awareness, dedication and capability to deal with emotional disturbances. They are found to be flexible, self-assured, focused, vigorous and prepared to undertake risks by holding an optimistic approach towards life and maintaining good interpersonal relations with others. Individuals, families and social surroundings involve both risk and protective factors. Resilience depends upon the way an individual recovers from risk and overcomes traumas by utilizing problem-solving skills in order to avoid harmful circumstances.

One of the most essential aspects of resilience is coping with stressful situations. Coping relates to an individual's attempt to trim down the effect of complex traumatic circumstances (Courbasson, Endler, Kocovski, & Kocovski, 2002). Research suggests a dynamic relationship between coping and resilience. Resilience relates to an adaptive behaviour with respect to complexities whereas coping refers to behaviour or reaction of an individual that weakens the effects of adversities of day-to-day living (Snyder & Dinoff, 1999). It takes into account the cognitive processes along with one's conduct of behaviour involved in dealing with stressors. As posited by Endler and Parker (1999), an individual generally adopts three kinds of approaches while coping with the adversities of life: task-oriented, emotion-oriented, and avoidance-oriented coping styles. Task-oriented coping focuses on reducing the effect of adverse situations. Emotion-oriented coping strategies deal with restricting the impact of stress that is emotion-provoking in nature rather than just resolving traumatic incidents. Avoidance-oriented coping attempts to use disruption and diversion for eliminating the impact of stress. Among the three approaches, task-oriented coping has been widely considered to be the best way for dealing with stress as compared to other approaches. Coping skills include both positive and negative modes of behaviour (Livneh, Livneh, Maron, & Kaplan, 1996). Individuals with positive coping skills display traits of flexibility and sensibility with future-driven personality that helps them in eliminating stress. Negative coping skills are reflected by traits associated with rigidity and reality distortion behaviour. Coping depends upon both the individual as well as the external resources that help in upholding high self-esteem, enhancing mental well-being and diminishing the detrimental effect of stressful situations.

Resources enhancing resilience

Resilience is a product of both personal and familial factors that help in averting negative influences and handling stressors on regular basis. It is the sum of those resources that are operative in nature, safeguard against the impact of risk factors and promote positive outcomes in people at menace. These resources, observed in the form of protective factors, take into account both the personal as well as external strengths. Personal strengths relate to the individual competencies, and external strengths are external resources involving strong social networks, family cohesion, warmth and support systems. Some of the effective resources that are found responsible for enhancing resilience include internal locus of control, self-efficacy, willpower, self-awareness, altruistic behaviour, sense of purposeful living, finding meaning in adverse situations, strong social bonds with others and availability of both personal and social resources in dealing with traumatic events (Wilson, 1995). All these factors intermingle towards generating resilience. For example during traumatic experiences, individuals with an internal locus of control are likely to look for means to deal with setbacks (Zakin, Solomon, & Neria, 2003). At the same time, they are able to form a strong social network that upholds strong self-disclosure along with displaying altruistic behaviour and positive emotions for coping with trauma. Resilient individuals are able to utilize resources in a way that serves as an effective tool to prosper and grow from experiences.

Personal strengths as protective factors

Personal strengths are the assets possessed by an individual that are innate, leading to one's overall growth and prosperity. Personal assets relate to internal traits possessed by an individual that helps in buffering negative events (Wayman, 2002). Resilient individuals show a high prevalence of positive relationships with family members, social intelligence, self-esteem, personal control,

95

perseverance, positive coping skills, goal–oriented behaviour and effective problem-solving skills. These traits of resilience can be enhanced in an individual early by showing care during their childhood and establishing a positive relationship with parents, which in turn will leave a positive impact on their behaviour. Described here are some of the essential personal strengths that serve as protective factors for enhancing resilience among individuals.

Self-efficacy: Albert Bandura, a pioneer in the area of self-efficacy, has defined self-efficacy as a belief in one's own abilities in order to attain certain goals that are seen as the basis for human agency (Bandura, 1999). It is basically a belief system that a person holds about himself regarding his capability in handling difficult circumstances. Individuals high on self-efficacy are likely to persist in their efforts and overcome negative thoughts. Self-efficacious people are adaptable and flexible and display perseverance under challenging circumstances. It also involves one's will-ingness to look for challenging tasks by engaging thoroughly in it and inculcating a feeling of self-worth. A belief towards having a control over one's life plays a significant role in successful adaptation towards traumatic events. Holding such beliefs serves as a vital component in build-ing resilience (Aspinwall & Richter, 1999). People with high self-efficacy hold a strong faith in their ability about completing a task productively and having a control over their behaviour. A higher sense of self-efficacy affects an individuals' performance on assignments they undertake along with their perseverance and diligence in accomplishing it. A stronger sense of self-efficacy results in consistent and focused efforts put forth in attaining task. There has been vast research that depicts relationship between resilience and self-efficacy (Earvolino-Ramirez, 2007). Resilient individuals are rated high on self-efficacy and are generally found to be more capable of using effective coping strategies under difficult situations. Coping style depends upon the availability of resources lying within an individual. There is a strong association between resilience and cop-ing, as coping relates to looking for means towards utilizing personal resources and resilience is a constructive result of successful coping. Coping skills are essential towards maintaining positive adaptation to stressors (Compas, Connor-Smith, Saltzman, Thomsen, & Wadsworth, 2001). High self-efficacy equips an individual in dealing with the challenges of life, which in turn increases resilience.

Social competence: Social competence, as a skill, focuses on drawing positive responses from others so that it helps in enhancing healthy social relationships. It refers to easy temperament that envisages an individual's adjustment to the surroundings (Werner & Smith, 2001). High social competence promotes sociability by connecting well and sharing a mutual gratifying bond of relationships. It focuses on building resilience and good communication skills that helps in managing conflicting situations, thereby reducing risk-prone behaviours. Empathy, compassion and altruism are essential components of social competence that facilitate positive emotions in social relationships. Empathy is a distinctive feature of resilience that relates to comprehending and sharing others' feelings. Compassion emphasizes humanity and the means for reducing the distress of other people. Altruism focuses on helping behaviour without any motive. Individuals with low social competence tend to have poor social skills with the highest rates of relapse and severe psychiatric problems (Lerner, 1984).

Spirituality: Spirituality and religious faith are two important factors that promote resil-iency among individuals. Spirituality relates to inner, subjective experience that makes an individual feel a strong interest in understanding the meaning of things in life (Ellens, 2009). It is the capability of an individual to develop an innovative way of understanding one's own life. It is a universal phenomenon that has a direct impact on psychological well-being. Research shows a strong association between spirituality and mental health. Those who have stronger spiritual beliefs show better adjustment to life satisfaction (Peres, Moreira-Almeida, Nasello, & Koenig, 2007). They are also able to maintain good psychological well-being and have the capacity to recover more quickly from stressful events by using effective coping strategies in order to cope with stress (Singh & Pareek, 2007). According to Vaughan (2002), spiritual intelligence helps in contributing to psychological well-being and promoting overall healthy human development.

Hardiness: Hardiness, as a personality variable, exhibits a significant relationship with coping behaviour and resilience under stressful situations. It relates to an individual's problem-solving skills and the capability to organize resources for attaining desired goals. As described by Kobasa (1979), hardiness is a personality trait that focuses on both coping strategies and appraisal. It covers three aspects: faith in one's ability to have a control over events, dedication and willingness to keep oneself occupied in activities and acceptance of change in life as a challenge to learn and grow. It serves as an important aspect of resilience for PTSD (Agaibi & Wilson, 2005). A study carried out by Maddi and Hightower (1999) revealed that hardy individuals depicted better planning and more dynamic coping patterns. Hardiness is observed to have a negative correlation with behavioural disengagement and tendency for alcohol consumption in order to deal with stressors. At the same time, it also has a significant positive association with the dimensions of social support. Individuals high on hardiness are observed to be more enthusiastic, display satisfaction in life, have strong social bonding and exhibit high symptoms of well-being. Hardy people turn stressful situations into opportunities that help towards enhancing their performance and growth.

Self-worth and self-esteem: Self-worth and self-esteem are two important intrapersonal personality attributes residing within an individual that play a significant role towards promoting resilience. As per the most widely accepted definition of 'self', it is a favourable or unfavourable attitude towards the self (Rosenberg, 1965). Self-worth has been observed to be one of the most prominent characteristics of resilient individuals that relates to an optimistic feeling about oneself and others. Varied studies have highlighted that resilient individuals display high self-esteem (Buckner, Mezzacappa, & Beardslee, 2003). Those rated high on self-esteem are likely to remain happy, vigorous and creative by putting relentless efforts to conquer intricacies whereas people low on self-esteem are observed to remain negative and tensed with depressing thoughts regarding the future (Coleman & Hendry, 1990). As an individual strength of resilience, when self-esteem is taken in conjunction with external support systems and environmental factors, then it serves to play an influential role towards mental health. Resilient individuals exhibit an elevated intensity of self-esteem, an optimistic outlook towards life and high self-efficacy (Visser, 2007). People with low self-esteem display feelings of worthlessness, unhappiness, discontent, incompetence and disappointment as compared to people with high self-esteem.

Problem-solving skills: Problem-solving skills play a vital role towards the enhancement of resiliency and are generally developed during childhood. It takes into account the ability to plan, think abstractly, remain flexible and seek unconventional ways of solving problems. Individuals who lack problem-solving skills display poor mental health problems. High resiliency brings more capability towards problem-solving skills. These skills not only promote adaptive coping but also help in dealing with complexities and challenges of life. Problem-solving strengths are related to enhanced adaptability, reduced intensity of depression, higher levels of optimism and healthier ways of coping with adversities (Heppner & Lee, 2002). Insight, a problem-solving skill, contributes towards resiliency. It refers to the "mental habit of asking penetrating questions of oneself and, subsequently, providing honest answers" (Wolin & Wolin, 1993, p. 71). Individuals with better insights are able to adjust more socially, don't go by inexperienced assumptions and always remain cautious about their surroundings (Rubin, 1996). Having insight enhances one's ability to look for alternative ways for solving problems and conflicts in routine lives.

Internal locus of control: Locus of control can be either internal or external. Individuals with internal locus of control display the tendency to take responsibility of the consequences of their actions whereas those with an external locus of control blame outside forces and believe that others are responsible for whatever happens to them. Internal locus of control depends on one's accomplishments and setbacks rather than the presence of external resources. Internal locus of control and resilience are observed to be interlinked as they share many traits altogether. For example both these traits involve certain characteristics that are common to both, like having a better ego functions, helping others and displaying healthy coping behaviour. According to Wilson (1995), internal locus of control, self-efficacy, coping resources, altruistic behaviour and social bonding are found to be significant predictors of resilience. The use of coping strategies depends upon the way how an individual evaluates the stressors. For example when the stressors are considered to be controllable, the individual takes it as a challenge rather than recognizing it as a menace. Under such circumstances, it is the sense of control that serves as an important component towards task-oriented coping strategies being adopted by the person. It is the internal locus of control that results in positive coping strategies, thus reducing the chances of risk.

Sense of purpose and bright future: A sense of purpose means finding meaning in one's life. It is found to be highly effective in enhancing healthy outcomes despite complexities (Werner & Smith, 1992). Werner and Smith (1992) carried out studies on children and observed that efficient coping depends upon an individual's level of self-confidence, along with their belief that they can envisage both the internal as well as the external factors, which helps in dealing with the stressors of life. A sense of anticipation that focuses on one's ability to ascertain the future is one of the factors that contribute towards the mental health and well-being (Vaillant, 2000). An optimal level of performance depends upon an individual's level of intrinsic motivation, determination, drive, commitment and dedication. A strong sense of constructive future leads to high rate of success, optimistic approach towards life and good mental health. Watt, David, Ladd and Shamos (1995) have opined that goal-oriented behaviour, persistent attempts to complete the task and strong determination to sustain in adverse situations are some of the traits associated with resilient behaviour. A sense of purpose and bright future enhances an individual's ability to foresee the consequences of their actions and plan a bright future in order to endure the negativities of life.

Optimism: Optimism is a major motivational state related to elevated mental health and enhanced well-being. It relates to positive faith and conviction that are associated with positive sentiments. It focuses on an individual's capability to sustain hope regarding futuristic outcomes. Optimism is positively related to good health and well-being. Optimistic outlook is an important factor that contributes towards resilience and finding positive meaning in life. It serves as an important resilient factor towards adapting to adversities. For example holding an optimistic feeling in order to recapitulate from stressful conditions is found to be related to higher level of resilience (Connor & Davidson, 2003). Such an attitude raises one's level of hope by reducing the symptoms of depression. Positive thinking is another way for enhancing resilience that helps an individual to have a broader outlook in reframing a situation in a positive and productive manner. A study carried out by Gilbar, Ben-Zur and Lubin (2010) on military personnel revealed that certain personal strengths like optimism, self-confidence and feelings of control are positively related to resilience. During stressful situations, these positive traits help soldiers towards optimal performance and sustenance under pressure. Resilient soldiers remain focused on their assignments by displaying determination, firmness and motivation. They are also beneficial in creating a positive outlook towards life, reinstating their self-esteem, recuperating from traumas, adapting to deployments, making use of adaptive coping strategies and enhancing social bonds.

Social strengths as protective factors

Social factors are considered imperative for individuals to be resilient. Social resilience relates to the ability to connect and maintain constructive relationship with others in order to deal with traumatic life experiences. It emphasizes altering the adversities into growth by enhancing interpersonal resources and capacities. Towards this end, family remains the main source of strength for fostering resilience. Resilient people have close network of emotional ties with family members that cultivate caring and supportive relationships with them. An individual's behavioural outcome is best reflected through the social bonding shared by the family members (Feldman, Stiffman, & Jung, 1987). The quality of relationship in a family leads to a stable and supportive environment that is essential towards developing resilience. High degree of family cohesion, adaptability and positive communication strengthens resilience in family during crisis. The resilience of an individual depends upon the intensity of bonding being shared by family members. The more the family is able to adapt to the situational demands, the better will be their ability to bounce back from adversities. The strong family ties lead to a stronger and richer relationship among members at the time of setbacks. Stressful life events can take a shape of positive growth if families are resilient. Family resilience depends upon the persistence, strong willpower, diligence and innovative ways of taking initiative in order to overcome challenges. Prevalence of certain family traits in the form of social support and family flexibility brings emotional stability and makes an individual resilient, safeguard against stressors and enhances their growth and psychosocial adjustment during distress (Carson, Swanson, Cooney, Gillum, & Cunningham, 1992). Establishing a resilient attitude involves a strong social support system, effective problem–solving skills and personal resources for adapting to the adversities. Families who value and respect their children's concern are more likely to encourage resiliency.

The interaction among family members helps in contributing towards coping and building resilience. Cooperation and flexibility is seen in those families who hold a positive attitude towards others. Certain family traits that are found to be responsible for enhancing positivity and dealing effectively with hardships include accepting stressors as a part and parcel of life, working as a team towards resolving issues and assigning a leadership role to parents by letting them remain flexible and empathetic towards the concerns of their children. Therefore, families who join hands at the time of stress, collaborate towards solving problems and value each other thus promoting resilience. As compared to non–resilient families, resilient families tend to find ways to deal with and adapt to challenges. Families serving as protective factors enhance the altruistic behaviour of an individual and increase their resistance to stress and negative events of life. Resilient families impart a flexible environmental condition that broadens the success level and health of the individual. Families with unhealthy environmental conditions result in depression and failure to cope with stressors. Resilient families affect the personality as well as the stress resistance level of an individual. Warm parenting helps in counteracting risk by enhancing coping resources and interpersonal skills. Parents who are themselves resilient during stressful situations are more likely to serve as effective role models for their children. Also, parents displaying reduced levels of depression, family cohesiveness and strong social networks contribute towards enhancing resiliency in children.

Parents play a significant role in teaching, guiding, mentoring, controlling, helping, supporting and encouraging their children. All these skills are possible only if there is a healthy interaction and effective communication between parents and their children. The enhanced quality of interpersonal communication between parents and their children helps in overcoming the constant pressures and strains faced by family. The amount of love, warmth and nurturance expressed by the parents assists in development of resilience in children. Parents can foster resilience in children by creating a steady and secure relationship in family; maintaining high quality of interpersonal skills; serving as a good role model; instilling social values and inculcating feelings of care, belongingness and warmth. As a result of these traits, children are able to grow positively, get along with others effectively and develop a sense of being cared and valued in the family.

Parents play a vital part towards childhood outcomes. Ineffective parenting and marital discord results in unhealthy outcomes. Proper supervision and care by parents reduces the prevalence of risk factors. The presence of protective factors observed in the form of parenting style often results in competence building. Parental control is one of the key determinants of resilience among adolescents. Baumrind (1968) and Maccoby and Martin (1983) focuses on four styles of parental control: the permissive parenting style (parents displaying high in warmth and low in controlling/supervision), the authoritarian style (high on control and low in warmth), the authoritative style (high in both control and warmth) and the indulgent style also referred to as the neglecting or rejecting parenting style (low in both control and warmth). All these styles of parenting leave a huge impact on the academic performance of adolescents and are found to be associated with both adaptive and maladaptive strategies used by them in achievement contexts (Aunola, Stattin, & Nurmi, 2000). For example adolescents from authoritative families display adaptive task-oriented strategies whereas families with the indulgent and authoritarian style use maladaptive strategies. However, permissive families reflect self-enhancing attributes as compared to other styles.

Besides personal traits and family networks, there are environmental factors prevailing in the community that affect the personality of an individual. Environmental factors are "external influences that provide support and protect against negative factors threatening the resilient person" (Wayman, 2002, p. 168). People who get respect and support from the outer world are the ones who are able to perform well under hardships. Schools provide the base for boosting the motivation and enhancing the self-esteem of adolescents. Since resilience is a developmental process, it takes into account both the internal as well as the external resources that facilitate them in developing strengths. The personal resources that are innate and the interpersonal resources observed in the form of social support received from both the family and the environment reinforces adolescent behaviour and enhances their coping skills and resiliency.

Conclusion

Resilience is a dynamic process that enhances the capability of an individual to have strong control over unfavourable situations. It focuses on specific traits and coping skills that help an individual to rebound from the detrimental disputes of life. Resilience is not entirely an inborn trait, since everyone is born with certain personality traits that can be developed over a period of time. During life-threatening situations, individuals with resilient outlook are more likely to adapt effectively and display reduced poor mental health outcomes. The varying life experiences help them to learn, prosper and develop intervention strategies for dealing with the hardships of life. Resilience can be attained through multiple pathways that aim at capitalizing personal and social resources. Personal resources are those dispositional attributes of the individual that forms the part of an overall personality. It includes factors like; self-efficacy, internal locus of control, problem-solving ability, optimism, spirituality and self-esteem. Social resources, on the other hand, emphasizes an individual's skills to work with others; to form social networks and to seek social support from family, peers and the outer world. Resilience is a strength-based approach that doesn't completely eliminate the probability of risk factors but helps in shifting the attention towards identifying those protective factors that contribute towards human growth and development. The balance and interaction between risk and protective factors depends upon the rate and extent of recurrence along with the developmental phases at which they take place. Protective factors lead to positive outcomes despite the elevated risk for maladjustment and serves as a buffer against risk factors, thereby promoting resilience and developing resilient personalities.

References

Agaibi, C. E., & Wilson, J. P. (2005). Trauma, PTSD and resilience: A review of literature. *Trauma Violence Abuse, 6*(3), 195–216.

Annalakshmi, N. (2007). Resilience in relation to extraversion-introversion, psychoticism, and neuroticism. *Indian Journal of Psychometry & Education, 38*(1), 51–55.

Aspinwall, L. G., & Richter, L. (1999). Optimism and self-mastery predict more rapid disengagement from unsolvable tasks in the presence of alternatives. *Motivation and Emotion, 23*(3), 221–245.

Aunola, K., Stattin, H., & Nurmi, J. (2000). Parenting styles and adolescent's achievement strategies. *Journal of Adolescence, 23*(2), 205–222.

Bandura, A. (1999). A social cognitive theory of personality. In L. A. Pervin & O. P. John (Eds.), *Handbook of personality* (2nd ed., pp. 154–196). New York: Guilford.

Baumrind, D. (1968). Authoritarian vs. authoritative parental control. *Adolescence, 3*(11), 255–272.

Bonanno, G. A. (2005). Resilience in the face of potential trauma. *Current Directions in Psychological Science, 14*(3), 135–138.

Buckner, J. C., Mezzacappa, E., & Beardslee, W. R. (2003). Characteristics of resilient youths living in poverty: The role of self-regulatory processes. *Development and Psychopathology, 15*(1), 139–162.

Carson, D. K., Swanson, D. M., Cooney, M. H., Gillum, B. J., & Cunningham, D. (1992). Stress and coping as predictors of young children's development and psychosocial adjustment. *Child Study Journal, 22*(4), 273–302.

Cloninger, C. R., Salloum, I. M., & Mezzich, J. E. (2012). The dynamic origins of positive health and well-being. *International Journal of Person-Centred Medicine, 2*(1), 1–9.

Coleman, J. C., & Hendry, L. (1990). *The nature of adolescence* (2nd ed.). London: Routledge.

Compas, B. E., Connor-Smith, J. K., Saltzman, H., Thomsen, A. H., & Wadsworth, M. E. (2001). Coping with stress during childhood and adolescence: Problems, progress, and potential in theory and research. *Psychological Bulletin, 127*(1), 87–127.

Compas, B. E., Hinden, B. R., & Gerhardt, C. A. (1995). Adolescent development: Pathways and processes of risk and resilience. *Annual Review of Psychology, 46*, 265–293.

Connor, K. M., & Davidson, J. R. T. (2003). Development of a new resilience scale: The Connor-Davidson resilience scale (CD-RISC). *Depression and Anxiety, 18*(2), 76–82.

Courbasson, C., Endler, M. A., Kocovski, N. S., & Kocovski, N. L. (2002). Coping and psychological distress for men with substance use disorders. *Current Psychology, 21*(1), 35–50.

Earvolino-Ramirez, M. (2007). Resilience: A concept analysis. *Nursing Forum, 42*(2), 73–82.

Ellens, J. H. (2009). Introduction to healing spirituality and religion. In J. H. Ellens (Ed.), *The healing power of spirituality: How faith helps humans thrive* (Vol. 1, pp. 1–5). Santa Barbara, CA: Praeger Press.

Endler, N. S., & Parker, J. D. A. (1999). *Coping inventory for stressful situation* (2nd ed.). North Tonawanda, NY: Multi-Health Systems.

Feldman, R., Stiffman, A., & Jung, K. (1987). *Children at risk: In the web of parental mental illness.* New Brunswick, NJ: Rutgers University Press.

Frogge, S. (2000). The resiliency factor. *Driven, 3*(2), 18–19.

Gilbar, O., Ben-Zur, H., & Lubin, G. (2010). Coping, mastery, stress appraisals, mental preparation, and unit cohesion predicting distress and performance: A longitudinal study of soldiers undertaking evacuation tasks. *Anxiety Stress Coping, 23*(5), 547–562.

Henry, D. L. (1999). Resilience in maltreated children: Implications for special needs adoption. *Child Welfare, 78*(5), 519–540.

Heppner, P. P., & Lee, D. G. (2002). Problem-solving appraisal and psychological adjustment. In C. R. Snyder & S. J. Lopez (Eds.), *Handbook of positive psychology* (pp. 288–298). New York: Oxford University Press.

Hurtes, K. P., & Allen, L. R. (2001). Measuring resiliency in Youth: The resiliency attitudes and skills profile. *Therapeutic Recreation Journal, 35*(4), 333–347.

Jew, C. J., Green, K. E., & Kroger, J. (1999). Development and validation of a measure of resiliency. *Measurement and Evaluation in Counseling and Development, 32*(2), 75–89.

Kim-Cohen, J., Moffitt, T. E., Caspi, A., & Taylor, A. (2004). Genetic and environmental processes in young children's resilience and vulnerability to socioeconomic deprivation. *Child Development, 75*(3), 651–668.

Kobasa, S. C. (1979). Stressful life events, personality and health: An inquiry into hardiness. *Journal of Personality and Social Psychology, 37*(1), 1–11.

Lerner, J. (1984). Difficult temperament and drug use: Analysis from the New York Longitudinal Study. *Journal of Drug Education, 14*(1), 1–7.

Lerner, R. M., Dowling, E. M., & Anderson, P. M. (2005). Positive youth development, a developmental systems view. In C. B. Fisher & R. M. Lerner (Eds.), *Encyclopedia of applied developmental science* (pp. 859–862). Thousand Oaks, CA: Sage Publications.

Livneh, H., Livneh, C. L., Maron, S., & Kaplan, J. (1996). A multidimensional approach to the study of the structure of coping with stress. *The Journal of Psychology, 130*(5), 501–512.

Luthar, S. S. (2006). Resilience in development: A synthesis of research across five decades. In D. Cicchetti & D. J. Cohen (Eds.), *Developmental psychopathology: Risk, disorder, and adaptation* (pp. 740–795). New York: Wiley.

Maccoby, E. E., & Martin, J. A. (1983). Socialization in the context of the family: Parent-child interaction. In P. H. Mussen & E. M. Hetherington (Eds.), *Handbook of child psychology: Vol. 4: Socialization, personality, and social development* (pp. 1–101). New York: John Wiley & Sons.

Maddi, S., & Hightower, M. (1999). Hardiness and optimism expressed in coping patterns. *Consulting Psychology Journal: Practice and Research, 51*(2), 95–105.

Masten, A. S., & Reed, M. J. (2002). Resilience in development. In C. R. Snyder & S. J. Lopez (Eds.), *Handbook of positive psychology* (pp. 74–88). London: Oxford University Press.

Miller, L. H., Smith, A. D., & Rothstein, L. (1993). *The stress solution: An action plan to manage the stress in your life.* New York: Pocket Books.

Mrazek, P. J., & Mrazek, D. (1987). Resilience in child maltreatment victims: A conceptual exploration. *Child Abuse and Neglect, 11*(3), 357–365.

Nakaya, M., Oshio, A., & Kaneko, H. (2006). Correlations for Adolescent Resilience Scale with big five personality traits. *Psychological Reports, 98*(3), 927–930.

O'Rourke, N. (2004). Psychological resilience and the well-being of widowed women. *Ageing International, 29*(3), 267–280.

Peres, J., Moreira-Almeida, A., Nasello, A., & Koenig, H. (2007). Spirituality and resilience in trauma victims. *Journal of Religion & Health, 46*(3), 343–350.

Reich, J. W., Zautra, J. W., & Hall, J. S. (2010). *Handbook of adult resilience.* New York: Guilford Press.

Rosenberg, M. (1965). *Society and the adolescent self-image.* Princeton, NJ: Princeton University Press.

Rubin, L. (1996). *The transcendent child: Tales of triumph over the past.* New York: Harper-Collins.

Seligman, M. E. P. (1992). *Helplessness: On depression, development and death.* New York: Freeman.

Singh, S., & Pareek, R. (2007). Positive predictors of health. *Journal of Indian Health Psychology, 2*(1), 10–19.

Smith, C., & Carlson, B. (1997). Stress, coping and resilience in children and youth. *Social Service Review, 71*(2), 231–256.

Snyder, C. R., & Dinoff, B. L. (1999). Coping where have you been? In C. R. Snyder (Ed.), *Coping: The psychology of what works* (pp. 3–19). New York: Oxford University Press.

Vaillant, G. E. (2000). Adaptive mental mechanisms: Their role in a positive psychology. *American Psychologist, 55*(1), 89–98.

Vaughan, F. (2002). What is spiritual intelligence? *Journal of Humanistic Psychology, 42*(2), 16–33.

Visser, W. A. (2007). *Daily hassles, resilience, and burnout of call centre staff* (Unpublished Doctorate Thesis). North-West University, Potchefstroom, South Africa.

Watt, N., David, J., Ladd, K., & Shamos, S. (1995). The life course of psychological resilience: A phenomenological perspective on deflecting life's slings and arrows. *Journal of Primary Prevention, 15*(3), 209–246.

Wayman, J. C. (2002). The utility of educational resilience for studying degree attainment in school dropouts. *The Journal of Educational Research, 95*(3), 167–178.

Werner, E. E. (2000). Protective factors and individual resilience. In S. J. Meisels & J. P. Shonkoff (Eds.), *Handbook of early childhood intervention* (pp. 115–132). New York: Cambridge University Press.

Werner, E. E., & Smith, R. S. (1992). *Overcoming the odds: High-risk children from birth to adulthood.* Ithaca, NY: Cornell University Press.

Werner, E. E., & Smith, R. S. (2001). *Journeys from childhood to midlife: Risk, resilience and recovery.* Ithaca, NY: Cornell University Press.

Wilson, J. P. (1995). Traumatic events and PTSD prevention. In B. Raphael & E. D. Barrows (Eds.), *The handbook of preventative psychiatry* (pp. 281–296). Amsterdam, the Netherlands: Elsevier North-Holland.

Wolin, S. J., & Wolin, S. (1993). *The resilient self: How survivors of troubled families rise above adversity*. New York: Villard Books.

Zakin, G., Solomon, Z., & Neria, Y. (2003). Hardiness, attachment style and long term psychological distress among Israeli POWs and combat veterans. *Personality and Individual Differences, 34*(5), 819–829.

9

Hardiness as a pathway to resilience under stress

Salvatore R. Maddi

Some people think that the best life involves avoiding whatever stressful circumstances may come your way. They believe that life should be predictable and consistent and that differences of opinion and beliefs can only make things worse.

The weaknesses of this position were made clear by existential psychology. Kierkegaard (1954), a founder of this position, theorized that everything we do or think in life is a result of the decisions we are constantly making. He argued that these decisions can be for the future (i.e. change) or the past (i.e. consistency). Thinking of choosing the future brings anxiety (as you cannot predict what will happen), and choosing the past brings guilt (as you are losing possibility and are stuck with a sense of missed opportunity). For Kierkegaard, what is important in the process of living is to grow and develop by choosing the future rather than the past. In order to do this, one has to be able to moderate the resulting anxiety. And, if one is able to do this, at least one will not be overwhelmed by the growing guilt of missed opportunity, and lack of fulfillment in living.

This existential approach has been very helpful to Maddi in his research, theorizing, counseling, and consulting. Early in his career, he was studying the aspects of personality that would lead to creativity (Maddi, 1965). What he was finding is that people who are interested in variety and change are most likely to achieve creativity. Then, in the early 1970s, a student of his brought him an article she had found in *Family Circle* magazine about how you should stay away from stressful circumstances, as they might kill you. Maddi and his research team talked about this and decided to study whether people who perform better under stress are also more provoked by change and motivated by this to be more creative. This interest in individual differences under stress led us to the Illinois Bell project.

The Illinois Bell project

In the mid-1970s, the US telephone industry was still a federally regulated monopoly, because it had been thought important that reliable and inexpensive telephone service was in the public interest. So, Illinois Bell Telephone (IBT), for which Maddi was a consultant, did not need to worry about its bottom line. But, the newly developing internet was changing this situation, and it was becoming clear that the government would at some point deregulate the telephone industry, in order to encourage competition in the US and around the world.

With the cooperation of IBT decision-makers, Maddi and his research team began collecting data on 450 managers in 1974, assuming that deregulation would occur before too many years went by. Every year, the managers in the sample were interviewed and were administered a number of relevant personality tests. In addition, their job performance measures and evaluations were also available.

Six years into the research project, deregulation occurred, and its effects are still regarded as a major disruption for the company and its employees. Indeed, between 1980 and 1981, almost 50 % of the sample was terminated, as IBT struggled to try to survive and compete effectively with new companies in the internet era. The data collection process already mentioned continued for another six years, in order to see the effects of the upheaval on managers in the sample. Fortunately, it was possible to continue data collection even on the managers who had been terminated and who needed to find and fulfill jobs in other (sometimes new) companies. This study has been regarded as a classical natural experiment and has led to many findings.

The results of this study showed that, in the six years following the deregulation of the telephone industry, roughly two-thirds of the sample fell apart in various ways. There were definite signs of anxiety, depression, and anger, undermining not only performance at work but in home life as well. Indeed, there were divorces, violence, substance abuse, and even suicides. But, the other third of the sample, not only survived, but also thrived following deregulation. At work, they either rose up in the ranks, or if they were among those terminated, they found significant jobs in other organizations or even started their own companies. They were also to give to and get social support from their significant others and were able to grow and develop by dealing effectively with the stress of deregulation.

Of special significance was the comparison of attitudes and beliefs in the managers before the disruptive deregulation occurred (Maddi & Kobasa, 1984). The clear differences between the managers who thrived after the deregulation and those who fell apart led to the definition of hardiness. All along, those who thrived on deregulation were much stronger in the attitudes of commitment, control, and challenge. No matter how bad things might get, they wanted to stay involved with people and contexts (commitment), to continue to struggle to have an influence on outcomes (control), and to learn how to grow and develop by trying to deal effectively with stresses (challenge). In contrast, the managers who fell apart under deregulation had even before it believed in playing it safe by avoiding stresses and, if unsuccessful in this, by sinking into alienation and powerlessness. These results led to conceptualizing hardiness as attitudes (the 3Cs of commitment, control, and challenge) and strategies (problem solving rather than avoidance coping, socially supportive rather than conflictual interactions, and beneficial rather than overindulgent self-care). We considered hardy attitudes to provide the courage and motivation to be able to do the hard work of turning stresses to growth advantages. This is quite consistent with the existential view, summarized well by Nietzsche (1969, p. 254) as "whatever doesn't kill me makes me stronger."

Also done with the IBT data was a study (Khoshaba & Maddi, 1999) on the early life experiences of managers, measured by interviews and questionnaires administered before deregulation took place. Then, following deregulation, managers who thrived on it were compared to those who fell apart. Content analyses of the interview and questionnaire data showed that the managers who subsequently thrived on the deregulation were higher in remembering a disruptive, stressful early family life and having been selected by their parents to be successful nonetheless. They accepted this role as the hope of the family and worked hard to justify this. These results are consistent with the assumption that hardiness can be learned, rather than be inborn. It also

105

indicates that parents can help their children grow in hardiness by having them understand that life is by its nature stressful and that involving themselves in this, rather than running away from it, is the way to grow and develop toward a better life. In contrast, parents who are overprotective and controlling jeopardize their children's growth toward hardiness.

Further development of the hardiness approach

By now, there are more than a thousand hardiness references over the last thirty-five years. In this process, our various versions of the hardiness questionnaire have been translated into more than fifteen Asian and European languages, to say nothing of the numerous countries that use it in English. There have been some reviews of this body of work (e.g. Funk, 1992; Maddi, 1990; Orr & Westman, 1990; Ouellette, 1993). In summary, hardiness research has shown that the hardiness attitudes (the 3Cs of commitment, control, and challenge) are positively related to the hardiness strategies of problem-solving (rather than avoidance) coping, socially supportive (rather than conflictual) interactions, and beneficial (rather than overindulgent) self-care. This hardiness pattern has been positively associated with performance, conduct, mood, and health in samples of college and high school students and of working adults in military, firefighting, sports, and business contexts (Maddi, 2002). Specific topics and studies will be presented in the following sections.

An important consideration is the systematic improvement of the measurement of hardy attitudes. The original questionnaire for the 3Cs of commitment, control, and challenge was fifty items in length. Over the years, the measure has been shortened and improved. The current version (Maddi & Khoshaba, 2001) is the eighteen Likert-item Personal Views Survey, III-R (third edition, revised). Examples of items are, for commitment, "I often wake up eager to take up life wherever it left off"; for control, "When I make plans, I'm certain I can make them work"; and for challenge, "Changes in routine provoke me to learn." Cronbach's alpha coefficients for all three Cs range in the .70s, and for total hardiness, even higher. The 3Cs are positively correlated, and each of them shows a high correlation with the total hardiness score. It has also been found (e.g. Sinclair & Tetrick, 2000) that factor analysis of the hardiness test items yields the three empirically related first-order factors of commitment, control, and challenge and that these factors are positively related to the second-order factor of hardiness. This pattern has supported using a total hardiness score, as all three first-order factors are needed for the existential courage conceptualization of this measure (Maddi, 2002, 2006). In another study (Maddi & Harvey, 2005), no cross-cultural or demographic differences were found in hardiness.

Now summarized will be some especially important studies on the role of hardiness in various performance, conduct, and health activities. For example similar results to those obtained at IBT have been reported for samples of people working in other occupations, such as bus drivers (Bartone, 1989), lawyers (Kobasa, 1982), and nurses (Keane, Ducette, & Adler, 1985). In all three occupations, hardiness is positively correlated with measures of performance and satisfaction and negatively correlated with anxiety and depression. Similar findings have also been obtained in samples of American employees experiencing culture shock on work missions abroad (Atella, 1989) and of foreign immigrants to the United States (Kuo & Tsai, 1986). As to effectiveness in sports activities, there is a study by Maddi and Hess (1992). They measured hardiness levels of male, high school varsity basketball players in the summer and then obtained from their coaches the objective statistics of the players' performance throughout the ensuing season. Hardiness predicted six out of seven indices of performance in the expected direction, showing that, even among players good enough to be on the varsity team, hardiness predicted performance excellence.

Also, a number of studies have been done concerning hardiness and military personnel. For example Bartone (1999) found that soldiers who were high in hardiness adjusted better than those who were low in several ways, including health and life stresses. Further, there is also evidence that soldiers high in hardiness, not only adapted better during operational deployments than did their less hardy counterparts, but they also responded more favourably in the months following their return from deployments (Britt, Adler, & Bartone, 2001). Johnsen, Jarle, Pallesen, Bartone, and Nissestad (2009) have found a positive relationship between hardiness and leadership behaviour among US Navy cadets. Hardiness has also been found to be predictive of performance success in soldiers undergoing special-forces training in Norwegian Naval Academy cadets (Bartone, Johnsen, Eid, Brun, & Laberg, 2002). Similarly, there was a positive correlation between hardiness and both retention and performance excellence in West Point cadets undergoing training to become officers (Maddi, Matthews, Kelly, Villarreal, & White, 2012).

In addition to studies of the relationship of hardiness to performance are other studies concerning the expected negative relationship of hardiness with conduct problems, such as alcohol and gambling abuse. For example Maddi, Wadhwa, and Haier (1996) considered alcohol and drug use among high school graduates about to enter college. Whereas a family risk factor index was positively correlated with self-report of whether alcohol or drugs were tried, hardiness was negatively related to self-report of frequency with which these substances were used. As to more objective measurement, drugs and alcohol use were assessed through urine screens, which were also negatively related to hardiness.

Similar results were obtained in a study of Norwegian military defense personnel, showing a negative relationship between hardiness and alcohol abuse (Bartone, Hystad, Eid, & Brevik, 2012). Also found in a sample of college students is a negative relationship between hardiness and gambling (Maddi et al., in press).

Comparison of hardiness and other possible predictors

Understandably enough, some questions have arisen as to whether hardiness is little more than some other personality variable. This has led to several empirical studies comparing hardiness and some other possible predictors of performance.

One other possible predictor that has been proposed is negative affectivity, or neuroticism (e.g. Funk & Houston, 1987; Hull, Van Treuren, & Virnelli, 1987). Hardiness findings cannot be explained away as no more than negative affectivity. This is indicated by a study (Maddi & Khoshaba, 1994) in which hardiness and an accepted measure of negative affectivity were entered into regression analyses as independent variables in the attempt to predict the clinical scales of the Minnesota Multiphasic Personality Inventory (MMPI) as dependent variables. With the effects of negative affectivity controlled, hardiness was still a pervasive negative predictor of MMPI clinical scale scores.

Another alternative predictor that could be confounding hardiness results is optimism. In considering this possibility, Maddi and Hightower (1999) did three related studies, which compared the relative influence of hardiness and optimism on transformational and regressive coping. Involving undergraduate students with a wide range of everyday experiences, the first two studies differed in the tests used to assess transformational and regressive coping styles. Nonetheless, the results were the same: by comparison with optimism, hardiness was a more powerful positive predictor of transformational coping and a negative predictor of regressive coping than was optimism. In the third study, the same approach was used in a sample on women who had breast lumps and were arriving at a specialty clinic for diagnosis of whether or not the lumps were cancerous. Under this life-threatening stressor, optimism finally showed as many coping effects as did hardiness, but it was still true that only hardiness was a negative predictor of regressive coping. Taken together, these three studies show that hardiness is a better predictor of effective coping, and that optimism, by comparison, may be laced with naive complacency.

Another alternative to hardiness that has been proposed is grit, which is considered the courage of having a definite goal that affects performance under stress and will never be given up (Duckworth & Quinn, 2009). By comparison, hardiness is the existential courage to continue to learn from and change under life's stresses (Maddi, 2002).

To investigate this, a sample of cadets at the US Military Academy were tested for hardiness and grit some weeks before their training began, and then their performance evaluations were followed during the four years of the intentionally stressful training. The results of the study showed that hardiness was a better predictor than grit of cadet retention and performance (Maddi et al., 2012; Maddi, Matthews et al., in press; Maddi, Savino et al., in press).

Current practice applications of the hardiness approach

There is now a growing, practical need for hardiness assessment and training. This practical need is growing due to the increasing rate of change that is making life more turbulent, what some think of as chaos (Naisbitt, 1982; Peters, 1988). Change is fueled by our transition from industrial to information societies, with everyone scurrying to keep up with the continual, dramatic advances in computer and internet technologies and the changes they introduce into everyday life. Trying to adapt to the pressures of change, companies are continually restructuring (e.g. decentralizing, merging, downsizing, upsizing), which certainly influences the lives of employees. In the attempt to help individuals deal well and grow with all this change, Maddi and Khoshaba (2005) have developed hardiness assessment and training procedures that can be used in consulting with individuals and organizations.

As to hardiness assessment, there is now the HardiSurvey III-R, a valid and reliable sixty-five-item questionnaire that measures the vulnerability factors of high stress, strain, and regressive coping along with the resilience factors of high hardiness attitudes, problem-solving coping, and supportive social interactions (Maddi & Khoshaba, 2001). Vulnerability and resilience factors are compared with each other, and with available norms, leading to a wellness ratio. This test can be taken on our website (www.HardinessInstitute.com), which will generate a comprehensive report for you about your resilience or vulnerability under stress.

As to hardiness training, there is now a comprehensive workbook (Khoshaba & Maddi, 2008) that includes instructions, exercises, case studies, and evaluation procedures concerning how to engage in problem-solving (rather than avoidance) coping, socially supportive (rather than conflictual) interactions, and beneficial (rather the overindulgent) self-care. You are also shown how to use what is learned to deepen your hardy attitudes of commitment, control, and challenge, so that once the training is over, you will have the courage and the strategies to do the hard work involved in improving your functioning in everyday living. This workbook can be used by trainees on their own or with the supervision of a certified hardiness trainer.

There are some studies showing the effectiveness of the hardiness training procedure. In a study utilizing an earlier version of the training procedure, Maddi, Kahn, and Maddi (1998) trained managers at IBT in the year following the deregulation of the telephone industry. The results of the study showed that after the training was over, these managers performed more effectively and felt less anxious and overwhelmed, despite the huge disruption of the company. Similarly, in a waiting-list control study of IBT managers (Maddi, 1987), those who went through the training, not only increased in their hardy attitudes, but also in job satisfaction and social support, while simultaneously decreasing in both self-report an objective indices of strain. These beneficial results were still present at a six-month follow-up testing. In another study (Maddi et al., 2002), a sample of high-risk undergraduates went through hardiness training when they arrived at college and showed higher retention rates than did other high-risk undergraduates who did not experience the training.

Further, a more recent study (Maddi, Harvey, Khoshaba, Fazel, & Resurreccion, 2009) showed that undergraduate students who went through a hardiness training course based on the work-book, by comparison with a carefully developed control group, not only increased in hardiness, but also in grade point average at graduation.

Concluding remarks

In terms of conceptualization and empirical support, it appears that the hardiness approach has had growing validity over the years. This encourages its use in assessment and training to increase the likelihood that individuals and organizations will be able to turn stressful circumstances from potential disasters into growth opportunities instead.

References

Atella, M. (1989). *Crossing boundaries: Effectiveness and health among Western managers living in China* (Unpublished Doctoral Dissertation). Chicago: University of Chicago.

Bartone, P. T. (1989). Predictors of stress related illness in city bus drivers. *Journal of Occupational Medicine, 31*(8), 657–663.

Bartone, P. T. (1999). Hardiness protects against war-related stress in army reserve forces. *Consulting Psychology Journal: Practice and Research, 51*(2), 72–82.

Bartone, P. T., Hystad, S. W., Eid, J., & Brevik, J. I. (2012). Psychological hardiness and coping style as risk/resilience factors for alcohol abuse. *Military Medicine, 177*(5), 517–524.

Bartone, P. T., Johnsen, B. H., Eid, J., Brun, W., & Laberg, J. C. (2002). Factors influencing small-unit cohesion in Norwegian Navy officer cadets. *Military Psychology, 14*(1), 1–22.

Britt, T. W., Adler, A. B., & Bartone, P. T. (2001). Deriving benefits from stressful events: The role of engagement in meaningful work and hardiness. *Journal of Occupational Health Psychology, 6*(1), 53–63.

Duckworth, A. L., & Quinn, P. D. (2009). Development and validation of the short grit scale. *Journal of Personality Assessment, 91*(2), 166–174.

Funk, S. C. (1992). Hardiness: A review of theory and research. *Health Psychology, 11*(5), 335–345.

Funk, S. C., & Houston, B. K. (1987). A critical analysis of the hardiness scale's validity and utility. *Journal of Personality and Social Psychology, 53*(3), 572–578.

Hull, J. G., VanTreuren, R. R., & Virnelli, S. (1987). Hardiness and health: A critique and alternative approach. *Journal of Personality and Social Psychology, 53*(3), 518–530.

Johnsen, B. J., Jarle, E., Pallesen, S., Bartone, P. T., & Nissestad, O. A. (2009). Predicting transformational leadership in naval cadets: Effects of personality hardiness and training. *Journal of Applied Social Psychology, 39*(9), 2213–2235.

Keane, A., Ducette, J., & Adler, D. (1985). Stress in ICU and non-ICU nurses. *Nursing Research, 34*(4), 231–236.

Khoshaba, D. M., & Maddi, S. R. (1999). Early experiences in hardiness development. *Consulting Psychology Journal: Practice and Research, 51*(2), 106–116.

Khoshaba, D. M., & Maddi, S. R. (2008). *Hardi training: Managing stressful change* (4th ed.). Newport Beach, CA: Hardiness Institute.

Kierkegaard, S. (1954). *The sickness unto death.* New York: Doubleday.

Kobasa, S. C. (1982). Commitment and coping in stress resistance among lawyers. *Journal of Personality and Social Psychology, 42*(4), 707–717.

Kuo, W. H., & Tsai, Y. (1986). Social networking, hardiness, and immigrant's mental health. *Journal of Health and Social Behavior, 27*(2), 133–149.

Maddi, S. R. (1965). Motivational aspects of creativity. *Journal of Personality, 33*(3), 330–347.

Maddi, S. R. (1987). Hardiness training at Illinois Bell Telephone. In J. P. Opatz (Ed.), *Health promotion evaluation* (pp. 101–115). Stevens Point, WI: National Wellness Institute.

Salvatore R. Maddi

Maddi, S. R. (1990). Issues and interventions in stress mastery. In H. S. Friedman (Ed.), *Personality and disease* (pp. 121–154). New York: Wiley.

Maddi, S. R. (2002). The story of hardiness: Twenty years of theorizing, research, and practice. *Consulting Psychology Journal: Practice and Research, 54*(3), 175–185.

Maddi, S. R. (2006). Hardiness: The courage to grow from stresses. *Journal of Positive Psychology, 1*(3), 160–168.

Maddi, S. R., & Harvey, R. H. (2005). Hardiness considered across cultures. In P. T. Wong & L. C. J. Wong (Eds.), *Handbook of multicultural perspectives on stress and coping* (pp. 403–420). New York: Springer.

Maddi, S. R., Harvey, R. H., Khoshaba, D. M., Fazel, M., & Resurreccion, N. (2009). Hardiness facilitates performance in college. *Journal of Positive Psychology, 4*(6), 566–577.

Maddi, S. R., & Hess, M. (1992). Personality hardiness and success in basketball. *International Journal of Sports Psychology, 23*(4), 360–368.

Maddi, S. R., & Hightower, M. (1999). Hardiness and optimism as expressed in coping patterns. *Consulting Psychology Journal, 51*(2), 95–105.

Maddi, S. R., Kahn, S., & Maddi, K. L. (1998). The effectiveness of hardiness training. *Consulting Psychology Journal, 50*(2), 78–86.

Maddi, S. R., & Khoshaba, D. M. (1994). Hardiness and mental health. *Journal of Personality Assessment, 63*(2), 265–274.

Maddi, S. R., & Khoshaba, D. M. (2001). *HardiSurvey III-R: Test development and internet instruction manual.* Newport Beach, CA: Hardiness Institute.

Maddi, S. R., & Khoshaba, D. M. (2005). *Resilience at work: How to succeed no matter what life throws at you.* New York: Amacom.

Maddi, S. R., Khoshaba, D. M., Jensen, K., Carter, E., Lu, J. H., & Harvey, R. H. (2002). Hardiness training for high-risk undergraduates. *NACADA Journal, 22*(1), 5–55.

Maddi, S. R., & Kobasa, S. C. (1984). *The hardy executive: Health under stress.* Homewood, IL: Dow Jones-Irwin.

Maddi, S. R., Matthews, M. D., Kelly, D. R., Villarreal, B., Gundersen, K., & Savino, S. C. (in press). The continuing role of hardiness and grit on performance and retention in West Point cadets. Military Psychology.

Maddi, S. R., Matthews, M. D., Kelly, D. R., Villarreal, B., & White, M. (2012). The role of hardiness and grit in predicting performance and retention of USMA cadets. *Military Psychology, 24*(1), 19–28.

Maddi, S. R., Savino, S. C. M., Bach, S. C., Saifabad, N., Shirmohammadi, M., & Brown, S. D. (in press). Hardiness is negatively related to gambling. *Journal of Personality.*

Maddi, S. R., Wadhwa, P., & Haier, R. J. (1996). Relationship of hardiness to alcohol and drug use in adolescents. *The American Journal of Drug and Alcohol Abuse, 22*(2), 247–257.

Naisbitt, J. (1982). *Megatrends: Ten new directions transforming our lives.* New York: Warner Books.

Nietzsche, F. (1969). *The will to power.* W. Kaufmann (ed.). New York: Vintage.

Orr, E., & Westman, M. (1990). Hardiness as a stress moderator: A review. In M. Rosenbaum (Ed.), *Learned resourcefulness: On coping skills, self-control, and adaptive behavior* (pp. 64–94). New York: Springer-Verlag.

Ouellette, S. C. (1993). Inquiries into hardiness. In L. Goldberger & S. Bresnitz (Eds.), *Handbook of stress: Theoretical and clinical aspects* (2nd ed., pp. 77–100). New York: Free Press.

Peters, T. (1988). *Thriving on chaos.* New York: Knopf.

Sinclair, R. R., & Tetrick, L. E. (2000). Implications of item wording for hardiness structure, relations to neuroticism, and stress buffering. *Journal of Research in Personality, 34*(1), 1–25.

10

Collective resilience and social support in the face of adversity

Evidence from social psychology

Chris Cocking

An alien observer of the global media coverage of disasters emanating from planet Earth could be forgiven for thinking that humanity is facing an increasingly precarious existence. Indeed, the Centre for Research on the Epidemiology of Disasters (CRED), which maintains an Emergency Events Database[1] (EM-DAT), recorded 6,873 natural disasters worldwide between 1994 and 2013 (an average of nearly 1 per day), claiming 1.35 million lives and affecting over 218 million people in total. However, what is often neglected is that, despite these privations, people and communities often cope much better than they are usually given credit for and can show remarkable resilience instead. This chapter will illustrate the possibility for such resilience in the face of adversity and document how the concept itself has evolved from initially individualist perspectives, to more group-oriented approaches that explore how community cohesion can be maintained in the face of disruption and upheaval. Recent evidence from studies of mass emergencies that support the notion of collective resilience emerging from a sense of shared threat will also be considered and the implications of such findings for emergency planning and response, as well as considerations of recent critiques of resilience.

Individual/developmental resilience

The term 'resilience' is almost ubiquitous in current popular and academic discourses,[2] and in the 2015 UK TV election debate between the party leaders, the term was mentioned within five minutes of the debate starting.[3] There has also been considerable discussion in recent years over what the term actually means,[4] and Jackson, Firtko, and Edenborough (2007) illustrate the different conceptualisations that have been attributed to resilience: "Resilience has been constructed as a trajectory, a continuum, a system, a trait, a process, a cycle, and a qualitative category" (p. 1). While the term itself has most probably been in use for centuries, academic studies of 'resilience' are comparatively more recent, having begun within the last half century (Masten, Gewirtz, & Sapienza, 2013). It was initially used to describe the resilience of physical, ecological and organisational systems to 'bounce back' after systemic shocks or external attacks and is now also used to explain how people and communities can cope with the challenges they may face through their day-to-day existence (Norris, Stevens, Pfefferbaum, Wyche, & Pfefferbaum, 2008). It is currently used in developmental fields to look at children and young people's development from both academic (Ungar, 2012) and practitioner[5] perspectives, although resilience in adults has also been explored (e.g. Reich, Zautra, & Hall, 2010). Ungar (2012) described how five different recognised phases (or 'waves') have emerged from resilience research. The first phase focussed on exploring possible individual genetic or psychological factors that made certain children more resilient than others (e.g. Ungar, 2006). However, these approaches that considered individual resilience in isolation to other factors have been countered by research (e.g. Rutter, 1987) showing the protective factors that external social influences (such as family, school etc.) can also have on children. This led to a second wave that explored such protective factors and then a third wave that looked at how positive development under stress could help children develop resilience in response to personal challenges or harmful environments (Ungar, Brown, Liebenberg, Cheung, & Levine, 2008). As research began to consider these varied influences, resilience models became increasingly complex, thus leading to a fourth wave that tried to incorporate such complexity and that introduced four related concepts to consider within such models: decentrality, complexity, atypicality and cultural sensitivity. While resilience models that emerged from this wave can be quite detailed and reflect great complexity within their structure (e.g. Hart, Blincow, & Thomas, 2007), there was a concern that wider social and community influences on resilience still needed to be considered in more depth, leading to a fifth wave that is increasingly guiding current related academic research – that of community resilience.

Community resilience

In response to this perceived bias towards individualised perspectives on resilience, there has been a shift to consider in more detail, not only the wider social and cultural influences on individual development, but also how communities in general deal with adversity. This fifth wave of resilience has been applied to considering the healthy development of children and adolescents (Hart et al., in press; Ungar, 2012) and different possible cultural influences on resilience models. Ungar (2008) highlights the need to be aware of context-specific influences on resilience rather than assuming a 'one-size-fits-all' approach, as it can be problematic to try to impose culturally specific resilience models in situations where they may be less relevant or even duplicate pre-existing support networks. For instance, Nguyen-Gillham, Giacaman, Naser, and Boyce (2008) explored resilience in Palestinian youths and suggested that the concept has largely been developed from Western perspectives, which tend to prioritise individualised approaches and ignores the potential for communal care and support (a concept known locally as *sumud* or steadfastness, p. 292).

There is also a growing recognition of the need to explore broader applications of resilience beyond developmental perspectives and how communities can support each other in times of crisis. This is especially relevant in the case of mass emergencies (such as flooding, disease outbreaks, terrorist attacks etc.) as, while individuals may perceive and experience events from their own unique perspectives, they are by definition a collective phenomenon. For instance, Kaniasty and Norris (2004) argued that disasters are "community-level events that bring harm, pain and loss to large numbers of people simultaneously" (p. 200). Such community resilience could be considered as a qualitatively distinct concept from individual resilience because, as Norris et al. (2008) argued, there is often more to community resilience than a mere collection of resilient individuals. The UK Cabinet Office (2011) described community resilience as "communities and individuals harnessing local resources and expertise to help themselves in an emergency, in a way that complements the response of the emergency services" (p. 4), and suggested that different communities that can be affected by mass emergencies. For instance, four different conceptual communities are described when considering emergency planning and response: 'geographical communities', where people are in close proximity with each other; 'interest communities', where members have an existing shared interest (such as faith groups, sports clubs, online communities etc.); 'circumstance communities', where people are brought together by being affected by a similar incident (a train crash, terrorist attack etc.); and 'supporter communities', those who plan for, and respond to emergencies, both professional and voluntary (such as the emergency services). There can also be overlap between these different communities, as supporters may come from the same geographical location or have the same shared interest, although communities of circumstance could also comprise of people who were previously complete strangers (UK Cabinet Office, 2011, p. 12).

Early psychological 'panic' models of mass emergencies (e.g. La Piere, 1938; Smelser, 1962; Straus, 1944) assumed collective vulnerability during disasters, such as selfish, irrational behaviour ('mass panic', looting etc.). However, such models have been criticised by later work (e.g. Cocking, 2013 a, b; Drury, Cocking, & Reicher, 2009 a, b) as being overly polemical and unsupported by evidence from studies of numerous historical emergencies since World War II (e.g. Fritz, 1996; Quarantelli, 2001). They report a wealth of evidence that contradicts the traditional clichéd assumptions of societal breakdown and irrational, selfish behaviour during disasters and instead provide compelling support for the idea that social attachment bonds endure even during life-threatening emergencies (e.g. Mawson, 2005), which can also be the basis for general community cohesion and resilience in the face of shared adversity. Furthermore, the common fear of social collapse after disasters is rarely supported by detailed examination of the available evidence, but this does not stop often sensational coverage of 'social collapse' after disasters. For instance, in the aftermath of Hurricane Katrina, there were lurid media descriptions of alleged anti-social behaviours in New Orleans, but Voorhees, Vick and Perkins (2007) explored in detail the events behind such coverage and found that descriptions of survivors' behaviours as 'looting' or 'gathering essential supplies' often depended on the ethnicity and/or social class of the people doing it. Furthermore, more generalised reports of anti-social behaviour in the media were contradicted by research conducted by the University of Delaware's Disaster Research Center (Barsky, Trainor, & Torres, 2006; Rodriguez, Trainor, & Quarantelli, 2006) that found pro-social behaviour was the norm instead. This general maintenance of social order has been described as the concept of social capital (Aldrich, 2013; Dynes, 2006), whereby social bonds endure, even if physical infrastructure (such as health services, transport links, food distribution networks etc.) is compromised:

> Recovery of societies depends on their internal social networks, which create the bonds called social capital. These bonds . . . determine the recovery and resilience of any society. Through bridging individuals beyond ethnicity and other social boundaries, places such as public schools, and clubs, all contribute to building societal resilience. All these factors link social capital, creating good neighbourliness and eventually contributing to the general wellbeing and recovery of any society in case of disasters. This bonding, bridging and linking of individual are essential in creating social capital which is critical after disaster It is social infrastructure and not physical infrastructure that drives recovery and resilience of any community.
>
> *(Aldrich, 2013, pp. 16–17)*

There are also tangible, practical benefits for communities that have existing social capital networks. For instance, Perez-Sales, Cervellon, Vazquez, Vidales, and Gaborit's (2005) study of community resilience after the 2001 El Salvador earthquake, found that, when the earthquake shelters for survivors reflected characteristics of their own local community, then there was more participation in community activities, and participants reported more positive emotional memories.

Emergent resilience and the Social Identity Model of Collective Resilience (SIMCR)

The concept of community resilience explains well how existing social bonds can endure in communities under threat, However, there is also the possibility that new links may be created when such communities face adversity, as people come together to face a common threat and experience a sense of unity that they may not have previously felt. This idea has been developed by recent work exploring mass emergencies by social psychologists who propose that mass emergencies can be a source of emergent collective resilience (Cocking, 2013a, b; Drury et al., 2009a, b). Consequently, Drury (2012) formulated the Social Identity Model of Collective Resilience (SIMCR), which suggests the following psychological processes that often occur during a mass emergency. First, collective resilience emerges from the shared experience of facing a common threat, which can develop even amongst crowds of complete strangers where there may be minimal pre-existing social attachment bonds (as often happens in spontaneous mass emergencies, such as the terrorist attacks of 9/11 or 7/7). Drury (2012) explains this seemingly counter-intuitive notion by detailing the theoretical position of the SIMCR in terms of the possible psychological antecedents leading to both psychological and behavioural consequences. Thus, individuals can experience a cognitive shift so that they begin to see themselves as a psychological crowd rather than a physical aggregate of people (see Figure 10.1). This happens in crowd emergencies

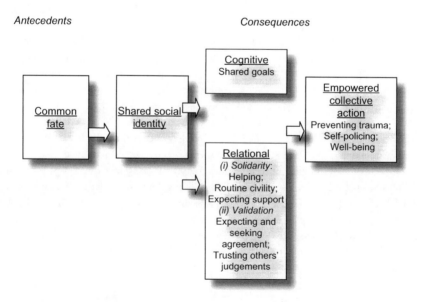

Figure 10.1   The Social Identity Model of Collective Resilience
Source: Adapted from Drury, 2012, p. 201.

when a common fate results in a sense of unity from the perception of a shared threat (e.g. 'We're all in this together'). This can cause a psychological change whereby people begin to see themselves in more collective (rather than individual) terms that promotes a relational transformation in the ways that people interact with each other. This creates more social solidarity as crowd members develop a shared sense of psychological unity with each other, meaning that the boundaries between the self and others are less salient, and people become more likely to identify (and so empathise) with others in need. Finally, empowered collective action becomes more likely, as those affected begin to engage in co-operative and/or altruistic behaviour (as opposed to selfish, uncooperative behaviour), as they not only feel able to help others whose needs they are more likely to empathise with, but they also feel that they can draw upon collective support from others if necessary. Such support is not always manifested by individual heroism (although this can also happen) but tends to manifest itself in what has been termed the routine civility of everyday social cohesion (Reicher & Haslam, 2010). So, for instance, during emergency evacuations, even if people do not help others themselves, they will tend to stand back to let others pass and not obstruct others who are helping those in greater need. This support manifests itself during the acute phases of an emergency but also in its aftermath as people begin to rebuild their communities and provide mutual psychosocial support that can help shield survivors from possible psychological trauma (Williams & Drury, 2009).

It is also perhaps worth considering a brief caveat here before assuming that *all* crowd behaviour during emergencies is necessarily pro-social and that *no one* behaves in selfish and/or anti-social ways. The picture is often more nuanced, and it is possible that people will behave competitively in crowds if a common identity is less salient (e.g. the 'Black Friday' retail phenomenon that developed in the US whereby shoppers compete for limited deals on reduced goods[6]). What appears to happen is that social norms develop amongst those in emergency crowds whereby co-operative behaviour predominates. Therefore, those that behave co-operatively would be considered as representative of others within the situation, and any instances of selfish and/or anti-social behaviour towards others would be considered as anti-normative and consequently rejected or even sanctioned by other crowd members. So, for instance, Connell's (2001) study of collective behaviour on 9/11 found that, during the evacuation of the World Trade Center, behaviour was generally calm and orderly with people helping others. But if anyone behaved selfishly by trying to 'cut in line' (p. 14), they were quickly berated by others and made to wait their turn.

Recent evidence

Evidence to support the SIMCR comes from studies (Drury et al., 2009a, b) of various mass emergencies (such as the 1989 Hillsborough football disaster,[7] and the 7/7/2005 London bombings[8]), where survivors' accounts often contradicted clichéd stereotypes of selfish or 'panicked' behaviour and instead reported a generalised sense of shared identity and co-operation amongst survivors and eye-witnesses, even during life-threatening emergencies. More recent work has developed these findings to explore in more detail the following myths that are often associated with mass emergency behaviour, such as the notion of 'stampedes' (Cocking, 2013a); the assumption that survivors of emergencies will be so stunned into inaction during the acute phases of emergencies that they would be unable to support each other before outside help arrives (Cocking, 2013b); and the common usage of the term 'panic' to describe emergency behaviour (Cocking & Drury, 2014). Each phenomenon will now be explored in turn.

1 Stampede myths

'Stampede' is a term commonly used to describe crowd crush disasters (such as in Shanghai, China, 31 December 2014[9]), when there have been injuries and/or fatalities involved, implying that people have fled in a mindless, animalistic way, without any regard for their fellow human beings. However, detailed studies of such incidents rarely match with this assumption, with fatalities usually resulting from compressive asphyxia (because of sheer crowd density), as opposed to people being deliberately trampled by other crowd members as they try to escape (e.g. Fruin, 1993; Helbing & Mukerji, 2012). People also tend to help each other, and if this doesn't happen, it is usually because they are physically unable to do so due to physical pressures in the crowd (Johnson, 1987). Furthermore, Cocking's (2013a) interview study of crowd flight during disorder found that, while crowds can scatter after being charged by the police, they maintained co-operative social ties (such as helping others who had fallen over). Participants also often reported an enhanced sense of psychological unity that increased crowd militancy and escalated crowd disorder. Therefore, the term 'stampede' is considered inadequate in explaining crowd behaviour in emergencies, and its use has been rejected in academic fora.[10]

2 Bystander apathy

A common assumption within populist narratives is that people in crowds are less likely to help others in need. This has become known in social psychology as the 'bystander effect' (Darley & Latané, 1970) and has been used to illustrate crowd vulnerability in emergencies, as those affected will be too 'panicked' or shocked to help each other and would need direction from professional responders. However, Manning, Levine and Collins (2007) highlight the all-encompassing (and somewhat contradictory) nature of such a position, as it assumes that people in mass emergencies will either 'panic' and behave irrationally or will be frozen into inaction. Recent research into mass emergencies, such as the 7/7/2005 London bombings (Cocking, 2013b; Drury et al., 2009b), has found that such crowd apathy is unsupported by the numerous examples of cooperation amongst survivors and witnesses in the immediate aftermath of the explosions before the emergency services arrived. The concept of spontaneous crowd co-operation has been labelled 'zero responders' and can be utilised as a potential force multiplier for the emergency services (Cole, Walters, & Lynch, 2011), especially during siege situations where there can be delays in victims receiving outside help (such as the terrorist attack on the Westgate shopping mall in Kenya, 25 September 2013[11]).

3 The pervasiveness of 'panic' narratives

The term 'panic' has been broadly rejected in academic circles as it is not supported by evidence (e.g. Quarantelli, 2001) but is still used in descriptions of emergency behaviour – even amongst those who would have good reason to reject its implications (such as the survivors of disasters). For instance, Cocking and Drury (2014) found that survivors of the 1989 Hillsborough football disaster used the term in their accounts, despite the controversies around the disaster and its causation. They concluded that these survivors certainly rejected the implications of the term 'panic' (such as the false assumption that they were somehow to 'blame' for the tragedy) but still used the term because it is so deeply embedded in wider social discourse. Indeed, some problematised the term in their accounts but felt they were constrained by the language available to them ('[T]he only way I can describe it is panic' p. 93). So, the term is not only inaccurate to describe human behaviour in emergencies but is also deeply ideological. Therefore, 'panic' should not be used to describe such situations, and discourses that better reflect collective resilience should be encouraged.

Enduring or temporary nature of collective resilience?

There is considerable evidence to support the notion of emergent collective resilience during the acute phases of an emergency, and in a previous overview of the literature, Cocking (2013c) argued that individuals (and even whole communities) affected by disasters could come together to provide mutual social support, and this support could have a role in shielding survivors from psychological trauma. However, whether such resilience can endure and remain in the aftermath and recovery phase is a topic of debate. For instance, Kaniasty and Norris (2004), argued that while there is often 'instantaneous post-disaster mobilization of help and support' (p. 202), both suffering and assistance can also be distributed inequitably in a way that mirrors pre-existing structural inequalities (as it is usually socially and economically disadvantaged communities that are disproportionately affected by disasters). Furthermore, such spontaneous mobilisations of support can deteriorate once the immediate threat from the disaster dissipates – especially if resources are depleted. Therefore, they suggested the Social Support Deterioration Deterrence (SSDD) model to capture these nuances in post-disaster social support (Kaniasty & Norris, 2004 p. 206), although they felt that deterioration in support was not inevitable, and survivors could continue to benefit from social support that could shield them from emotional distress under the right conditions. Fritz (1996) suggested that disasters can cause a 'societal shock, which disrupts habitual, institutionalized patterns of behavior and renders people amenable to social and personal change' (p. 55). So, perhaps disasters create a brief period of time where previous social and economic inequalities become less salient (as there are more immediate concerns to address), thus creating the possibility for brief post-disaster utopias to emerge (as suggested by Solnit, 2009) before such communities are disrupted by the re-imposition of 'normal' social structures (and consequently the reappearance of pre-existing economic and political inequalities).

Critiques of resilience, and is it more than mere sociological Prozac?

The frequent usage of resilience in academic and popular discourse means that it is perhaps not surprising that the concept has come under critical scrutiny, with social and cultural theorists (e.g. Bottrell, 2013; de Lint & Chazal, 2013) attacking resilience for its potential to place responsibility for dealing with social inequality with the individual, rather than challenging the social inequalities that can threaten individual resilience. However, Hart et al. (in preparation) address such attacks by suggesting that resilience perspectives that conduct more co-produced research can help empower people to challenge and overcome social injustice rather than perpetuating them (Bolzan & Gale, 2012). They also recognise the need to consider resilience within its broader contexts, rather than locating it within one's own individual responsibility, so that issues of social injustice and inequality can be addressed and challenged. Others (e.g. Furedi, 2007; Harrison, 2012) have argued that, while the concept of resilience in itself may not necessarily be problematic, the way that it can influence political narratives can be, as it can shift the emphasis away from understanding and challenging existing structural inequalities that could hinder long-term resilience, and as a consequence, it could be used as a justification for minimising governmental and/or corporate responsibility to address such inequalities. For instance, Harrison's (2012) study of social hardship in

UK towns found that individual families adopted what could be perceived as 'resilient' moves to deal with their own financial hardships (such as spending less from their weekly family budgets on essentials), but to assume that these are facets of a broader long-term community resilience could reduce pressure on local and national authorities to tackle the root causes of the structural inequalities that give rise to such deprivation. She concluded that, while the concept of vulnerability is often seen in terms of broader economic and political power relationships, resilience 'tends to characterize as individual that which should be understood to be a result of collective effort' (p. 110).

There are also broader possible ideological implications with the concept of resilience, in that, if local and national authorities assume that communities will be able to cope no matter what disaster befalls them, then this could negatively affect resource allocation for emergency management planning and response budgets. This has especially been an issue for resilience research in the UK, as in 2010, the newly elected coalition government introduced the idea of the 'Big Society',[12] which was intended to empower local communities to provide services and support. However, this initiative attracted criticism from Ishkanian and Szreter (2012) who argued that seeking increased involvement from the voluntary sector could be used as a justification for covering the gaps in public spending that have developed as a result of recent austerity measures. In 2013, the Civil Exchange think-tank even argued that the concept of the 'Big Society' was not suitable for communities where there was existing deprivation (despite these being the communities that would arguably benefit more from increased voluntary activity) and concluded it was "a policy better suited to the leafy suburbs".[13] It is easy to see how such concerns over the 'Big Society' can emerge, as the UK Cabinet Office (2011) National Framework on Community Resilience explicitly refers to the concept: "This programme is part of the Government's 'Big Society' commitment to reduce the barriers which prevent people from being able to help themselves and to become more resilient to shocks" (p. 3).

Some take a more overtly polemical view, such as Evans and Reid (2014), who suggest that the term resilience is a neo-liberal deception that can disempower threatened communities. They suggest we should instead embrace humanity's inherent vulnerability in an uncertain world and 'live dangerously', because it is impossible to live in a world entirely free of risk, and insecurity is a necessary part of the human condition. Diprose (2015) felt that promoting resilience also had the potential for quite reactionary consequences, as it could encourage people to pursue their own personal gain over the interests of others and could even be used to perpetuate inequality and/or social injustice or as justification for imposing measures that further exacerbate inequality (see Figure 10.2). She concluded that 'resilience is no basis for contentious politics, and its circulation as a dominant idea may do more harm than good' (p. 45).

These critiques of resilience raise some legitimate concerns about how the concept can be misused in ways that could negatively impact upon long-term individual and community well-being if wider social contexts and potential threats to resilience are not considered in sufficient detail. However, there are two potential issues worth considering that illustrate possible nuances between different possible conceptualisations of resilience.

First, there could be clearer conceptual distinctions drawn between how individuals and/or family units may seek their own personal strategies to achieve resilience that by definition may not be available to all (such as competing with others to achieve comparatively greater economic, social, or political status) and the emergent collective resilience of empowered communities coming together to respond to specific short-term threats and then perhaps challenge the unequal structures that can make some communities more vulnerable to hazards than others in the long term. It could be argued that the concept of emergent collective resilience is less vulnerable to

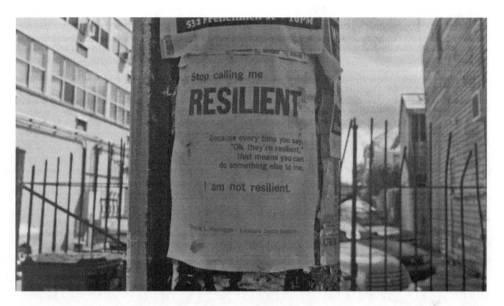

Figure 10.2   Poster published by the Louisiana Justice Institute, New Orleans, USA
Source: http://candychang.com/resilient/. Printed here by kind permission of artist Candy Chang, http://candychang.com.

the critiques that have been directed at individual resilience models, as it is much better placed to explore and critique the social contexts (and existing social inequalities) that can influence or even hinder individual resilience and well-being.

Second, advocates of emergent collective resilience approaches (e.g. Drury, 2012; Furedi, 2007) assert that the evidence showing how communities can unite and support each other in the face of sudden upheavals should never be used as justification for local and national governments to cut back on resource allocation and/or excuse public spending cuts – something that Harrison (2012) implies could happen if local and national governments assume that people will inevitably 'bounce back' from adversity. This has direct implications for pre-disaster preparedness and post-disaster response mitigation, as people can only behave resiliently if they are given the capacity and resources to do so, and if such resources are lacking, any consequent collective resilience may be less likely to emerge. So for instance, a fundamental theoretical tenet of the SIMCR is that people need to feel a shared sense of threat in order for them to develop a common psychological identity, and so the mere exposure to traumatic events may not necessarily promote collective resilience. Therefore, if the threat is not considered to be shared equitably within the affected community (e.g. if there are individuals and/or groups that are perceived to be less adversely affected or perceived to enjoy greater post-disaster support), then this could hamper the development of such a shared identity, which would make unified collective action to support others less likely. For instance, Klein (2007) argues that disasters often create new opportunities for exploitation by the private sector, which can exacerbate economic inequality, and highlights the disturbing dystopian potential of what she termed 'disaster apartheid', whereby access to support and medical aid in New Orleans post-Hurricane Katrina, was divided along economic and racial lines (p. 408).

Implications

There are also more specific implications for emergency planning and response when considering whether communities exposed to threat behave in vulnerable or resilient ways. For instance, if those in authority assume that those affected by disasters are susceptible to 'panic' and/or anti-social behaviour, then more paternalistic or even authoritarian measures are likely to be adopted. Consequently, this could mean that the focus of the authorities' disaster response could be more influenced by the desire to maintain 'law and order' rather than ensuring public safety and efficient evacuation. This can have implications for the allocation of resources and may also have fatal consequences. For instance, Tierney, Bevc and Kuligowski (2006) argued that the exaggerated media accounts of 'looting' and reports of gang-rapes and multiple murders (which later turned out to be false) in New Orleans after Hurricane Katrina, led the local police department to re-allocate police resources to deal with 'lawbreakers' rather than helping people in danger, and this reduced the chances of survival of stranded residents, some of whom may not have perished had they been rescued earlier. Therefore, Drury (2012) suggested that, rather than being seen as part of the problem, crowds could be viewed as a 'social cure' (p. 25). Previous examples of the potential contribution that zero-responders can make (e.g. Cocking 2013b; Cole et al., 2011) could be recognised by emergency responders as a way of involving communities in emergency planning and response and not assuming that they will 'panic' at the first sign of danger.

Conclusion

Despite some potential theoretical problems with overly individualistic interpretations of the broader theoretical paradigm, the concept of collective resilience still appears to have some utility. However, such utility may depend upon its associated theoretical models being able to consider the social context in which resilience can emerge (as well as the structural inequalities that may hinder such resilience from emerging), ensuring responsibility for achieving resilience is not placed with the individual and not prioritising the attainment of individual resilience over the collective well-being of the community as a whole. Recent theoretical advances in resilience research are currently addressing such issues, with some seeing greater theoretical synergy between individual and collective resilience approaches, as well as the potential to address and challenge inequality that may be responsible for a lack of resilience. For instance, Hart et al. (in preparation) suggest that 'bringing resilience research and practice with a social justice approach with giving an equal and simultaneous emphasis on individual and the wider system is possible' (p. 2).

Therefore, a dual approach to advancing collective resilience theory and research could perhaps guide further work in this area. First, continued efforts to explore and celebrate the strength of the human spirit in the face of continued adversity would be most welcome. However, it is also vital to maintain an ongoing emphasis on how such collective resilience can best be encouraged, so that communities are not only able to support each other but are also empowered to question (or even resist) the structural inequalities that can influence whether such resilience emerges or not. Then we will be closer to developing concepts of resilience that better serve those communities around the world that are often described as such and empowering them to better prepare for, and respond to, the threats we can all face in this uncertain world.

Notes

1 www.emdat.be/.
2 A recent Google Scholar search for 'resilience' scored over 1,160,000 hits: https://scholar.google.co.uk/scholar?hl=en&q=Resilience&btnG=&as_sdt=1%2C5&as_sdtp.

3 https://twitter.com/DrChrisCocking/status/583707246040875009.
4 Hart et al. (in press) list nearly twenty different possible definitions currently in use in resilience theory and research.
5 The University of Brighton–sponsored website (www.boingboing.org.uk/) is a good example of academic research collaborating with community practitioner and service user groups in the field of resilience.
6 http://dontpaniccorrectingmythsaboutthecrowd.blogspot.co.uk/2014/11/black-friday-incidents-are-not.html.
7 http://en.wikipedia.org/wiki/Hillsborough_disaster.
8 http://news.bbc.co.uk/1/shared/spl/hi/uk/05/london_blasts/what_happened/html/.
9 http://dontpaniccorrectingmythsaboutthecrowd.blogspot.co.uk/2015/01/shanghai-crowd-crush-tragedy.html.
10 http://drury-sussex-the-crowd.blogspot.co.uk/2011/01/why-do-stampedes-happen-at-crowd-events.html.
11 http://dontpaniccorrectingmythsaboutthecrowd.blogspot.co.uk/2013/09/zero-responders-nairobi-shopping-mall.html.
12 www.gov.uk/government/publications/building-the-big-society.
13 www.theguardian.com/politics/2013/dec/09/big-society-deprived-david-cameron-charitable-wealthy.

References

Aldrich, D. (2013). *Building resilience: Social capital in post disaster recovery*. A symposium on major disaster and resilience for society: Lessons learnt from the past, for the future. Dept of Civil Engineering, University of Tokyo, Retrieved from www.civil.t.u-tokyo.ac.jp/FSO/pdf/FSO_Symposium_2013_Booklet.pdf#page=18

Barsky, L., Trainor, J., & Torres, M. (2006). *Disaster realities in the aftermath of Hurricane Katrina: Revisiting the looting myth*. University of Delaware Disaster Research Center MISCELLANEOUS REPORT #53. Retrieved from http://udspace.udel.edu/bitstream/handle/19716/2367/Misc+Report+53.pdf?sequence=1

Bolzan, N., & Gale, F. (2012). Using an interrupted space to explore social resilience with marginalized young people. *Qualitative Social Work, 11,* 502–516.

Bottrell, D. (2013). Responsibilised resilience? Reworking neoliberal social policy texts. *M/C Journal of Media and Culture, 16*(5), 16.

Cocking, C. (2013a). Crowd flight during collective disorder-a momentary lapse of reason? *Journal of Investigative Psychology & Offender Profiling, 10*(2), 219–236.

Cocking, C. (2013b). Crowd resilience during the 7/7/2005 London bombings: Implications for the emergency services. *International Journal of the Emergency Services, 2*(2), 79–93.

Cocking, C. (2013c) Collective resilience versus collective vulnerability after disasters-a social psychological perspective. In R. Arora (Ed.), *Disaster management: A medical perspective* (pp. 449–463). Oxford, UK: CABI.

Cocking, C., & Drury, J. (2014). Talking about Hillsborough: "Panic" as discourse in survivors' accounts of the 1989 football stadium disaster. *Journal of Community and Applied Social Psychology, 24*(2), 86–99.

Cole, J., Walters, M., & Lynch, M. (2011). Part of the solution, not the problem: The crowd's role in emergency response. *Contemporary Social Science, 6*(3), 361–375.

Connell, R. (2001). *Collective behavior in the September 11, 2001 evacuation of the World Trade Center*. University of Delaware, Disaster Research Center. Preliminary paper #313. Retrieved from http://dspace.udel.edu/bitstream/handle/19716/683/PP313.pdf?sequence=1

Darley, J. M., & Latané, B. (1970). *The unresponsive bystander: Why doesn't he help?* New York, NY: Appleton Century Crofts.

De Lint, W., & Chazal, N. (2013). Resilience and criminal justice: Unsafe at low altitude. *Critical Criminology, 21*(2), 157–176.

Diprose, K. (2015). Resilience is futile. *Soundings: A Journal of Politics and Culture, 58,* 44–56.

Drury, J. (2012). Collective resilience in mass emergencies and disasters: A social identity model. In J. Jetten, C. Haslam, & S. A. Haslam (Eds.), *The social cure: Identity, health and well-being* (pp. 195–215). Hove, UK: Psychology Press.

Drury, J., Cocking, C., & Reicher, S. (2009a). Everyone for themselves? A comparative study of crowd solidarity among emergency survivors. *British Journal of Social Psychology, 48*(3), 487–506.

Chris Cocking

Drury, J., Cocking, C., & Reicher, S. (2009b). The nature of collective resilience: Survivor reactions to the 2005 London bombings. *International Journal of Mass Emergencies and Disasters, 27*(1), 66–95.

Dynes, R. (2006). Social capital: Dealing with community emergencies. *Homeland Security Affairs, 2*(2), 1–26.

Evans, B., & Reid, J. (2014). *Resilient life: The art of living dangerously.* Cambridge, UK: Polity Press.

Fritz, C. E. (1996). *Disasters and mental health: Therapeutic principles drawn from disaster studies.* University of Delaware, Disaster Research Center, Historical and comparative disaster series #10 (original work published 1961).

Fruin, J. (1993). *The causes and prevention of crowd disasters.* Originally presented at the First International Conference on Engineering for Crowd Safety, London, England, March 1993. Revised exclusively for crowdsafe.com, January 2002. Retrieved from www.crowdsafe.com/FruinCauses.pdf

Furedi, F. (2007). *Invitation to terror.* London, UK: Continuum Press.

Harrison, E. (2012). Bouncing back? Recession, resilience and everyday lives. *Critical Social Policy, 33*(1), 97–113.

Hart, A., Blincow, D., & Thomas, H. (2007). *Resilient therapy with children and families.* London: Buunner Routledge.

Hart, A., Gagnon, E., Eryigit-Madzwamuse, S., Cameron, J., Aranda, K., Heaver, B. (in press). Uniting resilience research and practice with a health inequalities approach. *Health: An Interdisciplinary Journal for the Social Study of Health, Illness and Medicine.*

Helbing, D., & Mukerji, P. (2012). Crowd disasters as systemic failures: Analysis of the love parade disaster. *EPJ Data Science, 1,* 1–7.

Ishkanian, A., & Szreter, S. (2012). *The big society debate: A new agenda for social policy?* Cheltenham, UK: Edward Elgar Publishing.

Jackson, D., Firtko, A., & Edenborough, M. (2007). Personal resilience as a strategy for surviving and thriving in the face of workplace adversity: A literature review. *Journal of Advanced Nursing, 60*(1), 1–9.

Johnson, N. (1987). Panic at "The who concert stampede": An empirical assessment. *Social Problems, 34*(4), 362–373.

Kaniasty, K., & Norris, F. (2004). Social support in the aftermath of disasters, catastrophes, and acts of terrorism: Altruistic, overwhelmed, uncertain, antagonistic, and patriotic communities. In R. J. Ursano & C. S. Fullerton (Eds.), *Bioterrorism: Psychological and public health interventions* (pp. 220–229). Cambridge, UK: Cambridge University Press.

Klein, N. (2007). *The shock doctrine.* London, UK: Penguin Books.

LaPiere, R. (1938). *Collective behavior.* New York, NY, USA: McGraw Hill.

Manning, R., Levine, M., & Collins, A. (2007). The Kitty Genovese murder and the social psychology of helping: The parable of the 38 witnesses. *American Psychologist, 62*(6), 555–562.

Masten, A. S., Gewirtz, A. H., & Sapienza, J. (2013). Resilience in development: The importance of early childhood. In R. E. Tremblay, R. G. Barr, & R. De V. Peters (Eds.), *Encyclopedia on early childhood development* (pp. 1–6). Montreal, Quebec: Centre of Excellence for Early Childhood Development.

Mawson, A. R. (2005). Understanding mass panic and other collective responses to threat and disaster. *Psychiatry, 68*(2), 95–113.

Nguyen-Gillham, V., Giacaman, R., Naser, G., & Boyce, W. (2008). Normalising the abnormal: Palestinian youth and the contradictions of resilience in protracted conflict. *Health and Social Care in the Community, 16*(3), 291–298.

Norris, F., Stevens, S., Pfefferbaum, B., Wyche, K., & Pfefferbaum, R. (2008). Community resilience as a metaphor, theory, set of capacities, and strategy for disaster readiness. *American Journal of Community Psychology, 41*(1–2), 127–150.

Perez-Sales, P., Cervellon, P., Vazquez, C., Vidales, D., & Gaborit, M. (2005). Post-traumatic factors and resilience: Shelter management and survivors' attitudes after the earthquakes in El Salvador (2001). *Journal of Community and Applied Social Psychology, 15*(5), 368–382.

Quarantelli, E. L. (2001). The sociology of panic. In N. J. Smelser & P. B. Baltes (Eds.), *International encyclopedia of the social and behavioural sciences* (pp. 11020–11023). New York, NY, USA: Pergamon Press.

Reich, J., Zautra, A., & Hall, J. (2010). *Handbook of adult resilience.* London, UK: Guilford Press.

Reicher, S., & Haslam, S. A. (2010). Beyond help: A social psychology of collective solidarity and social cohesion'. In M. Snyder & S. Sturmer (Eds.), *The psychology of helping: New directions in the study of intergroup prosocial behavior* (pp. 289–309). Oxford, UK: Blackwell.

Rodriguez, H., Trainor, J., & Quarantelli, E. (2006). Rising to the challenges of a catastrophe: The emergent and pro-social behaviour following Hurricane Katrina. *The Annals of the American Academy of Political Science, 604*(1), 82–101.

Rutter, M. (1987). Psychosocial resilience and protective mechanisms. *American Journal of Orthopsychiatry,* *57*(3), 316–331.

Smelser, N. J. (1962). *Theory of collective behavior.* London, UK: Routledge and Kegan Paul.

Solnit, R. (2009). *A paradise built in hell: The extraordinary communities that arise in disaster.* New York, US: Viking.

Straus, A. L. (1944). The literature on panic. *Journal of Abnormal and Social Psychology, 39*(3), 317–328.

Tierney, K., Bevc, C., & Kuligowski, E. (2006). Metaphors matter: Disaster myths, media frames and their consequences in Hurricane Katrina. *Annals of the American Academy of Political and Social Science, 604*(1), 57–81.

UK Cabinet Office. (2011). *Strategic national framework on community resilience.* Retrieved from www. cabinetoffice.gov.uk/sites/default/files/resources/Strategic-National-Framework-on-Community-Resilience_0.pdf

Ungar, M. (2006). Nurturing hidden resilience in at-risk youth in different cultures. *Journal of Canadian Academic Child Adolescent Psychiatry, 15*(2), 53–58.

Ungar, M. (2008). Resilience across cultures. *British Journal of Social Work, 38*(2), 218–235.

Ungar, M. (2012). *Enhancing the development of resilience in early adolescents: Literature review.* The Learning Partnership, Canada. Retrieved from www.thelearningpartnership.ca/what-we-do/knowledge-mobilization/research-and-insight-reports

Ungar, M., Brown, M., Liebenberg, L., Cheung, M., & Levine, K. (2008). Distinguishing differences in pathways to resilience among Canadian youth. *Canadian Journal of Community Mental Health, 27*(1), 1–13.

Voorhees, C. W., Vick, J., & Perkins, D. D. (2007). "Came hell and high water": The intersection of Hurricane Katrina, the news media, race and poverty. *Journal of Community and Applied Social Psychology, 17*(6), 415–429.

Williams, R., & Drury, J. (2009). Psychosocial resilience and its influence on managing mass emergencies and disasters. *Psychiatry, 8*(8), 293–296.

11

The Applied Metatheory of Resilience and Resiliency

Glenn E. Richardson

The Metatheory of Resilience and Resiliency (MRR) (Richardson, 2002a) provided a theoretical foundation upon which educational and counseling interventions could be built. The assumption with the MRR is that people can be taught and have the agency to become more resilient. Some confusion exists within the study of resiliency in that some resilience professionals are studying the discovery pathway of resilience inquiry and others are attempting to educate and counsel people along the applied resilience pathway. The intent of this chapter is to first distinguish between the discovery pathway of resiliency inquiry and the applied pathway of resiliency inquiry. The chapter will then focus on the five waves of applied resiliency inquiry, which includes:

- Identification of resilient qualities
- The resiliency journey or process
- Resilient drives
- Resonation and quickening
- Self-mastery

The chapter concludes with a discussion of the assumptions necessary for helping those that professionals serve.

Divergent paths of resilience inquiry: discovery and application

Attempts to define and explore the construct of resilience and resiliency are often frustrated by numerous variances in definitions, the roles of protective factors versus risk factors, genetic limitations, and the degree of adversity that either diminishes resilience or enhances it. Confusing even more are the numerous social, ecological, genetic, and personal variables that may or may not predict whether a person will be resilient or not. In brief, the discovery pathway is wrought with some disagreement and confusion, making it challenging for helping professionals to help foster resilience in the audiences they serve.

It is with the second wave of inquiry that the discovery pathway and the applied pathway began to diverge. The discovery pathway produced a second wave of inquiry that embraced the developmental systems approach and positive adaptation in the context of adversity. The third wave investigated interventions that changed developmental pathways with a focus on young people. The fourth wave from the perspective of discovery was to understand and integrate resilience "across multiple levels of analyses with growing attention to epigenetics and neurobiological processes" (Wright, Masten, and Narayan, 2013).

Resilience educators and counselors required a more practical and intervention-based construct than merely "adapting well" or "bouncing back" or attempts to alter developmental pathways in order to teach students how to become more resilient. The applied pathway focuses on the detail of the personal experience of "adaptation" or "bouncing back". The assumption that everyone can discover innate resilient qualities through the resiliency process has application to individuals, families, organizations, and communities. To differentiate the discovery and applied waves of resilience inquiry, the MRR will be referenced as the Applied Metatheory of Resilience and Resiliency (AMRR) (Richardson, in press).

Resilient qualities: the first wave of resilience and resiliency inquiry

Common to both the discovery and applied resiliency inquiry was the identification of resilient qualities. The first wave of resiliency inquiry did not emerge from academic grounding in theory but rather through the phenomenological identification of characteristics of survivors, mostly young people, living in high-risk situations. Foundational studies (Werner & Smith, 1982; Garmezy, 1985; Rutter, 1987) cited in most of the phenomenological resilience literature identified qualities that predicted the capacity to thrive in the face of personal and social challenge. The outcome of the first wave, which continues to this day, is the identification of dozens of these resilient qualities. It is interesting that, in the academic discipline of positive psychology, the most studied qualities are the same as the resilient qualities. Qualities include adaptability, good communication skills, self-esteem, courage, self-mastery, problem-solving skills, integrity, self-efficacy, internal locus of control, happiness, optimism, faith, self-determination, wisdom, creativity, self-control, gratitude, forgiveness, hope, and humility, among others (Seligman, 2011).

The focus on positive resilient qualities has tremendous implications to helping professionals who now, rather than identifying and attempting to fix problems, can build strengths, gifts, and talents to thrive through adversity. These strengths are then built upon with the expected result of seeing problems diminish.

Resiliency: the second wave of resilience and resiliency inquiry

The mechanism for acquiring the resilient qualities identified in the first wave is the essence of the second wave of resiliency inquiry and describes the process for accessing resilient qualities. Flach (1988) first described the process as the "Law of Disruption and Reintegration", which detailed the experience of "bouncing back" or "adapting well". It was detailed even further in the "Resiliency Model" (Richardson, Neiger, Jensen, & Kumpfer, 1990) and again in the Metatheory of Resilience and Resiliency (Richardson, 2002b). The detailed process of acquiring resilient qualities or protective factors is called resiliency, which occurs with each new life experience, good or bad.

> Applied resiliency is the process and experience of being disrupted by life events, adversity, or challenges, and, in the humbling trough of introspective enlightenment, accessing innate self-mastering strengths to grow stronger through the disruption.
>
> *(Richardson, 2016)*

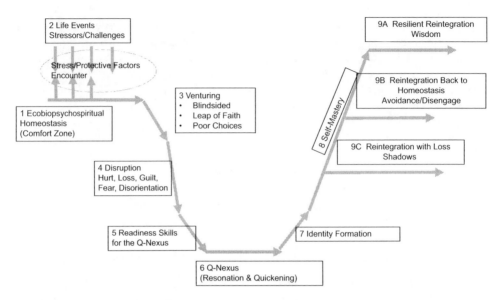

Figure 11.1 The Resiliency Model
Source: Richardson (2016).

Understanding the disruptive and reintegrative process or journey that accompanies every new life experience provides an opportunity for people to resiliently map life experiences. Helping professionals should be aware that with each new experience or new information, people experience a minor or major disruption with an opportunity to learn and enhance their capacities. Metaphorically, in a state of homeostasis, each person has an intact view of the world. With each new experience, a new piece of the puzzle is available to add to the world view. It requires that the puzzle disrupt and fall apart and rebuild with the new piece of the puzzle. The world view continues to expand with each new experience that people choose to add to their world view. The AMRR applies the stages of the Resiliency Model to help people embrace life events. Figure 11.1 (Richardson, in press) describes the applied resiliency process with description of each stage by number.

1   Ecobiopsychospiritual homeostasis (comfort zone)

Homeostasis is a moment in time when a person has adapted to their life situation. Homeostasis suggests balance and normalcy. It is a state of physical, mental, spiritual, and life adaptation. Ecobiopsychospiritual homeostasis emphasizes the multidimensional nature of comfort zones including ecological, biological, psychological, and spiritual homeostasis.

Ecological homeostasis: Ecological homeostasis suggests an adaptation to one's environment. People live where they live, work where they work, and play where they play. People choose or are compelled to live in a certain place. The environment may be enriching or less than enriching, but a person has adapted to it.

Biological homeostasis indicates that people have adapted to a state of physical health and appearance. They look like they look. They may be underweight or overweight. They may have certain physical conditions to which they have adapted. They may be aware of biological talents such as singing, coordination, or physical appearance.

Intellectual (mental) homeostasis implies that people know what they know at a point in time. They have learned enough math to do a budget. They have learned to read. They have learned enough to perform duties as a student or an employee. They have learned to use electronic devices. They have developed a personality that best helps them to optimize their life.

Spiritual homeostasis suggests that a person has adjusted to his/her beliefs. People may have identified a source of spiritual strength and are content with the degree of closeness and intimacy with that source.

2 Life events, stressors, and challenges

Life events are experiences that come from external sources or from the perception of external stressors. Many life events are stressors that "blindside" and force someone out of the adapted state of homeostasis. Life events may come as physical, mental, spiritual, or ecological external opportunities. Sometimes an event is internal, and assumptions are made that may affect one's life, but in reality, it does not and only becomes worry. Life events may occur by living out of character when thoughts and actions are in conflict with a sense of what is right and wrong. For example lying, cheating, or stealing are actions that likely violate one's moral framework resulting in leaving the peace of homeostasis.

Opportunities are the most desirable means to leave homeostasis. Encountering opportunities emerges from innate resilient drives to progress and improve life experiences. People have innate drives to play, to learn, to serve, and to have new experiences.

Figure 11.1 shows the downward arrows for the life events and then has opposing arrows that point upward representing the resilient qualities and factors a person has developed in one's life. Encountering similar life experiences to those in the past may allow a person to resist disruptions because of the skills that were learned previously. Notice that there is an arrow coming down from life events that has no opposing arrow. The arrow represents a new event for which one has no experience or resilient qualities with which to cope. The encounter between the new experience and lack of coping skills for the experience will likely result in a disruption. The disruption may be an opportunity, or it may be something that is undesirable.

3 Venturing

The stressor and resilient quality exchange may result in venturing or leaving homeostasis in light of a choice or life event. Optimal venturing occurs when people seek opportunities to learn and improve themselves. Being forced into new experiences from external life events or the perception of a life event also compels a person to disruption. The third mechanism for venturing is by making choices outside of one's character code, resulting in feelings of guilt.

4 Disruptions

The outcome of being blindsided by life events, leaping into new adventures, or stepping outside of one's moral framework is disruption. As people leave homeostasis and find themselves in uncharted waters, a range of mixed emotions may surface. Stage 4 of the resilient journey shows a disruption after having been taken from the state of homeostasis.

When blindsided by life events, disruptions will be sensed as hurt, loss, fear, or some other sense of disorientation. In disagreements with loved ones, there is a sense of loss of closeness. A person may feel a loss of predictability or comfort when moving to a new place. Even when unexpected opportunities arrive, there is still some discomfort. When venturing into new experiences, there is a sense of fear or discomfort along with the excitement in the new adventure but still sensing a loss of homeostasis. Thinking or behaving outside of one's moral framework will be experienced as guilt.

5   Readiness skills for the resonation and quickening

When disruptions occur, people ready themselves for insights that come from beyond normal thinking capacity. Humility and openness ready a person because their ego is diminished and their resonating capacity increases. There are many techniques, practices, and skills that help people to prepare to receive answers to questions. Integrative skills such as meditation, art therapy, music therapy, journaling, storytelling, aerobic exercise, and reading inspiring literature are skills that help people gain insights and energy to resiliently thrive through adversity.

6   Resonation and quickening

In the trough of disruption, people find themselves in optimal states of openness and humility. Resonation is a gentle prompt that lets people know that thoughts and actions are on the right path. Quickening is more forceful when someone has a sudden insight, a burst of understanding, or a Gestalt. These are moments of synchronicity when everything comes together. This is a time of infusions of knowing what to do and how to do it. This is a moment of guidance and direction. People are filled with confidence and courage. The insights may be labeled intuition, gut feelings, synchronicity, or even impactful dreams. It may be feelings that come in response to a fervent prayer. It may be a moment of clarity or insightfulness. Resonation will be described with more detail in the discussion of postulates later in this chapter.

7   Identity formation

Quickening gives people insights and peace to move forward. With each new resonating or quickening moment, people have the opportunity to create a new identity. The new identity is one that is a product of the insight someone has received from the quickening moment. It is the identity that will most effectively deal with the current life event or venture. With disruptions, people may need to discover the warrior, the peacemaker, the protector, the leader, the follower, the teacher, or the student that will thrive most effectively in the life event. Applied resiliency provides instruction and skills to create new identities.

8   Self-mastery

Once an identity is formed, it may take a few moments or perhaps days and weeks to have that identity become part of one's nature. Self-mastery embraces the powerful qualities of persistence, drive, and a strong work ethic. It is the ability to overcome undesirable behaviors and thoughts that impede progression. Self-mastery persists until the task of personal change is complete. Skills of self-mastery include work ethic, persistence, and habit breaking.

9   Reintegration

With insight received from the resonation and quickening and the drive and persistence of self-mastery, people can celebrate the creation of a new identity. For example someone can transform a self-centered identity into an altruistic identity. A person may change from being a sedentary person to an active person. People can see it, feel it and know how to live the new identity. Still people have agency and the choice to give up and return to previous habits and identities. One can resiliently reintegrate, reintegrate back to homeostasis, or reintegrate with loss.

9A   Resilient reintegration

Optimally, people embrace adversity, change, opportunity, or life events and gain the desired qualities and virtues described in the first wave of resiliency inquiry. Persistence in the new identity will harvest qualities indicative of resilient reintegration. Resilient reintegration implies that, in the aftermath of disruptions and leaving homeostasis, one will rebound stronger with more resilient qualities. Resilient reintegration enables people to progress in life. Each new experience is an opportunity, creating new identities and growth.

9B   Reintegration back to homeostasis

Reintegration back to the comfort zone is to ignore the insight and direction received during the resonating and quickening moment. It is not persisting during the self-mastery stage but rather giving up and going back to what one knows even though it may be undesirable. People recognize that a new identity would make them stronger but lost the vision or decided it was too difficult. A person may have even tried to assume the new identity but then disengaged. Sometimes, even though people know what they can become in the wake of a disruption, they decide to just get past the experience and not embrace the life lesson. Each time a person just tries to "get past it" without growth, the result is stagnation in that dimension of life.

9C   Reintegration with loss

Often times when people encounter life events, they are not open to the insights that can come through resonation. Rather, they give up resilient qualities. They find themselves losing hope, courage, and optimism because of the disruption. Sometimes they turn to secondary emotions such as anger, jealously, or vengeance. Reintegration with loss is also exemplified by those who may envision new identities that will help them resiliently reintegrate but instead give up and resort to alcohol, drugs, or habits that are not progressive.

Figure 11.1 is a simplistic model. People experience the resilient journey many times a day with new information and new challenges and being blindsided with life events. They may be able to resiliently reintegrate in a short amount of time, such as with new information, or it may take extensive time, such as in the case of divorce or financial crises. People can resiliently reintegrate immediately or simply get past the experience and learn from the disruption after time has passed. The resilient journey applies to every role and experience in one's life whether it be with physical setbacks, social challenges, emotional strain, or conflicts with morals. The resilient journey can be mapped and outcomes charted using the model in Figure 11.1.

Resilience: the third wave of resilience and resiliency inquiry

Resiliently mapping the resilient journey provides a roadmap of choices to travel and resiliently reintegrate, but the journey requires motivation and energy. The third wave of resilience inquiry is the discovery of innate motivation and driving forces. Resilience is a force or yearning within everyone that drives him/her to thrive through the resiliency process. It is the drive to fulfill innate yearnings and drives to self-actualize. It is the drive to fulfill a person's childlike, character, noble, ecological, universal, essential, and intellectual resilience (Richardson, 2012). Helping professionals need to understand that housed within every soul are common resilient drives and yearnings and that the energy produced by these forces are motivators used to progress through the resiliency process. Intrinsic motivation or resilience is key to thriving through the resilient journey. Postmodern, multidisciplinary identification of motivational forces may include several of the following descriptions that are potentially most helpful in thriving through adversity.

Childlike resilience is an innate energy producing source within most people. Although many people may have buried their childlike natures deep within themselves in the wake of pain and difficult life experiences, the energy source is innate. When reflecting upon one's childlike nature, one can sense the drive or yearning to have fun, to play, to be creative, to find humor and laugh, to be spontaneous, to take risks, to be genuine, to be curious, to be open, and to have pleasure. People can learn to face their challenges with a childlike attitude making life challenges more tolerable.

Character resilience is the yearning to live within a chosen moral framework. Most people resonate to concepts such as integrity, honesty, trustworthiness, kindness, loyalty, and honor. These principles carry across cultures, genders, and the life span. A sense of freedom and energy result when living within one's chosen character qualities. Stepping outside of a character code, the result is likely feelings of guilt and regret. Guilt is an energy drain and compromises energy to resiliently reintegrate.

Noble resilience is the yearning and drive to feel valued and important. Self-esteem, self-efficacy, and self-worth all reflect noble resilience. Feeling good about oneself is generally a product of having a purpose and meaning in life. Where noble resilience is the drive to feel valued and worthy, the natural yearning to help others through altruistic acts of service becomes the mechanism to feel that nobility. People that feel nobility are also more likely to be more resilient.

Ecological resilience is the drive to connect with energy from one's surroundings. Candace Pert (1999) describes how vibrations that come from nature activate neuropeptides in the body. The receptive neuropeptides connect with receptors in the cells and send messages of resilient qualities through the communicative mechanism of vibrations. Soft, life-enriching, and healing vibrations come from natural settings. Plant therapy, pet therapy, music therapy, and other sources of soothing vibrations help people thrive through adversity.

Synergistic resilience is the yearning and drive to connect with others. The drive to connect is in essence love. Another chapter could be written about resilient relationships, but space limitations mandate a brief overview of social support in resiliency. As loved ones speak optimistically, instill hope, and generate courage in their relationships, the resilient qualities may emerge, which, according to the field of psychoneuroimmunology, will help promote optimism, courage, and other resilient qualities.

Universal resilience is the yearning and drive to connect to a strength, power, and energy beyond normal capacity. Studies have demonstrated that faith facilitates optimism, drive, and success in overcoming health problems. Agnostics and atheists can be educated regarding the vast wisdom of the collective unconscious mind, which reflects a universal wisdom. They may also be instructed regarding string theory and other forms of theoretical physics that suggests that we are walking, breathing in an energy field. Most people believe in a form of deity. The techniques and skills required of a person to access peace, energy, and comfort from a higher power may be through integrative health modalities. Helping professionals can help students by encouraging practices such as meditation, Tai Chi, yoga, prayer, and other evidence-based techniques and skills.

Essential resilience is the most primitive and basic drive to live and survive. Helping professionals often focus on essential needs to help people. There is no question that aerobic movement, optimal sleep, and prudent eating patterns fortify the body to better deal with life challenges. Skills such as intuitive eating, sensing when a body needs to move and be active, or sleeping when a person wants sleep will help energize the soul to thrive.

Intellectual resilience is the drive to understand and plan experiences and identities to optimize the human experience. The role of intellectual resilience is to sense innate drives and yearnings including childlike, noble, character, and universal resilience. The role of intellectual resilience is to listen and then plan to fulfill the basic drives. Personality evolves based upon the way the mind determines the best thoughts and actions to fulfill resilient drives. It is the force behind thinking, deciding, learning and planning. Intellectual resilience brings to consciousness the resilient drives.

Resonation and quickening: the fourth wave of resilience and resiliency inquiry

Perhaps the fourth wave of resiliency inquiry has the most history in time but has emerged recently as a skill-based experience to help foster resiliency. Humankind has longed to have insights to know what to do in times of decision or times of needed emotional strength. Resonation and quickening are the experiences to know what to do, when to do it, have confidence that it is the right thing to do, and have the energy to make it happen. Resonation and quickening skills are labeled as complementary and alternative medicine (Micozzi, 2015). The complementary or integrative health skills are the same skills that people can use to thrive through adversity. In the trough of disruption in the resiliency process, people are encouraged to practice integrative health skills to ready themselves for insights or "Ah, ha!" moments. Readiness practices such as finding meaning in art, music, literature, and theater may inspire insights. People can ready themselves for quickening by practicing journal writing, meditation, imagery, poetry, storytelling, reminiscence, prayer, self-hypnosis, or vision quests. Readiness for answers as to how to be resilient can also be experienced in nature, with aromas, colors, and other ecological resilience strategies described earlier. People may receive moments of inspiration when doing psychomotor activities that allow for the mind and spirit to ponder. Aerobic exercise, Tai Chi, driving a car, or even showering offer opportunities to ponder life's challenges in preparation for and allow for quickening.

Quickening the experience of receiving insights or inspiration that fills one's entire soul with an answer, or courage, or whatever resilient quality (first wave) is needed. These quickening moments are almost magical as they fill one's heart and mind with direction and confidence to do what one needs to do, or feel how one needs to feel, based upon a wisdom that comes from these moments. These moments can also be taught as part of resiliency education. The quickening experience may be described as having bursts of understanding, renewed energy, moments of enlightenment and inspiration, renewed hope and optimism, synchronicity, feelings of rightness, intuition, gut feelings, envisioning a new identity, peace melting confusion, hunches, Gestalts, and feelings of rightness.

Self-mastery: the fifth wave of resilience and resiliency inquiry

The fifth wave of applied resiliency inquiry is to learn self-mastery. Self-mastery is taking advantage of defining moments of enlightenment and using them for motivation and drive to experience resilient reintegration. Self-mastery is a conscious choice to resiliently reintegrate from disruptions by creating a new identity to effectively deal with the health choice. Smokers create a new identity as a non-smoker. An inactive person creates a new active identity. A person who has been lazy creates a new identity as a hard worker. Other examples of among hundreds of identities are listed here. Note, that depending upon the situation, each identity may be useful in dealing with life challenges. These are presented as opposites, but both may be needed depending upon the nature of each disruption.

- Warrior or peacemaker
- Giver or receiver
- Teacher or student
- Romantic or pragmatic
- Loyalist or rebel
- Introvert or extravert
- Creator or destroyer
- Believer or skeptic
- Optimist or pessimist
- Humble or proud
- Powerful or vulnerable
- Flexible or immoveable

In the fifth wave of resiliency inquiry, self-mastery embraces theories such as self-determination theory (Ryan & Deci, 2000), self-efficacy from social cognitive theory (Bandura, 1977), and hardiness (Kobasa, Maddi, & Kahn, 1982) among others.

Self-mastery is a critical wave of inquiry because of the importance for resilient reintegration. It involves the positive psychological concept of persistence. Persistence or grit is the ability to continue to maintain the new identity in spite of challenges. The core of persistence is to continue to access the resilience drives of the third wave. When students can make an adventure with the new identity, make it fun, if possible, and find humor in the identity as per the childlike nature, it will be easier to persist. If students will stay within their sense of character, they will more likely have the energy to persist. If the new identity provides service, the resulting feelings of self-worth will help with persistence. If students feel as though they have guidance from universal sources of strength, they will likely persist.

Becoming more resilient often requires people to overcome thoughts and behaviors that are undesirable. Self-mastery provides guidelines to help people overcome self-defeating thoughts and behaviors. Applied resilience provides guidelines as to how to strengthen resilience and follow the resiliency map to recovery and resilient reintegration while at the same time disarming the undesirable thoughts and behaviors. Richardson (2016) details the training to overcome undesirable actions through resilient strengthening and nurturing resilient drives.

Truths or postulates

The AMRR makes assumptions that, through counseling or education, people can become more resilient. If people were only able to resiliently reintegrate from life's challenges based upon genetics or social influences, then educators and counselors would be wasting their time in trying to help people. The assumptions that helping professionals can make in order to apply resiliency and resilience concepts are also called "postulates". The assumed truths are logical and consistent with common sense. The five postulates described here are implied in the previous discussions of resiliency and resilience. The five postulates are 1) innateness, 2) resonation, 3) progression, 4) faith/belief, and 5) agency.

1 The postulate of innateness

A constant among the many academic, philosophical, and religious thoughts is that housed within each person is a potential to access strength and insight well beyond normal capacities. In psychology, Carl Jung spoke of a collective unconscious mind that housed the wisdom of the ages. In Eastern philosophies, the thought is that people are walking in a sea of energy and insight as described as Qi. In physics, everyone is part of a sea of energy and wisdom that fills multiple universes called "strings." In Theism, many believe that God's Spirit fills the immensity of space and that their spirits can access His Spirit.

The fundamental postulate of innateness suggests that our conscious mind is a tiny percentage of our potential capacity. People have the potential, through different sources to access insights, strengths, and talents that are housed either within them or in the world in which they live. Helping professionals can assume that their students and clients have within them the resilient yearnings and drives of resilience. They have the mechanism and potential skills to access the truths in a universe of energy, wisdom, and strength. The postulate of innateness that has consumer appeal may be stated as follows:

> The solution to every problem, the means to every dream, and all that everyone ever needed, wanted or hoped for resides in the sea of energy, vitality, enlightenment, and power that dwells within them and within the world around them.

2 The postulate of resonation

To reinforce the importance of resonation, it is important to consider this as a truth. The language of the universe is really in a form of vibrations or frequencies. (Greene, 2003). To know a truth, a person will vibrate at the same frequency as the truth. Not everyone resonates to the same truth. The mechanism may be best explained as how a first grade teacher might explain resonation. The teacher may strike a tuning fork explaining how the sound waves are making our eardrums vibrate so that we heard the sound. She may again strike the tuning fork and bring up a second tuning fork that was not vibrating. Placing the new tuning fork near the vibrating tuning fork causes the new tuning fork to vibrate at the same frequency. In life, as people try to make good decisions, the best choice is the one to which he/she resonates. The person will feel the rightness of choice with soft gentle vibrations much like the second tuning fork. The insights people need to resiliency thrive through adversity are disclosed through the universal and subtle vibrational language of resonation.

3 The postulate of progression

Progression states that, through the resiliency process, one can progress or harvest resilient qualities (first wave) throughout a lifetime. Progression can be maximized by resiliently reintegrating through life experiences. This postulate may be questioned if thinking only of physical progression because it is obvious that people peak at midlife and see physical decline in later years. This postulate may also be challenged if only thinking of intellectual learning abilities. Mentally, people learn very quickly in the early years, but as they age, learning becomes slower. It is difficult

Glenn E. Richardson

to make a case for progression throughout a lifetime considering only physical and mental experiences. The dimension of life to be able to progress throughout a lifetime is by the harvesting of resilient qualities. Even in senior years, people can still harvest qualities of peace, joy, compassion, optimism, courage, integrity, happiness, and love. The postulate of progression suggests that the way to progress throughout a life is to harvest as many resilient qualities as possible through life experiences. Many people have had experiences visiting with loved ones in their final days of life. Some may be bitter and angry, but others show resilient qualities in their countenances. They can see in their eyes wisdom, compassion, caring, and peace.

4   The postulate of belief or faith

All of the good ideas, all of the desires, and all of the good intentions will fall by the wayside if people do not have the belief that they can resiliently reintegrate. The first step of the resiliency process is to take the leap of faith into the new experience to acquire resilient qualities. One of the most powerful concepts to help people to change their behaviors comes from Albert Bandura (1977) who identified the concept of self-efficacy as "our belief in our ability to succeed in certain situations." Faith is a similar construct, but rather than sensing that, a person can take leaps of faith by their own resilience; they believe that they can do it with the help from a force greater than themselves (universal resilience). The idea of faith has been an important postulate for centuries, with the earliest advocacy evident in spiritual literature throughout history. Faith is evident in all the Eastern philosophies and religions. The postulate of belief or faith is initiated with resonation (confirming rightness), then believing by creating a vision of accomplishment, sensing courage from resilient drives, and then taking action.

5   The postulate of agency

Central to the AMRR is the postulate of agency. People must understand that in any circumstance, they can still choose their attitude. Agency is best expressed from the wisdom of Viktor Frankl (1984), who after three years of suffering in a Nazi concentration camp in World War II stated:

> The last of the human freedoms is to choose one's attitude in any given set of circumstances . . . to choose one's own way. And there were always choices to make. Every day, every hour, offered the opportunity to make a decision, a decision which determined whether you would or would not submit to those powers which threatened to rob you of your very self, your inner freedom.

People can continue to harvest resilient qualities even in dismal circumstances. The postulate of agency recognizes that the mind is charged with the challenge of discerning between a progressive path that will harvest resilient qualities throughout a lifetime or giving up and stagnating. In a world of opposing forces, people have the power to choose their path.

Conclusion

The Applied Metatheory of Resilience and Resiliency provides a framework for helping professionals to provide resilience interventions in many educational and counseling situations. Resiliency-mapping life events can apply to almost every life experience. Discovering innate resilient drives within students and clients is an important experience to help them find the motivation and energy to become stronger from experience. Helping professionals can persist in identifying strengths and gifts in everyone by recognizing and embracing the resilient postulates.

Resiliency training has proven efficacious in worksites (Waite & Richardson, 2004) and with patients with Type 2 diabetes (Bradshaw et al., 2007). Guidelines have been recommended to families (Richardson & Hawkes, 1995), communities (Richardson, Neiger, Dunn, & Ross, 1996), public schools (Richardson & Nixon, 1997), and mental health programs (Richardson, 2002a). Applied resilience training helps people discover innate motivational and energy resources to thrive through challenges.

References

Bandura, A. (1977). Self-efficacy: Toward a unifying theory of behavior change. *Psychological Review, 84*(2), 191–215.

Bradshaw, B. G., Richardson, G. E., Kumpfer, K., Carlson, J., Stanchfield, J., Overall, J., . . . Kulkarni, K. (2007). Determining the efficacy of a resiliency training approach in adults with Type 2 Diabetes. *The Diabetes Educator, 33*(4), 650–659.

Flach, F. (1988). *Resilience: Discovering a new strength at times of stress.* New York: Ballantine.

Frankl, V. E. (1984). *Man's search for meaning* (3rd ed.). New York: Pocket Books.

Garmezy, N. (1985). Stress-resistant children: The search for protective factors. In J. E. Stevenson (Ed.), *Recent research in developmental psychopathology* (pp. 213–233). Oxford: Pergamon Press.

Greene, B. (2003). *The elegant universe.* New York: Vintage Books.

Kobasa, S. C., Maddi, S. R., & Kahn, S. (1982). Hardiness and health: A prospective study. *Journal of Personality and Social Psychology, 42*(1), 168–177.

Micozzi, M. S. (2015). *Fundamentals of complementary and alternative medicine* (5th ed.). St. Louis: Elsevier Sanders.

Pert, C. B. (1999). *Molecules of emotion: The science behind mind-body medicine.* New York: Simon & Schuster.

Richardson, G. E. (2002a). Mental health promotion through resilience and resiliency education. *International Journal of Emergency Mental Health, 4*(1), 65–75.

Richardson, G. E. (2002b). The metatheory of resilience and resiliency. *Journal of Clinical Psychology, 58*(3), 307–321.

Richardson, G. E. (2012). *The seven Q-Nexus experiences: Thriving through adversity and challenge.* Salt Lake City: Q-Nexus, LLC.

Richardson, G. E. (2016). *Living resiliently: 16 experiences to enhance personal resilience:* iuniverse, Bloomington, Indiana.

Richardson, G. E. & Hawks, S. R. (1995) A practical approach for enhancing resiliency in families. *Family Perspective, 29*(3), 235–250.

Richardson, G. E., Neiger, B., Dunn, D., & Ross, J. (1996). Helping communities to become resilient. *Resiliency in Action, 1*(3), 31–38.

Richardson, G. E., Neiger, B., Jensen, S., & Kumpfer, K. (1990). The resiliency model. *Health Education, 21*(6), 33–39.

Richardson, G. E., & Nixon, C. J. (1997). A curriculum for resiliency. *Principal, 77*(2), 26–28.

Rutter, M. (1987). Psychosocial resilience and protective mechanisms. *American Journal of Orthopsychiatry, 57*(3), 316–331.

Ryan, R. M., & Deci, E. L. (2000). Self-determination theory and the facilitation of intrinsic motivation, social development, and well-being. *American Psychologist, 55*(1), 68–78.

Seligman, M. E. P. (2011). *Flourish.* New York: Free Press.

Waite, P., & Richardson, G. E. (2004). Determining the efficacy of resiliency training in the worksite. *Journal of Allied Health, 33*(3), 178–183.

Wright, M. O., Masten, A. S., & Narayan, A. J. (2013). Resilience processes in development: Four waves of research on positive adaptation in the context of adversity. In S. Goldstein & R. B. Brooks (Eds.), *Handbook of resilience in children* (2nd ed., pp. 15–37). New York: Springer.

12

The resilience processes of Black South African young people

A contextualised perspective

Linda C. Theron

Positive adjustment to significant adversity, or resilience, is a complex, multi-level process that supports functional outcomes as defined by a given social system at a given point in time (Masten, 2014). Amongst others, this process demands constructive interplay between individuals and their social systems. Such interaction is typically comprised of universally occurring psychosocial processes including, amongst others, attachment, agency, and mastery; problem solving; and meaning making (see Masten & Wright, 2010, pp. 222–229 for details). Although they are common to young people's adjustment globally, these processes are necessarily shaped by contextual realities and by cultural expectations, values, and practices (Panter-Brick, 2015). This means that the form that these processes take, and which are likely to be prioritised, will depend on the sociocultural context in which young people are embedded (Ungar, 2011). For example along the Arctic Circle in Northern Norway, young men are more likely to draw on attachments to their uncles to support their adaptation (Nystad, Spein, & Ingstad, 2014), whereas on mainland China, Chinese youngsters will turn to their biological parents before considering any alternate source of support (Tian & Wang, 2015). Their choices are shaped by the prevailing cultural expectations and living arrangements. Moreover, resilience-supporting interventions that disrespect the cultural and contextual relativity of adaptive processes will probably be sub-optimal. Consequently, resilience theorists are urged to provide contextualised explanations of resilience – i.e. to account for how culture and context shape the psychosocial processes that protect young people against adversity (Masten, 2014; Panter-Brick, 2015; Ungar, 2011, 2015).

In response, I direct this chapter toward considering how traditionally African culture, and the realities of rural and/or township South African contexts, shape Black South African adolescents' interactive processes of adjustment to compound challenges. Similar to the definition of functional outcomes being relative to a given community at a given point in time, culture and context are fluid too. Thus, this chapter must be read with the understanding that whilst the argument it makes (i.e. to truly understand and subsequently champion resilience, contextualised accounts are crucial) is perennial, the findings reported will need to be periodically interrogated and probably adjusted.

For the purposes of this chapter, culture is defined as everyday practices that are common to a group of people and the *shared* beliefs, values, and expectations related to these practices (see Panter-Brick, 2015). Context is defined as the physical and social environment in which young people are nested (see Ungar, 2015). Resilience is conceptualised from an ecological systems perspective as an adaptive, dynamic process that draws on interactions between individuals and the systems they are part of (e.g. family, community, cultural group) (Masten, 2014; Ungar, 2011).

Traditional African ways-of-being

Although Africa is comprised of multiple countries and ethnicities, with associated cultural particularities, the presence of recurrent features across these countries and groups facilitates contemplation of a traditionally African way-of-being (Theron & Phasha, 2015). Experiencing the self as interconnected, or adopting a 'relational model of identity' (Eze, 2014, p. 237), is central to a traditionally everyday African way-of-being. Such interconnectedness is multi-faceted and includes a sense of respectful connection to a supreme power (i.e. God or gods); the dead (i.e. ancestors); a community of living others (i.e. family, tribe, race); and the physical environment (Botha & Moletsane, 2012; Mwamwenda, 2004). Connectedness to a supreme power/s and the dead is expressed as deep spirituality and includes ancestral and religious practices. Spirituality assuages hardship in that it affords a sense of security (e.g. the expectation that ancestors/God will enable positive outcomes) and inevitable mastery (e.g. the powers that be would not allow unmanageable life-experiences).

Experiencing the self as inter-related, and valuing this, is further expressed in the traditional cultural value of *Ubuntu* or *Botho* (among other synonyms), which encourages regarding all living others as dignified co-equals (Eze, 2014; Watson, McMahon, Mkhize, Schweitzer, & Mpofu, 2011). Allied to this is a sense of duty to the collective – in contributing to others, the individual is recognised as a person. In other words, traditional African ways-of-being are essentially socially responsible, or moral, ways-of-being (Pityana, 1999). This finds expression in, for example kinship systems of child-rearing and acceptance of shared responsibility for the well-being of community members (including children and the elderly). Among more traditional Black South African families, this duty is frequently interpreted as educational achievement (e.g. completing high school and tertiary education), given that educational achievement is associated with upward mobility from which the extended family stands to benefit. In addition, educational achievement reflects well on Black South Africans in general because it contradicts the menial identity that historical Apartheid policies crafted (Phasha, 2010; Theron & Phasha, 2015). In this way, educational progress, and all that is associated with it, represents a culturally valued goal, which according to Panter-Brick (2015, p. 237) is likely to be 'the leitmotiv that drives wellbeing trajectories towards specific pursuits'.

Salient contextual factors

Most Black South African children live in township[1] or rural communities. Although this generalisation has limitations, it is likely that Black South African young people, who grow up in townships and/or rural areas will have lived experiences of typical contextual realities. These tend to include pervasive poverty (Mathews & Benvenuti, 2014; Theron, 2015). For example in 2012, 56% of South African children lived below the lower poverty line (R635 per month or around $52). Black South African children were most likely to know poverty, with 37% living in homes where no adult was employed (compared with 7% of Indian and 2% of White children – see Hall & Sambu, 2014). Such poverty is directly related to historic Apartheid laws that segregated Black South Africans into structurally inferior township communities and/or structurally inferior rural areas, and the enduring legacy of this injustice. Linked to this is a reality of many young people growing up without knowing their biological fathers (Nduna & Sikweyiya, 2015). Young people are more likely to be living with their biological mothers or a mother figure (typically a grandmother or other female kin). Growing up apart from fathers/biological parents – because of, for example poverty, parental migration relating to employment, better education opportunities, teenage pregnancies, and/or cultural practices – characterises childhood in South Africa, particularly for Black children (Hall, Meintjes, & Sambu, 2014). Fewer than 29% of Black South African children live with both their biological parents (compared with 79% Indian and 78% White children), 26% do not live with either parent, and 42% live with their mothers.

From the perspective of Black South African young people themselves: understanding how culture and context shape the resilience processes

As noted in the introduction of this chapter, the resilience literature urges accounts of resilience processes that use emic perspectives (see, for example McCubbin & Moniz, 2015; Panter-Brick, 2015). But, it also urges accounts that privilege the perspectives of young people themselves (see, for example Liebenberg & Ungar, 2009; Wright, Masten, & Narayan, 2013). This begs the question: how do Black South African young people's accounts of their resilience reflect the traditionally African ways-of-being and the challenging realities that typify township and/or rural contexts (as summarised earlier)? This is the question that directs this chapter. Given the tendency to under-explain the resilience processes of South African young people in contextualised and youth-directed ways, it is currently an incompletely answered question (Theron & Phasha, 2015).

Method

A starting point for answering this question is a review of extant publications that provide youth-directed reports of what informs the resilience processes of Black South African young people. I limited my search to English-medium articles that were published in indexed journals. Using the search engines linked to Ebscohost, I searched for articles that reported the resilience processes of Black South African young people (i.e. children, but also youth up to the age of 35[2]). I excluded all articles that did not contain the word resilience/resiliency/resilient in the title, abstract, or keywords or that had not included young people themselves as participants. I further limited the search to articles published from 2000 onwards, given the tendency of earlier articles to neglect context and culture in explanations of the resilience processes of South African young people (see Theron & Theron, 2010). I scoped the articles and further excluded those that did not report results that would support an understanding of how culture and context informed the resilience processes of Black young people (e.g. Mampane & Bouwer, 2006). This resulted in the inclusion of twenty-seven articles (Barbarin, Richter, & deWet, 2001; Cook & White, 2006; Dass-Brailsford, 2005; Ebersöhn, 2007; Ebersöhn & Maree, 2006; Germann, 2005; Govender & Killian, 2001; Hlatshwayo & Vally, 2014; Kritzas & Grobler, 2005; Lau & Van Niekerk, 2011; Malindi, 2014a, b; Malindi & Theron, 2010; Odendaal, Brink, & Theron, 2011; Phasha, 2010; Pienaar, Beukes, & Esterhuyse, 2006; Pienaar, Swanepoel, van Rensburg, & Heunis, 2011; Pillay & Nesengani, 2006; Theron,

2007, 2013, 2015; Theron et al., 2011; Theron & Malindi, 2010; Theron & Theron, 2013, 2014; Van Breda, 2015; Wild, Flisher, & Robertson, 2011).

Next, I analysed the included articles deductively, using the psychosocial mechanisms associated with the resilience processes of Sesotho-speaking young people, as reported earlier by me and two co-researchers (i.e. Theron, Theron, & Malindi, 2013). To better understand emic perspectives of the psychosocial resources that support Sesotho-speaking young people to beat the odds associated with township and/or rural communities, we worked with a panel of adults – all of whom were well-acquainted with Black young people living in a rural part of South Africa. The detail of this study is reported in Theron et al. (2013), and thus for the purposes of this chapter, suffice it to say that, using a grounded theory approach, we theorised that six mechanisms informed the resilience of Sesotho-speaking South African young people. These entailed (1) having and drawing on active support systems (i.e. a network of support, including immediate and extended family, peers, community members, and service-providers/professionals); (2) being value-driven (i.e. allegiance to traditional African culture, including *Ubuntu* and spirituality); (3) making educational progress (i.e. commitment to education and educational aspiration); (4) being a dreamer (i.e. hopeful future-orientation); (5) demonstrating acceptance (i.e. tolerance of intractable hardship without reneging on a hopeful future-orientation); and (6) drawing on personal resources (i.e. being flexible, solution-focused, responsive, determined, assertive, communicative, and self-assured).

These mechanisms, therefore, offer a culturally relevant departure point for analysis and so became the *a priori* codes that I used to explore how traditionally African culture, and the realities of rural and/or township South African contexts, shape Black South African adolescents' interactive processes of adjustment to compound challenges. Additionally, my rationale related to the six mechanisms as being adult-informed. This prompted our call for future iterations that foreground the perspectives of young people themselves (see Theron et al., 2013). Using the mechanisms as a framework for analysis of existing youth-directed accounts of resilience would facilitate an understanding of how well this adult-directed explanation fits with that of young people's and allow nascent comment on inter-generational understandings of resilience processes.

Once I had sorted the present publications according to the six adult-driven facets of resilience, I interpreted how the detail reported by young people reflected their culture and context. I also considered how well young people's accounts fitted with that of the adult-panel (as reported in Theron et al., 2013). I asked an independent, experienced resilience-focused researcher to critically consider my analysis. I used his comments to make minor changes.

Results

The young people who participated in the included studies were mostly adolescents (twelve studies compared with four that included young adults and one that included children only). A number of the studies included participants that ranged from childhood to adolescence (seven studies) or adolescence to young adulthood (three studies). There was a similar mix in terms of context: fourteen studies included both rural and urban township communities, seven urban townships only, and six rural communities only. The resilience processes of participating Black South African young people occurred in the face of chronic adversity, including violence (family, community, political, sexual); poverty, orphanhood, and/or neglect; HIV- and AIDS-related challenges (including social stigma); substance-abusing families/communities; streetism; high mobility/migrancy; and/or physical disability.

My analysis of the literature suggested that, regardless of the nature of the risk, all six adult-identified mechanisms of resilience contributed to a lesser/greater extent to why/how young people adjusted well to adverse life circumstances.[3] A frequency count showed that being value-driven and having and drawing on active support systems were reported more often than the other four resilience-supporting mechanisms (i.e. making educational progress, being a dreamer, drawing on personal resources, demonstrating acceptance). Also, young people's accounts suggested that being a dreamer was intertwined with educational aspirations and progress in this regard (and accordingly reported as such in the following).

Being value-driven[4]

The traditionally African values that young people had been socialised to and adhere to, and that they have made their own, directed their everyday practices.

Essentially, youth-informed accounts of resilience placed emphasis on the protective nature of these values that they had internalised and acted on. This included the protective value of Christian religious beliefs and practices (e.g. church attendance, prayer) and ancestral beliefs and practices (e.g. communing with ancestors). It also included *Ubuntu* values (e.g. respect, reciprocity) and cultural practices/rites as integral to how and why they adjusted to hardship.

Spirituality (i.e. religious and/or ancestral beliefs and practices) supported meaning making and/or hope (e.g. Dass-Brailsford, 2005) and access to a community of supportive others (e.g. Germann, 2005; Pillay & Nesengani, 2006). It encouraged a tendency to behave in more normative ways and in doing so supported regulation (i.e. conforming to societal order – see Malindi & Theron, 2010; Pienaar et al., 2006; Pienaar et al., 2011). It also prompted emancipation, in that spiritual values, such as forgiveness or conceptualising God as a father figure, encouraged young people to forgive, adopt new identities, and move on (e.g. Odendaal et al., 2011; Phasha, 2010).

Allegiance to *Ubuntu* values translated into young people directing their agency toward serving their families and community at some point in the future (e.g. Dass-Brailsford, 2005; Theron, 2013; Theron & Theron, 2013). In the interim, allegiance to *Ubuntu* dictated respectful interaction with others, which in turn secured attachments and provided a sense of belonging (e.g. Lau & van Niekerk, 2011; Theron et al., 2011). When young people came from families or communities that enacted ancestral practices or rites of passage, or encouraged culturally appropriate forms of emotional expression (e.g. via music), this facilitated a sense of mastery, group identity, and belonging (e.g. Cook & White, 2006; Malindi, 2014a, b; Theron, 2015; Theron & Malindi, 2010).

Importantly, young people's accounts included reference to family and community members (also service providers and professionals) behaving in ways that aligned with *Ubuntu* values (e.g. Theron et al., 2011). For example young people who told their life stories to Theron and Theron (2014) described teachers who enacted a sense of duty to their students and whose everyday actions were similar to those of caring kin. The same was reported by the Sesotho-speaking young people living in the rural district where the Pathways to Resilience Study took place (see Theron, 2015). They also included accounts of kin and elders actively passing on cultural heritage, in the form of stories, rituals, and/or songs (Cook & White, 2006; Pienaar et al., 2011; Theron & Malindi, 2010).

Having and drawing on active support systems[5]

Unlike in North American and European accounts of the psychosocial supports of resilience (see Werner, 2013), nuclear family structures were underemphasized in what Black South African young people reported – they emphasized kinship, or extended family, systems (see Theron

& Theron, 2013, for a detailed explanation of kinship systems). Within kinship systems, mothers and grandmothers were generally prioritized (e.g. Barbarin et al., 2001; Dass-Brailsford, 2005; Germann, 2005; Govender & Killian, 2001; Malindi, 2014b; Phasha, 2010; Theron, 2015). For example of the 172 isiZulu-speaking participants in the study by Govender and Killian (2001), 60% reported living with their mothers. Kin facilitated resilience processes by offering secure attachments (that provided access to basic resources needed for survival and pragmatic and emotional support), supporting young people to make meaning of hardship and in doing so accommodate hardship, and urging culturally relevant agency such as educational aspirations and being a role model for younger peers (e.g. Dass-Brailsford, 2005; Phasha, 2010; Theron, 2007; Theron & Theron, 2013). Although there was mention of supportive community members (e.g. neighbours – e.g. Phasha, 2010; Theron, 2007) and of supportive civil organisations or service providers/professionals (e.g. Hlatshwayo & Vally, 2014; Malindi, 2014b; Theron & Theron, 2014; Van Breda, 2015), most young people relied on kin. For example in the study by Wild et al. (2011) with young people who were orphans, 96% of younger adolescents (aged 10–14) and 85% of older adolescents (15–19) lived with biological kin. Significantly, when community-affiliated adults were included in accounts of resilience, these accounts suggested that these adults behaved in kin-like ways, such as providing food and clothing, encouraging school attendance, or forming caring bonds with young people (e.g. Malindi, 2014b; Theron, 2015; Theron & Theron, 2014).

Making educational progress and being a dreamer[6]

As explained next, these two mechanisms were interwoven in young people's accounts of what informed their resilience. There were exceptions (e.g. Malindi, 2014a; Van Breda, 2015 reported optimistic future aspirations without linking these to education). Mostly though, youth-directed accounts of resilience illustrated that young people dreamed of an improved and/or purposeful future, one that was enabled by having completed high school, college, and/or university. Young people associated the latter with opportunity for meaningful employment and status. They perceived that the associated benefits would profit the collective – their families or communities – too (e.g. Dass-Brailsford, 2005; Hlatshwayo & Vally, 2014; Phasha, 2010; Pienaar et al., 2011; Theron, 2015; Theron & Theron, 2013). Young people's families and communities reinforced an intermingling of dreaming and educational aspiration directly (e.g. via high expectations) and indirectly (e.g. via others role-modelling educational and subsequent lifestyle success) by (Dass-Brailsford, 2005; Ebersöhn, 2007; Theron, 2007, 2015; Theron & Malindi, 2010; Theron & Theron, 2013, 2014). For example in the study by Dass-Brailsford (2005), one young man (with the pseudonym of Cedric) voiced this as: 'I am my family's hope' (p. 582). Similarly, in the study reported by Theron and Theron (2014), Atile (also a pseudonym) reported how his teachers' expectations drove him: 'I thought that they saw potential in me, and so I have to reveal, take out, that potential and show them that I can, not let them down. Yeah, they believed a lot in me' (p. 300).

Drawing on personal resources[7]

Young people's accounts of their resilience occasionally included reference to personal attributes and strengths that they harnessed. As originally suggested by the adult panel that informed Theron et al.'s study (2013), these included being flexible, solution-focused, responsive, determined, assertive, communicative, and self-assured (Dass-Brailsford, 2005; Ebersöhn, 2007; Ebersöhn & Maree,

2006; Germann, 2005; Malindi, 2014a; Malindi & Theron, 2010; Theron, 2007; Theron & Malindi, 2010; Van Breda, 2015). What young people added to this was appreciation and use of humour (e.g. Ebersöhn, 2007; Malindi, 2014a; Malindi & Theron, 2010).

Demonstrating acceptance[8]

Being tolerant of hardship and simultaneously being hopefully future-oriented was reported, but infrequently so (Germann, 2005; Lau & Van Niekerk, 2011; Odendaal et al., 2011; Theron, 2013, 2015; Theron & Malindi, 2010; Theron & Theron, 2013; Van Breda, 2015). In some instances, acceptance flowed from meaning-making processes that suggested that hardship was pervasive and therefore something that needed to be accommodated (e.g. Theron, 2015). In others, it related to young people reframing difficulties as opportunities for growth (e.g. Lau & van Niekerk, 2011; Theron, 2013). Alternatively (e.g. Germann, 2005; Theron & Malindi, 2010), young people were stoical about life's challenges because they believed that they had already coped with more difficult ones.

Drawing tentative conclusions

As noted at the outset of this chapter, culture and context are fluid. Consequently the conclusions here will need to be periodically updated and revised as necessary. Nevertheless, at this point in time and as detailed here, the earlier review prompts a contextualised understanding of the psychosocial mechanisms (such as attachment, agency and mastery, and meaning making) that characteristically informed the resilience processes of Black South African young people who participated in research studies during 2000–2015.

The influence of traditionally African culture on the resilience processes of Black South African young people

With the exception of drawing on personal resources – which, following Werner (2013), appear to be generic enough to fit the personal resources of young people globally – the mechanisms described earlier fit with the traditionally African cultural maxims of harmoniously interrelated ways-of-being, including valuing kinship systems (see Mkhize, 2006), spiritually oriented ways-of-being, and honouring a duty to the collective. The review earlier included multiple examples of this being a bi-directional process – young people and their social ecologies showed allegiance to traditional African culture. Accordingly, the universally occurring attachment process was expressed as being connected to extended family and/or to adults who behave in kin-like ways (see also Theron, 2015; Theron & Phasha, 2015). Similarly, young people were sustained by resources and meaning making that traditional Africans value, namely religious and ancestral beliefs and practices. Tolerant acceptance, coupled with forgiveness, is part of this spiritual belief system (Phasha, 2010). Hope too was not an individually focused construct: it was aligned with what the cultural group valued (i.e. education), actively reinforced, and intertwined with an education-enabled future that would, potentially, uplift the collective.

Interestingly, Hlatshwayo and Vally (2014) considered that investment in education, given its likely long-term gains, offered migrant young people a form of resistance against xenophobia. It is possible, that educational progress enables young people to defy the many derogatory labels that were imposed on Black South Africans during Apartheid and to disrupt entrenched cycles of poverty. In many ways, this is what archetypal Black South African leaders, such as Biko and Mandela, aspired to in their urging of young people to valorise education (see Theron, 2015; Theron & Phasha, 2015). Nevertheless, I suggest that being invested in education is a gentle form of resistance – one that adheres to traditionally African expectations of harmonious inter-relatedness.

There is a cautionary note to this. Although the vast majority of studies detailed how cultural values, practices, and expectations enabled resilience processes, there were isolated accounts of the opposite. For example Dass-Brailsford (2005) noted instances of an absence of *Ubuntu*-informed responses to her participants' educational success: in some cases, community members were jealous. Theron and Theron (2014) reported the disillusionment of young people when teachers failed to live up to *Ubuntu* values and, instead, put young people down or turned a blind eye to social injustice or, worse, perpetrated injustice themselves. Phasha (2010) noted that some mothers and extended family behaved in toxic ways that jeopardized young women's resilience. Similarly, Theron (2013) commented on how cultural expectations curtailed participants' freedom to choose alternate life-paths or act in their own best interests. In other words, understandings of how culture informs the resilience processes of young people should not be blind to the potential of cultural expectations to 'entrap' (Panter-Brick, 2015, p. 239) young people or to the potential for young people to be disappointed when cultural belief systems (e.g. religion) fail to protect them from tragedies, calamities, and other negative experiences (Masten, 2014).

The influence of context on the resilience processes of Black South African young people

Again, with the exception of personal resources, the mechanisms described earlier fit with the contextual reality of most Black South African young people living with their mothers or other non-biological parent figures (Hall et al., 2014). Given this, the pre-eminence of mothers and grandmothers in young people's accounts of resilience makes sense. So too does the prominence of teachers, given that most Black South African young people have no/limited access to other service providers/professionals (Theron & Theron, 2014).

As argued in Theron (2015), the contextual reality of structurally inferior communities in which human suffering is so wide-spread that appears normative could explain tolerant acceptance. An alternative would be an activist resistance (see, for example Honwana, 2013). The fact that acceptance was least well reported (compared with the other five mechanisms) illustrates a possible difference in the perspectives of adults and young people about what informs resilience. It is possible that the perspectives of the adult panel that informed the theorising reported by Theron et al. (2013) were shaped by their lived experiences of being young people during the Apartheid regime. The viciousness of the then government against activists – see for example Mandela (1995) – could easily have conditioned people to endorse stoic acceptance of hardship and to dissuade resistance. Many younger Black Africans are responding less passively, but it is unclear how their activism can be sustained and whether sustained activism will support mean-ingful outcomes (Honwana, 2013). Thus, contextual understandings of resilience come with a cautionary note too: it is insufficient to document how context shapes resilience processes (see Theron, 2015). Resilience-focused researchers have a moral responsibility to draw attention to the ways in which contexts place young people at risk and to advocate for structural and social change that will make it less necessary for young people to engage in resilience processes (be they tolerant or activist).

Linda C. Theron

Way forward

Understanding that resilience is a contextualised process instructs resilience-supporting interactions between young people and their social ecologies – in particular mental health practitioners and other service providers. In the case of Black African young people, social ecologies are advised to recognise what is apparently a 'leitmotiv' (Panter-Brick, 2015, p. 237): investment in education for the good of the self and the collective. Because the extant literature reviewed in this chapter excluded accounts of whether such investment pays off, it is crucial that resilience research follows up on how young people's education-intertwined dreams play out, and if/how this leitmotiv changes. Equally importantly, to champion resilience in the meantime, social ecologies need to draw on, and sustain, what young people themselves prioritise: kinship systems, service providers who behave in kin-like ways, inter-related ways-of-being, and an *Ubuntu* ethic. Simultaneously, mental practitioners and other service providers need to campaign for change that will transform physical and social ecologies into spaces that are less likely to jeopardize the well-being of young people.

Notes

1 Townships residential areas were specifically created by the Apartheid government (i.e. 1948–1994) to segregate black South Africans. Similar to favelas in Rio de Janeiro or ghettos in urban America, townships are structurally inferior and poorly serviced (Swartz & Scott, 2014).
2 The African Charter considers 35 to be the upper age limit for youth – see Unesco (no date).
3 Given the number of studies that included participants that ranged across developmental stages and/or that came from both rural and urban contexts, it is not possible to comment on if/how the mechanisms varied according to developmental stage/context.
4 Nineteen of the twenty-seven (or 70% of) articles included traditional African values as having a protective influence.
5 Sixteen of the twenty-seven (or 59% of) articles included relationships as having a protective influence.
6 Twelve of the twenty-seven (or 44% of) articles included educational aspirations and dreams of a better life as having a protective influence.
7 Nine of the twenty-seven (or 33% of) articles included personal resources as having a protective influence.
8 Eight of the twenty-seven (or 30% of) articles included personal resources as having a protective influence.

References

Barbarin, O. A., Richter, L., & deWet, T. (2001). Exposure to violence, coping resources, and psychological adjustment of children. *American Journal of Orthopsychiatry, 71*(1), 16–25.
Botha, K., & Moletsane, M. (2012). Western and African aetiological models. In A. Burke (Ed.), *Abnormal psychology: A South African perspective* (2nd ed., pp. 56–83). Cape Town, RSA: Oxford University Press.
Cook, P., & White, W. (2006). Risk, recovery and resilience: Helping young and old move together to support South African communities affected by HIV/AIDS. *Journal of Intergenerational Relationships, 4*(1), 65–77.
Dass-Brailsford, P. (2005). Exploring resiliency: Academic achievement among disadvantaged black youth in South Africa. *South African Journal of Psychology, 35*(3), 574–591.
Ebersöhn, L. (2007). Voicing perceptions of risk and protective factors in coping in a HIV & AIDS landscapes reflecting on capacity for adaptiveness. *Gifted Education International, 23*(2), 149–159.
Ebersöhn, L., & Maree, J. G. (2006). Demonstrating resilience in an HIV and AIDS context: An emotional intelligence perspective. *Gifted Education International, 22*(1), 14–30.
Eze, C. (2014). Rethinking African culture and identity: The Afropolitan model. *Journal of African Cultural Studies, 26*(2), 234–247.

Germann, S. E. (2005). I am a hero – Orphans in child-headed households and resilience. *Commonwealth Youth and Development, 3*(2), 39–53.

Govender, K., & Killian, B. J. (2001). The psychological effects of chronic violence on children living in South African townships. *South African Journal of Psychology, 31*(2), 1–11.

Hall, K., Meintjes, H., & Sambu, W. (2014). Demography of South Africa's children. In S. Mathews, L. Jamieson, L. Lake, & C. Smith (Eds.), *South African child gauge 2014* (pp. 90–93). Cape Town, RSA: Children's Institute, University of Cape Town.

Hall, K., & Sambu, W. (2014). Income poverty, unemployment and social grants. In S. Mathews, L. Jamieson, L. Lake, & C. Smith (Eds.), *South African child gauge 2014* (pp. 94–98). Cape Town, RSA: Children's Institute, University of Cape Town.

Hlatshwayo, M., & Vally, S. (2014). Violence, resilience and solidarity: The right to education for child migrants in South Africa. *School Psychology International, 35*(3), 266–279.

Honwana, A. M. (2013). *Youth, waithood and protest movements in Africa.* International African Institute, Lugard Lecture. Retrieved from www.internationalafricaninstitute.org/downloads/lugard/Lugard%20 Lecture%20%202013.pdf

Kritzas, N., & Grobler, A. A. (2005). The relationship between perceived parenting styles and resilience during adolescence. *Journal of Child and Adolescent Mental Health, 17*(1), 1–12.

Lau, U., & van Niekerk, A. (2011). Restorying the self: An exploration of young burn survivors' narratives of resilience. *Qualitative Health Research, 21*(9), 1165–1181.

Liebenberg, L., & Ungar, M. (2009). Introduction: The challenges in researching resilience. In L. Liebenberg & M. Ungar (Eds.), *Researching resilience* (pp. 3–25). Toronto: University of Toronto Press.

McCubbin, L. D., & Moniz, J. (2015). Ethical principles in resilience research: Respect, relevance, reciprocity and responsibility. In L. C. Theron, L. Liebenberg, & M. Ungar (Eds.), *Youth resilience and culture: Commonalities and complexities* (pp. 217–229). Dordrecht, the Netherlands: Springer.

Malindi, M. J. (2014a). Swimming upstream in the midst of adversity: Exploring resilience-enablers among street children. *Journal of Social Sciences, 39*(3), 265–274.

Malindi, M. J. (2014b). Exploring the roots of resilience among female street-involved children in South Africa. *Journal of Psychology, 5*(1), 35–45.

Malindi, M. J., & Theron, L. C. (2010). The hidden resilience of street youth. *South African Journal of Psychology, 40*(3), 318–326.

Mampane, R., & Bouwer, C. (2006). Identifying resilient and non-resilient middle-adolescents in a formerly black-only urban school. *South African Journal of Education, 26*(3), 443–456.

Mandela, N. (1995). *Long walk to freedom.* London, UK: Abacus.

Masten, A. S. (2014). *Ordinary magic: Resilience in development.* New York, NY: Guilford.

Masten, A. S., & Wright, M. O. (2010). Resilience over the lifespan: Developmental perspectives on resistance, recovery and transformation. In J. W. Reich, A. J. Zautra, & J. S. Hall (Eds.), *Handbook of adult resilience* (pp. 213–237). New York, NY: Guilford.

Mathews, S., & Benvenuti, P. (2014). Violence against children in South Africa: Developing a prevention agenda. In K. Hall., I. Woolard., L. Lake, & C. Smith (Eds.), *The South African child gauge* (pp. 26–34). Cape Town: Children's Institute, University of Cape Town.

Mkhize, N. (2006). African traditions and the social, economic and moral dimensions of fatherhood. In L. Richter & R. Morrell (Eds.), *Baba: Men and fatherhood in South Africa* (pp. 183–198). Cape Town, RSA: HSRC Press.

Mwamwenda, T. S. (2004). *Educational psychology: An African perspective.* Sandton, South Africa: Heinemann.

Nduna, M., & Sikweyiya, Y. (2015). Silence from young women's narratives of absent, unknown and undisclosed fathers from Mpumalanga, South Africa. *Journal of Child and Family Studies, 24*(4), 536–545.

Nystad, K., Spein, A. R., & Ingstad, B. (2014). Community resilience factors among indigenous Sámi adolescents: A qualitative study in Northern Norway. *Transcultural Psychiatry, 51*(5), 651–672.

Odendaal, I. E., Brink, M., & Theron, L. C. (2011). Rethinking Rorschach interpretation: An exploration of resilient black South African adolescents' personal constructions. *South African Journal of Psychology, 41*(4), 528–539.

Panter-Brick, C. (2015). Culture and resilience: Next steps for theory and practice. In L. C. Theron, L. Liebenberg, & M. Ungar (Eds.), *Youth resilience and culture: Commonalities and complexities* (pp. 233–244). Dordrecht, the Netherlands: Springer.

Phasha, T. N. (2010). Educational resilience among African survivors of child sexual abuse in South Africa. *Journal of Black Studies, 40*(6), 1234–1253.

Pienaar, A., Swanepoel, Z., van Rensburg, H., & Heunis, C. (2011). A qualitative exploration of resilience in pre-adolescent AIDS orphans living in a residential care facility. *Journal of Social Aspects of HIV/AIDS, 8*(3), 128–137.

Pienaar, J. M., Beukes, R. B., & Esterhuyse, K. G. (2006). The relationship between conservatism and psychological well-being in adolescents. *South African Journal of Psychology, 36*(2), 391–406.

Pillay, J., & Nesengani, R. I. (2006). The educational challenges facing early adolescents who head families in rural Limpopo Province. *Education as Change, 10*(2), 131–147.

Pityana, B. (1999). The renewal of African moral values. In M. Makgoba (Ed.), *African renaissance* (pp. 137–148). Cape Town, RSA: Tafelberg.

Swartz, S., & Scott, D. (2014). The rules of violence: A perspective from youth living in South African townships. *Journal of Youth Studies, 17*(3), 324–342.

Theron, L. C. (2007). Uphenyo ngokwazi Kwentsha ukumelana nesimo esinzima: A South African study of resilience among township youth. *Child and Adolescent Psychiatric Clinics of North America, 16*(2), 357–375.

Theron, L. C. (2013). Black students' recollections of pathways to resilience: Lessons for school psychologists. *School Psychology International, 34*(5), 527–539.

Theron, L. C. (2015). Towards a culturally- and contextually-sensitive understanding of resilience: Privileging the voices of black, South African young people. *Journal of Adolescent Research.* Ahead of print, doi: 10.1177/0743558415600072

Theron, L. C., Cameron, C. A., Didkowsky, N., Lau, C., Liebenberg, L., & Ungar, M. (2011). A "day in the lives" of four resilient youths: A study of cultural roots of resilience. *Youth & Society, 43*(3), 799–818.

Theron, L. C., & Malindi, M. J. (2010). Resilient street youth: A qualitative South African study. *Journal of Youth Studies, 13*(6), 717–736.

Theron, L. C., & Phasha, N. (2015). Cultural pathways to resilience: Opportunities and obstacles as recalled by black South African students. In L. C. Theron, L. Liebenberg, & M. Ungar (Eds.), *Youth resilience and culture: Commonalities and complexities* (pp. 51–66). Dordrecht, the Netherlands: Springer.

Theron, L. C., & Theron, A. M. C. (2010). A critical review of studies of South African youth resilience, 1990–2008. *South African Journal of Science, 106*(7–8), 1–8.

Theron, L. C., & Theron, A. M. C. (2013). Positive adjustment to poverty: How family communities encourage resilience in traditional African contexts. *Culture & Psychology, 19*(3), 391–413.

Theron, L. C., & Theron, A. M. C. (2014). Education services and resilience processes: Resilient black South African students' experiences. *Child and Youth Services Review, 47*(3), 297–306.

Theron, L. C., Theron, A. M. C., & Malindi, M. J. (2013). Towards an African definition of resilience: A rural South African community's view of resilient Basotho youth. *Journal of Black Psychology, 39*(1), 63–87.

Tian, G., & Wang, X. (2015). Cultural pathways to resilience: Informal social support of at-risk youth in China. In L. C. Theron, L. Liebenberg, & M. Ungar (Eds.), *Youth resilience and culture: Commonalities and complexities* (pp. 93–104). Dordrecht, the Netherlands: Springer.

Unesco. (no date). *What do we mean by "youth"?* Retrieved from www.unesco.org/new/en/social-and-human-sciences/themes/youth/youth-definition/

Ungar, M. (2011). The social ecology of resilience: Addressing contextual and cultural ambiguity of a nascent construct. *American Journal of Orthopsychiatry, 81*(1), 1–17.

Ungar, M. (2015). Resilience and culture: The diversity of protective processes and positive adaptation. In L. C. Theron, L. Liebenberg, & M. Ungar (Eds.), *Youth resilience and culture: Commonalities and complexities* (pp. 37–48). Dordrecht, the Netherlands: Springer.

Van Breda, A. D. (2015). A comparison of youth resilience across seven South African sites. *Child & Family Social Work* (ahead of print). doi: 10.1111/cfs.12222

Watson, M., McMahon, M., Mkhize, N., Schweitzer, R. D., & Mpofu, E. (2011). Career counselling people of African ancestry. In E. Mpofu (Ed.), *Counselling people of African ancestry* (pp. 281–293). New York, NY: Cambridge.

Werner, E. E. (2013). What can we learn about resilience from large-scale longitudinal studies? In S. Goldstein & R. B. Brooks (Eds.), *Handbook of resilience in children* (2nd ed., pp. 87–102). New York, NY: Springer.

Wild, L. G., Flisher, A. J., & Robertson, B. A. (2011). Risk and resilience in orphaned adolescents living in a community affected by AIDS. *Youth & Society, 45*(1), 140–162.

Wright, M. O., Masten, A. S., & Narayan, A. J. (2013). Resilience processes in development: Four waves of research on positive adaptation in the context of adversity. In S. Goldstein & R. B. Brooks (Eds.), *Handbook of resilience in children* (pp. 15–37). New York, NY: Springer.

13

Emotion flexibility and psychological risk and resilience

Karin G. Coifman and Shaima Y. Almahmoud

Psychological resilience is typically understood to involve a complex series of processes or behaviors that *together* contribute to high or normative levels of functioning within the context of highly aversive events. After decades of research, we now know convincingly that resilience is both common (Bonanno, 2004) and multi-faceted (Bonanno, Brewin, Kaniesty, & LaGreca, 2010). However, in this chapter, we propose that many processes commonly associated with resilient outcomes (e.g. adaptive coping and appraisals, supportive relationships) are those that are inherently influenced by emotion and, in particular, are likely grounded in flexible emotion processing. As such, we focus here on the constructs of emotion flexibility, examining links between emotion flexibility and psychological risk and resilience, providing evidence of the underlying neuro-anatomy and circuitry, and discussing influential factors and related research issues.

Most contemporary models of emotion posit that emotions evolved to serve discrete functions in order to facilitate survival and adaptation to specific environmental threats and demands, across species. Indeed, there is clear evidence for discrete functions for emotions such as fear (Ohman & Mineka, 2001), sadness (Bonanno, Goorin, & Coifman, 2008), anger (Lerner & Keltner, 2001), disgust (Tybur, Lieberman, Kurzban, & DeScioli, 2013), joy, and happiness (Gruber, Mauss, & Tamir, 2011) to facilitate survival as well as social living. In particular, there is research demonstrating the important role emotions play in relationships, facilitating connection, support, and shared values (Keltner, Haidt, & Shiota, 2006). Moreover, importantly, there is also considerable evidence demonstrating how emotions can facilitate cognitive processes that underlie individual and group coping efforts (e.g. problem solving: Gasper, 2003; persistence: He, Xu, & Degnan, 2012; empathy: Roberts, Strayer, & Denham, 2014). All in all, this considerable body of evidence suggests that discrete emotions serve unique functions that underlie multiple adaptive processes. However, implicit in theory and prior research is the notion that emotions are only adaptive within the context for which they evolved. For example fear is highly adaptive in the presence of a true threat (cf. Ohman & Mineka, 2001). Fear is associated with a number of physiological changes that facilitate efficient responses to threat for the individual (e.g. increases in sympathetic autonomic activity) as well as corresponding behavioral signals that are adaptive for the larger group. For example facial expressions of fear are highly recognizable across cultures (Russell, Suzuki, & Ishida, 1993) and species (Bloom & Friedman, 2013). Moreover, there are specific changes in cognitive processing associated with fear responses that can facilitate enhanced attention and perceptual clarity (Phelps, Ling, & Carrasco, 2006). However, when fear responses extend beyond the context of a true threat, they are typically maladaptive, and patterns of contextually insensitive or over-generalized fear responses have been consistently tied to poor psychological functioning, including damaging relationships (e.g. Rehman, Evraire, Karimiha, & Goodnight, 2015) and increasing risk of psychiatric disease (Graham & Milad, 2011). Similar evidence exists for most other emotions, including joy (Gruber et al., 2011). Indeed, embedded in most models of emotion, emotion regulation and emotion-related psychiatric disorders (i.e. depression, anxiety, stress, eating and substance disorders) is the notion that emotions are adaptive yet contextually bound (Cole, Michel, & Teti, 1994; Ekman, 1992; John & Gross, 2004; Kring, 2008; Nolen-Hoeksema & Watkins, 2011). Indeed, although specific emotions can serve important functions, they are only adaptive if they are flexibly and appropriately limited in response to contextual demands.

Given that emotions are functionally limited by context, it is reasonable then to assume that *adaptive emotional processing or responding must include frequent and flexible modulation* as circumstances and demands shift. As such, much of emotion processing is likely to proceed implicitly or automatically, so as to not deter an individual from more important activities that require deliberate or conscious action (Koole & Rothermund, 2011). Indeed, we can define emotion flexibility broadly as the ability to respond to shifting emotional contexts, including environmental contexts as well as internally elicited emotion (cf. Ochsner et al., 2009) with appropriate modulation of emotional responses, encompassing automatic, implicit as well as deliberate processing. This by definition would include the ability to generate or up-regulate emotions in response contextual factors as well as the ability to shift or down-regulate emotions as contextual parameters or features change (Coifman & Bonanno, 2009).

Flexible emotion processing has been studied either directly or relatedly across samples and circumstances. Indeed, there is a growing body of research specifically indexing emotion flexibility through lab paradigms and experience sampling. However, there are a number of related constructs that are important to also consider under this umbrella of emotion flexibility. For example the constructs of emotional reactivity, negative emotionality, threat sensitivity, or even neuroticism all to some degree capture the tendency of an individual to generate negative emotional responses in negative emotion-eliciting contexts.[1] Moreover, some views of emotion regulation encompass broadly the ability to generate *and* up-regulate emotions (e.g. Cole et al., 1994) whereas others have focused primarily on the ability to alter or down-regulate emotions (e.g. Gross, 2010). However, what differentiates specific study of emotion flexibility, versus the many related constructs, is that emotion flexibility demands repeated assessments of real-time emotion responding across multiple contexts or circumstances in order to afford the opportunity to index both the degree of responsiveness to contexts and the flexibility of responses to contextual change. Indeed, it is this considerable methodological demand that likely has limited the amount of specific research on emotion flexibility (as well as other related indices of flexibility, cf. Kashdan & Rottenberg, 2010). However, in this chapter, we will review neuro-biological evidence supporting the two primary underlying dimensions of emotion flexibility, growing evidence directly supporting the link between emotional flexibility and adaptation, and conversely emotional rigidity and maladjustment, as well as consider key elements that influence emotion flexibility including heritable, environmental, and lifestyle factors.

A two-dimensional model of emotion flexibility

Contemporary models distinguish *emotion* responses from enduring *affective* states (e.g. mood) by specifying that emotions are discrete entities, of brief duration, that evolved to facilitate specific responses to environmental threats (Ekman, 1992; Rosenberg, 1998). As such, emotion responses encompass specific behavioral, physiological (e.g. autonomic), and cognitive shifts that are often only loosely coupled or operate in only loosely concordant ways (Bonanno & Keltner, 2004). Conscious awareness of emotion is not necessary for emotional responses or even regulatory responses. Indeed, considerable evidence suggests that awareness of emotion processes is rare and only present a relatively small part of the time (Barge & Williams, 2007; Winkielman & Berridge, 2004). Emotion responses are produced or altered in response to contextual cues, either internal or external in origin. However, both the production of emotion responses and changes in these responses can be understood as occurring because of two closely interrelated processes that underlie emotion flexibility: 1) *emotion generation*, defined as the extent to which an individual is reactive or sensitive to emotional stimuli or context that influences the *degree* to which emotion responses (behavioral, physiological, and/or cognitive) emerge; and 2) *emotion regulatory control*, defined as the extent to which an individual is able to *shift* emotion in accordance with changing conditions, either internally or externally generated. Shifts indicating regulatory activities manifest as *changes* in behavioral, physiological, and/or cognitive indices of emotion. Although some dominant characterizations of emotion regulatory responses focus *only* on deliberate actions (e.g. reappraisal or suppression (Gross & John, 2003), we employ a broader definition based on the growing consensus that regulatory control of emotion is primarily automatic/implicit (Koole & Rothermunde, 2011; Mauss, Bunge, & Gross, 2007). Indeed, regulatory activity is commonly evidenced in specific brain regions associated with deliberate *and* automatic or implicit control of attention, working memory, and inhibition, all processes underlying emotion regulatory control (Kaplan & Berman, 2010; Pourtois, Notebaert, & Verguts, 2012; Shackman et al., 2011). Moreover, deliberate as well as automatic or implicit emotion regulatory strategies activate similar neural correlates and have similar effects on emotion responses (Payer, Baicy, Lieberman, & London, 2012; Williams, Bargh, Nocera, & Gray, 2009). As such, *emotion regulatory control,* from this broader perspective, includes actions undertaken deliberately, automatically, or implicitly to alter behavioral, physiological, or cognitive responses to emotion-evoking stimuli, circumstances, and/or events.

Emotion generation and regulatory control map closely onto neuroanatomical regions that have been shown to discretely influence these processes as well as to have extensive and highly complex interacting circuitry (Dennis & Chen, 2007; Hartley & Phelps, 2010; LeDoux & Phelps, 2008). For example considerable neuroimaging data implicate the limbic region in emotion generation, irrespective of valence, most notably involving the amygdalae (Cunningham & Brosch, 2012). By contrast, regulatory control involves the prefrontal cortex (Braver, Cole, & Yarkoni, 2010; Kane & Engle, 2002; Perlman & Pelphrey, 2010) in regions that influence traditionally higher-order "cognitive control" processing elements (i.e. attention, working memory, inhibition; see Hofmann, Friese, & Roefs, 2009; Kaplan & Berman, 2010; McRae, Jacobs, Ray, John, & Gross, 2012; Pourtois et al., 2012; Shackman et al., 2011). However, this classic bottom-up, top-down view has become increasingly murky. Most recent models of the neural circuitry of emotion, based on cross-species research, suggest a complex interaction between amygdala activity in response to sensory input that broadly project to cortical and subcortical regions. This is in contrast to activity originating in cortical regions (e.g. dorso-lateral prefrontal cortex) that may inhibit the amygdala through its connection with the medial prefrontal cortex (LeDoux & Phelps, 2008). For example there is considerable non-human primate and rodent research indicating that activity in the ventromedial prefrontal cortex is necessary for the extinction of fear through its inhibition of amygdala output (Pape & Pare, 2010; Quirk & Mueller, 2008). Moreover, some regions of the medial prefrontal cortex (prelimbic cortex vs. infralimbic cortex) are involved in *activating* fear versus others in *inhibiting* fear, and both of these regions have extensive reciprocal connections with the amygdalae (Pape & Pare, 2010). Indeed, there is increasing evidence of complex bi-directional controls over emotion responding (including both emotion generation and emotion regulatory control), and the complexity of these processes make them particularly challenging to disentangle in humans (LeDoux, 2012). *In sum, this evidence overwhelmingly suggests that, although emotion generation and emotion regulatory control can be considered distinct, they are highly interrelated.* Indeed, it seems one is never without the other.

In the course of daily life, one could argue for the importance of the interaction of emotion generation and emotion regulatory control in *adaptive* emotion processing. For example adaptive responses to negative events (e.g. a failed grade on a test) involve emotion generation (e.g. behavioral displays of anger, sympathetic autonomic arousal, and the verbal expression of frustration) as well as some degree of emotion regulatory control facilitated by automatic and/ or deliberate means (e.g. redirecting attention to evaluate future opportunities for remediation, which manifests as decreased displays of anger, decreased sympathetic autonomic activity and/or increased parasympathetic activity, and verbal expressions of acceptance and/or hope for change). Alternatively, adaptive responses to positive events (e.g. being selected for lead in the play) also involve emotion generation (e.g. behavioral displays of joy and excitement, sympthetic arousal, and verbal expressions of happiness) and often some degree of emotion regulatory control facilitated by automatic and/or deliberate means (e.g. in this case redirecting attention to less-fortunate cast members, which then decreases displays of joy, decreases arousal, and increases verbal expressions of empathy and support). As such, the *interaction* of emotion generation and emotion regulatory control can afford the individual the requisite flexibility to effectively to meet a wide range of contextual demands in daily life (Bonanno & Burton, 2013; Coifman & Bonanno, 2009). In the context of highly aversive life events, emotion flexibility would facilitate adaptive coping responses, the maintenance of relationships and occupational responsibilities by allowing the individual to *both engage and disengage from event-related emotions* in order to still meet the demands of daily life.

Evidence of this precise interaction has been relatively hard to capture in the laboratory, and much research has focused on examining contextually sensitive emotion generation *or* emotion regulatory control. In particular, researchers have employed lab paradigms that place implicit demands on participants to spontaneously shift emotional responses to adjust to shifting emotional contexts. These paradigms capitalize on the interdependence or reciprocal nature of emotion generation and emotion regulatory control, specifically, the notion that greater emotion generation demands greater emotion regulatory control and greater emotion regulatory control facilitates greater emotion generation. For example in Figure 13.1, the hypothetical situation of learning about a failing grade is depicted. In the first moment, greater generation of negative emotion in response to learning about the failing grade then demands greater regulatory control to mitigate that response in the service of adaptive cognitive processing. However, in this context emotion regulatory control can also service a shift to other, negative emotions (i.e. fear/worry) and positive emotions (i.e. hope). The greater the regulatory control, the greater the flexibility of emotion generation over time.

Karin G. Coifman and Shaima Y. Almahmoud

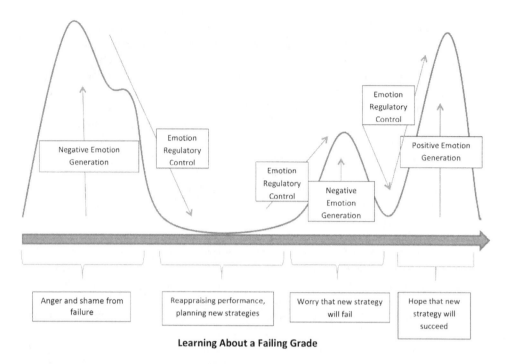

Figure 13.1 Emotion generation and emotion regulatory control sharing reciprocal influence over time

Emotion flexibility and psychological adjustment

Research focused on capturing emotion generation *and/or* emotion regulatory control is growing, demonstrating a compelling link between emotion flexibility and psychological adaptation. For instance, in a sample of bereaved adults, *both* contextually sensitive generation of negative emotion (in response to a query about recent negative events) *and* regulatory control of negative emotion (down-regulation of negative emotion when the context became explicitly positive) early after the loss, was predictive of psychological resilience eighteen months after the loss (Coifman & Bonanno, 2010). Importantly, participant emotion was assessed in real-time during an idiographic interview in which questions about the loss, coping, and recent positive and negative events created unique emotion-eliciting contexts. This paradigm then allowed for direct examination of emotion flexibility and adjustment to spousal bereavement in mid-life, a highly aversive event. Emotion flexibility has also been linked to adaptive discussion of stressful life events in a study of parent–child dyads (Hollenstein & Lewis, 2006). Methodologically, this investigation was quite distinct, indexing and analyzing emotional expressions from moment to moment during naturalistic discussions. However, the data clearly demonstrated the importance of both negative emotion generation and regulatory control in *adaptive* discussions and indicated a tight link between emotion generative ability and regulatory control (characterized as "flexibility" here).

In other populations, there has been research more explicitly focused on emotion generation *or* emotion regulatory control. For example there is evidence that contextually responsive negative emotion generation predicts treatment adherence in chronically ill patients (Harvey, Coifman, Ross, Kleinert, & Giardina, 2014), relationship adjustment in intimate partnerships, and responses to social threat in first-year college students (Coifman, Flynn, & Pinto, 2016). In addition, there is also evidence that contextually sensitive generation of positive emotion predicts long-term social adjustment in victims of childhood sexual abuse (Bonanno et al., 2007). Finally, other research has focused on examining specific evidence of emotion regulatory control in relation to adjustment. For example in first-year college students in New York City immediately following the 9/11 terrorist attacks, flexible up- and down-regulation of emotional expressions (negative and positive) predicted psychological resilience two years later (Bonanno, Papa, Lalande, Westphal, & Coifman, 2004). Together, these data amount to a compelling body of work demonstrating the importance of emotion flexibility in psychological adjustment.

However, not all interactions of emotion generation and emotion regulatory control are adaptive. Indeed, there is increasing evidence suggesting *maladaptive interactions* between these two dimensions that may be critical to understanding the emergence of symptoms of psychiatric illness, most notably emotional disorders. For example deficits in prefrontal processing consistent with areas involved in regulatory control appear to result in prolonged emotional generation (although this generation is not necessarily heightened, just more enduring; cf. Dannlowski et al., 2009). This particular interaction of poor regulatory control with presumably normative emotion generation has been implicated in patients with depression (Erk et al., 2010). In contrast, heightened amygdala responses to emotional stimuli (i.e. heightened emotion generation) have been shown to influence and likely interfere with prefrontal regulatory processes (Dennis & Chen, 2007). This particular interaction of heightened emotion generation with presumably normative regulatory control has most often been implicated in individuals with anxiety (Shackman et al., 2006).

There is now a convincing body of evidence demonstrating some fairly straightforward associations between heightened emotion generation and anxiety (Craske et al., 2009; Craske et al., 2012) versus decreased emotion generation and depressive disorders and/or dysphoria (Bylsma, Morris, & Rottenberg, 2008). For example recent work by Peeters, Berkhof, Rottenberg & Nicolson (2010) has consistently associated a lack of emotion generation (both negative and positive emotions) with depressive symptoms. Indeed, this particular association has proven useful in predicting the persistence of depression (Peeters, Berkhof, Rottenberg, & Nicolson, 2010).

With regard to regulatory control the data is more complex, particularly with regard to specific symptom clusters. For example there is a large body of work linking deficits in regulatory control processes to anxiety and depression, in particular, difficulty with inhibitory processes in emotional contexts (Joorman, Levens, & Gotlib, 2011). The evidence for regulatory deficits in non-emotional contexts appears to be limited primarily to depressive pathology (Hammar & Ardal, 2009; Levin, Heller, Mohanty, Herrington, & Miller, 2007), suggesting that in anxiety, regulatory deficits could be attributed to an individual's *heightened emotion generation that interferes with emotion regulatory control.* However, disentangling these dimensions in current clinical samples is particularly complex given the very clear limitations of current diagnostic systems (Insel et al., 2010). Nevertheless, it is clear that emotion generation and emotion regulatory control are key dimensions that have a lot to offer in clinical research, particularly research focused on more effectively modelling emotion-related disease. Moreover, it is clear that emotion *in*-flexibility, or perhaps more aptly "emotion rigidity", may be frequent in emotional disorders, although much more work here is warranted.

Factors underlying emotion flexibility

It is increasingly evident that there are a number of factors, inherited and learned, that can strongly influence emotion processing differences across individuals, including in particular processes that underlie emotion flexibility. Together, these factors likely account for a considerable portion of the variability evident in emotion processing. As such, they are highly relevant in models of psychological risk and resilience. Although reviewing this entire literature is beyond the scope of this chapter, we will review examples of evidence supporting the influence of some key factors.

Over the last two decades there has been an increasing proportion of research focused on explicating genetic influences on psychiatric risk and disease. This research is complicated and has been fraught with controversy over weak methodology and replication. However, in one particular area, hundreds of articles have now been published examining the link between variation in the serotonin transporter (5-HTT) gene (*SLC6A4*) and psychological risk. Recent reviews have been able to integrate and synthesize basic research findings across species suggesting links between variation in *SLC6A4* and emotion processing that are driven by changes in neural circuitry (cf. Hariri & Holmes, 2006). In particular, there is evidence that individuals carrying two copies of the functional short (S') allele show deficits in emotion regulatory control (Gilman et al., in press). This may be because of reduced or inefficient connectivity between the prefrontal cortex and the amygdala (Beevers, Pacheco, Clasen, McGeary, & Schnyer, 2010; Pezawas et al., 2005). Although variation in *SLC6A4* is highly promising, it is one gene, and there are likely hundreds of heritable genetic factors that influence the processes and/or circuitry that underlie emotion flexibility. Importantly, we can point to twin studies that have broadly demonstrated the heritability of emotional responsivity (typically measured in terms of sensitivity or reactivity to negative emotional content; cf. Steptoe, van Jaarsveld, Semmler, Plomin, Wardle, 2009) as well as regulatory resources (typically measured as higher-order neurocognitive resources; cf. Tucker-Drob & Briley, 2014). Indeed, it is quite clear that individuals are born with varying levels of emotion generative and regulatory control resources that are then influenced by what occurs in life.

Despite the increasing evidence linking specific inherited genetic variation to emotion flexibility, there is even more compelling evidence suggestive of epigenetic effects, which may be highly influential in emotion processing. Epigenetic variation is defined as changes to the genome that occur as a result of *experience* and then are passed on to subsequent generations. An excellent example of epigenetic variation highly relevant to psychological risk and resilience (and also to emotion flexibility), is research examining the influence of high-contact mothering in rats (e.g. high licking and grooming mothers) on subsequent generations. For example there is evidence that maternal behavior influences stress reactivity in offspring, such that greater licking and grooming produces greater activation of the glucocorticoid receptor gene thereby lowering circulating glucocorticoid (stress hormone) levels as more receptors remove it from circulation (Meaney, 2001). The resulting effect is greater approach-related behavior (e.g. greater exploration, less fearfulness) as well as cognitive processing benefits that facilitate greater regulatory control (Blair, 2010). Most important, however, is the evidence, now also suggested in human samples (Diamond & Amso, 2008), of the intergenerational transmission of these benefits, such that offspring of high-contact mothers have offspring who show similar benefits.

Considerable developmental research has also demonstrated the role of parenting on emotion regulatory control resources and emotion generative responses through behavioral mechanisms (Pollack, 2012). For example there is research demonstrating alterations in early emotion attentional processing (e.g. biases towards negative emotional content) resulting in greater negative emotion generation in individuals who experienced maltreatment (Shackman & Pollack, 2014; Shackman, Shackman, & Pollack, 2007). These alterations have been tied to later increased risk for emotion-related disorders. In addition, there is evidence suggestive of the influence of parenting and attachment on emotion regulatory control. For example multiple investigations of severely maltreated children have demonstrated a strong link to deficits in higher-order cognitive processes underlying regulatory control (e.g. Nolin & Ethier, 2007). In addition, there is also evidence demonstrating ways in which parenting might enhance emotion regulatory control. One example would be research examining attachment and parenting influences on the development of emotional language (Denham & Kochanoff, 2002). For example in children, it is has been well established that greater emotion knowledge and understanding is associated with better adjustment and reduced risk (Denham et al., 2002; Ensor, Spencer, & Hughes, 2011). Indeed, there is evidence demonstrating the beneficial influence of emotion-related discussion between parents and children (Van Bergen & Salmon, 2010) as well as evidence breaking down parent-related and other factors that influence emotion language development (Beck, Kumschick, Eid, & Klann-Delius, 2012; Martin, Williamson, Kurtz-Nelson, & Boekamp, 2015; Salmon et al., 2013). Finally, in adults, richer use of emotion language and more complex conceptualization of emotional experience has been directly tied to emotion regulatory benefits (Lieberman et al., 2007) as well as increased adaptive behavior during stress (Coifman, Ross, Kleinert & Giardina, 2014) and resilient outcomes (Coifman, Bonanno, & Rafaeli, 2007).

Finally, there is a growing literature demonstrating the influence of contemporary lifestyle factors that influence emotion processing and ultimately emotion flexibility. For example there is new research examining how interpersonal emotion regulatory processes occur within intimate partnerships, suggesting that stable and supportive close relationships might enhance emotion flexibility (Zaki & Williams, 2013). In addition, there is evidence that sleep directly influences the efficiency of the circuitry underlying emotion regulatory control, such that deficits in sleep result in less emotion flexibility (e.g. Yoo, Gujar, Hu, Jolesz, & Walker, 2007). Moreover, there is evidence demonstrating that increased physical activity enhances emotion flexibility, including both emotion generation and emotion regulatory control (Shields, Matt, & Coifman, 2015). Together, these factors suggest that there is much to be better understood in models of emotion flexibility and certainly should be considered in models of psychological risk and resilience.

Methodological challenges to consider in the study of emotion flexibility

Given the potential significance of emotion flexibility in adaptive behavior, and psychological processes leading to resilience, it is of great importance that research in this area continues to increase. However, testing the link between emotion flexibility and psychological adjustment is complicated for a number of reasons. First, and perhaps most importantly, the nature of emotion and the emotion response system demands real-time measurement (emotions are rapidly produced and resolved) on multiple channels of responding. Emotions are multi-dimensional with emotion-related behavior, autonomic activity and reported experience only "loosely coupled" (Bonanno & Keltner, 2004). As such, dimensions can serve differing functions, can operate on different time scales (Bulteel et al., 2014), and be under varying influences often not accessible to the individual. Indeed, it is likely that heavy reliance on self-reported emotion has led some research astray, given the vulnerability of that particular response channel to other influence. For example self-reported emotion can be easily altered by demand characteristics (e.g. Dubitsky, Weber, & Rotton, 1993) or environmental circumstances (e.g. Messner & Wanke, 2011) notwithstanding how dispositional tendencies can also bias *reporting* of emotion relative to other response dimensions (e.g. Coifman, Bonanno, Ray, & Gross, 2007).

Next, measurement of emotion flexibility demands that individuals are assessed, not just in real time, but also *across varying contexts* in order to index both emotion generation as well as emotion regulatory control. In addition, the context and type of assessment must be designed so as to minimize demand characteristics and allow for naturalistic responses. For example although there has been a proliferation of research on emotion regulation in which participants are instructed to engage in one or more regulatory techniques (e.g. Gruber, Hay, & Gross, 2014), this cannot by definition capture emotion flexibility. In those particular paradigms, individuals are following explicit instructions and deliberately engaging in a strategy that they may or may not have otherwise enacted. As such, responses that result are not indicative of emotion flexibility (no matter how successful) but instead are indicative of responses associated with a strategy, or an individual's ability to respond to the paradigm in question. We might recommend that researchers interested in capturing emotion flexibility focus on using paradigms that implicitly place demands on participants to engage in different emotional contexts in turn (e.g. a series of films, interview questions, social interaction tasks). This allows for naturalistic and spontaneous emotion processing in response to shifting emotional content that may encompass all varieties of action in emotion generation and regulatory control (deliberate, automatic, implicit) on multiple dimensions of responding.

Finally, although there has been a proliferation of imaging studies examining emotion generation and/or emotion regulatory control processes, these methods also can fall prey to many of the same challenges of non-imaging studies. Indeed, most imaging studies in humans cannot differentiate or disentangle emotion generation from emotion regulatory processes *both* because of the extent of the interacting circuitry (e.g. the direction of the activity of neurons in the structures themselves is not evident; cf. Hartley & Phelps, 2010; LeDoux, 2012) *and* because of the nature of the tasks typically used. For example recent neuro-imaging investigations of resilient versus non-resilient individuals have revealed mixed findings (cf. van der Werff, Pannekoeke, Stein, & van der Wee, 2013), some suggesting differences in underlying emotion-related circuitry (e.g. Cisler et al., 2013) and others not (e.g. Shin et al., 2011). It is likely that much of the murkiness of this literature may be due to these important methodological limitations.

Summary and conclusion

Emotion flexibility is a key element in psychological resilience. Emotions are known to influence nearly every psychological process, and adaptive emotion processing is clearly essential for survival and healthy adjustment. In this chapter, we defined emotion flexibility as the balanced interaction of emotion generation and emotion regulatory control that is responsive to contextual, environmental, or other circumstantial change. Indeed, when there is an imbalance in these processes (e.g. heightened emotion generation and/or reduced emotion regulatory control), there is growing evidence that psychopathology emerges. Conceptually and clinically, there may be a clear advantage to considering each dimension as unique *and* as interacting and these dimensions offer a lot for better understanding processes that influence psychological resilience as well as processes that influence the development of psychological disease. Broadly, it is our hope that greater research attention will be focused on understanding emotion flexibility, including the many factors that may influence, in order to continue to build precise models of the processes that underlie both psychological risk and resilience.

Note

1   Although typically all of these constructs are negatively associated with psychological health, the constructs themselves are capturing a potentially adaptive process (e.g. generating negative emotion). However, as these constructs are often used, it is extreme scores that are maladaptive, potentially characterizing either heightened negative emotion generation or contextually insensitive or over-generalized negative emotion generation.

References

Barge, J. A., & Williams, L. A. (2007). *The nonconscious regulation of emotion*. New York: Guilford Press.

Beck, L., Kumschick, I. R., Eid, M., & Klann-Delius, G. (2012). Relationship between language competence and emotional competence in middle-childhood. *Emotion, 12*(3), 503–514.

Beevers, C. G., Pacheco, J., Clasen, P., McGeary, J. E., & Schnyer, D. (2010). Prefrontal morphology, 5-HTTLPR polymorphism and biased attention for emotional stimuli. *Genes, Brain and Behavior, 9*(2), 224–233.

Blair, C. (2010). Stress and the development of self-regulation in context. *Child Development Perspectives, 4*(3), 181–188.

Bloom, T., & Friedman, H. (2013). Classifying dogs' (Canis familiaris) facial expressions from photographs. *Behavioural Processes, 96*, 1–10.

Bonanno, G. A. (2004). Loss, trauma, and human resilience: Have we underestimated the human capacity to thrive after extremely aversive events? *American Psychologist, 59*(1), 20–28.

Bonanno, G. A., Brewin, C. R., Kaniasty, K., & La Greca, A. M. (2010). Weighing the costs of disaster: Consequences, risks, and resilience in individuals, families, and communities. *Psychological Science in the Public Interest, 11*(1), 1–49.

Bonanno, G. A., & Burton, C. L. (2013). Regulatory flexibility: An individual differences perspective on coping and emotion regulation. *Perspectives on Psychological Science, 8*(6), 591–612.

Bonanno, G. A., Colak, D. M., Keltner, D., Shiota, M. N., Papa, A., Noll, J. G., . . . Trickett, P. K. (2007). Context matters: The benefits and costs of expressing positive emotion among survivors of childhood sexual abuse. *Emotion, 7*(4), 824–837.

Bonanno, G. A., Goorin, L., & Coifman, K. G. (2008). Sadness and grief. In M. Lewis, J. M. Haviland-Jones, & L. F. Barrett (Eds.), *Handbook of emotions* (3rd ed., pp. 797–810). New York: Guilford Press.

Bonanno, G. A., & Keltner, D. (2004). The coherence of emotion systems: Comparing "online" measures of appraisal, facial expressions, and self-report. *Cognition and Emotion, 18*(3), 431–444.

Bonanno, G. A., Papa, A., Lalande, K., Westphal, M., & Coifman, K. G. (2004). The importance of being flexible the ability to both enhance and suppress emotional expression predicts long-term adjustment. *Psychological Science, 15*(7), 482–487.

Braver, T. S., Cole, M. W., & Yarkoni, T. (2010). Vive les differences! Individual variation in neural mechanisms of executive control. *Current Opinion in Neurobiology, 20*(2), 242–250.

Bulteel, K., Ceulemans, E., Thompson, R. J., Waugh, C. E., Gotlib, I. E., Tuerlinckx, F., & Kuppens, P. (2014). DeCon: A tool to detect emotional concordance in multivariate time series data of emotional responding. *Biological Psychology, 98*, 29–42.

Bylsma, L. M., Morris, B. H., & Rottenberg, J. (2008). A meta-analysis of emotional reactivity in major depressive disorder. *Clinical Psychology Review, 28*(4), 676–691.

Cisler, J. M., James, G. A., Tripathi, S., Mletzko, T., Heim, C., Hu, X. P., . . . Kilts, C. D. (2013). Differential functional connectivity within an emotion regulation neural network among individual resilient and susceptible to the depressogenic effects of stress. *Psychological Medicine, 43*(3), 507–518.

Coifman, K. G., & Bonanno, G. A. (2009). Emotion context sensitivity in adaptation and recovery. In A. Kring & D. Sloan (Eds.), *Emotion regulation and psychotherapy* (pp. 157–173). New York: Guilford.

Coifman, K. G., & Bonanno, G. A. (2010). When distress does *not* become depression: Emotion context sensitivity and adjustment to bereavement. *Journal of Abnormal Psychology, 119*(3), 479–490.

Coifman, K. G., Bonanno, G. A., & Rafaeli, E. (2007). Affect dynamics, bereavement and resilience to loss. *Journal of Happiness Studies, 8*(3), 371–392.

Coifman, K. G., Bonanno, G. A., Ray, R. D., & Gross, J. J. (2007). Does repressive coping promote resilience? Affective-autonomic response discrepancy during bereavement. *Journal of Personality and Social Psychology, 92*(4), 745–758.

Coifman, K. G., Flynn, J. J., & Pinto, L. A. (2015). When context matters: Negative emotions predict psychological health and adjustment. *Motivation and Emotion*. Online first: DOI: 10.1007/s11031-016-9553-y

Coifman, K. G., Ross, G. S., Kleinert, D., & Giardina, P. (2014). Negative affect differentiation and adherence during treatment for Thalassemia. *International Journal of Behavioral Medicine, 21*(1), 160–168.

Cole, P. M., Michel, M. K., & Teti, L. O. (1994). The development of emotion regulation and dysregulation: A clinical perspective. *Monographs of the Society for Research in Child Development, 59*(2–3), 73–100.

Craske, M. G., Rauch, S. L., Ursano, R., Prenoveau, J., Pine, D. S., & Zinbarg, R. E. (2009). What is an anxiety disorder? *Depression and Anxiety, 26*(12), 1066–1085.

Craske, M. G., Wolitzky-Taylor, K. B., Mineka, S., Zinbarg, R., Waters, A. M., Vrshek-Schallhorn, S., . . . Ornitz, E. (2012). Elevated responding to safe conditions as a specific risk factor for anxiety versus depressive disorders: Evidence from a longitudinal investigation. *Journal of Abnormal Psychology, 121*(2), 315–324.

Cunningham, W. A., & Brosch, T. (2012). Motivational salience: Amygdala tuning from traits, needs, values, and goals. *Current Directions in Psychological Science, 21*(1), 54–59.

Dannlowski, U., Ohrmann, P., Konrad, C., Domschke, K., Bauer, J., Kugel, H., . . . Suslow, T. (2009). Reduced amygdala-prefrontal coupling in major depression: Association with MAOA genotype and illness severity. *The International Journal of Neuropsychopharmacology, 12*(1), 11–22.

Denham, S. A., Caverly, S., Schmidt, M., Blair, K., DeMulder, E., Caal, S., . . . Maston, T. (2002). Preschool understanding of emotions: Contributions to classroom anger and aggression. *Journal of Child Psychology and Psychiatry, 43*(7), 901–916.

Denham, S. A., & Kochanoff, A. T. (2002). Parental contributions to preschooler's understanding of emotion. *Marriage & Family Review, 34*(3–4), 311–343.

Dennis, T. A., & Chen, C. C. (2007). Neurophysiological mechanisms in the emotional modulation of attention: The interplay between threat sensitivity and attentional control. *Biological Psychology, 76*(1–2), 1–10.

Diamond, A., & Amso, D. (2008). Contributions of neuroscience to our understanding of cognitive development. *Current Directions in Psychological Science, 17*(2), 136–141.

Dubitsky, S., Weber, R., & Rotton, J. (1993). Heat, hostility, and immune function: The moderating effects of gender and demand characteristics. *Bulletin of the Psychonomic Society, 31*(6), 534–536.

Ekman, P. (1992). An argument for basic emotions. *Cognition and Emotion, 6*(3–4), 169–200.

Ensor, R., Spencer, D., & Hughes, C. (2011). You feel sad? Emotion understanding mediates effects of verbal ability and mother-child mutuality on pro-social behaviors: Findings from 2 years to 4 years. *Social Development, 20*(1), 93–110.

Erk, S., Mikschl, A., Stier, S., Ciaramidaro, A., Gapp, V., Weber, B., & Walter, H. (2010). Acute and sustained effects of cognitive emotion regulation in major depression. *Journal of Neuroscience, 30*(47), 15726–15734.

Gasper, K. (2003). When necessity is the mother of invention: Mood and problem solving. *Journal of Experimental Social Psychology, 39*(3), 248–262.

Gilman, L., Latsko, M., Matt, L., Flynn, J., Cabrera, O., Douglas, D., . . . Coifman, C. (in press). *Variation of 5-HTTLPR and deficits in emotion regulation: A pathway to risk?* Manuscript submitted for publication.

Graham, B. M., & Milad, M. R. (2011). The study of fear extinction: Implications for anxiety disorders. *American Journal of Psychiatry, 168*(12), 1255–1264.

Gross, J. J. (2010). The future's so bright, I got a wear shades. *Emotion Review, 2*(3), 212–216.

Gross, J. J., & John, O. P. (2003). Individual differences in two emotion regulation processes: Implications for affect, relationships, and well-being. *Journal of Personality and Social Psychology, 85*(2), 348–362.

Gruber, J., Hay, A. C., & Gross, J. J. (2014). Rethinking emotion: Cognitive reappraisal is an effective positive and negative emotion regulation strategy in bipolar disorder. *Emotion, 14*(2), 388–396.

Gruber, J., Mauss, I. B., & Tamir, M. (2011). A dark side of happiness? How, when, and why happiness is not always good. *Perspectives on Psychological Science, 6*(3), 222–233.

Hammar, A., & Ardal, G. (2009). Cognitive functioning in major depression – a summary. *Frontiers in Human Neuroscience, 3*, 26.

Hariri, A. R., & Holmes, A. (2006). Genetics of emotional regulation: The role of the serotonin transporter in neural function. *Trends in Cognitive Science, 10*(4), 182–191.

Hartley, C. A., & Phelps, E. A. (2010). Changing fear: The neurocircuitry of emotion regulation. *Neuropsychopharmacology, 35*(1), 136–146.

Harvey, M. M., Coifman, K. G., Ross, G., Kleinert, D., & Giardina, P. (2014). Contextually appropriate emotion-word use predicts adaptive health behavior: Emotion context sensitivity and treatment adherence. *Journal of Health Psychology, 1–11.* doi: 10.1177/1359105314532152

He, J., Xu, Q., & Degnan, K. A. (2012). Anger expression and persistence among young children. *Social Development, 21*(2), 343–353.

Hofmann, W., Friese, M., & Roefs, A. (2009). Three ways to resist temptation: The independent contributions of executive attention, inhibitory control, and affect regulation to the impulse control of eating behavior. *Journal of Experimental Social Psychology, 45*(2), 431–435.

Hollenstein, T., & Lewis, M. D. (2006). A state space analysis of emotion and flexibility in parent-child interactions. *Emotion, 6*(4), 656–662.

Insel, T., Cuthbert, B., Garvey, M., Heinssen, R., Pine, D. S., Quinn, K., . . . Wang, P. (2010). Research Domain Criteria (RDOC): Toward a new classification framework for research on mental disorders. *American Journal of Psychiatry, 167*(7), 748–751.

John, O. P., & Gross, J. J. (2004). Healthy and unhealthy emotion regulation: Personality processes, individual differences, and life span development. *Journal of Personality, 72*(6), 1301–1333.

Joorman, J., Levens, S. M., & Gotlib, I. H. (2011). Sticky thoughts: Depression and rumination are associated with difficulties manipulating emotional material in working memory. *Psychological Science, 22*(8), 979–983.

Kane, M. J., & Engle, R. W. (2002). The role of prefrontal cortex in working memory capacity, executive attention, and general fluid intelligence: An individuals-differences perspective. *Psychonomic Bulletin & Review, 9*(4), 637–671.

Kaplan, S., & Berman, M. G. (2010). Directed attention as a common resource for executive functioning and self-regulation. *Perspectives on Psychological Science, 5*(1), 43–57.

Kashdan, T. B., & Rottenberg, J. (2010). Psychological flexibility as a fundamental aspect of health. *Clinical Psychology Review, 30*(7), 865–878.

Keltner, D., Haidt, J., & Shiota, M. N. (2006). Social functionalism and the evolution of emotions. In M. Schaller, J. A. Simpson, & D. T. Kenrick (Eds.), *Evolution and Social Psychology* (pp. 115–142). Madison, CT: Psychosocial Press.

Koole, S. L., & Rothermund, K. (2011). "I feel better but I don't know why": The psychology of implicit emotion regulation. *Cognition & Emotion, 25*(3), 389–399.

Kring, A. (2008). Emotion disturbances as transdiagnostic processes in psychopathology. In M. Lewis, J. M. Haviland-Jones, & L. F. Barrett (Eds.), *Handbook of emotions* (3rd ed., pp. 691–708). New York: Guilford Press.

LeDoux, J. (2012). A neuroscientist's perspective on debates about the nature of emotion. *Emotion Review, 4*(4), 375–379.

LeDoux, J., & Phelps, E. (2008). Emotional networks and the brain. In M. Lewis, J. M. Haviland-Jones, & L. F. Barrett (Eds.), *Handbook of emotions* (3rd ed., pp. 159–179). New York: Guilford Press.

Lerner, J. S., & Keltner, D. (2001). Fear, anger, and risk. *Journal of Personality and Social Psychology, 81*(1), 146–159.

Levin, R. L., Heller, W., Mohanty, A., Herrington, J. D., & Miller, G. A. (2007). Cognitive deficits in depression and functional specificity of regional brain activity. *Cognitive Therapy and Research, 31*(2), 211–233.

Lieberman, M. D., Eisenberger, N. I., Crockett, M. J., Tom, S. M., Pfeifer, J. H., & Way, B. M. (2007). Putting feelings into words: Affect labelling disrupts amygdala activity in response to affective stimuli. *Psychological Science, 18*(5), 421–428.

McRae, K., Jacobs, S. E., Ray, R. D., John, O. P., & Gross, J. J. (2012). Individual differences in reappraisal ability: Links to reappraisal frequency, well-being, and cognitive control. *Journal of Research in Personality, 46*(1), 2–7.

Martin, S. E., Williamson, L. R., Kurtz-Nelson, E. C., & Boekamp, J. R. (2015). Emotion understanding (and misunderstanding) in clinically referred preschoolers: The role of child language and maternal depressive symptoms. *Journal of Child and Family Studies, 24*(1), 24–37.

Mauss, I. B., Bunge, S. A., & Gross, J. J. (2007). Automatic emotion regulation. *Social and Personality Psychology Compass, 1*(1), 146–167.

Meaney, M. J. (2001). Maternal care, gene expression, and the transmission of individual differences in stress reactivity across generations. *Annual Review of Neuroscience, 24*(1), 1161–1192.

Messner, C., & Wanke, M. (2011). Good weather for Schwarz and Clore. *Emotion, 11*(2), 436–437.

Nolen-Hoeksema, S., & Watkins, E. R. (2011). A heuristic for developing transdiagnostic models of psychopathology: Explaining multifinality and divergent trajectories. *Perspectives on Psychological Science, 6*(6), 589–609.

Nolin, P., & Ethier, L. (2007). Using neuropsychological profiles to classify neglected children with or without abuse. *Child Abuse & Neglect, 31*(6), 631–643.

Ochsner, K. N., Ray, R. R., Hughes, B., McRae, K., Cooper, J. C., Weber, J., . . . Gross, J. J. (2009). Bottom-up and top-down processes in emotion generation: Common and distinct neural mechanisms. *Psychological Science, 20*(11), 1322–1331.

Ohman, A., & Mineka, S. (2001). Fears, phobias, and preparedness: Toward an evolved module of fear and fear learning. *Psychological Review, 108*(3), 483–522.

Pape, H. C., & Pare, D. (2010). Plastic synaptic networks of the amygdala for the acquisition, expression, and extinction of conditioned fear. *Physiological Reviews, 90*(2), 419–463.

Payer, D. E., Baicy, K., Lieberman, M. D., & London, E. D. (2012). Overlapping neural substrates between intentional and incidental down-regulation of negative emotions. *Emotion, 12*(2), 229–235.

Peeters, F., Berkhof, J., Rottenberg, J., & Nicolson, N. A. (2010). Ambulatory emotional reactivity to negative daily life events predicts remission from major depressive disorder. *Behaviour Research and Therapy, 48*(8), 754–760.

Perlman, S. B., & Pelphrey, K. A. (2010). Regulatory brain development: Balancing emotion and cognition. *Social Neuroscience, 5*(5–6), 533–542.

Pezawas, L., Meyer-Lindenberg, A., Drabant, E. M., Verchinski, B. A., Munoz, K. E., Kolachana, B. S., . . . Weinberger, D. R. (2005). 5-HTTLPR polymorphism impacts human cingulate-amygdala interactions: A genetic susceptibility mechanism for depression. *Nature Neuroscience, 8*(6), 828–834.

Phelps, E. A., Ling, S., & Carrasco, M. (2006). Emotion facilitates perception and potentiates the perceptual benefits of attention. *Psychological Science, 17*(4), 292–299.

Pollack, S. D. (2012). The role of parenting in the emergence of human emotion: New approaches to the old nature-nurture debate. *Parenting: Science and Practice, 12*(2–3), 232–242.

Pourtois, G., Notebaert, W., & Verguts, T. (2012). Cognitive and affective control. *Frontiers in Psychology, 3*, 1–2.

Quirk, G. J., & Mueller, D. (2008). Neural mechanisms of extinction learning and retrieval. *Neuropsychopharmacology, 33*(1), 56–72.

Rehman, U. S., Evraire, L. E., Karimiha, G., & Goodnight, J. A. (2015). Actor-partner effects and the differential roles of depression and anxiety in intimate-relationships: A cross-sectional and longitudinal analysis. *Journal of Clinical Psychology, 7*(7), 715–724.

Roberts, W., Strayer, J., & Denham, S. (2014). Empathy, anger, guilt: Emotions and prosocial behavior. *Canadian Journal of Behavioral Science, 46*(4), 465–474.

Rosenberg, E. L. (1998). Levels of analysis and the organization of affect. *Review of General Psychology, 2*(3), 247–270.

Russell, J. A., Suzuki, N., & Ishida, N. (1993). Canadian, Greek, and Japanese freely produced emotion labels for facial expressions. *Motivation and Emotion, 17*(4), 337–351.

Salmon, K., Evans, I. M., Moskowitz, S., Grouden, M., Parkes, F., & Miller, E. (2013). The components of young children's emotion knowledge: Which are enhanced by adult emotion talk. *Social Development, 22*(1), 94–110.

Shackman, A. J., Salomons, T. V., Slagter, H. A., Fox, A. S., Winter, J. J., & Davidson, R. J. (2011). The integration of negative affect, pain and cognitive control in the cingulate cortex. *Nature Reviews Neuroscience, 12*(3), 154–167.

Shackman, A. J., Sarinopoulos, I., Maxwell, J. S., Pizzagalli, D. A., Lavric, A., & Davidson, R. J. (2006). Anxiety selectively disrupts visuospatial working memory. *Emotion, 6*(1), 40–61.

Shackman, J. E., & Pollack, S. D. (2014). Impact of physical maltreatment on the regulation of negative affect and aggression. *Development and Psychopathology, 26*(4), 1021–1033.

Shackman, J. E., Shackman, A. J., & Pollack, S. D. (2007). Physical abuse amplifies attention to threat and increases anxiety in children. *Emotion, 7*(4), 838–842.

Shields, M., Matt, L. M., & Coifman, K. G. (2015). Physical activity and negative emotion during peer-rejection: Evidence for emotion context sensitivity. *Journal of Health Psychology*. doi: 10.1177/1359105315587139

Shin, L. M., Bush, G., Milad, M. R., Lasko, N. B., Brohawn, K. H., Hughes, K. C., . . . Pitman, R. K. (2011). Exaggerated activation of dorsal anterior cingulate cortex during cognitive interference: A monozygotic twin study of posttraumatic stress disorder. *American Journal of Psychiatry, 168*(9), 979–985.

Steptoe, A., van Jaarsveld, C. H. M., Semmler, C., Plomin, R., & Wardle, J. (2009). Heritability of daytime cortisol levels and cortisol reactivity in children. *Psychoneuroendocrinology, 34*(2), 273–280.

Tucker-Drob, E. M., & Briley, D. A. (2014). Continuity of genetic and environmental influences on cognition across the life span: A meta-analysis of longitudinal twin and adoption studies. *Psychological Bulletin, 140*(4), 949–979.

Tybur, J. M., Lieberman, D., Kurzban, R., & DeScioli, P. (2013). Disgust: Evolved function and structure. *Psychological Review, 120*(1), 65–84.

Van Bergen, P., & Salmon, K. (2010). Parent-child reminiscing: Associations between an elaborative style and emotion knowledge. *New Zealand Journal of Psychology, 38*, 51–56.

Van der Werff, S., Pannekoeke, J. N., Stein, D. J., & Van der Wee, N. J. A. (2013). Neuroimaging of resilience to stress: Current state of affairs. *Human Psychopharmacology, 28*(5), 529–532.

Williams, L. E., Bargh, J. A., Nocera, C. C., & Gray, J. R. (2009). The unconscious regulation of emotion: Nonconscious reappraisal goals modulate emotional reactivity. *Emotion, 9*(6), 847–854.

Winkielman, P., & Berridge, K. C. (2004). Unconscious emotion. *Current Directions in Psychological Science, 13*(3), 120–123.

Yoo, S. S., Gujar, N., Hu, P., Jolesz, F. A., & Walker, M. P. (2007). The human emotional brain without sleep: A prefrontal amygdala disconnect. *Current Biology, 17*(20), 877–878.

Zaki, J., & Williams, W. C. (2013). Interpersonal emotion regulation. *Emotion, 13*(5), 803–810.

14

Meaning making and resilience

Crystal L. Park

Resilience refers to bouncing back – returning relatively quickly to one's pre-trauma levels of mental health or even remaining relatively un-distressed – following a traumatic experience (Bonanno, Brewin, Kaniasty, & La Greca, 2010). Many psychosocial factors that facilitate resilience have been identified, including previous trauma exposure and social support (Bonanno et al., 2010; King et al., 2012). However, much less is known about the actual *processes* through which people achieve resilience. This chapter takes a meaning-making perspective to illustrate what we know about *how* people recover their mental health and well-being following traumatic experiences.

From this perspective, trauma results when events are appraised as violating individuals' deeply held global beliefs and goals. Meaning making involves either reappraising the traumatic event to perceive it as more consistent with their pre-trauma global beliefs and goals (changing situational meaning) or revising their global beliefs and goals to accommodate their experience (changing global meaning). These changes in meaning, or *meanings made*, decrease individuals' perceptions of violations between their global beliefs and goals and the event, facilitating psychological adjustment to the trauma and promoting resilience. Following a brief introduction to the meaning-making model, this chapter reviews the evidence regarding meaning-making processes in the context of resilience.

The meaning-making model

The meaning-making model focuses on two levels of meaning, global and situational. Global meaning comprises people's fundamental beliefs about themselves and the world, their hierarchies of goals and values, and their sense of meaning and purpose. Situational meaning refers to one's interpretation of and subsequent reactions to a given situation, including assigning meanings to one's experiences and determining the potential discrepancies between one's global and appraised meaning as well as attempts to reconcile those discrepancies (termed "meaning making"), which result in changes in either appraised or global meaning (termed "meaning made"). See Figure 14.1 for a depiction of this process.

People appraise or assign meanings to situations to understand their personal significance (Folkman & Lazarus, 1984). These appraised meanings are formed by individuals' global meaning

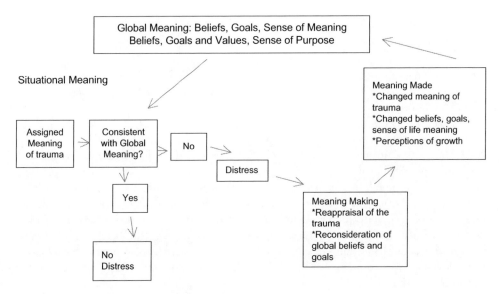

Figure 14.1 The meaning-making model
Source: Park, 2010.

combined with the specific details of a particular situation. For example those with a strong sense that stressful situations are amenable to change may try to understand an event in terms of which aspects can be modified, while someone who believes that events are distributed fairly might seek to understand what prior mistake or offense he or she committed to deserve the present adversity.

Following appraisal of the meaning of an event, individuals determine the extent to which that assigned meaning is congruent with their global beliefs about the world and themselves and their desires and goals. Traumatic events may violate or even "shatter" global beliefs and goals. Such violations or discrepancies may initiate individuals' cognitive and emotional processing efforts – "meaning making" – to rebuild their meaning systems in a way that incorporates their understanding of the trauma (Park & Folkman, 1997).

Meaning making may result in a variety of outcomes, including changes in appraisals of a stressful event (e.g. coming to see it in a more positive light), changes in global meaning (e.g. changing one's global beliefs, spiritual or religious values, or overarching life goals), and perceived stress-related or post-traumatic growth (e.g. perceptions of increased appreciation for life, stronger connections with family and friends, or greater awareness of one's strengths; Park, 2009). Successfully making meaning reduces perceived discrepancies between appraised and global meanings and restores a sense of a meaningful world and a worthwhile life.

Meaning making and resilience following trauma

The meaning-making model has been used to frame research following a variety of highly stressful or traumatic events, including serious illness, bereavement, terrorist attacks, natural disasters, and combat (Park, 2010). These studies have endeavored to identify elements of meaning that mitigate distress following traumatic exposures and that promote a faster and more complete recovery. Such studies add to our understanding the experiences of trauma survivors and may be useful in developing future prevention and intervention efforts.

Global meaning and resilience

Research has examined relations between a range of global meaning and individuals' responses to and recovery from traumatic events to determine whether some kinds of global meaning promote resilience. Global beliefs, such as having a sense of the world as benevolent and fair, have been linked to better adjustment. For example in a sample of 396 Israeli veterans of the 1973 Yom Kippur War, beliefs in self-worth, the benevolence of other people, and the orderliness (as opposed to randomness) of the world were related to less distress and post-traumatic stress disorder (PTSD) symptomatology (Dekel, Solomon, Elklit, & Ginzburg, 2004). In a study of German flood victims, a belief that the universe metes out negative events in a predictable and fair way was associated with lower levels of anxiety, depression, and general psychological distress (but not PTSD symptomatology) (Otto, Boos, Dalbert, Schöps, & Hoyer, 2006). Similarly, high levels of belief in controllability were associated with lower levels of general distress in a sample of survivors of the Marmara earthquake in Turkey (Sumer, Karanci, Berument, & Gunes, 2005). These studies suggest that global beliefs that the world is controllable and fair can be adaptive in the aftermath of trauma. Such beliefs may allow survivors to feel more agency and thus cope more effectively with the trauma and its aftermath.

Having a strong sense of meaning or purpose in life also facilitates post-traumatic resilience. For example in a sample of military veterans, meaning in life was related to lower levels of depression and PTSD symptoms (Owens, Steger, Whitesell, & Herrera, 2009). In a sample of survivors of the 2005 Pakistan earthquake, nearly two-thirds of whom met criteria for likely PTSD, purpose in life was associated with fewer PTSD symptoms and more positive emotions (Feder et al., 2013). In a prospective study of mostly non-Hispanic Black, low-income mothers living in the New Orleans area, purpose in life assessed one year prior to Hurricane Katrina predicted perceived post-traumatic growth – but not PTSD – one and two years after the hurricane (Lowe, Manove, & Rhodes, 2013). Trauma survivors' ability to maintain a sense that their lives mattered and that they had valuable purposes to accomplish appears to help trauma survivors persevere and maintain more positivity, leading to resilience.

Religiousness and spirituality have also been implicated in resilience. In another sample of survivors of the 2005 Pakistani earthquake, assessed three years following it, being "religious-minded" was independently related to lower PTSD symptoms (Ali, Farooq, Bhatti, & Kuroiwa, 2012), suggesting a salutary effect of a global religious life. Findings on religiousness/spirituality and adjustment are inconsistent, however, and some studies have not found a relationship between them, such as a study of a large sample of college students in the areas affected by Hurricanes Katrina and Rita in 2005, for whom religiousness was unrelated to trauma symptoms (Pecchioni, Edwards, & Grey, 2011). Further, another analysis of the prospective data collected from low-income mothers following Hurricane Katrina (described earlier) found that pre-disaster religiousness did not have a direct effect on post-disaster distress, although it did predict less post-disaster distress through a heightened sense of purpose and optimism (Chan, Rhodes, & Pérez, 2012).

Situational meaning and resilience

According to the meaning-making model, myriad aspects of survivors' appraised meanings of the trauma will influence their perceptions of violations of global meaning and subsequent trauma. One recent national survey found that individuals who did not have diagnosable PTSD following any of a number of highly stressful experiences – compared to those who did – were less likely to appraise the event as having occurred because of something they did wrong or that they should have been able to prevent it, and they were less likely to blame themselves and others for the traumatic event (Cox, Resnick, &Kilpatrick, 2014). These findings are consistent with the large literature on appraisals of stressors that generally show that perceiving a stressful event as less threatening and more controllable leads to resilience. For example among 69 bereaved family members and close friends who perished in the Mount Saint Helens volcanic eruption, not seeing the death as preventable predicted decreased distress at one and three years after the eruption (Chenell & Murphy, 1992). A study of survivors of the 2011 Japanese earthquake/tsunami/nuclear disaster found that higher challenge appraisals and lower appraisals of threat were related to less distress and higher perceptions of growth from the disaster and quality of life three months afterwards (Kyutoku et al., 2012).

Much of the research on trauma appraisals and resilience has focused on a specific type of appraisal, causal attributions, one's understanding of why a given event occurred. Attributions can be naturalistic, supernatural/religious, or both. For example naturalistic explanations for the occurrence of a serious car accident may involve weather, driver inattention, or road conditions, while religious attributions may include God's efforts to teach, challenge, or punish the afflicted or to teach a lesson to others (Spilka, Hood, Hunsberger, & Gorsuch, 2003). Individuals often make naturalistic attributions for the immediate or proximal cause of an event but also invoke religious or metaphysical explanations for the more distal, metaphysical cause (see Park & Folkman, 1997).

Religious attributions are often related to better recovery. Nearly half of a sample of women surveyed near the site of the South East Anatolian (Turkey) earthquake explained the quake as the will and guidance of God, while 41% considered it a natural event, and 9% blamed human irresponsibility. Women who blamed other humans for the disaster reported higher levels of distress than did those explaining it as God's will or as a natural event (Sezgin & Punamäki, 2012). In a sample of women survivors of the 2004 Indonesian tsunami, studied three years after the disaster, attributions to karma were negatively related to depressive or PTSD symptoms (Banford, Wickrama, & Ketring, 2014). Similarly, in the study of undergraduates after Katrina and Rita, those who appraised such disasters as God's plan, a random natural event, and a result of the law of averages had significantly lower levels of posttraumatic depreciation (PTD) than did those who saw it as a freak of nature or due to moral karma or payback (Pecchioni et al., 2011).

Not all religious attributions are associated with resilience, however, and the specifics of the attribution influence its associations with recovery. For example in the sample of survivors of the Pakistani earthquake mentioned earlier, one type of religious appraisal for the disaster, feeling punished by God for one's sins or lack of spirituality, was, perhaps not surprisingly, associated with higher symptom levels and negative emotions (Feder et al., 2013). Similarly, survivors of the 1993 Midwest (US) Flood who attributed the flood to God's love or reward was associated with better psychological adjustment and higher religious well-being, while those who saw the flood as due to God's anger or punishment experienced greater distress (Smith, Pargament, Brant, & Oliver, 2000).

Trauma attributions have important implications for resilience in terms of the degree of global meaning violation. Some types of attributions may help survivors maintain a view of the world as predictable and comprehensible and of God as loving, while others may leave survivors feeling vulnerable and without a sense of control. Importantly, attributions often change over time through the processes of meaning making, reconsidering the traumatic event and seeing it in more benevolent ways (Park, 2010).

Perceived violations and resilience

According to the meaning-making model, following initial event appraisal, individuals determine the fit or discrepancy between their appraised meaning of the event and their global meaning. Perceptions of discrepancy (e.g. with one's sense of the controllability or comprehensibility of the world) create the distress, which in turn drives meaning-making efforts (Carver & Scheier, 1998; Dalgleish, 2004; Horowitz, 1975; Janoff-Bulman & Frieze, 1983; Watkins, 2008). Further, the *extent* of discrepancy between the appraised meaning of the event and one's global meaning determines the level of distress experienced. Traumatic impact results from large discrepancies between appraised and global meaning (e.g. Everly & Lating, 2004; Koss & Figueredo, 2004).

Although most meaning-making theorists emphasize violations of global beliefs as the most potent aspect of discrepancy, the violation of goals (e.g. the extent to which the event is not what the person wants to have had happen or to which other goals are rendered less attainable) and concomitant loss of sense of purpose in life may be even more powerful in generating distress (Dalgleish, 2004; Rasmussen, Wrosch, Scheier, & Carver, 2006). Indeed, recent research with college students who had experienced a variety of traumas (Park, Mills, & Edmondson, 2012) and with combat veterans (Steger, Owens, & Park, 2015) has shown that violation of both global beliefs and global goals predicts post-traumatic distress and, further, that goal violation appears to be more distressing than does belief violation.

Meaning-making processes and resilience

The meaning-making model posits that recovering from traumatic events involves reducing the discrepancy between the appraised meaning of the trauma and one's global meaning (Park, 2010a). *Meaning making* refers to the processes through which people reduce this discrepancy. Following a traumatic exposure, people often engage in problem-focused and emotion-focused coping (Aldwin, 2007). However, by its nature, trauma involves a situation in which loss or damage has already taken place, and thus, problem solving is less relevant. In the aftermath of trauma, meaning making – approach-oriented intrapsychic efforts to reduce discrepancies between appraised and global meaning – is particularly relevant and potentially more adaptive (Mikulincer & Florian, 1996).

Through meaning making, individuals attempt to restore their global meaning when it has been disrupted or violated or to resolve those violations by developing an acceptable understanding of the traumatic event consistent with their global meaning. Meaning making thus aims to reduce discrepancy by changing either the very meaning of the stressor itself (appraised meaning) or by changing one's global meaning system. Meaning making involves coming to see or understand the situation in a different way and reviewing and reforming one's beliefs and goals in order to regain consistency among them (Davis, Wortman, Lehman, & Silver, 2000). Following stressful events, people more commonly attempt to change their situational appraisals to incorporate them into their global meaning (i.e. assimilation), such as coming to see the event as less damaging or, perhaps, even in some ways fortuitous or beneficial.

When the appraisal of an event is so discrepant with global meaning that assimilation is very difficult, as in the case of trauma, meaning making may consist of efforts to change global meaning to accommodate the trauma. For example severe trauma can severely disrupt people's global meaning by exposing them to the unpredictable and darker sides of life and humanity, including human vulnerability and evil (Gray, Maguen, & Litz, 2007; Janoff-Bulman, 1989). Facing this darker side may necessitate changes in global meaning, such as in views of the balance of good and evil in the world or in beliefs about one's own power or control over one's life. Meaning making is essential to reduce discrepancies between of global meaning and appraised meanings of traumatic events (Fillip, 1999; Steger & Park, 2012).

Meaning making also involves deliberate efforts to deal with a traumatic event (e.g. Folkman, 1997), such as searching for answer to questions like "Why me?" (Bulman & Wortman, 1977) or for ways to understand the situation in more benign ways (Park, 2010). Meaning making refers to a broad category of efforts to cope with a situation by deliberately changing either appraised or global meaning. Meaning making is distinguished from problem- or emotion-focused coping efforts by its motive, to decrease the global meaning–appraised meaning discrepancy (Folkman & Moskowitz, 2007). Folkman (1997) identified meaning-making coping as "(a) using positive reappraisal, (b) revising goals and planning goal-directed problem-focused coping, and (c) activating spiritual beliefs and experiences" (p. 1216). Other meaning-making coping strategies include making downward comparisons with real or hypothetical others who are in relatively poorer straits (Buunk & Gibbons, 2007; Taylor, Wood, & Lichtman, 1983) or selectively focusing on positive attributes of an event and seeking to identify benefits or remind oneself of those benefits (Tennen & Affleck, 2002).

Reappraisal strategies are common and fairly effective following trauma (Aldwin, 2007). Through reappraisal, survivors can create new, less threatening ways of viewing the trauma and its consequences, and these reappraised meanings should facilitate the reduction of discrepancies with global meaning. For example in a study of firefighters who had experienced a work-related trauma, reappraisal was strongly associated with resilience in terms of fewer PTSD symptoms (Armstrong, Shakespeare-Finch, & Shochet, 2014).

Depending on the circumstances, meaning making may best promote mental health when employed along with more active coping strategies. For example in a longitudinal study, adult survivors of Hurricane Katrina who used both direct problem solving and seeking of social support along with acceptance and reappraisal had the most resilient trajectories of recovery (Wadsworth, Santiago, & Einhorn, 2009). Such findings make sense, given that, along with grappling with broad existential issues introduced by the trauma, individuals must often deal with many trauma-related practical problems that require direct action.

Religious coping, a set of meaning-making strategies involving actions related to God or a higher power used by individuals to deal with traumatic experiences, is very common following trauma (Park, 2013) and is associated with resilience (Park, 2013; Wadsworth et al., 2009). Importantly, religious coping with trauma is not just a US-based phenomenon but in fact is and has long been a common approach to understanding and coping with traumatic events around the world (Gaillard & Texier, 2010). Positive religious coping, which involves attempting to gain comfort, intimacy, and closeness with God, is generally associated with fewer symptoms of psychological distress and greater reports of psychological growth after traumatic events, although the effects are somewhat inconsistent (Harris et al., 2008; Pargament, Feuille, & Burdzy, 2011). On the other hand, negative religious coping, which includes reappraisals of the traumatic event as punishment from God and questioning God's power, is consistently related to higher levels of distress and poorer adjustment (Harris et al., 2008; Pargament et al., 2011).

Some studies have found religious coping to relate positively to post–trauma resilience. For example in a sample of survivors displaced by Hurricane Katrina, prayer was associated with lower stress symptoms (Spence, Lachlan, & Burke, 2007), and in the study of survivors of the 1993 Midwest (US) flood mentioned earlier, positive religious coping was associated with better psychological adjustment while negative religious coping was associated with greater distress

(Smith et al., 2000). However, findings regarding religious coping with trauma suggest it does not always lead to resilience. For example in a study of African-American women, using religious coping to deal with sexual assault was positively related to both depression and PTSD symptoms (Bryant-Davis, Ullman, Tsong, & Gobin, 2011).

Meanings made and resilience

These meaning-making efforts are attempts to generate satisfactory meanings that reduce discrepancies between situational and global meaning and thereby promote resilience by restoring a sense of the world as meaningful and one's own life as worthwhile (Michael & Snyder, 2005). *Meanings made* are the outcomes of this meaning-making process. There are many different types of meanings that survivors may make following trauma, some involving changes in the survivor's appraised meaning of the trauma and others of their global meaning. Perceptions of growth or positive change are also a common outcome of the meaning-making process.

Reappraised meaning of the trauma: Individuals often transform their appraisals of the trauma, rendering its meaning less aversive and more consistent with their pre-existing global beliefs and desires. For example survivors may come to see that the trauma or its implications is relatively less severe than those experienced by others (Taylor et al., 1983) or that they are fortunate that it was not worse (Thompson, 1985). They may also re-evaluate the implications of the event for their future in more positive ways (Resick et al., 2008). These more positive reappraisals are related to better post-traumatic adjustment. For example a study of writing to promote meaning making in college student trauma survivors found that reappraising the trauma in a more benign way (more controllable, less threatening) was associated with improvements in psychological distress and PTSD symptoms (Park & Blumberg, 2002).

Changed global meaning: Through meaning making, people can also change their global meaning. For example global beliefs may shift towards a view of life as less controllable or other people as less benevolent. One's view of God may shift towards a less powerful or benevolent deity (Cason, Resick, & Weaver, 2002; Park, 2005). Restoration of positive but realistic global beliefs is often an important part of therapeutic recovery efforts following trauma (e.g. Resick et al., 2008). *Perceptions of change* in global meaning following trauma are common and positively related to resilience. One recent national survey found that individuals who did not develop diagnosable PTSD following a highly stressful experience compared to those who did were less likely to report post-trauma changes on a variety of negative global beliefs (e.g. "The world is completely dangerous"; "I am a bad person"; "I can't trust anyone"; "My soul or spirit is permanently damaged"; "I have no chance for career, relationship, marriage or children") (Cox et al., 2014). Trauma survivors may also change their global goals through meaning making. For example following traumatic events, some survivors develop new goals, such as advocating for stricter drunk driving laws or greater resources for victims of violent crime (Armour, 2003; Grossman, Sorsoli, & Kia-Keating, 2006).

Perceived growth following trauma: Perhaps the most commonly studied outcome of meaning making is perceived post-traumatic growth. High levels of perceived growth have been reported following many traumatic events, including earthquakes (e.g. Xu & Liao, 2011), combat (Engelhard, Lommen, & Sijbrandij, 2014), assault (e.g. Kleim & Ehlers, 2009), and hurricanes (e.g. Lowe et al., 2013). The meaning of this perceived growth is unclear in spite of the hundreds of studies focusing on it (Park, 2010). Although often considered to be a positive outcome in and of itself, many studies, including those focused specifically on disaster survivors, have shown that post-traumatic growth is *positively* associated with PTSD symptoms and other symptoms of distress. For example in the prospective study of low-income mothers after Katrina, post-traumatic growth and PTSD symptoms were moderately strongly positively correlated both two and three years afterwards (Lowe et al., 2013). Similarly, post-traumatic growth was highly correlated with post-traumatic stress symptoms in adult survivors one year following the 2008 Sichuan earthquake (Xu & Liao, 2011), in Thai survivors six months after the 2004 tsunami (Tang, 2006), and in combat veterans (Engelhard et al., 2014). Perceived growth is not always adversely related to adjustment following trauma. For example in survivors of the Japanese earthquake tsunami/earthquake/nuclear disaster, perceived growth was positively related to anxiety but negatively to depressive symptoms and positively to quality of life, perhaps due to some underlying positivity or optimism factor (Kyutoku et al., 2012). This co-occurrence of high distress levels and high perceptions of growth are often interpreted as indicating that perceptions or reports of growth following traumatic events is an effort towards coping (i.e. wanting to believe in a positive outcome rather than reflecting actual positive change) (Maercker & Zoellner, 2004). These findings, however, do not mean that survivors do not grow or experience positive changes following trauma – many likely do – just that self-reporting measures are a poor way to assess post-traumatic growth (Frazier et al., 2009).

Future research and clinical implications

This brief review illustrates how meaning-making processes can promote resilience following trauma. Studies to date suggest that survivors' global meaning and the appraisals and meaning making in which they engage following trauma are important influences on their resilience. Findings to date are promising but far from conclusive. The nature of trauma – as unexpected and highly aversive – poses substantial challenges to researchers in conducting well-planned research close to the trauma. Thus, most studies reviewed here took place months or years following the trauma, after which much coping and meaning making has already taken place. Further, most studies are conducted cross-sectionally, a design that is ill-suited to determine temporal direction among the studied variables (e.g. do positive changes in global beliefs lead to resilience, or does resilience lead to positive changes in global beliefs?).

Further, to truly understand meaning making following trauma, one needs pre-trauma baseline data. For example studies of trauma survivors that have examined individuals' pre-trauma global beliefs, such as in a just or fair world, a benevolent God, or controllability, are virtually non-existent. Yet understanding which types of pre-existing global meaning lead to resilience and thriving would be extremely useful for developing prevention approaches. Some researchers have attempted to solve this problem by converting ongoing research projects into disaster-focused projects, thus having some relevant baseline data prior to the disaster (e.g. Chan et al., 2012). Finally, the present review focused only on individual meaning making. Clearly, meaning making occurs in the context of social relationships – families, congregations, communities – and more comprehensive research will be needed to examine these broader interrelations between individual and social processes of coping and meaning making.

The high rates of trauma exposure in the general population and the high rates of long-lasting trauma sequelae suggest that the need for a better understanding of how to help those affected to be resilience is strong. This understanding may comprise both intervention efforts following trauma to minimize its impact (e.g. McMackin, Newman, Fogler, & Keane, 2012) and prevention or preparedness efforts to facilitate resilience in the event of a future trauma (Park & Slattery, 2014; Woud, Postma, Holmes, & Mackintosh, 2013).

References

Aldwin, C. M. (2007). *Stress, coping, and development: An integrative approach.* New York: Guilford.

Ali, M., Farooq, N., Bhatti, M. A., & Kuroiwa, C. (2012). Assessment of prevalence and determinants of posttraumatic stress disorder in survivors of earthquake in Pakistan using Davidson Trauma Scale. *Journal of Affective Disorders, 136*(3), 238–243.

Armour, M. (2003). Meaning making in the aftermath of homicide. *Death Studies, 27*(6), 519–540.

Armstrong, D., Shakespeare-Finch, J., & Shochet, I. (2014). Predicting post-traumatic growth and post-traumatic stress in firefighters. *Australian Journal of Psychology, 66*(1), 38–46.

Banford, A. J., Wickrama, T., & Ketring, S. A. (2014). Physical health problem intrusion linking religious attributions to marital satisfaction in survivors of the 2004 tsunami. *Journal of Geography and Natural Disasters, 4*(1), 118.

Bonanno, G. A., Brewin, C. R., Kaniasty, K., & La Greca, A. M. (2010). Weighing the costs of disaster consequences, risks, and resilience in individuals, families, and communities. *Psychological Science in the Public Interest, 11*(1), 1–49.

Bryant-Davis, T., Ullman, S. E., Tsong, Y., & Gobin, R. (2011). Surviving the storm the role of social support and religious coping in sexual assault recovery of African American women. *Violence against Women, 17*(12), 1601–1618.

Bulman, R. J., & Wortman, C. B. (1977). Attributions of blame and coping in the "real world": Severe accident victims react to their lot. *Journal of Personality and Social Psychology, 35*(5), 351–363.

Buunk, A. P., & Gibbons, F. X. (2007). Social comparison: The end of a theory and the emergence of a field. *Organizational Behavior and Human Decision Processes, 102*(1), 3–21.

Carver, C. S., & Scheier, M. F. (1998). *On the self-regulation of behavior.* New York: Cambridge University Press.

Cason, D. R., Resick, P. A., & Weaver, T. L. (2002). Schematic integration of traumatic events. *Clinical Psychology Review, 22*(1), 131–153.

Chan, C. S., Rhodes, J. E., & Pérez, J. E. (2012). A prospective study of religiousness and psychological distress among female survivors of Hurricanes Katrina and Rita. *American Journal of Community Psychology, 49*(1–2), 168–181.

Chenell, S. L., & Murphy, S. A. (1992). Beliefs of preventability of death among the disaster bereaved. *Western Journal of Nursing Research, 14*(5), 576–594.

Cox, K. S., Resnick, H. S., & Kilpatrick, D. G. (2014). Prevalence and correlates of post-trauma distorted beliefs: Evaluating DSM-5 PTSD expanded cognitive symptoms in a national sample. *Journal of Traumatic Stress, 27*(3), 299–306.

Dalgleish, T. (2004). Cognitive approaches to posttraumatic stress disorder: The evolution of multi representational theorizing. *Psychological Bulletin, 130*(2), 228–260.

Davis, C., Wortman, C. B., Lehman, D. R., & Silver, R. (2000). Searching for meaning in loss: Are clinical assumptions correct? *Death Studies, 24*, 497–540.

Dekel, R., Solomon, Z., Elklit, A., & Ginzburg, K. (2004). World assumptions and combat-related posttraumatic stress disorder. *The Journal of Social Psychology, 144*(4), 407–420.

Engelhard, I. M., Lommen, M. J., & Sijbrandij, M. (2014). Changing for better or worse? Posttraumatic growth reported by soldiers deployed to Iraq. *Clinical Psychological Science* (online ahead of print). doi: 10.1177/2167702614549800

Everly, G. S. J., & Lating, J. M. (2004). *Personality-guided therapy for posttraumatic stress disorder.* Washington, DC: American Psychological Association.

Feder, A., Ahmad, S., Lee, E. J., Morgan, J. E., Singh, R., Smith, B. W., . . . Charney, D. S. (2013). Coping and PTSD symptoms in Pakistani earthquake survivors: Purpose in life, religious coping and social support. *Journal of Affective Disorders, 147*(1–3), 156–163.

Fillip, S. H. (1999). A three-stage model of coping with loss and trauma. In A. Maercker, M. Schutzwohl, & Z. Solomon (Eds.), *Posttraumatic stress disorder: A lifespan development perspective* (pp. 43–78). Seattle, WA: Hogrefe & Huber.

Folkman, S. (1997). Positive psychological states and coping with severe stress. *Social Science & Medicine, 45*(8), 1207–1221.

Folkman, S., & Lazarus, R. L. (1984). *Stress and coping.* New York: Springer.

Folkman, S., & Moskowitz, J. T. (2007). Positive affect and meaning-focused coping during significant psychological stress. In M. Hewstone, H.A.W. Schut, J.B.F. de Wit, K. Van Den Bos, & M. S. Stroebe (Eds.), *The scope of social psychology: Theory and applications* (pp. 193–208). New York: Psychology Press.

Frazier, P., Tennen, H., Gavian, M., Park, C. L., Tomich, P., & Tashiro, T. (2009). Does self-reported post-traumatic growth reflect genuine positive change? *Psychological Science, 20*, 912–919.

Gaillard, J. C., & Texier, P. (2010). Religions, natural hazards, and disasters: An introduction. *Religion, 40*(2), 81–84.

Gray, M. J., Maguen, S., & Litz, B. T. (2007). Schema constructs and cognitive models of posttraumatic stress disorder. In L. P. Riso et al. (Eds.), *Cognitive schemas and core beliefs in psychological problems: A scientist-practitioner guide* (pp. 59–92). Washington, DC: American Psychological Association.

Grossman, F. K., Sorsoli, L., & Kia-Keating, M. (2006). A gale force wind: Meaning making by male survivors of childhood sexual abuse. *American Journal of Orthopsychiatry, 76*(4), 434–443.

Harris, J. I., Erbes, C. R., Engdahl, B. E., Olson, R. H., Winskowski, A. M., & McMahill, J. (2008). Christian religious functioning and trauma outcomes. *Journal of Clinical Psychology, 64*(1), 17–29.

Horowitz, M. (1975). Intrusive and repetitive thoughts after experimental stress. *Archives of General Psychiatry, 32*(11), 1457–1463.

Janoff-Bulman, R. (1989). Assumptive worlds and the stress of traumatic events: Applications of the schema construct. *Social Cognition, 7*(2), 113–136.

Janoff-Bulman, R., & Frieze, I. H. (1983). A theoretical perspective for understanding reactions to victimization. *Journal of Social Issues, 39*(2), 1–17.

King, L. A., Pless, A. P., Schuster, J. L., Potter, C. M., Park, C. L., Spiro, A., III, & King, D. W. (2012). Risk and protective factors for traumatic stress disorders. In G. Beck & D. Sloan (Eds.), *Oxford handbook of traumatic stress disorders* (pp. 333–346). New York: Oxford University Press.

Kleim, B., & Ehlers, A. (2009). Evidence for a curvilinear relationship between posttraumatic growth and posttrauma depression and PTSD in assault survivors. *Journal of Traumatic Stress, 22*(1), 45–52.

Koss, M. P., & Figueredo, A. J. (2004). Change in cognitive mediators of rape's impact on psychosocial health across 2 years of recovery. *Journal of Consulting and Clinical Psychology, 72*(6), 1063–1072.

Kyutoku, Y., Tada, R., Umeyama, T., Harada, K., Kikuchi, S., Watanabe, E., . . . Dan, I. (2012). Cognitive and psychological reactions of the general population three months after the 2011 Tohoku earthquake and tsunami. *PloS One, 7*(2), e31014.

Lowe, S. R., Manove, E. E., & Rhodes, J. E. (2013). Posttraumatic stress and posttraumatic growth among low-income mothers who survived Hurricane Katrina. *Journal of Consulting and Clinical Psychology, 81*(5), 877–889.

McMackin, R. A., Newman, E. E., Fogler, J. M., & Keane, T. M. (2012). *Trauma therapy in context: The science and craft of evidence-based practice.* Washington, DC: American Psychological Association.

Maercker, A., & Zoellner, T. (2004). The Janus face of self-perceived growth: Toward a two-component model of posttraumatic growth. *Psychological Inquiry, 15*(1), 41–48.

Michael, S. T., & Snyder, C. R. (2005). Getting unstuck: The roles of hope, finding meaning, and rumination in the adjustment to bereavement among college students. *Death Studies, 29*(5), 435–458.

Mikulincer, M., & Florian, V. (1996). Coping and adaptation to trauma and loss. In M. Zeidner & N. Endler (Eds.), *Handbook of coping: Theory, research, applications* (pp. 554–572). Oxford, England: John Wiley & Sons.

Otto, K., Boos, A., Dalbert, C., Schöps, D., & Hoyer, J. (2006). Posttraumatic symptoms, depression, and anxiety of flood victims: The impact of the belief in a just world. *Personality and Individual Differences, 40*(5), 1075–1084.

Owens, G. P., Steger, M. F., Whitesell, A. A., & Herrera, C. J. (2009). Posttraumatic stress disorder, guilt, depression, and meaning in life among military veterans. *Journal of Traumatic Stress, 22*(6), 654–657.

Pargament, K., Feuille, M., & Burdzy, D. (2011). The brief RCOPE: Current psychometric status of a short measure of religious coping. *Religions, 2*(1), 51–76.

Park, C. L. (2005). Religion and meaning. In R. F. Paloutzian & C. L. Park (Eds.), *Handbook of the psychology of religion and spirituality* (pp. 295–314). New York: Guilford.

Park, C. L. (2009). Overview of theoretical perspectives. In C. L. Park, S. Lechner, M. H. Antoni, & A. Stanton (Eds.), *Positive life change in the context of medical illness: Can the experience of serious illness lead to transformation?* (pp. 11–30). Washington, DC: American Psychological Association.

Park, C. L. (2010). Making sense of the meaning literature: An integrative review of meaning making and its effects on adjustment to stressful life events. *Psychological Bulletin, 136*(2), 257–301.

Park, C. L. (2013). Religion and meaning. In R. F. Paloutzian & C. L. Park (Eds.), *Handbook of the psychology of religion and spirituality* (2nd ed., pp. 357–379). New York: Guilford.

Park, C. L., & Blumberg, C. J. (2002). Disclosing trauma through writing: Testing the meaning-making hypothesis. *Cognitive Therapy and Research, 26*(5), 597–616.

Park, C. L., & Folkman, S. (1997). The role of meaning in the context of stress and coping. *Review of General Psychology, 1*(2), 115–144.

Park, C. L., Mills, M., & Edmondson, D. (2012). PTSD as meaning violation: A test of a cognitive worldview perspective. *Psychological Trauma Theory, Research Practice, and Policy, 4*(1), 66–73.

Park, C. L., & Slattery, J. M. (2014). Resilience interventions with a focus on meaning and values. In M. Kent, M. C. Davis, & J. W. Reich (Eds.), *The resilience handbook: Approaches to stress and trauma* (pp. 370–382). New York: Routledge.

Pecchioni, L. L., Edwards, R., & Grey, S. H. (2011). The effects of religiosity and religious affiliation on trauma and interpretations following Hurricanes Katrina and Rita. *Journal of Communication & Religion, 34*(1), 37–58.

Rasmussen, H. N., Wrosch, C., Scheier, M. F., & Carver, C. S. (2006). Self-regulation processes and health: The importance of optimism and goal adjustment. *Journal of Personality, 74*(6), 1721–1747.

Resick, P. A., Galovski, T. E., Uhlmansiek, M. O., Scher, C. D., Clum, G. A., & Young-Xu, Y. (2008). A randomized clinical trial to dismantle components of cognitive processing therapy for posttraumatic stress disorder in female victims of interpersonal violence. *Journal of Consulting and Clinical Psychology, 76*(2), 243–258.

Sezgin, U., & Punamäki, R. L. (2012). Earthquake trauma and causal explanation associating with PTSD and other psychiatric disorders among South East Anatolian women. *Journal of Affective Disorders, 141*(2–3), 432–440.

Smith, B. W., Pargament, K. I., Brant, C., & Oliver, J. M. (2000). Noah revisited: Religiouscoping by church members and the impact of the 1993 Midwest flood. *Journal of Community Psychology, 28*(2), 169–186.

Spence, P. R., Lachlan, K. A., & Burke, J. M. (2007). Adjusting to uncertainty: Coping strategies among the displaced after Hurricane Katrina. *Sociological Spectrum, 27*, 653–678.

Spilka, B., Hood, R. W., Hunsberger, B., & Gorsuch, R. (2003). *The psychology of religion: An empirical approach* (3rd ed.). New York: Guilford.

Steger, M. F., Owens, G. P., & Park, C. L. (2015). Violations of war: Testing the meaning-making model among military veterans. *Journal of Clinical Psychology, 71*(1), 105–116.

Steger, M. F., & Park, C. L. (2012). The creation of meaning following trauma: Meaning making and trajectories of distress and recovery. In R. A. McMackin, T. M. Keane, E. Newman, & J. M. Fogler (Eds.), *Toward an integrated approach to trauma focused therapy: Placing evidence-based interventions in an expanded psychological context* (pp. 171–191). Washington, DC: American Psychological Association Press.

Sumer, N., Karanci, A. N., Berument, S. K., & Gunes, H. (2005). Personal resources, coping self-efficacy, and quake exposure as predictors of psychological distress following the 1999 earthquake in Turkey. *Journal of Traumatic Stress, 18*(4), 331–342.

Tang, C. S. K. (2006). Positive and negative postdisaster psychological adjustment among adult survivors of the Southeast Asian earthquake–tsunami. *Journal of Psychosomatic Research, 61*, 699–705.

Taylor, S. E., Wood, J. V., & Lichtman, R. R. (1983). It could be worse: Selective evaluation as a response to victimization. *Journal of Social Issues, 39*(2), 19–40.

Tennen, H., & Affleck, G. (2002). Benefit-finding and benefit-reminding. In C. R. Snyder & S. J. Lopez (Eds.), *Handbook of positive psychology* (pp. 584–597). New York: Oxford University Press.

Thompson, S. C. (1985). Finding positive meaning in a stressful event and coping. *Basic and Applied Social Psychology, 6*, 279–295.

Wadsworth, M. E., Santiago, C. D., & Einhorn, L. (2009). Coping with displacement from Hurricane Katrina: Predictors of one-year post-traumatic stress and depression symptom trajectories. *Anxiety, Stress, & Coping, 22*(4), 413–432.

Watkins, E. R. (2008). Constructive and unconstructive repetitive thought. *Psychological Bulletin, 134*(2), 163–206.

Woud, M. L., Postma, P., Holmes, E. A., & Mackintosh, B. (2013). Reducing analogue trauma symptoms by computerized reappraisal training: Considering a cognitive prophylaxis? *Journal of Behavior Therapy and Experimental Psychiatry, 44*(3), 312–315.

Xu, J., & Liao, Q. (2011). Prevalence and predictors of posttraumatic growth among adult survivors one year following 2008 Sichuan Earthquake. *Journal of Affective Disorders, 133*(1–2), 274–280.

15

Spiritual intelligence

A core ability behind psychosocial resilience

J. C. Ajawani

Stress is the response to events that threaten or challenge a person. Whether it be a task deadline, a family problem, or even daily hassles, life is full of circumstances and events, known as stressors, that produce threats to one's well-being.

Resilience in psychology refers to the idea of an individual's tendency to cope with stress and adversity. This coping may result in the individual 'bouncing back' to a previous state of normal functioning or using the experience of exposure to adversity to produce a 'steeling effect' and function better than expected (Masten, 2009). Most research now shows that resilience is the result of individuals being able to interact with their environments and the processes that either promote well-being or protect them against the overwhelming influence of risk factors (Zautra, Hall, & Murray, 2010). In this sense, 'resilience' occurs when there are cumulative 'protective factors'.

Resilience is a two-dimensional construct concerning the exposure of adversity and the positive adjustment outcomes of the adversity (Annunzianta, Hogue, Faw, & Liddle, 2006). This two-dimensional construct implies two judgments: one about a 'positive adaptation' and the other about the significance of risk or adversity (Luthar & Cicchetti, 2000).

Resilience is better understood as the opportunity and capacity of individuals to navigate their way to psychological, social, cultural, and physical resources that may sustain their well-being, and their opportunity and capacity to negotiate individually and collectively for these resources to be provided and experienced in culturally meaningful ways (Ungar et al., 2007).

Spirituality is considered as basic knowledge that increases environmental adaptability of people and has at least five efficiencies that lead to adaptive behaviour: capability to subsume deeds in order to orient with integration of the world, experiencing a high level of self-consciousness, investigating and purifying daily experiences about individual and spiritual and religious feelings, using spiritual resources to solve life problems and virtuous deeds such as forgiveness, self-acceptance etc. (Bakhtiarpoor, Heidarie, & Alipoor, 2011), all of which are protecting factors for psychosocial resilience. Kaplan, Marks, and Mertens (1997) and Pargament (1997) also observed that higher levels of religious faith and spirituality were associated with more adaptive coping responses, a more optimistic life orientation, greater perceived social support, lower levels of anxiety, and thus higher resilience among recovering individuals. Certain aspects of spirituality may, hypothetically, promote or hinder certain psychological virtues that increase resilience.

With the advent of twenty-first century, there is growing evidence that there is third 'Q' – 'SQ', or spiritual intelligence, apart from IQ and EQ. Thus, the full picture of human intelligence can be completed with this third 'Q', that is spiritual intelligence. Spiritual intelligence has been described as the ultimate intelligence by Zohar and Marshall (2000), who place it at the top of a hierarchy, with emotional intelligence (EQ) below and rational intelligence (IQ) below that. The research of Persinger (1996) and Ramchandran (1999) led to an identification of a 'God-spot' in the human brain. The 'God-spot' is an area in the brain that functions like a built-in spiritual centre located within neural connections in the temporal lobes. Examination of various brain scans, taken with positron emission topography, reveals that these natural areas light up whenever subjects are exposed to discussion of spiritual motifs. These findings strongly suggest that the brain is wired for cognitive constructs that produce meaning-making reflection, that is humans are naturally predisposed to think in spiritual terms.

Zohar and Marshall (2000) stress the utility of spiritual intelligence in solving problems of meaning or value and those of an existential nature. It also facilitates decision making and the recognition of choices that will be more meaningful, suggesting a potential means of adaptation and problem solving. They relate spiritual intelligence to moral reasoning, suggesting that it gives people moral sense and is used to wrestle with questions of good and evil. It further allows them to be creative, to change the rules, and to alter situations. According to Zohar and Marshall (2000), indications of a highly developed spiritual intelligence include the capacity to be flexible (actively and spontaneously and adaptive), a high degree of self-awareness, a capacity to face suffering and pain and to transcend, the quality of being inspired by vision and values, a reluctance to cause unnecessary harm, a tendency to see the connections between diverse things (being holistic), a marked tendency to ask 'why?' or 'what if?' questions and to seek 'fundamental' answers, and a facility for working against convention.

Emmons (2000a) defines spiritual intelligence as the adaptive use of spiritual information to facilitate everyday problem solving and goal attainment. He proposed five core components of spiritual intelligence: (a) the capacity for transcendence; (b) the ability to enter into heightened spiritual states of consciousness; (c) the ability to invest everyday activities, events, and relationships with a sense of the sacred; (d) the ability to utilize spiritual resources to solve problems in living; and (e) the capacity to engage in virtuous behaviour or to be humble to display compassion. The fifth component of this model was later removed by Emmons (2000b).

Emmons' (2000b) model of spiritual intelligence was supported and expanded by Noble (2000, 2001). Describing spiritual intelligence as an innate human ability, Noble (2001) added two additional core abilities: (1) the conscious recognition that physical reality is embedded within a larger, multi-dimensional reality with which people interact, consciously and unconsciously, on a moment-to-moment basis and (2) the conscious pursuit of psychological health, not only for themselves, but for the sake of the global community. Noble (2000) further added that spiritual intelligence includes an openness to unusual and diverse experiences broadly labeled 'spiritual' as well as a continuous attempt to understand the meaning of these experiences in the various aspects of one's life and the awareness that the whole is always greater than the sum of its parts, no matter how cherished a part might be.

Noble (2001) also stressed the importance of a high level of spiritual intelligence for one's psychological health. In particular, she noted its ability to increase resilience, suggesting that those with higher spiritual intelligence are better able to adapt and overcome adversity by relying on inner strengths.

Vaughan (2003) agrees with Noble's (2000, 2001) contention that phenomenological experiences of a spiritual nature may contribute to the development of spiritual intelligence. Vaughan (2003) views spiritual intelligence as involving the capacity for a deep understanding of existential issues and questions such as, 'Who am I?', 'Why I am here?', and 'What really matters?'; the capacity to recognize multiple levels of consciousness; and the awareness of spirit as the ground of being and the awareness of one's relationship to the transcendent, to all people and to the earth. She believes that spiritual intelligence exists as a potential in all people and can be cultivated by a variety of practices or training. She also emphasizes the relationship between spiritual intelligence and adaptation to stressful events.

More recently, a grounded theory approach was undertaken by Aram (2007) in order to investigate spiritual intelligence. His underlying assumptions reflected that spiritual intelligence can be differentiated from spiritual experience (e.g. a belief in God). He identified seven major themes on the basis of his preliminary research involving interviews of individuals who were described as adaptively embodying spirituality in daily life. These themes are (1) meaning (experiencing meaning and purposes in daily activities); (2) consciousness (trans-rational knowing, mindfulness, and practice); (3) grace (trust, love, and reverence for the sacred); (4) transcendence (holism, nurturing relationships and connections); (5) truth (acceptance, forgiveness, and openness to all truth); (6) peaceful surrender to self (egolessness, accepting one's true nature); and (7) inner-directed freedom (liberation from attachments and fears, discernment, integrity).

A lot about spiritual intelligence has been reiterated in Indian religious script – *The Bhagavad Gita.*

Luthar (1991) observed that people who had higher spiritual intelligence were more flexible, self-conscious, capable of intention, and holistic toward the universe; sought answers for his basic questing about life; and criticized traditions and cultures. Crichton (2008) also found that spiritual intelligence easily enabled people to change and evolve.

Narayanan and Jose (2011) also found that some of the dimensions of spiritual intelligence, i.e. truth, equanimity, joy, synthesis, and discernment, were strong predictors of resilience. Alex and Ajawani (2011) observed that spiritual intelligence was a crucial factor in marital happiness, that is, highly spiritually intelligent couples showed higher levels of marital happiness. Similarly, Chhawchharia, Ajawani, and Verma (2011) found that highly spiritually intelligent older adults were happier than less spiritually intelligent older adults. Ajawani (2013, 2014a) found that highly spiritually intelligent people showed higher resilience than less spiritually intelligent people.

In general, fifteen core components can be proposed to comprise spiritual intelligence, namely (1) compassion, (2) critical existential thinking, (3) divinity, (4) egolessness, (5) equanimity, (6) flexibility, (7) forgiveness, (8) gratitude, (9) meaning and purpose in life, (10) openness to experience, (11) self-acceptance, (12) self-actualization, (13) self-awareness, (14) spiritual practice, and (15) transcendental awareness (Ajawani, Sethi, & Chhawchharia, 2009).

Compassion

Compassion is one of the core components of spiritual intelligence, which can be considered to play its vital role in psychosocial resilience. It is the ability of reaching out to others in a spirit of love and respect. It is fundamentally a humane quality and acts as a form of medicine that dissolves away the hard-hearted and selfish attitudes that are true known sources of stress for the person who carries them. In the Bhagavad Gita (2012), Lord Krishna also asserts that it is due to loving compassion felt by Him for those persons who dedicate and devote their lives to Him, that He always manifest in their hearts and minds as the paramount object of their thoughts, plans, and activities, accompanied by the realization of His transcendental qualities and attributes.

Having comprehended the qualities, attributes, and character of Supreme Lord regarding His phenomenal, transcendental potencies manifesting throughout all of the creation and His 'yoga', or the science of the individual consciousness, attains communion with His ultimate consciousness, eternally. This knowledge will mature into appreciation, which will evolve into loving devotion for Him, and subsequently, bliss will naturally arise within the hearts and minds of His devotees and thus eventually resilience.

Buddha also says that the quality of being compassionate leads a man to have good health, success in life, and happiness, which are the contributory factors to his psychosocial resilience.

Ajawani (2013, 2014a) also observed that compassion leads to a decrease in biological markers of stress and an increase in indices of adaptive immune function. Along with this, compassion adds to psychological well-being, all of which help an individual to be better resilient.

It seems that quality of being compassionate improves one's physical and psychological health, leading to being more resilient, as both the factors contribute to one's resilience.

Critical existential thinking

Critical existential thinking refers to thinking about one's existence, i.e. the capacity of a person to critically contemplate the nature of existence, reality, the universe, space, time, death, and other existential thinking and IQ (Shearer, 2006). High IQ can be viewed as an important contributor to one's resilience as it helps a person to examine stress situations logically, protecting him from inappropriate responses that otherwise can prove stress provoking. In fact, it is the intellectually disciplined process of actively and skillfully conceptualizing, applying, analyzing, synthesizing, and/or evaluating information, which in turn help a person to prepare him to deal with stress situations without being perturbed by them and thus remain stress free.

In the Bhagavad Gita (2012), it is asserted that Vedic knowledge alone destroys spiritual ignorance. That is why Lord Krishna used the word *jnana* or, knowledge referring to knowledge of the Vedas, which gives actual awareness of the ultimate reality. Here the word *jnana* denotes a supra-conscious experience. It does not mean expertise in intellectual empirical knowledge, nor does it mean proficiency in mundane analytical knowledge.

Similarly, in reply to Arjuna's query, Lord Krishna explains that when one has achieved *atma tattva* or realization of the soul and experienced its spiritual existence then one will be cognizant of their physical body merely as a house within which the *atma* inhabits, and this *atma* is a distinct entity separate from the physical and subtle bodies, which leads to a resilient state as one frees himself from all agonies that his body feels.

Ajawani (2013, 2014a) observed that overcoming the existential crisis aids in the resolution of the larger crisis within which it occurs by strengthening the will of the individual and cultivating hardiness or existential courage.

It seems that critical existential thinking can serve as multi-faceted source of adaptation, coping, problem solving, and abstract reasoning, particularly in crises of an existential nature, thereby increasing psychosocial resilience and thus decreasing the adverse effects of stresses in an individual's life.

Divinity

Divinity always carries connotations of goodness, beauty, beneficence, justice, and other positive pro-social attributes. Helliswell (2003) found that faith in a higher power or energy positively correlated with life satisfaction and happiness, which are true contributors in an individual's resilience.

It can be reasoned that quality of divinity is transcendental in its origin and demonstrates a range of indicators of religious commitments, including feelings of closeness to a divine entity and certainty of belief, which may contribute to increased life satisfaction and thus increases resilience (Ajawani, 2013, 2014a).

In the Bhagavad Gita (2012) Lord Krishna reveals that He is '*bijam mam sarva bhutanam*', that is the original seed of all existence. This means that Thy (God) manifested the original seed for all being that possesses the potency for all species that are moving or stationary to produce effects in the same species uninterruptedly for all successive issues of procreation indefinitely and not subject to any modification or decay nor is it ever destroyed with each individual being. The pure fragrance is thus to show the pleasure of Lord Krishna as the origin of the wonderful scent of the earth. In the world of meritorious and virtuous creations, law of external righteousness is enjoyed. The law of creation known as *rita* represents universal order, truth, and righteousness as well as perennial principles from time immemorial, which are auspicious activities for the benefit of all living being. Thus, the Supreme Lord abides in the earth as its fragrant essence, which can only be meritorious, yet He awards all merits and demerits. Abiding in fire is its brilliant energy; abiding in humans, He is the *atma*, the bequeather of life itself, abiding in the spiritually intelligent. He is wisdom, abiding in the splendid. He is exalted splendour and by the act of manifestation, He is the eternal seed for all existence.

Believing this fact may lead an individual to surrender to the ultimate divine power for all his acts and outcomes and thus be resilient.

Egolessness

Egolessness can be referred to as an emotional state where one feels no ego (or self), of having no distinct being apart from the world around oneself. In its literal sense, egolessness inculcate altruistic acts in an individual, which in turn is a source of great social support. This predisposed social support helps the individual to be psychosocially resilient during social crises, a common experience during various stages of a life span as the natural outcomes of undesirable social interactions. Alex and Ajawani (2012) observed that there was greater marital happiness in egoless couples.

In reply to Arjuna's query, Lord Krishna explains that one endowed with spiritually purified intelligence is naturally predominated with *sattva guna*, the mode of goodness. The mind is controlled by not indulging in positive or negative thoughts and illusory conceptions, and the control of senses is neutrality towards them without aversion or attraction towards their objects. Adopting spirituality leads an individual with high spiritual intelligence to be completely eradicated from all egoism and from conceptions that one is a physical body and thus be more psychosocially resilient than an individual with egoistic attitudes.

Lord Krishna also speaks about the non-binding effects that the actions of the spiritually intelligent ensure. They are without egoism and unattached to the doership of actions. Being completely satisfied, by the bliss they experience within their consciousness, they maintain their bodily existence by accepting what comes on its own accord. They are no longer affected by the dualities of life such as good and evil, the state that promotes psychosocial resilience in such individuals with high egolessness.

Equanimity

Equanimity is an evenness of mind under stress. It is the controlling of emotional or mental agitation through will and habit. It is a practice most often discussed in Buddhist and Sufi traditions. The Buddha described a mind filled with equanimity as abundant, exalted, and immeasurable, without hostility and without ill-will. In the Bhagavad Gita (2012), Lord Krishna asserts that those who are factually situated in spiritual intelligence, perform activities as a matter of duty, free from conceptions of gain and loss, unconcerned about the resultant rewards. They are assuredly delivered from the bondage of birth and death in the material existence and are liberated to the spiritual realms and thus remain psychosocially resilient. This information is well documented in the Vedic scriptures also.

The Bhagavad Gita (2012) quotes that equanimity, a spiritual state, can be gained by yoga and meditation. A person who believes in *karma* may practice in his duty with evenness of mind, nonchalant about the *karma-phal*, or outcomes. A *gyani*, or wise person, preaches his wisdom in firmness detached from all emotions. Such a 'knower of self' is a *samdarshi*, or one who finds everyone equal, who envisions the supreme 'self' in all being and all beings in the self. A *dhyan yogi,* one who is on the path of meditation, for whom the Supreme is the object of realization, holding pleasures and pains in the same balance. For a *bhakti yogi,* one who is on the path of devotion, equanimity is obtained through his compassion towards all and in him removing himself from all dualities. Thus, the undiluted reach the eternal abode, the freedom from worldly bondage, the *nirvana.* Worldly bondages are true sources of stress in modern life, and thus a state such like *nirvana* can help a person to be psychosocially resilient.

Flexibility

Flexibility applies to one's overall ability to adapt to unfamiliar, unpredictable, and changing circumstances. Because of their attitude, freedom from rigidity, flexible people have the readiness to react towards varying environmental situations, as per their demands, in a non-whimsical manner leading to being well adjusted even in stressful situations where non-flexible or rigid people get perturbed easily. Lawton (1951) described a well-adjusted person as one who can compromise when encountered with difficulties. Thus, it is quite reasonable to believe that flexible people are resilient because they readily adapt personally, emotionally, and socially and enjoy life at all stages of their lives. In contrast, rigid people continue to practice old behaviour patterns in new settings where they may prove ineffective and inefficient. Such people are resistant to new ideas and are unable to adjust with changes of the specific period of life span and are unable to use more appropriate ways that are required. This inevitably intensifies the severity of stressors.

Nolen-Hoeksema, Wisco, and Lyubomirsky (2008) demonstrated that an absence of flexibility was linked to certain variants of psychopathology while the presence of flexibility leads to more versatile and more adept behaviour, which in turn can be reasoned to lead to higher psychosocial resilience.

Forgiveness

Forgiveness may be considered in terms of the person who concludes resentment, indignation, or anger as a result of perceived offense, difference, or mistake or ceasing to demand punishment or restitution to others as well as himself. Most world religions include teachings on forgiveness, and many of these teachings provide an underlying basis for varying modern-day traditions and practices of forgiveness. Some religious doctrines or philosophies also place greater emphasis on the need for humans to find some sort of divine forgiveness, for their own humans to practice forgiveness of one another, and for yet others to make little or no distinction between divine and human forgiveness as, in either case, the resulting outcome is a relief from stress that otherwise places havoc on individuals' psychological well-being. Thus, forgiveness can be considered a resilience booster. By forgiving others, one frees himself spiritually and emotionally. The Bhagavad Gita (2012) quotes that forgiveness is an act of one's personal will in obedience and of submission to God's will, trusting God to bring emotional healing. Forgiving others takes moral courage. It ends the illusion of separation, and its power can change misery into happiness in an instant, which is a vital source for psychosocial resilience.

Friedman and Toussaint (2009) observed that people who kept on forgiving oneself and others were happier and thus more stress free than those who kept grudges against others.

In her book entitled *The Journey*, Bays (1999) has presented empirical evidence of emotional and physical healing through forgiving oneself, others, and even God. She also quotes W. B. Yeats who expresses the tranquillity that comes in after forgiving: "We can make our mind so like still water that beings gather about us to see their own images, and so for a moment live a clearer, perhaps even fiercer, life because of our quiet". There is a Sanskrit word that is often used to describe this phenomenon. It is called *satsang*: '*sat*' means 'truth', and '*sang*' means 'in the called company of truth' or in the presence of, or in the community of truth. Here people are resting in peace, in stillness, in the company of truth itself. It is clear that forgiveness brings in the true state of *statsang*, which makes a person be resilient.

Gratitude

Gratitude is a feeling, emotion, or attitude acknowledging the benefit that one has received or will receive. Almost all religious manuscripts are filled with the idea of gratitude and encourage their followers to be grateful and express thanks to God in all circumstances. McCullough, Emmons, and Tsang (2002) found that people who were more grateful had higher levels of subjective well-being. Grateful people were found to be happier, less depressed, less stressed, and more satisfied with their lives and social relationships, which form a fertile platform for psychosocial resilience.

DeSteno, Bartlett, Baumann, Williams, and Dickens (2010) observed that grateful people had more positive ways of coping with difficulties they experienced in their lives, being more likely to seek support from other people, to reinterpret and grow from the experience, and to spend more time planning how to deal with problems. Such people were more likely to have lower levels of stress and depression and thus to have higher levels of psychological well-being. All these situations can easily be reasoned to inculcate a higher level of psychosocial resilience in those who practice gratitude.

Byrne (2012) devoted her whole book *The Magic* to the importance of gratitude in human life. She has modified the passages from the gospel of Matthew in Holy Scriptures, such as "Whoever has gratitude will be given more, and he or she will have an abundance. Whoever does not have gratitude, even what he or she has will be taken from him or her". She asserts that gratitude operates through a universal law that governs one's whole life. According to the law of attraction, which governs all the energy in the universe, from the formation of an atom to the movement of the planets, like attracts like. It is because of the law of attraction that the cells of every living creature are held together, as well as substance of every material object. In a human's life, the law operates on his thoughts and feelings, because they are energy too, and so whatever one thinks, whatever one feels, he attracts to him.

Dating back thousands and thousands of years to the earliest recordings of humankind, the power of gratitude was preached and practiced and, from there, was passed on through the centuries, sweeping across the continents, permeating one civilization and culture to the next. The major religions of Christianity, Islam, Judaism, Buddhism, Sikhism, and Hinduism all have gratitude at their core to lead one's life in a resilient manner.

Meaning and purpose of life

Meaning and purpose of life is defined as the ability to construct personal meaning and purpose in all physical and mental experiences, including the capacity to create and master a life purpose.

Meaning and purpose play valuable and adaptive roles when an existential crisis, existential neurosis, or existential frustration has a sense of meaninglessness. Therefore, it is quite reasonable to suggest that a high capacity for personal meaning production would be quite adaptive in dealing with such existential problems. In fact, if this ability is cultivated at high level, it will likely prevent such a crisis or vacuum from even fully developing, as it will provide an individual with seemingly endless sources of personal meaning and purpose, which will enhance an individual's capability of psychosocial resilience.

Mascaro and Rosen (2005, 2006) found positive correlations between measures of hope and both implicit and explicit measurers of personal meaning and negative correlations between personal meaning and both depression and neuroticism. These findings clearly suggest that meaning and purpose make a person hopeful, which predisposes him to be resilient as such a person's faith for good things to happen always makes him to feel assured even in stressful situations of life. It is argued that, in order for meaning to reach a level at which it acts as a buffer against stress, an individual must demonstrate a high capacity for personal meaning and purpose within stressful situations, thereby transforming the stressor and reducing its negative impact. Once meaning is derived from a stressful situation, further distress is likely to be averted. Similarly, when faced with dilemmas, personal meaning can lead to a meaning-based solution, i.e., a solution that considers the meaning and purpose of the dilemma and therefore acts as a method of problem solving as well. Attaching purpose to problems and decisions deepens their meaning and provides additional direction, increasing the likelihood that an individual will attain present goals leading to psychosocial resilience.

There are enumerable places in the Bhagavad Gita (2012) wherein Lord Krishna has elaborated the importance of meaning and purpose of life, which can be reasoned to play its vital role in psychosocial resilience. Lord Krishna has revealed the eternal truth that he is the *atma*, or soul within all beings in existence, be they human, animal, aquatic, plant, demi-gods, or any species of life that was not cloned. He is the maintainer, sustainer, and monitor of all beings through the medium of the *atma* and all of its impulses come from Him. All souls emanate from the Supreme Lord and, because of Him, are completely spiritual and eternal. Whoever does not avail himself and conformably acts to this eternal truth, or takes this eternal truth seriously in earnest, should be understood to be completely destitute of knowledge and unable to evolve spiritually and to be incapable of achieving *atma tattva*, that is knowledge of the soul becomes lost. Spiritual intelligence is what determines the light of knowledge in material existence. In the absence of spiritual knowledge, darkness and ignorance prevails, and knowledge becomes erroneous and defective. Thus, it has been illustrated that doership transpires due to union of *prakriti*, that is material nature and the physical body being influenced by the *gunas* or modes of goodness and conscience, and this is dependent ultimately upon the Supreme Lord.

In the Bhagavad Gita (2012), it is further depicted that the virtuous who still possess desires and worship the Supreme Lord for the fulfillment of these desires get them and eventually they gradually attain *moksha*, that is liberation from material existence, the ultimate truth of life, and thus are resilient. But those who are not devoted to the Supreme Lord are overtly in *raja guna*, that is the mode of passion, as well as those who are situated in *tama guna*, that is modes of ignorance being overwhelmed by their expectations to gratify their desires, remain in bondage continuously revolving in *sansara*, that is the endless cycle to birth and death, and thus destined to severe stresses and sufferings – a state of poor resilience.

Lord Krishna sets the parameters for practicing *karma yoga* or prescribed Vedic activities. Accordingly, *karma yoga* leads to knowledge because performing Vedic activities purifies the mind. But once the mind is purified, one advances to *yoga*, that is the science of the individual consciousness attaining communion with the ultimate consciousness, then one leaves *karma yoga* and becomes devoted to meditation, absorbed internally with no inclination for external activities that otherwise impede and distract introspection and reflection. This is said to be the means for spiritual knowledge to mature and thus a resilient way of living life. That is the knowledge that one is completely dependent upon the Supreme Lord and that He alone is the actual performer of all actions and guarantees that all reactions to actions are neutralized by the fire of wisdom.

Openness to experience

Openness to experience is one of the components of spiritual intelligence, expected to play its vital role in psychosocial resilience. People who score low on this component are considered to be closed to experience. They tend to be conventional and traditional in their outlook and behaviour. They prefer familiar routines to new experiences and generally have a narrower range of interests. Deprivation from experiences leads to a poorer state of achievements, which may be quite dissatisfying to these people with low level of openness to experience, a source of low subjective well-being. Apart from it, since such people lack new experiences in fast-changing perspectives, their perceived stress is very high, being not able to cope with constant failures. This makes such people be poor in psychosocial resilience. In contrast, people who are open to experience are privileged due to their experience-seeking attitudes, which in fact, helps them to work on desired goals in new ways and take up every chance of seeking experience, which ultimately leads them to be highly resilient.

Openness to experience helps people to understand and accept their criticism with an open mind, which leads them to have a comfortable state of mind for themselves. They manage good inter-personal relationships with other people. Openness to experience also helps these people in the course of changes, which are essential due to modernization. Apart from it, openness to experience also helps people to share their own feelings with others easily leading to greater peace of mind in moments of stress, due to greater level of social support.

Vaughan (2003) and Nasel (2004) are of the view that an open and contemplative mindset that tolerates uncertainty, paradox, and mystery is beneficial to the growth of spiritual intelligence. In contrast, a rigid, closed, and definitive acceptance of a particular belief system may hinder its development, which ultimately be the cause of low resilience.

Self-acceptance

Self-acceptance refers to an individual's satisfaction or happiness with himself and is thought to be necessary for good mental health (Shepard, 1979). It can be achieved by ceasing to criticize, solving the defects of one's self, and then accepting them to be existing within one's self, that is tolerating oneself to be imperfect in some parts. Everyone has strengths and weaknesses. Knowing one's weaknesses is always more important than knowing the strengths. Once a person knows himself, it becomes easier for accepting the self. His strengths provide him confidence for being victorious while his weaknesses do not dishearten him as nobody on this earth.

Self-acceptance is a springboard of lasting success without getting negative feelings of failure. On a broader scale, self-acceptance is accepting things and persons as they are today because the self is part of circumstance and of everything around it, and nothing remains isolated and inconsiderable. Unless one accepts what is right here and right now, one can't make a right move for a change if needed. Acceptance is best exercised when one makes his assessing mind a real friend of one's personality and is made to accept it as it is in reality. In such a situation, the mind provides its best services to the personality and is made to accept it as it is in reality without insisting on having some particular attributes, and this changes the personality for the better. This gives happiness to the person because he has achieved it without any external intervention. Thus, self-acceptance truly paves way to become or provides a genuine fertile ground for psychosocial resilience as it is not a matter of any stress when one accepts his strengths and weaknesses as they are.

Wayne (1993) assert that self-acceptance helps a person to lead a stress-free life in contrast to self-rejecting person who is usually stressed and thus unable to form and maintain good relationship, i.e., depriving himself from a powerful source of social support that would have helped him in becoming resilient.

Self-actualization

Self-actualization is manifested by becoming involved in pursuits leading to a meaningful, rich, and full life and hence has been considered a vital factor in psychosocial resilience.

Excitement about one's interests energizes and motivates a person to continue his interests. Thus, self-actualization is correlated with feelings of self-satisfaction in the course of life. A self-actualized person enjoys happiness at high level as he is able to achieve the developmental goals. Maslow (1943) asserts that self-actualization also involves being satisfied with one's overall achievement at play, at work, and in relationships. According to Maslow (1943), self-actualized people have a healthy balance between multiple activities to keep their lives in a truly stress-free and happy state. Such people live life to the fullest. They do what they truly love to do, and as a consequence, their work becomes a pleasure, which leads to a sense of subjective well-being, contentment, and happiness leading them ultimately to be resilient.

It is clear that a self-actualized person easily adapts emotionally, is able to control his impulses, and is persistently effortful in achieving his goals due to acknowledgement about his own potentialities and life goals. His emotional adeptness also helps him to act out in desirable manners bringing equilibrium between his needs and desires and goal-satisfaction. Consequently, he becomes more resilient than a person who is unable to self-actualize.

In the Bhagavad Gita (2012) it is asserted that by becoming immersed in the wisdom that Lord Krishna is prepared to reveal, that is the *jiva* or embodied being attains identification with the Supreme Lord and is no longer subject to *sansara* or the perpetual cycle of birth and death. In his book *Many Lives, Many Masters*, Weiss (1988) evidenced this aspect of self-actualization.

Self-awareness

Self-awareness is crucial for success in every sphere of life. It is the ability to recognize one's feelings, to differentiate between them, and to know what one is feeling. Kerr, Johnson, Gans, and Krumrine (2004) found that those who had difficulty in identifying their own emotional reactions reported greater problems in personal and social adjustment and thus were unable to establish loving and trustful relationships without awareness of the impact of their behaviour on others. This may lead to feeling stress all the time and thus poor psychosocial resilience.

In contrast, a self-aware person finds better scope to adjust in various spheres of life and remains happy because his self-awareness helps him to behave in an appropriate manner, as the time and situation demand, and seeking happiness for self and others too. He is an emotionally adept person who behaves in an adaptable manner in his personal emotional life in family, work, and other situations while interacting with others. His reactions during social interactions provide a compatible and soothing environment and provide social support during crises, thus making the individual more psychosocially resilient. Self-awareness adds to his experience to deal all these in appropriate manner enabling him to achieve success, a top priority during all stages of life. A natural outcome of this is that higher levels of psychological well-being all around lead to higher levels of psychosocial resilience. However, the lack of self-awareness leads a person to react in whimsical and impulsive ways, causing stressful states for himself and others too.

In the Bhagavad Gita (2012), Lord Krishna states that, by imbibing and actualizing attributes, one assumes the nature of *brahman*, the spiritual substratum pervading all existence. The mind is friendly to those who are able to restrain it from flowing externally outwards after sense objects, but if one is unable to subdue the mind, it will harass and aggravate one to satisfy the senses and becomes its worst enemy. Lord Krishna has conveyed that an ungoverned and uncontrolled mind being attached to sense of gratification interposes obstructions and deviations in a way that deviates and hinders one from attaining *atma tattva*, that is realization of the soul. Sage Parasara, the father of Vedavyasa, states that mind itself is the sole cause of bondage in the material existence as well as the sole cause of *moksha* or liberation from the material existence. A mind infatuated with desire for sense objects constitutes a state of bondage and a mind free from the delusion of desire for sense objects constitutes the way to *moksha* – the resilient way of leading the life.

Spiritual practice

Spiritual practice is one's personal journey of going inward beyond the five senses, the mind, and mental acts to experience the transcendental awareness within oneself. By performing individual and collective spiritual practices, a person is able to transform one's perspective about the world around. As an individual performs spiritual practices he feels more in the 'flow' of life and more connected to 'source' and everything around, which may lead him to overcome stresses easily and to transform oneself as psychosocially resilient. Wong, Rew, and Slaikeu (2006) observed a positive relationship between spiritual practices and happiness, which can be predictive of future resilience after facing severe stressful situations in one's life. Similarly, Purohit and Ajawani (2011) observed the positive role of spiritual practices in resilience.

In the Bhagavad Gita (2012), Lord Krishna has emphasized the importance of spiritual practices. He says that eating foods that are of *sattvaguna* – the mode of goodness is pleasurable. But when foods are excessively bitter, spicy, salty, sour, pungent, etc., the result is discomfort and misery culminating in sickness and disease. They are of *raja guna* the mode of passion. In reply to a query from Arjuna pertaining to spiritual practice, Lord Krishna says that by *karma yoga*, which is performed surrendering all actions to the Supreme Lord, there is spiritual intelligence that, when bequeathed, gives single-minded determination that is resolute in spiritual consciousness. But in the case of those enacting actions with desires of fruitive rewards, their thoughts are endless due to their desires being endless. Performance of daily rituals enjoyed by the Vedic scripture, such as meditation on the Supreme Lord and occasional rituals performed on special occasions, are never done in vain even if there is some defect present. But fruitive actions motivated by rewards are always tainted by the imperfection of fruitive desires, which is binding to fruitive reaction, as well as the defect of not surrendering their actions to the Supreme Lord. Thus, spiritual practices aimed at surrendering to the Supreme Lord lead to psychosocial resilience by way of freeing oneself from desire fulfillment urges.

Transcendental awareness

Transcendental awareness is defined as going beyond physical human experience or existence apart from and not subject to the material universe (Oxford University Press, 2001). Noble (2001) defined it as the ability to recognize physical reality embedded within a larger, multi-dimensional reality.

Coward and Reed (1996) proposed that the process of self-transcendence leads to physical and psychological well-being by awareness of wholeness and integration among dimensions of one's being, providing additional sources of personal meaning. Transcendental awareness leads to personal growth, positive relations with others, purpose in life, and life satisfaction, all leading to enhancement in one's psychological well-being and thus making the individual psychosocially resilient, eventually.

In the Bhagavad Gita (2012), Lord Krishna says that, if one is unable to practice detachment by himself, then one should mentally dedicate all actions to the Supreme Lord, entrusting himself to Him as the doer and offer all prescribed 'Vedic' activities as well as worldly activities in renunciation. This includes surrendering all ordinances, injunctions, and prohibitions as well as one's daily mundane duties along with the resultant hopes, aspirations, and rewards unto the Supreme Lord who becomes the only goal. One who after due reflection makes this resolve, has perceived that Lord Krishna is the supreme reality to attain and thus leading to resilient life.

Ellermann and Reed (2001) observed a positive association between self-transcendence and subjective well-being that may prove to be a strong source of psychosocial resilience.

Thus, it is quite clear that an individual with high spiritual intelligence is inculcating his psychosocial resilience through nurturance of protecting and promoting factors both while interacting with his environment.

Here, it is pertinent to note that spiritual intelligence can be enhanced as a matter of learning experiences. It is reasonable to believe that enhanced spiritual intelligence through appropriate intervention programme, will eventually makes a person to behave in resilient manner (Ajawani, 2014b). Chhawchharia (2012) found that spiritual intelligence training enhanced happiness of people. Similarly, Ajawani and Verma (2012) too observed that spiritual intelligence intervention programme enhanced need level of individuals that can be considered as vital in resilience.

References

Ajawani, J. C. (2013). Stress resilience during old age as the function of need level and spiritual intelligence. *DMV Journal, 6*(1), 130–136.
Ajawani, J. C. (2014a). *Stress resilience during various stages of life span as the function of need level and spiritual intelligence: An intervention programme in perspective of the Bhagavad Gita* (Unpublished Post-Doctoral (D. Lit.) Dissertation). Hindu University of America, Florida.
Ajawani, J. C. (2014b). Stress resilience as the function of spiritual intelligence training. *Indo-Indian Journal of Social Science Researches, 10*(1), 4–8.
Ajawani, J. C., Sethi, A., & Chhawchharia, K. (2009). *Spiritual intelligence scale.* Raipur (C.G.), India: F. S. Management India Pvt. Ltd., F. S. House, Maruti Vihar.
Ajawani, J. C., & Verma, S. (2012). Impact of spiritual intelligence intervention programme on need level. *Indo-Indian Journal of Social Science Researches, 8*(1), 122–126.
Alex, M., & Ajawani, J. C. (2011). Marital happiness as the function of spiritual intelligence. *International Multi-Disciplinary Research Journal, 1*(9), 6–7.

Alex, M., & Ajawani, J. C. (2012). *Marital happiness as the function of egolessness.* Paper presented at National Seminar on Globalization and Changing Role of Women, Raipur, held on 20th & 21st Nov. 2012.

Annunzianta, D., Hogue, A., Faw, L., & Liddle, H. A. (2006). Family functioning and school success in at-risk, inner-city adolescents. *Journal of Youth and Adolescence, 35*(1), 100–108.

Aram, J. Y. (2007). *The seven dimensions of spiritual intelligence: An ecumenical, grounded theory.* Paper presented at the 115th Annual Conference of the American Psychological Association, San Francisco, CA.

Bakhtiarpoor, S., Heidarie, A., & Alipoor, K. S. (2011). The relationship of the self-focused attention, body image concern and generalized self-efficacy with social anxiety in students. *Life Science Journal, 8*(4), 704–713.

Bays, B. (1999). *The journey.* London: Harper Element, Harper Collins Publishers Ltd.

The Bhagavad Gita. (2012). Retrieved from www.bhagavad-gita.org

Byrne, R. (2012). *The magic.* London: Simon & Schuster UK Ltd.

Chhawchharia, K. (2012). *Happiness during middle age as the function of spiritual intelligence and gender* (Unpublished Doctoral Dissertation). Pt. R.S. University, Raipur (C.G.).

Chhawchharia, K., Ajawani, J. C., & Verma, S. (2011). Happiness in old age as the function of spiritual intelligence and gender. *Journal of Psychology, Applied to Life and Work, 3*, 12–17.

Coward, D., & Reed, P. G. (1996). Self-transcendence: A resource for healing at the end of life. *Issue in Mental Health Nursing, 17*(3), 275–288.

Crichton, J. S. (2008). *A qualitative study of spiritual intelligence in organizational leaders* (Dissertation). The Marshall Goldsmith School of Management, Alliant International University, San Francisco, CA.

DeSteno, D., Bartlett, M. Y., Baumann, J., Williams, L. A., & Dickens, L. (2010). Gratitude as a moral sentiment: Emotion guided cooperation in economic exchange. *Emotion, 10*(2), 289–293.

Ellermann, C. R., & Reed, P. G. (2001). Self-transcendence and depression in middle age adults. *Western Journal of Nursing Research, 23*(7), 698–713.

Emmons, R. A. (2000a). Spirituality and intelligence: Problems and prospects. *The International Journal for the Psychology of Religion, 10*(1), 57–64.

Emmons, R. A. (2000b). Is spirituality an intelligence? Motivation, cognition, and the psychology of ultimate concern. *The International Journal for the Psychology of Religion, 10*(1), 3–26.

Friedman, P. H., & Toussaint, L. L. (2009). The relationship between forgiveness, gratitude, and well-being: The mediating role of affect and beliefs. *Journal of Happiness Studies, 10*(6), 635–654.

Helliswell, J. F. (2003). How's life? Combining individual and national variables to explain subjective well-being. *Economic Modeling, 20*, 331–360.

Kaplan, M. S., Marks, G., & Mertens, S. B. (1997). Distress and coping among women with HIV infection: Preliminary findings from a multiethnic sample. *American Journal of Orthopsychiatry, 67*(1), 80–91.

Kerr, S., Johnson, V. K., Gans, S. E., & Krumrine, J. (2004). Predicting adjustment during the transition to college: Alexithymia, perceived stress and psychological symptoms. *Journal of College Student Development, 45*(6), 593–611.

Lawton, G. (1951). *Aging successfully.* New York: Columbia University Press.

Luthar, S. S. (1991). Vulnerability and resilience: A study of high risk adolescents. *Child Development, 62*(3), 600–616.

Luthar, S. S., & Cicchetti, D. (2000). The construct of resilience: Implications for interventions and social policies. *Development and Psychopathology, 12*(4), 857–885.

McCullough, M. E., Emmons, R. A., & Tsang, J. (2002). The grateful disposition: A conceptual and empirical topography. *Journal of Personality and Social Psychology, 82*(1), 112–127.

Mascaro, N., & Rosen, D. H. (2005). Existential meaning's role in the enhancement of hope and prevention of depressive symptoms. *Journal of Personality, 73*(4), 985–1014.

Mascaro, N., & Rosen, D. H. (2006). The role of existential meaning as a buffer against stress. *Journal of Humanistic Psychology, 46*(2), 168–190.

Maslow, A. H. (1943). A theory of human motivation. *Psychological Review, 50*, 370–396.

Masten, A. S. (2009). Ordinary magic: Lessons from research on resilience in human development. *Education Canada, 49*(3), 28–32.

Narayanan, A., & Jose, T. P. (2011). Spiritual intelligence and resilience among Christian youth in Kerala. *Journal of the Indian Academy of Applied Psychology, 37*(2), 263–268.

Nasel, D. D. (2004). *Spiritual orientation in relation to spiritual intelligence: A consideration of traditional Christianity and new age/individualistic spirituality* (Unpublished Doctoral Dissertation). University of South Australia, South Australia, Australia.

Noble, K. D. (2000). Spiritual intelligence: A new frame of mind. *Spirituality and Giftedness, 9*, 1–29.

Noble, K. D. (2001). *Riding the windhorse: Spiritual intelligence and the growth of the self.* Cresskill, NJ: Hampton Press.

Nolen-Hoeksema, S., Wisco, B. E., & Lyubomirsky, S. (2008). Rethinking rumination. *Perspectives on Psychological Science, 3*(5), 400–424.

Oxford University Press. (2001). *Oxford dictionary of current English* (3rd Ed.). Oxford: Oxford University Press.

Pargament, K. I. (1997). *The psychology of religion and coping: Theory, research, practice.* New York, NY, USA: Guilford Publications, Inc.

Persinger, M. A. (1996). Feelings of past lives as expected perturbations within neuro-cognitive processes that generate the sense of self: Contributions from limbic labiality and vectorial hemisphericity. *Perceptual and Motor Skills, 83*(2), 1107–1121.

Purohit, A., & Ajawani, J. C. (2011). Impact of spiritual practices on happiness in middle-agers. *International Multi-Disciplinary Research Journal, 1*(9), 1–3.

Ramchandran, V. S. (1999). *Phantoms in the brain: Exploring the mysteries of the human brain.* London: Fourth Estate.

Shearer, C. G. (2006). *Development and validation of a scale for existential thinking.* Unpublished manuscript. Kent State University, Ohio, USA.

Shepard, L. A. (1979). Self-acceptance: The evaluative component of the self-concept construct. *American Educational Research Journal, 16*(2), 139–160.

Ungar, M., Brown, M., Liebessberg, L., Othman, R., Kwong, W. M., Armstrong, M., & Gilgun, J. (2007). Unique pathways to resilience across cultures. *Adolescence, 42*(166), 287–310.

Vaughan, F. (2003). What is spiritual intelligence? *Journal of Humanistic Psychology, 42*(2), 16–33.

Wayne, M. (1993). *Acceptance of self and others.* North Carolina Cooperative Extension Service as HE-276–2. North Carolina State University, North Carolina, USA.

Weiss, B. (1988). *Many lives, many masters.* New York: Simon & Schuster Inc.

Wong, Y. J., Rew, L., & Slaikeu, K. D. (2006). A systematic review of recent research on adolescent religiosity/spirituality and mental health. *Issues in Mental Health Nursing, 27*(2), 161–183.

Zautra, A. J., Hall, J. S., & Murray, K. E. (2010). Resilience: A new definition of health for people and communities. In J. W. Reich, A. J. Zautra, & J. S. Hall (Eds.), *Handbook of adult resilience* (pp. 3–34). New York: Guildford Press.

Zohar, D., & Marshall, I. (2000). *S.Q.: Connecting with our spiritual intelligence.* New York: Bloomsbury Publishing House.

Section III
Applied evidence

16

Resilience and countering violent extremism

Stevan Weine

Resilience-centered approaches

The concept of resilience, borrowed from engineering, has been used to underlie a wide spectrum of interventions in the social, psychological, psychosocial, and health domains. It refers to "positive or adaptive outcomes in the presence of some type (or types) of risk, stress, adversity, daily life challenges, or trauma" (Criss, Henry, Harrist, & Larzelere, 2015, p. 4). These include disaster response, violence reduction, and cancer prevention (Aisenberg & Herrenkohl, 2008; Luthar & Goldstein, 2004; McEntire, 2014; Paton, Smith, & Violanti, 2000; Wenzel et al., 2002). In these endeavors, resilience has been used to refer to resilience at one or more of individual, family, community, organization, and societal levels.

In the case of countering violent extremism (to be defined in the subsequent section), the dimensions of resilience that are most relevant are community and family resilience. According to Norris et al. (2008), community resilience is "a process linking a network of adaptive capacities to adaptation after a disturbance or adversity". This definition emphasizes that it is not just the resources but also those resources' dynamic attributes (e.g. their robustness, redundancy, and rapidity) that are essential. Community resilience emerges from four primary sets of adaptive capacities – economic development, social capital, information and communication, and community competence. Two examples of community resilience are shared problem solving and safe community spaces for youth to gather under adult supervision (White House, 2011b).

According to Froma Walsh (2003), family resilience consists of characteristics of family belief systems, family organization, and family communication processes (Walsh, 2003). Family resilience research has also pointed to such characteristics as connectedness, values, flexibility, family cohesion, family adaptability, family coherence, family hardiness, and valuing of family time and routines (Ahlert & Greeff, 2012; Deist & Greeff, 2015; Greeff & Nolting, 2013; Henry, Sheffield Morris, & Harrist, 2015; Patterson, 2002).

Resilience may also be viewed from the perspective of protective resources, which are social and psychological factors that can stop, delay, or diminish negative outcomes (Weine et al., 2014). Protective resources encompass not only resilience (e.g. bouncing back) but also resistance (e.g. preventing). Protective resources can reside in families, communities, and institutions. Thus, family protective resources include family capacities that can promote positive youth psychosocial well-being across a range of outcomes.

It is important to consider the links between family and community resilience and protective resources. Community protective resources work either by building family protective resources or by working directly upon the youth to promote psychosocial well-being. A range of different kinds of actors in a community can provide protective resources, such as teachers, clergy, coaches, and elders. One implication of this is that there is need for thinking about how community and/or family resilience may be changed through prevention, intervention, and/or policy initiatives.

Though resilience has been increasingly cited by terrorism experts and policymakers as an essential consideration when developing programs to counter violent extremism, research on resilience has not yet been systematically applied to this context (Aly, Taylor, & Karnovsky, 2014; Coaffee, 2006; Munton et al., 2011; Nasser-Eddine, Garnham, Agostino, & Caluya, 2011). However, over the past ten years, there has been an explosion of interest in resilience in the clinical, community, and family sciences concerning a broad range of adversities (Cutter et al., 2008; Eloff et al., 2014; Gewirtz & Edleson, 2007; Gordon, Rowe, & Garcia, 2015; Lennon & Heaman, 2015; Markovitz, Schrooten, Arntz, & Peters, 2015). What does this emerging knowledge of resilience tell us that is potentially relevant to countering violent extremism? First, resilience is neither entirely individual nor entirely social but an interactive combination (Luthar & Zigler, 1991). To understand resilience, it is necessary to look beyond individual characteristics and also examine multi-level characteristics at the peer, family, community, societal, state, and global levels. Second, people can be resilient to some risks but not to others (Luthar & Zigler, 1991). Third, when young people face risks from socio-economic and socio-cultural adversities, their family is often the strongest buffer against the associated risks (Weine & Siddiqui, 2009).

Countering violent extremism

Countering violent extremism (CVE) is "a realm of policy, programs, and interventions designed to prevent individuals from engaging in violence associated with radical political, social, cultural, and religious ideologies and groups" (Holmer, 2013, p. 2). While the overall goal of CVE is "to stop those most at risk of radicalization from becoming terrorists" (Benjamin, 2010), CVE focuses on individuals who are not engaging in criminal activities.

CVE is intended to encompass both prevention and intervention activities. Prevention activities are programs and policies that promote inclusion, engage youth and communities, diminish exposure to broad risk factors that threaten healthy development, and increase access to resources that promote well-being. Intervention activities are programs and policies that serve youth who demonstrate early risk markers of poor adjustment, which can include (but are not limited to) mental health problems, alienation, aggression/bullying, and/or delinquency, as well as individuals who may be increasingly drawn to violent extremist ideology and/or activities.

The government's vision for CVE in the United States was articulated in two documents written by the Obama White House. In August 2011, the White House released a brief document entitled "Empowering Local Partners to Prevent Violent Extremism in the United States," which was the country's first attempt at a strategy to build community resilience to counter violent extremism (White House, 2011a). Four months later, the White House released the more detailed "Strategic Implementation Plan for Empowering Local Partners to Prevent Violent Extremism in the United States" (White House, 2011b).

The Strategic Implementation Plan (SIP) recommends several practical steps for prevention through empowering local partners (White House, 2011b). One recommendation highlights the need to "foster community-led partnerships and prevention programming" through "expanding community-based solutions" (White House, 2011b, p. 10). Another recommendation is to provide communities with "information and training, access to resources and grants, and connections with the philanthropic and private sectors" (White House, 2011b, p. 10).

These documents describe how the US National Security Strategy's approach to countering violent extremism (CVE) should be grounded in resilience, which the SIP actually mentions twenty-one times. Emphasizing resilience highlights the positive attributes of communities and persons that have often been highly stigmatized in public discourses and could help to open doors to community–government collaboration. But what exactly is resilience in CVE? Can building it really prevent violent extremism? And, if so, how can we develop programs and policies that will empower communities to build resilience so as to prevent violent ideologies from taking root and to stop individuals from committing violent acts?

In order for these efforts to succeed, what are also needed are models and interventions that are well supported by theory and empirical evidence and that are feasible, acceptable, and appropriate to communities and their members. To this end, the authors conducted ethnographic research in the Somali-American community in Minneapolis-St. Paul in order to 1) characterize how social experiences impact involvement in violent extremism for diaspora youth and young adults; 2) understand how resilience might prevent violent extremism in communities under threat; and 3) inform the development of prevention strategies that incorporate both security and psychosocial dimensions and are based on theory, evidence, and community collaboration.

Somali-American study

Through a governmental–academic–community collaborative effort, we used ethnographic methods to study fifty-three youths, parents, and community providers in the Somali-American community. We conducted open-ended interviews so as to better understand what the components of resilience to violent extremism are and what strategies could help to further build resilience. Our research derived an empirical model, Diminishing Opportunities for Violent Extremism (DOVE), which is described in the following section (Weine & Ahmed, 2012).

Because it is important to look at resilience in relation to risks, our interviews also focused on characterizing risks in relation to the potential for violent extremism. Overall we identified a total of thirty-seven risk factors (see Table 16.1). These consisted of seventeen family and youth risks; twelve community risks; and eight global, state, and societal risks. No one risk factor explained involvement in violent extremism. Rather it was the interaction of multiple risk factors at the peer, family, community, global, state, and societal levels. Two examples of risk factors are summarized here with illustrative quotations.

Being passionate about Somalia

Somali-American youth reported caring deeply about Somalia and wanting to help make it better in their lifetimes. One youth said, "We were the generation that was going to help Somalia become a better country." This attitude predisposed some youth to solutions proposed by violent extremists to restore Somalia.

Being uninformed about Islam

Somali-Americans reported that youth did not know enough about Islam to question or resist extremist views and some parents did not know enough to talk to their children about these issues. One community service provider said, "Life is written in the book . . . how you should

Table 16.1 Risk factors combined to create an opportunity structure for violent extremism

Levels	Risk Factors	Opportunities
Global, State & Societal	• Secondary migration • Being an underserved U.S. refugee community	
Community	• Lack of support for youth • Unsafe neighborhoods • Social exclusion • Unmonitored spaces in community forums	
Family and Youth	• Family separation or loss • Weak parental support • Absolute trust in everyone who attends mosque • Mistrust of law enforcement • Overemphasis on government power • LACK OF AWARENESS OF VIOLENT RADICALIZATION AND RECRUITMENT • Lack of accurate info on violent radicalization and recruitment • Little parental involvement in education • Lack of opportunities • Lack of warning signs	**Youth's Unaccountable Times & Unobserved Spaces**
Global, State & Societal	• Viewing Somalia as a failed state • Violent extremism on the Internet • PERCEPTION OF A NEW THREAT TO SOMALIA • Objections to U.S. government foreign policy	
Community	• COMMUNITY SUPPORT FOR AL SHABAAB • Hearing bad news about Somalia • Social exclusion • Being a divided community • Remittance sending • Having a Normadic heritage • Interaction with migration brokers	**Perceived Social Legitimacy Of Violent Extremism**
Family and Youth	• Little family talk about war • Identity issues among members of Generation 1.5 • Being passionate about Somalia • Being uninformed about Islam • Being uninformed about Somalia • Social identity challenges • Indirect and direct traumas	
Global, State & Societal	• Terrorist organization's recruitment • Violent extremism on the Internet	
Community	• Sources of radical ideology	**Presence Of Recruiters Or Associates**

Source: Weine & Ahmed (2012).

CAPS = Transient risk

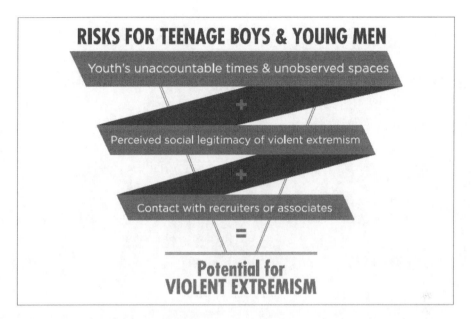

RISKS FOR TEENAGE BOYS & YOUNG MEN

Youth's unaccountable times & unobserved spaces

+

Perceived social legitimacy of violent extremism

+

Contact with recruiters or associates

=

**Potential for
VIOLENT EXTREMISM**

Figure 16.1   Risk for teenage boys and young men
Source: Weine & Ahmed, 2012.

value things, respect others, and appreciate others. If people followed it, then I believe there wouldn't be a big problem as there is now."

Moreover, we found that these risk factors combined to create an opportunity structure (Clarke & Newman, 2006) for violent extremism with three levels of opportunity (see Figure 16.1): 1) youth's unaccountable times and unobserved spaces, 2) the perceived social legitimacy of violent extremism, and 3) contact with recruiters or associates. Involvement in violent extremism depended on the presence of all three, with decreasing proportions of adolescent boys and young men exposed to the latter two.

Further, we found that efforts to increase resilience should involve strengthening protective resources that we described in the DOVE model (see Figure 16.2). Furthermore, family and youth, community, and government can help to strengthen protective resources at each of the three levels of opportunity. Priorities include diminishing 1) youth's unaccountable times and unobserved spaces, 2) the perceived social legitimacy of violent extremism, and 3) the potential for contacts with terrorist recruiters or associates.

Overall, we identified a total of forty-nine protective resources that can reduce the opportunities for entry into violent extremism (see Table 16.2). These consisted of sixteen family and youth protective resources, twenty community protective resources, and thirteen government protective resources. The table was organized in relation to both sectors and to the risk factors identified as mentioned earlier. Two examples of protective resources are summarized in the following section.

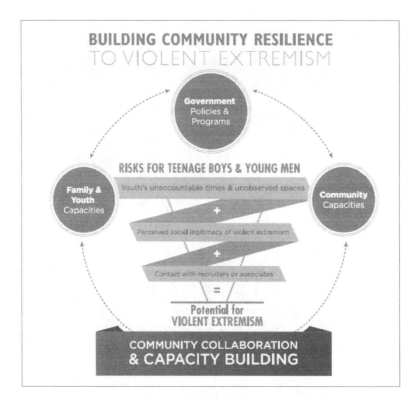

Figure 16.2 Building community resilience to violent extremism
Source: Weine & Ahmed, 2012.

Parental monitoring and supervision

Some Somali-American parents reported now more actively and consistently looking after their teenage children. One parent said,

> I show them we are friends. I try to have direct contacts all the time. I don't act that only I am a parent but also that I am their friend. At home, at school, and outside. Let me give you an example. When my kids want to hang around sports activities, I try to offer a time to go with them and know their friends, what they like, and stay most of the time, unless they are in class.

Youth civic engagement

Some Somali-American youth have become active in addressing issues of public concern, such as child protection, youth development, crime prevention, and electoral politics. One youth said,

> They actually train us to become leaders. And they give us lessons. And we go from one community to others, and we have campaigns against violence, and so the whole deal is poverty and justice, we have to do all these things to go against poverty.

The DOVE model represents that preventive initiatives should be directed at all three risk levels contributing to potential involvement in violent extremism. The goals are to diminish

Table 16.2 Resilience as strengthening protective resources

Sector	Aims	Protective Resources
Family and Youth	Diminish Youth's Unaccountable Times and Unobserved Spaces	• Awareness of risks and safeguards • Parental monitoring and supervision • Family confidants • Family social support • Family involvement in education • Access to services and helpers • Parental and youth help-seeking • Parental involvement in mosques & religious education
	Diminish the Perceived Social Legitimacy of Violent Extremism	• Focus on youth's future in the U.S. • Parental support for youth socialization • Rejecting tribalism and war • Parental talk with youth regarding threats • Youth civic engagement • Youth political dialogue
	Diminish Recruiters and Associates Presenting Opportunities	• Parents informing law enforcement • Parental messaging in community re youth protection
Community	Diminish Youth's Unaccountable Times and Unobserved Spaces	• Trusted accurate information sources • Increased activities in supervised community spaces • Mentoring of youth • Increased civilian liaisons to law enforcement • Interactions with community police • Social entrepreneurship • Interfaith dialogue • Social support networks
	Diminish the Perceived Social Legitimacy of Vioent Extremism	• Islamic education & Imam network • Community support for youth socialilization • Understanding of Islam as a peaceful religion • Youth civic engagement • Youth political dialogue • Youth opportunities for peace activism • Messaging to challenge legitimacy of violent extremism

(Continued)

Table 16.2 (Continued)

Sector	Aims	Protective Resources
	Diminish the Potential for Contacts with Recruiters and Associates	• Cooperation with law enforcement • Monitoring by community members • Messaging to warn off recruiters • Bloggers and websites against violent extremism • Critical voices in the community
Government (in part through supporting community-based NGOs)	Diminish Youth's Unaccountable Times and Unobserved Spaces	• Trusted accurate information sources • Community policing • Support for parenting and parent education • Support for after-school programs and mentoring • Support for youth and family social services
	Diminish the Perceived Social Legitimacy of Violent Extremism	• Empowering critical voices • Support for youth community services • Support for youth leadership training • Support for parenting and parent education
	Diminish Recruiters and Associates Presenting Opportunities	• Community policing • Training for community leaders and providers • Support for community messaging • Support for bloggers and websites

Source: Weine & Ahmed (2012).

youth's unaccountable times and unobserved spaces, the perceived social legitimacy of violent extremism, and the potential for contact with terrorist recruiters or associates. At every risk level, the researchers' found protective resources from the three partnership groups – youth and family, community, and government. What has been of concern to parents, community leaders, and government is that a great many youth are exposed to Level 1, and decreasing but still substantial proportions of youth are exposed to Levels 2 and 3.

Furthermore, it indicates that those efforts should involve the cooperative and collaborative efforts within and between the partnership levels of youth and family, community, and government. None can do it alone. What those efforts looked like would depend upon whether or not the protective resources of interest were either existent and strong, existent and weak, or nonexistent and modifiable.

The DOVE model can inform how to approach assessing risk and protection in different communities. With respect to risk and protection, it guides us 1) to acknowledge community members' concerns that violent extremism will not disappear from Somali-American communities anytime soon; 2) to shift to multi-level analyses of risk factors and protective resources that are well supported by theory, empirical evidence, and community collaboration; and 3) to understand why some communities provide more opportunities than others for involvement violent extremism and how to approach prevention.

With respect to intervention, it suggested the need to 1) intervene on all three opportunity levels, not just one; 2) involve government, community, and families working collaboratively to improve each other's capacities to address each level; and 3) sustain interventions over time. Finally, it suggested that resilience approaches to prevention should be well supported by theory, empirical evidence, and community collaboration.

The DOVE model indicates that building community resilience to violent extremism should involve sustaining, strengthening, or initiating the aforementioned protective resources at each of the three risk levels. This requires significant and sustainable cooperation and collaboration among youth and family, community, and government. At every risk level, all partners should both strengthen those protective resources modifiable by them and work with other partners to enhance their capacity to do the same.

There are multiple ways for prevention programming to diminish the risk of violent extremism. The following four strategies focused on youth and young adults devised from the study of Somali-Americans in Minneapolis-St. Paul but may also apply to other communities.

Supplying information and advice on risks and safeguards

Many parents and youth need help recognizing current risks and strategies to mitigate them. Parents need to know how to talk with their children about the dangers of violent extremism. For many, new parenting strategies are necessary, particularly in managing common urban problems. Somali-American community members reported that parents typically do not rely on mainstream media, which they regard as inaccurate, incomplete, and biased against their community. Information and advice for most parents and youth comes from the Somali media or word-of-mouth. New ideas and knowledge could be disseminated in part through these sources.

Changing norms regarding violent extremism

Community members suggested providing logistical support and training to elders and other critical voices. These initiatives could develop messaging to challenge the desire of young people to return to Somalia to fight. Support and coordination would be essential to ensure that efforts were targeted, focused on at-risk youth and young adults, effective, and sustainable. The goal would be to reframe these young people's passion for helping Somalia into other ways to serve the Somali-American community.

Enhancing support and services

Prior to the mobilization of youth to Somalia, community members and academics identified the need for youth services, housing, employment, and reduction of violence (French & Diaz, 2013). Youth and families face obstacles in accessing services and often must fend for themselves. To address these problems, new and expanded services from law enforcement and other community-based providers – mutual assistance associations, schools, and resettlement agencies – are needed. Alleviating pressing problems could reduce the risks for violent radicalization for some youth, and could improve community-wide perceptions about American society and government.

Stevan Weine

Providing young people opportunities for community involvement

Prevention programming could provide the means for young people to engage in public service. Community members critiqued several small-scale initiatives for insufficient opportunities and lack of sustainability. Somali community advocates have called for an expansion of humanitarian and peace work opportunities (Horst, 2006). New programs for diasporic youth create alternatives for channeling their passion for their homeland and people.

Implementing CVE

Since the completion of the Somali-American Minneapolis-St. Paul study, the terrorist threat has changed with the rise of ISIS, and the practice of CVE has evolved. Through 2015, US efforts to counter violent extremism domestically centered on the three "pilot" cities of Los Angeles, Minneapolis, and Boston. In February 2015, the White House held a Summit on Countering Violent Extremism (White House, 2015a). Each of the three pilot cities presented their CVE achievements, frameworks, and future plans. All reported major steps forward in engagement and partnership between law enforcement and communities. All shared preliminary plans to develop more targeted prevention and intervention components of multi-level CVE programs.

But community resistance to CVE has also risen. Advocacy groups, from the ACLU, to CAIR, and Stop LAPD Spying, have channeled grassroots suspicions and outrage over actual civil rights violations into opposition to CVE policies and practices (CAIR, 2012; Osman, 2013). Far from being central partners in CVE, some community members questioned the very premise of CVE, asserting, "We are not who you say we are." They cited the low prevalence of Muslims committing terrorist acts and they perceived CVE as a government program that put communities' civil liberties at risk. Even some in the community who believed in CVE shied away from using the term because to stand behind CVE was to jeopardize one's own standing in the community.

Even though CVE was introduced as an alternative to counter-terrorism, it has thus far failed to get far enough away and to show that it can do good. Has it really helped to build healthier communities? Can it truly be positioned as a partnership with communities when it is run by the US Attorney's office, the same office charged with prosecuting terrorists? Can community-based prevention and intervention really fit under a criminal justice framework? And is it possible to do CVE without significantly exacerbating the stigmatization of Muslim Americans? Community reaction suggests the answers to these questions are a resounding "no".

The authors of the SIP chose to focus on resilience because it offered a non-stigmatizing framework for empowering local communities to make changes that could diminish their vulnerability and increase their protection. However, this choice also introduced several key challenges that do not appear to have been much anticipated by the SIP. First, some of the targeted communities (Somali Americans in Minneapolis-St. Paul) were low-resource settings in ways that significantly compromised their abilities to build community resilience. Second, the CVE pilot program did not come with funding for communities or with a clear mandate for capacity building of community-based organizations. Third, when focusing on the terrorist threat, it becomes the primary focus, and other problems were backgrounded, but for community members, those other problems may be higher priorities. Lastly, the CVE program had no clear communication or operational strategies for building resilience, such as developing a train-the-trainer program whereby community leaders could be taught knowledge and skills that they could then pass on to other community members. The difficulty surmounting these challenges through policies and programs also made it harder to defend CVE against its critics. Building community and

198

family resilience itself is at risk of being dismissed along with CVE as being not good for the community.

One remedy for this situation is to approach building family and community resilience not simply as a means for achieving CVE, but as a strategy for building healthy, resilient communities and which addresses a spectrum of threats to community well-being, including radicalization to violence, but also other more common threats such as targeted violence, school failure, drugs, and suicide. In other words, we need to change the whole approach of CVE, not just the terminology.

One starting point is that communities often know best what they need to make them stronger and healthier. For some, this could be violence prevention more generally; for others, it could be youth mental health promotion or protection against distortions of religion. When communities are allowed to define their own needs, they are more likely to own the solutions and, in turn, the solutions are more likely to work.

Another starting point is that communities need ways to help those who are radicalizing to violence well before they cross the line to criminal behavior. To do this, they need programs run by multi-disciplinary community-based teams who draw upon criminal justice, mental health, public health, and education frameworks and remedies. When communities are able to build these capacities, there will be meaningful alternatives to using hard counterterrorism strategies when other strategies are called for.

Drawing upon community resilience theory and practice knowledge, we identified several other key considerations (Norris, Stevens, Pfefferbaum, Wyche, & Pfefferbaum, 2008). First, to increase resilience, communities need to diminish the real and perceived inequalities concerning economic resources, employment, and housing. This is clearly an issue for Somali-Americans, who have high rates of poverty, but also for some other group of Muslim immigrants and refugees and for some Black Muslims. Second, to increase resilience, CVE efforts must build social capital by engaging more people in CVE prevention and intervention processes. The practitioners of CVE to date are mostly from law enforcement, with smaller numbers coming from the community. One way to change this is to get community-based professionals from mental health and education involved in CVE (Schwartz, 2015; White House, 2015b). Third, prevention strategies are needed that boost already occurring opponents of radicalization, many of which are not known or acknowledged by those outside the community, especially given the tendency in the media to not cover such stories.

With respect to resilience, it is necessary to better understand and positively impact the interactions between family resilience and community resilience. In order to help in CVE, community resilience has to be able to reach into families and increase parental capacities to support, monitor, and supervise their youth. But the current usage of building community resilience does not seem to incorporate building family resilience in the ways implied in the SIP. Family resilience would appear to offer a very necessary and sound counterpart to community resilience for promoting youth well-being. Policies and programs should aim not only to better equip communities but to better equip families as well. This requires drawing, not only on criminal justice strategies, but on mental health and education approaches to strengthening communities and families.

Conclusion

Resilience has emerged as a key construct for developing, implementing, and evaluating CVE initiatives in impacted communities. However, CVE initiatives would be strengthened by better adhering to resilience theory and resilience-focused interventions as part of broader strategy of building healthy, resilient communities.

References

Ahlert, I. A., & Greeff, A. P. (2012). Resilience factors associated with adaptation in families with deaf and hard of hearing children. *American Annals of the Deaf, 157*(4), 391–404.

Aisenberg, E., & Herrenkohl, T. (2008). Community violence in context risk and resilience in children and families. *Journal of Interpersonal Violence, 23*(3), 296–315.

Aly, A., Taylor, E., & Karnovsky, S. (2014). Moral disengagement and building resilience to violent extremism: An education intervention. *Studies in Conflict & Terrorism, 37*(4), 369–385.

Benjamin, D. (2010, March 10). Testimony before the emerging threats and capabilities subcommittee of the senate armed services committee, Washington, DC.

CAIR. (2012). *CAIR-CA: LAPD abandons plan to map Muslims.* Retrieved from www.cair.com/press-center/cair-in-the-news/5280-cair-ca-lapd-abandons-plan-to-map-muslims.html

Clarke, R. V., & Newman, G. R. (2006). *Outsmarting the terrorists.* New York: Praeger Publishers.

Coaffee, J. (2006). From counterterrorism to resilience. *The European Legacy: Toward New Paradigms, 11*(4), 389–403.

Criss, M. M., Henry, C. S., Harrist, A. W., & Larzelere, R. E. (2015). Interdisciplinary and innovative approaches to strengthening family and individual resilience: An introduction to the special issue. *Family Relations, 64*(1), 1–4.

Cutter, S. L., Barnes, L., Berry, M., Burton, C., Evans, E., Tate, E., & Webb, J. (2008). A place-based model for understanding community resilience to natural disasters. *Global Environmental Change, 18*(4), 598–606.

Deist, M., & Greeff, A. P. (2015). Resilience in families caring for a family member diagnosed with dementia. *Educational Gerontology, 41*(2), 93–105.

Eloff, I., Finestone, M., Makin, J. D., Boeving-Allen, A., Visser, M., Ebersöhn, L., . . . & Forsyth, B. W. (2014). A randomized clinical trial of an intervention to promote resilience in young children of HIV-positive mothers in South Africa. *AIDS, 28*, S347–S357.

French, R., & Diaz, K. (2013, February 15). Mary Jo Copeland receives presidential medal. *Star Tribune.*

Gewirtz, A. H., & Edleson, J. L. (2007). Young children's exposure to intimate partner violence: Towards a developmental risk and resilience framework for research and intervention. *Journal of Family Violence, 22*(3), 151–163.

Gordon, R. A., Rowe, H. L., & Garcia, K. (2015). Promoting family resilience through evidence-based policy making: Reconsidering the link between adult–infant bedsharing and infant mortality. *Family Relations, 64*(1), 134–152.

Greeff, A. P., & Nolting, C. (2013). Resilience in families of children with developmental disabilities. *Families, Systems, & Health, 31*(4), 396–405.

Henry, C. S., Sheffield Morris, A., & Harrist, A. W. (2015). Family resilience: Moving into the third wave. *Family Relations, 64*(1), 22–43.

Holmer, G. (2013). *Countering violent extremism: A peacebuilding perspective.* Special Report 336. Washington, DC: United States Institute of Peace.

Horst, C. (2006). *Connected lives: Somalis in Minneapolis: Family responsibilities and the migration dreams of relatives.* Geneva.

Lennon, S. L., & Heaman, M. (2015). Factors associated with family resilience during pregnancy among inner-city women. *Midwifery, 31*(10), 957–964.

Luthar, S. S., & Goldstein, A. (2004). Children's exposure to community violence: Implications for understanding risk and resilience. *Journal of Clinical Child and Adolescent Psychology, 33*(3), 499–505.

Luthar, S. S., & Zigler, E. (1991). Vulnerability and competence: A review of research on resilience in childhood. *American Journal of Orthopsychiatry, 61*(1), 6–22.

McEntire, D. A. (2014). *Disaster response and recovery: Strategies and tactics for resilience.* Hoboken, NJ: John Wiley & Sons.

Markovitz, S. E., Schrooten, W., Arntz, A., & Peters, M. L. (2015). Resilience as a predictor for emotional response to the diagnosis and surgery in breast cancer patients. *Psycho-Oncology, 24*(12), 1639–1645.

Munton, T., Martin, A., Lorenc, T., Marrero-Guillamon, I., Jamal, F., Lehmann, A., & Sexton, M. (2011). Understanding vulnerability and resilience in individuals to the influence of al Qaida violent extremism. Croydon: Great Britain Home Office. Retrieved from https://scholar.googleusercontent.com/scholar?q=cache:ErbmcoLHxXkJ:scholar.google.com/&hl=en&as_sdt=0,5

Nasser-Eddine, M., Garnham, B., Agostino, K., & Caluya, G. (2011). *Countering Violent Extremism (CVE) literature review* (No. DSTO-TR-2522). Defence Science and Technology Organisation Edinburgh (Australia).

Norris, F. H., Stevens, S. P., Pfefferbaum, B., Wyche, K. F., & Pfefferbaum, R. L. (2008). Community resilience as a metaphor, theory, set of capacities, and strategy for disaster readiness. *American Journal of Community Psychology, 41*(1–2), 127–150.

Osman, A. (2013). *A review: The terror factory and the FBIs manufactured war on terrorism.* The CAIR for New York Blog. Retrieved from https://cair-ny.org/blog/a_review_the_terror_factory__the_fbis_manufactured_war_on_terrorism.html

Paton, D., Smith, L., & Violanti, J. (2000). Disaster response: Risk, vulnerability and resilience. *Disaster Prevention and Management: An International Journal, 9*(3), 173–180.

Patterson, J. M. (2002). Understanding family resilience. *Journal of Clinical Psychology, 58*(3), 233–246.

Schwartz, B. (2015). *START hosts conference on mental health, education, and countering violent extremism.* National Consortium for the Study of Terrorism and Responses to Terrorism. Retrieved from www.start.umd.edu/news/start-hosts-conference-mental-health-education-and-countering-violent-extremism

Walsh, F. (2003). Family resilience: A framework for clinical practice. *Family Process, 42*(1), 1–18.

Weine, S., & Ahmed, O. (2012). *Building resilience to violent extremism among Somali-Americans in Minneapolis-St. Paul.* Final Report to Human Factors/Behavioral Sciences Division, Science and Technology Directorate, US Department of Homeland Security. College Park, MD: START.

Weine, S., & Siddiqui, S. (2009). Family determinants of minority mental health and wellness. In Sana Loue & Martha Sajatovic (Eds.), *Determinants of minority mental health and wellness* (pp. 1–33). New York: Springer.

Weine, S. M., Ware, N., Hakizimana, L., Tugenberg, T., Currie, M., Dahnweih, G., . . . Wulu, J. (2014). Fostering resilience: Protective agents, resources, and mechanisms for adolescent refugees' psychosocial well-being. *Adolescent Psychiatry, 4*(4), 164–176.

Wenzel, L. B., Donnelly, J. P., Fowler, J. M., Habbal, R., Taylor, T. H., Aziz, N., & Cella, D. (2002). Resilience, reflection, and residual stress in ovarian cancer survivorship: A gynecologic oncology group study. *Psycho-Oncology, 11*(2), 142–153.

The White House. (2011a). *Empowering local partners to prevent violent extremism in the United States.* Retrieved from www.whitehouse.gov/the-press-office/2011/08/03/empowering-local-partners-prevent-violent-extremism-united-states

The White House. (2011b). *Strategic implementation plan for empowering local partners to prevent violent extremism in the United States.* Retrieved from www.whitehouse.gov/the-press-office/2011/12/08/strategic-implementation-plan-empowering-local-partners-prevent-violent-

The White House. (2015a). *Fact sheet: The White House summit on countering violent extremism.* Retrieved from www.whitehouse.gov/the-press-office/2015/02/18/fact-sheet-white-house-summit-countering-violent-extremism

The White House. (2015b). *Statement from the press secretary on the White House summit on countering violent extremism.* Retrieved from www.whitehouse.gov/the-press-office/2015/01/11/statement-press-secretary-white-house-summit-countering-violent-extremism.

17

Medical and social models of orphanhood

Resilience of adopted children and adoptive families[1]

Alexander V. Makhnach

Through all 140 years of its history, scientific psychology was focused on what was going wrong with the human being. That emphasis explains the major role of clinical psychology that was traditionally focused on the treatment of mental illnesses. Scientific research and the practice of the pioneers of the field aimed to cure psychopathology. The practice of treating mental illnesses triggered the development of independent methods and forms of pharmacological and psychotherapeutic approaches. Some of them proved efficient in treating certain types of illnesses. However, regarding mental illnesses as diseases fostered the medical model of treatment, which in its turn inspired further scientific research in the area of mental illnesses and psychiatric disorders. Yet the psychological functioning of a sane person and the question of the normal well-being were disregarded (Seligman, 2003). The term *medical model*, coined by R. D. Laing, is an umbrella notion that implies the whole set of procedures to be studied in universities by the future physicians, medical psychologists and psychotherapists (Laing, 1971). This set presupposes the case-record, analyses and necessary clinical procedures. In this case, the prognosis for a proper treatment is made from the perspective of deficiency. The medical model is a dominant approach to the person and its illness (physical suffering, mental disorder, social problems) with the major goal of unveiling symptoms and syndromes and treating the body (individual or social) as a highly complex mechanism. According to S. Curtis and A. Taket (1996), the medical model is now dominating the world of science. Within this model, the body is regarded as an operative machine, and disorders are compared to disrepairs that should be fixed, i.e. cured. The emphasis is put on diagnosis and treatment, not prevention, which in itself can be a deterioration factor (Curtis & Taket, 1996). Even the language of the medical model reflects its nature: the most commonly used words are *diagnosis, disease, illness, symptoms* and *intervention*. The results can be attained only with the help of interventions, procedures and tests, which may improve health or cure illness through medication, hospitalization or surgery.

Backed by much fundamental research, scientific conventions and figures of authority, the medical model is highly influential; however, it can distort reality by offering only one limited viewpoint on data, observations, phenomena and theories. Today, this model can be seen, not only as a set of procedures carried out on patients, but as a world model, which has proven highly influential among medical science theoreticians, psychologists, philosophers and anthropologists in the broadest sense of the term. Assisted by literature, mass media, cinema and prevailing ideology, this model of illness boosts and helps to internalize a person's negative self-perception, blocking development. Nowadays health services in most countries are based on the medical model, though it is said that the social model, implying more integral view on person and its health, is becoming more general.

There are two approaches present in modern psychology, as in social sciences in general, that can be compared to the models mentioned earlier, the medical model and the social model. The basic concept of the social model (positive socialization model), which initially emerged as a response to social segregation, is the notion of the equality of both normal and destitute people. Equal rights give a person, being in subject–subject relations with the closer environment, opportunity to decide independently and to live a full life, which is reminiscent of the definition of resilience: "Live well, work well and love well" (Garmezy, 1976). Social activity leads to social changes manifesting in attitudes towards this or that social group, in accessibility of the information in the forms suitable for all types of persons, in forming of the attitudes free from prejudices and, in the long run, in positive socialization. The model is focused on health, and all associated research is aimed at prevention of illness, promotion of healthy lifestyle and reducing the risk of falling ill.

In psychology, the medical model implies the idea that all abnormal patterns of behavior are caused by somatic problems that require purely medical approach. Researchers that are advocating the social model tend to have more integrative view, putting emphasis on embedded systems of social disease in the complex interplay of extended family links, social organization's involvement and cultural and historical contexts (Fergusson, Horwood, Shannon, & Lawton, 1989; Ungar & Liebenberg, 2005). Within the conceptual framework of the social model, improvements in health and well-being are achieved by directing effort towards addressing the social, economic and environmental determinants of health. The model demands social, economic and environmental determinants to be addressed so that health gains can occur. Since the social model provides for a person's health, the research cannot be carried out without regard to its ecology. That's why both the scope (health, person's healthy performance) and the subject (individual in its social environment) overlap with the U. Bronfenbrenner's ecological approach in developmental psychology of (Bronfenbrenner, 1979). In fact, the modern socio–cultural (ecological) perspective in developmental studies includes inter alia the interdisciplinary approach to the process of human socialization. U. Bronfenbrenner's ecological model, describing the structure of child's habitat, identifies four contexts of human development: familial, social, cultural and historic. With respect to children and adolescents, this approach implies research of the interconnection between possible developmental disorders as age progresses and the potential of positive children's socialization that can be promoted by proper use of habitat facilities, resources and resilience factors. The child in this case acts as the subject of possible changes and modifications. Positive socialization as an interplay of inner and outer factors (habitat in the widest sense of the word, cultural context, interrelation with the "significant other"), which makes each orphan more resilient.

On this research basis, with its fundamental ecological approach centered on children, the last few decades have been marked by research on child, adolescent and family resilience. Among the best known studies of resilience is the work of E. Werner (1993) and her colleagues. We must also mention the study of the same phenomena, carried out by M. Bleuer, who within forty years had watched more than 184 children with schizophrenic parents and had described their functioning in family, in communication with peers and relatives and in moments of joy and sorrow. In the majority of cases, parents produced a negative impact on these children. However, regardless of difficult environmental conditions and negative genetic background, surprisingly, many of these children demonstrated the ability to lead a "normal" or "almost normal" life. Less than 10% of the sample groups were diagnosed as schizophrenics as they aged. The evident resilience of the majority of children is of undeniable scientific interest and can be encouraging both for scientists and common citizens (Bleuer, 1978). M. Bleuer's observations are perhaps one of the first longitudinal studies, showing the interdependence between social and family risks and resilience of certain family members. Being a psychiatrist, M. Bleuer, however, deviates from the medical model of deficiency and lays an extrinsic emphasis on the potentials and resources of the family and individual (without naming them) that give a person the opportunity to change his life regardless of adverse conditions. Bleuer dissuades his patients from following the imposed script – to become as insane as their parents – and paradoxically invites them to look for potential reserves and resources in their families, in communication with peers and relatives, i.e. to become an active source of all necessary changes, to use the relations with others as an important resource. These resources are regarded as a necessary condition that helps the child to withstand and move on without destroying oneself. Interestingly it was not until some decades later that the first up-to-date theoretical study of resilience appeared, basing on relational competence theory (L'Abate, 1994). Within this approach, relational resilience is regarded as a relational competence (on emotional, cognitive and social levels) that is changing depending on cultural context, gender and changes, which occur over the periods of life cycles (Gianesini, 2013).

Medical and social models in respect to the orphanhood

Now we are going to show that the opposition of the *medical and social models* is valid in respect to the field of orphanhood as well. It should be pointed out that actually the medical model dominates both in public and professional discourse. Professionals in the field of orphanhood for a number of reasons prefer to stick to this model, as it allows regarding the orphan as a patient with medical and behavioral problems that can be diagnosed in terms of deficiency. The model still dominates the minds of experts and is highly influential among lawmakers in the field. The social model of orphanhood hasn't yet become basic for working with stigmatized children; it isn't widespread in the areas of orphans' upbringing, development, socialization, education, career choice etc. It is noteworthy that even the orphan's transfer to the substitute family can comply with the medical model of deficiency. The way in which the substitute family is guided after the adoption is of great importance; it must imply the closest interaction with experts, relatives and the community. Unfortunately, child protection and guardianship services continue to regard substitute families as potentially disadvantaged, thus working within the deficiency approach. This situation is frequent as far as destitute families that are unable to bring up children are concerned. For instance, a heavy-drinking (or drug-addicted) mother who leaves her child right after the birth or destitute parents who are being deprived of their child and their rights have to take the child to the orphanage – in both cases, the situation is considered "socially unhealthy", thus calling for procedures typical of the medical model. Often the so-called "treatment" of the social disease – alcoholism, drug addiction – and further socialization of parents constitute part of the medical model of orphanhood: this kind of parents are treated as ill, socially unfit and as those who can only act as passive recipients of help. Unfortunately, the medical model of orphanhood in these cases is being taken over by children, boosting their trans-generational dependency and parasitism. In terms of the phenomenology of the orphanhood, this model regards orphan's environment as made up of "symptoms" and "syndromes" of ill-being, which results in the reproduction of the circle of ill-being: children that never experienced the building-up of subject–subject relations will become ill parents themselves and will raise identical children and so on. This circle of ill-being is manifested in unstable self-esteem, dependence (as a person's characteristic, including permanent need of love and acceptance), as well as the negative self-perception as a person, member of family and member of society. From our viewpoint, the deficiency-based approach to the substitute family and the orphan is inherent to the medical model. And the social model implies the approach that is based on development and use of family's resources and potentials.

In order to analyze medical and social models of orphanhood in their historical perspective in Russia, let's consider how these models are marked in public and social discourses. In Russia, before World War II, orphanhood wasn't studied, although the number of orphans was great (because of the 1917 Revolution, the civil war of 1917–1923, collectivization and the resulting famine of 1927–1932). The little research that was carried out would never touch the problem of finding a new family for orphans. Starting in the 1930s, scientists had been mainly focusing on questions of deprivation and hospitalism of orphans in the process of their development. Because of country's isolation, Russian psychologists, both theoreticians and practitioners, knew nothing about the Western phenomenology of orphanhood, which had been developing within child psychoanalysis and developmental psychology. The second wave of orphans that came after the World War II didn't raise as much scientific interest in the USSR as it did in Europe. A scarce number of studies of the period, carried out mainly by pediatricians and educators and rarely by psychologists (Figurin & Denisova, 1949; Schelovanov & Aksarina, 1955), can be explained by political causes. There were no reasons to study those who had "happy childhood", which is "the must" in Communist society, particularly for orphans, who guarded by the state with its "children-are-our-future" declarations.

The *first period* can only be associated with the medical model that neglected the issues of adaptation and adoption. The emphasis was laid on health: good diet, sport, summer camps, cold training and etc. Thus, between 1917 and 1980s, the country had been suffering endless social disruptions – revolution, civil war, famine, World War II, post-war ruins – which resulted in two huge waves of orphans. This time range we will call the *first period*. As I have already mentioned, all studies of that time were closely associated with the principles of the medical model.

Within the *second period* of orphanhood studies, there appeared those focused on adoptive families (both adoption and guardianship), children from family-type orphanages. However, the results of these studies were rarely published (Prikhozhan & Tolstykh, 1980) and were also associated with the medical model, though certain elements of the socially oriented approach were beginning to take shape.

The *third period* is related to the new forms of orphans' family placement and can be outlined by the 1990s–early 2000s. During this period, a number of studies were already associated with the social model. This short period coincided with the new flow of orphans that took place in Russia in early 1990s. As for studies, the new terminology, the subject-oriented approach, the means and the forms of cooperation with adoptive families were the signs of gradually emerging features of the social model. Unfortunately, only a few research papers and data are left of this period. It is even sadder for us today, as we realize that the big wave of orphans was left without professional examination, care and support. Faced with social disruptions and witnessing so many orphans still alive but leading an asocial life, parents and psychologists began to recognize social roots of orphanhood and to look for social means of dealing with it. Some researchers "have passed through" the third period of studying new forms of orphans' family placement (family-type orphanages, SOS Kinderdorf villages, foster care families) far too quickly. It is regrettable that there were only few studies, touching the problem of putting in place of these new forms of family placement and comparing them with traditional ones.

The last *fourth period* is predominantly associated with the social model of orphanhood. The researchers take mainly foster families as case studies. This period is marked by interest in the new social institution of professional foster-family care.

Thus, history and economic conditions that determined the development of Russian psychology, as well as many other factors, prevented the experts from paying attention to the problems of orphanhood. Many questions described here are still left without answers, though they directly concern the need in changing the model of orphanhood.

These are the problems in the orphanhood domain associated with public and general social attitudes:

- Actual stigmatization of orphans; the widespread image of orphans as suffering from various illnesses and mental disorders and being unable to establish close reliable relationships
- The idea that the majority of orphans don't have a fine family life and professional career ahead of them
- Low level of society's involvement in the direct interaction with foster care homes
- Society's irresponsible attitude towards the family placement problem of its little members (orphans)
- Low level of society's (including professional community) support for the new forms of family placement, misunderstanding and rejection of the idea of professional care for orphans
- Unwillingness of public organizations to make timely and flexible decisions, to respond efficiently on all the changes in the field of orphanhood
- Health organization's collecting and analysis of data, privacy of information and statistics on orphans, their placement, the adoptive families, rights violation, cases of illnesses, infections and etc.

As to the professional community, the problems are:

- A narrow "esoteric" circle of experts, who stick to the same models of the private orphanhood institutions
- Lack of scientific interest to the problems of orphanhood and professional impotence in rendering assistance to the orphans and adoptive families
- The absence of the special estimator of preferable form of family placement for each orphaned child
- The low level of expertise as far as the adequate training of adoptive and foster parents is concerned
- The absence of longitudinal psychological studies, providing both state and society with data on benefits and drawbacks of orphans' placement, peculiarities of different adoptive and foster families, the phenomenology of orphanhood in general.

Most of these questions are left unanswered, but time and again they are being discussed by the members of society, where the medical model is dominating over the social one. Hence, all the answers and decisions, both professional and non-professional, are rooted in the medical model of orphanhood.

Today in Russia, the two models coexist *inter alia* in orphanhood discourse. Based on discourse analysis, M. S. Astoyants concluded that orphans are regarded as subjects of social exposure and also as part of the modern culture or social entity and characteristic of a certain historical period. She identifies three types of orphanhood discourses: the discourse of *social danger*, the discourse of *social self-justification* and the discourse of *social integration*. We believe that the first two types explicitly represent the medical model of orphanhood, while the last one represents the social model, including the subject relations between the orphan and the family (society). The discourse of *social danger* presents the orphan as someone excluded from society, as a potentially criminal element. The discourse of *social self-justification* is concerned with finding culprits, claiming that troubled families were guilty. The discourse of *social partnership* (social integration in solving the problems of orphans) acknowledges the problem of family's ill-being: "The child is considered to be a dynamic developing personality, while the problem of orphans is to be solved by the means of social integration and cooperation of public institutions, social agencies and organizations, professional unions and mass-media" (Astoyants, 2007). The understanding of one's orphanhood is a negative experience. It is known that the impact of experiences like that touches inner and outer determinants, which evaluate them. There, determinants become the markers of the discourse. A person's subjective attitude towards experiences and events is of great importance, as it can evaluate (mark) them as stress-producing or not in this or that setting (Dikaya & Makhnach, 1996). That is why the discourse of *social self-justification* sustains the medical model of orphanhood. In this context, the importance of life events in the investigation of the stress process in children from this focus seems very relevant. It connects with importance of developmental issues such as children's response to parental separation, coping in achievement contexts, repression or sensitization and developing resilience (Robson, 1997). This understanding of the role of negative experiences and events is especially important for adoptive families, both parents and children, as it can help to find the ways of coping with the aftermath by using orphan's individual and family's and society's in general collective resources. Children and parents learn new strategies for processing, managing and integrating their thoughts and feelings related to traumatic life events, leading to increased feelings of safety, improved communication, better parenting skills and healthier family relationships (Dorsey & Deblinger, 2012). This kind of work introduces adoptive families to the discourse of *social integration*, which is associated with the social model of orphanhood.

Both society and the orphan become the subjects of interaction. The research shows that in the field of orphanhood two types of discourse, the discourse of *social danger* and the discourse of *social partnership*, coexist and contradict each other. We believe that the shift from dominating the medical model towards the social model is almost absent in the phenomenology of orphanhood. It is noteworthy that the use of terms like *help* or *social service* is associated with the medical model and presupposes subject–object relationship. It means that the orphan as a person with special demands (physical, social) is in need of support. That makes him a problem, although the real problem lies in social barriers, created by the family and the public in general. The words *support, service* and *care* are often used by psychologists and social workers in their work with orphans and adoptive families. That is why the socialization of the orphan is a process of establishing his relations with the world around him by developing his life perspective, acquiring an education, specialization and finally self-fulfillment. For instance, it is important to take into account how the adoptive or foster family feels about the social support. D. Ghate and N. Hazel coined the notion of "negative support", emphasizing the subtle difference between aid and intervention, which can result in the loss of control over your own life and the life of a child (Ghate & Hazel, 2002). That's why many experts describe the instance of interaction between care services and substitute parents. The latter don't want to become the target of the intervention, as the rendering of assistance in this context means treatment in terms of deficiency, assuming that someone is "socially ill" and needs support (which is the typical medical model of the patient). Research associated with the social model of health focuses on actual social attitudes that are manifesting in stigmatization of children, orphans included (Mason, 1994). The process of the child's development is being linked to the degree of social acceptance of his advantages and disadvantages. This factor becomes crucial for the child's future.

In Russia, the system of guardianship causes a strong feeling of dependence among children from the very moment they come to the orphanage. Little orphans are told again and again that the state will take care of them. This results in gradually increasing dependence. According to M. Mason (1994), the medical model focuses on illness and boosts labeling, while the estimation, monitoring and therapy are imposed. That is true for orphans being treated paternalistically by orphanage workers and other public caretakers. It is known that orphans develop a special psychological pattern, the so-called "we of the orphanage". According to A. Prikhozhan and N. Tolstykh, child orphans divide world between "us" and "them". Orphans detach themselves from others, tend to act aggressively and have separate groups even within the orphanage (Prikhozhan & Tolstykh, 2007). In after-orphanage life, they reproduce the same patterns. They usually rent a flat or marry with their kin. In other words, they reproduce the model of segregation imposed to them by society. The closedness of the social institutional space, the limited access to social connections and the imposed social role (orphan's role) result in a specific asocial and sometimes even criminal way of life for the orphans or, on the contrary, push them to become the victims of various offences. The closedness of orphanages also limits the professional perspectives of the orphans. This is backed by the low self-rating as compared to normal children of the same age (Abelbeysov, 2011). This situation indicates the predominance of the discourse of *social danger*. That's why we believe that interrelations as an environmental factor are number one for orphans' resilience (Laktionova & Makhnach, 2009). A life in an orphanage doesn't require certain personality functions necessary for a normal life (Prikhozhan & Tolstykh, 2007). That's why, not having the skills of social behavior, necessary for successful adaptation and formation of socially acceptable behavior, orphans can take on only the patterns of their peers. The social environment beyond their group of peers doesn't suggest them a proper pattern of interaction, so socially stigmatized orphans fail to establish appropriated relation with other people on different levels. That's why the role of significant others (neighbors, incidental acquaintances, schoolmates, teachers, guardians) is crucial for orphans, as with their help they fill, by pity or support, the empty gaps in their emotional and social personality structures (Radina & Pavlycheva, 2010). This environment can be a risk factor or a defense factor, depending on who and to what extent becomes a significant other. Thus, the environment becomes a relational factor of resilience. The role of peers and schoolmates is important because it can promote positive socialization. An orphan can also take on the set of rules for his future life by following the only example taken from social interaction. Orphans, like any other teenagers, create their subculture that helps them to conceptualize the world and their lives. They tend to idealize certain phenomena, which are regarded by them as portals to the normal civilized life. We have already shown that orphans tend to support informal youth movements and to communicate with those addicted to alcohol. Unfortunately, this kind of behavior stands for a defensive response, which is a marker of inability of their subculture to form resilience (Laktionova & Makhnach, 2009).

It is known that only a few can discard overprotection and hothouse conditions by themselves as it requires certain inner and outer conditions. By inner, we mean character traits, for example the inner locus of control that helps to move towards one's resilience. Our research shows that teenage orphans with emotional and behavioral problems have their inner locus of control associated with social adaptation and resilience, but only in case of their *positive attitude towards oneself and others*. Only in this case can they feel emotionally at ease and can admit responsibility for what is going on (inner locus of control); they long for achievements (motivation) and dominance

(Makhnach & Laktionova, 2013). The mere fact of losing contact with habitual environment and establishing relations not only with peers show the potential resilience. Unfortunately, however, the social orphanhood system isn't aimed to encourage independent life attitude. It's not just the absence of everyday social skills but the inability to act and make decisions independently. As a result, orphans cannot lead an autonomous life; they are unable to foresee the consequences of their deeds, plan their activity, predict future, set an aim and gradually move towards its attainment (Iovchuk, Severnyy, & Morozova, 2008). This leads to incomplete or insufficient socio-psychological adaptation, inadaptability, school disadaptation and deviant behavior (Prikhozhan & Tolstykh, 2007).

We can't say that this situation is acceptable for the actual Russian social care system. But any system can preserve itself only by increasing inactivity of its elements. Each one, who wants to break through the limits of the system, constitutes a potential threat. That's why orphans' training can be oriented towards the independent attitude, as only inactive children can guarantee the system's stability. The orphan can hardly become independent and responsible in the context of passive consumption of services (educational, health-preserving). This system isn't aimed at producing socialized individuals; it forms a passive, dependent child that cannot survive without support and guardianship of the medical model.

If we consider adoptive families, they can also become the part of medical model after adopting an orphan. The families must always remember that orphans constitute a marginalized group. This image is most likely the fruit of predominance of the medical model. So, the adoptive family can become a special element, thus an excluded one (the medical model pattern again). So the members of adoptive family and those who render them professional assistance should look for intrafamilial and environmental resources as the social model presupposes. Thus, our research showed that successful family placement highly depends on the individual resilience of adoptive parents, fruitful intrafamilial communication, advanced skills of problem solving, reasonable resource management and a realistic view of the financial situation. All these factors reduce the risk of psychopathology in both parents (for example depression associated with adoption difficulties) and a child; they also provide for interaction, closer communication and proper adaptation of the orphan (Makhnach, Laktionova, & Postylyakova, 2015).

It is also important to realize that the former orphans reproduce the system of closedness in their subculture, importing them to the new family, especially when they have siblings. Sibling adoptions are often unsuccessful and lead to so-called de-adoption. T. Reilly and L. Platz showed that biological siblings adopted by the same family are more problematic that separated ones (Reilly & Platz, 2003). In a comparative study, R. Hegar showed that factor of joint sibling placement stays highly problematic (Hegar, 2005). R. Stryker made an interesting observation, having attracted attention to one peculiarity of orphans:

It didn't ever cross my mind to ask an adult to help me with things. If you needed help it meant that you were dumb. Stupid, because I didn't want to be put in a worse place, I asked (friends) Sergei and Erik to help. We helped each other get what we wanted.

(Stryker, 2000, p. 82)

This idea, articulated by the American, who had adopted a Russian child, demonstrates that orphans are not used to turn to their family for help, while familial help and support is one of the major factors of resilience. The "we of the orphanage" determines orphans' deeds and their life in general. The fact of being associated with an impotent and resourceless "we" demonstrates the social frailty of orphans (Prikhozhan & Tolstykh, 2007). There is the same phenomenon as we can observe, in another vulnerable group – a segregated ethnic one. Kumar, Mukherjee, and

Parkash (2012) analyzing the social perspective emphasize the fact that the opposition of "us" and "them" can lead to segregation and then even to the involvement in terrorism. They find that, often, perceived or existing socio-economic differences create "ethnicity-based conflicts" and results in "us vs. them" groups, which often take recourse to conflict (Kumar et al., 2012). In our case the opposition of "us" and "them" also causes social conflict, the distance between "us" and "them", which determines the whole subsequent life of the individual.

Russian folklore, acting as a container of discourses in their historical perspective, is of great interest in this context. As far as orphanhood is concerned, folklore, expressing a traditional philosophy of life, contains many proverbs and sayings that reflect the whole range of attitudes towards this social phenomenon. It is known that proverbs are cultural clichés that explain general laws and prescribed patterns of behavior. Out of the whole range of generalized, culture-bound principles, the individual "privatizes" only a few, which don't contradict each other and would lay a foundation of his behavior (Leontiev & Tarvid, 2005). In this respect, individually experienced proverbs that constitute an image of orphans and orphanhood reflect the attitude towards this social phenomenon. We choose twenty-five Russian proverbs about orphans and orphanhood. Then we grouped them according to the type of discourse they represent. Thus, nine proverbs were associated with exclusion of orphans from the society, eleven justified orphanhood and only five of them suggested that society itself is responsible for current state of affairs. In Russian proverbs, the terms used to define an orphan and orphanhood include loss of parents, the rupture of social bonds, lack of family support, the process and situation of deprivation and want and the lack of money or means of livelihood. Some of these are, indeed, the effects of orphanhood. However, the Russian equivalents of orphanhood treat these as integral parts of the totality of the process of orphanhood. Proverbs, advocating this viewpoint, we associate with the discourse of *social danger* (an orphan's childhood is a life-long heritage; the orphan is not noble). *Social self-justification,* which translates into orphanhood, is stretched to include poverty, physical and mental weakness and society's irresponsibility and is reflected in the following proverbs: "God granted the orphan a mouth, so he will give him some food as well" and "Only God would come to the orphan's defense". Proverbs like "Orphan's childhood is a life-long heritage" and "Orphan is not noble" fix the viewpoint that stigmatized orphans are not full members of society. The stigmatization of children and teenagers, who are enjoying a period of acquiring social skills, suspends this process and leaves no chance to quit the medical model of orphanhood. Orphanhood is regarded as a negative fact, as the *status quo* of an orphan's life with the discourse of social danger permanently looming nearby. The fixation of this fact in the orphan's personal discourse and the adoptive family's discourse leads to the consolidation of the discourse of social danger. This evidently doesn't add to the resilience of the child, his family or society in general. We believe that the proverbs reflecting the discourse of *social integration* ("The one who takes pity on the orphan will be rewarded by God", "The world still exists due to the orphans") are associated with the social model that correlated to society's resilience and its responsibility for its illnesses orphanhood included.

Conclusion

We believe that U. Bronfenbrenner's theory of ecological systems provides us with the best possible methodology for studying resilience. A gradual shift from the medical model of deficiency towards the social model has determined the principles and accents: more and more studies are focused on inner and outer factors of person's resilience, including well-being, hope, potential resources and meaning of life, which constitute the basis for positive socialization. This change also touched the socially inadaptive group of teenage orphans. However, the emerging discourse of *social partnership* embedded in the social model is far from being predominant in Russia both in public and professional circles. Problems of orphanhood are still examined in the context of the medical model. Inner and outer factors are rarely regarded as important for resilience, though the role cultural, familial impact, as well as the role of "significant others", can be crucial. The example of orphans as an inadaptive group can be the case for the shift from the discourse of social danger and the discourse of social self-justification towards the discourse of social partnership. This, however, can lead to the misunderstanding and underestimation of the role of significant others in orphans' resilience.

Present psychological developmental theories (psychogenetic, biochemical and stress theories) are based on the medical model of subject–object interaction between the agent and the recipient. The rejection of this model in favor of the social one leads to the subject–subject interaction between people.

The comparison of two models of orphanhood made us conclude that the medical approach is historically traditional for Russia. The medical model of deficiency is indispensable at certain stages of an orphan's education as it helps to diagnose this or that developmental deficit. But we must be aware that the paradigm of the medical model imposes a one-sided approach: the deficient proves to be sufficient. In fact, by using the deficiency model, the social caretaker limits himself. The social model examines orphan's resources, those personality characteristics that can be used as guidelines and call for further development. An orphan, as any other person, has both deficiencies and potentialities. The notion of resilience unites these opposites as we begin to examine, not only risk factors in the context of bigger family, society, peers and culture, orphan's health and personal behavioral features, but also the factors of resilience in above-named areas. Thus, the resilience approach in fact unites two models, the medical and the social. If resilience factors compensate for risk factors, the child will pass through each and every step of positive socialization. Moreover, as is known from the longitudinal experiments, it is not true for every developmental context (Anthony, 1987; Fergusson et al., 1989; Garmezy, 1976; Rutter, 1979; Sroufe, 2005; Ungar et al., 2008; Werner, 1993). This approach allows us to expose deficiency in an orphan's development and intentionally compensate for it, basing on his inner resources and resources of the family, society and culture. This can be considered the most balanced, reasonable and efficient strategy in the process of orphans' positive socialization.

Note

1   This study funded by the State task of FANO RF, № 0159–2016–0007.

References

Abelbeysov, V. A. (2011). Socialization of orphans and abandoned children in the orphanages: A sociological analysis of the problem. *Sociosphere, 1*, 53–68. [Abel'beysov, V. A. (2011). Sotsializatsiya detey-sirot i detey, ostavshikhsya bez popecheniya roditeley v detskom dome: Sotsiologicheskiy analiz problemy. *Sotsiosfera, 1*, 53–68] (in Russian).

Anthony, E. J. (1987). Risk, vulnerability, and resilience: An overview. In E. J. Anthony & B. J. Cohler (Eds.), *The invulnerable child* (pp. 3–48). New York: Guilford Press.

Astoyants, M. S. (2007). *Social orphanhood: Conditions, mechanisms and dynamic of exclusion (sociocultural interpretation)* (Thesis Synopsis, Doctor of Sociological Sciences). Rostov-on-Don: Pedagogical Institute, South Federal University. 44 p. [Astoyants, M. S. (2007). Sotsial'noye sirotstvo: Usloviya, mekhanizmy i dinamika eksklyuzii (sotsiokul'turnaya interpretatsiya). Avtoref. dis. . . . d-ra sotsiol. nauk. Rostov-n/D.] (in Russian).

Bleuer, M. (1978). *The schizophrenic disorders: Long term patient and family studies.* New Haven: Yale University Press.

Bronfenbrenner, U. (1979). *The ecology of human development.* Cambridge, MA: Harvard University Press.

Curtis, S., & Taket, A. (1996). *Health and societies: Changing perspectives.* London: Hodder Arnold.

Dikaya, L. G., & Makhnach, A. V. (1996). The relation of human being to adverse life events and factors of its formation. *Psikhologicheskiy zhurnal, 17*(3), 137–148. [Dikaya, L. G., & Makhnach, A. V. (1996). Otnosheniye cheloveka k neblagopriyatnym zhiznennym sobytiyam i faktory yego formirovaniya. *Psikhologicheskiy zhurnal, 17*(3), 137–148] (in Russian).

Dorsey, S., & Deblinger, E. (2012). Children in foster care. In J. Cohen, A. Mannario, & E. Deblingher (Eds.), *Trauma-focused CBT for children and adolescents: Treatment applications* (pp. 49–72). New York: Guilford Press.

Fergusson, D. M., Horwood, L. J., Shannon, F. T., & Lawton, J. M. (1989). The Christchurch Child Development Study: A review of epidemiological findings. *Paediatric & Perinatal Epidemiology, 3*(3), 302–325.

Figurin, N. L., & Denisova, M. P. (1949). *Development stages of children from birth to one year age.* Moscow: Medgiz. [Figurin, N. L., & Denisova, M. P. (1949). Etapy razvitiya povedeniya detey v vozraste ot rozhdeniya do odnogo goda. M.: Medgiz] (in Russian).

Garmezy, N. (1976). Vulnerable and invulnerable children: Theory, research and intervention. *Catalog of Selected Documents in Psychology, 6*(4), 1–23.

Ghate, D., & Hazel, N. (2002). *Parenting in poor environments: Stress, support and coping.* London: Jessica Kingsley Publishers.

Gianesini, G. (2013). Negotiating family challenges by transforming traditional gender roles in new identities: Patterns of resilience and parenthood in a sample of Italian couples. *Visions of the 21st Century Family: Transforming Structures and Identities. Contemporary Perspectives in Family Research, 7,* 277–316.

Hegar, R. L. (2005). Sibling placement in foster care and adoption: An overview of international research. *Children and Youth Services Review, 27*(7), 717–739.

Iovchuk, N. M., Severnyy, A. A., & Morozova, N. B. (2008). *Child social psychiatry for non-psychiatrists.* Sankt Petersburg: Piter. [Iovchuk, N. M., Severnyy, A. A., & Morozova, N. B. (2008). Detskaya sotsial'naya psikhiatriya dlya nepsikhiatrov. SPb.: Piter] (in Russian).

Kumar, U., Mukherjee, S., & Parkash, V. (2012). Sociocultural aspects of terrorism. In U. Kumar & M. K. Mandal (Eds.), *Countering terrorism: Psychosocial strategies* (pp. 47–73). New Delhi: Sage Publications.

L'Abate, L. (1994). *A theory of personality development.* New York: Wiley.

Laing, R. D. (1971). *The politics of the family and other essays.* London: Tavistock Publications Ltd.

Laktionova, A. I., & Makhnach, A. V. (2009). Resilience of orphaned adolescent. In E. G. Koblik (Ed.), *Children' projective activities as a resource for the development of their resilience* (pp. 6–32). Moscow: Women and Children First Charitable Foundation. [Laktionova, A. I., & Makhnach, A. V. (2009). Zhiznesposobnost' podrostkov-sirot. *Proyektnaya deyatel'nost' detey kak resurs razvitiya zhiznestoykosti* (pp. 6–32). M.: «Zhenshchiny i deti prezhde vsego»] (in Russian).

Leontiev, D. A., & Tarvid, E. V. (2005). The choice of proverbs as a world outlook projection. *Izvestiya of Southern Federal University. Engineering, 51*(7), 70–72. [Leont'yev, D. A., & Tarvid, Ye. V. (2005). Vybor poslovits kak mirovozzrencheskaya proyektsiya. *Izvestiya Yuzhnogo federal'nogo universiteta. Tekhnicheskiye nauki, 51*(7), 70–72] (in Russian).

Makhnach, A. V., & Laktionova, A. I. (2013). Individual and behavioral characteristics of adolescents as a factor of their resilience and social adaptation. *Psikhologicheskiy zhurnal, 34*(5), 69–84. [Makhnach, A. V., & Laktionova, A. I. (2013). Lichnostnyye i povedencheskiye kharakteristiki podrostkov kak faktor ikh zhiznesposobnosti i sotsial'noy adaptatsii. *Psikhologicheskiy zhurnal, 34*(5), 69–84] (in Russian).

Makhnach, A. V., Laktionova, A. I., & Postylyakova, Y. V. (2015). The role of family resourcefulness in the selection of the candidates for adoptive parents. *Psikhologicheskiy zhurnal, 36*(1), 108–122. [Makhnach, A. V., Laktionova, A. I., & Postylyakova, Yu. V. (2015). Rol' resursnosti sem'i pri otbore kandidatov v zameshchayushchiye roditeli. *Psikhologicheskiy zhurnal, 36*(1), 108–122] (in Russian).

Mason, M. (1994). *From father's property to children's rights.* New York: Columbia University Press.

Prikhozhan, A. M., & Tolstykh, N. N. (1980). Study of readiness for school children who raised up outside the family. In I. V. Dubrovina (Ed.), *Psychological and pedagogical problems of children education in the family and preparing youth for family life* (pp. 113–125). Moscow: USSR Academy of Pedagogical Sciences. [Prikhozhan, A. M., & Tolstykh, N. N. (1980). Izucheniye gotovnosti k shkol'nomu obucheniyu u detey, vospityvayushchikhsya vne sem'i. In I. V. Dubrovina (Ed.), *Psikhologo-pedagogicheskiye problemy vospitaniya detey v sem'ye i podgotovki molodozhi k semeynoy zhizni* (pp. 113–125). Moscow: APN SSSR] (in Russian).

Prikhozhan, A. M., & Tolstykh, N. N. (2007). *Psychology of orphanhood.* Sankt Petersburg: Piter. [Prikhozhan, A. M., & Tolstykh, N. N. (2007). *Psikhologiya sirotstva.* SPb.: Piter] (in Russian).

Radina, N. K., & Pavlycheva, T. N. (2010). "Significant others" in the life stories of graduates from boarding orphanages. *Sotsial'naya psikhologiya i obshchestvo, 1*, 124–135. [Radina, N. K., & Pavlycheva, T. N. (2010). «Znachimyye drugiye» v istoriyakh zhizni vypusknikov internatnykh sirotskikh uchrezhdeniy. *Sotsial'naya psikhologiya i obshchestvo, 1*, 124–135] (in Russian).

Reilly, T., & Platz, L. (2003). Characteristics and challenges of families who adopt children with special needs: An empirical study. *Children and Youth Services Review, 25*(10), 781–803.

Robson, M. A. (1997). *An exploration of stress and its perception in childhood.* Durham theses, Durham University. Retrieved from Durham e-theses online: http://etheses.dur.ac.uk/5061/

Rutter, M. (1979). Protective factors in children's responses to stress and disadvantage. In M. W. Kent & J. E. Rolf (Eds.), *Primary prevention in psychopathology: Social competence in Children* (Vol. 8, pp. 49–74). Hanover, NH: University Press of New England.

Schelovanov, N. M., & Aksarina, N. M. (Eds.). (1955). *Educating young children in child care centers: For medical schools.* Moscow: Medgiz. [Shchelovanov, N. M., & Aksarina, N. M. (Eds.) (1955). Vospitaniye detey rannego vozrasta v detskikh uchrezhdeniyakh: Dlya meditsinskikh uchilishch. M.: Medgiz] (in Russian).

Seligman, M. E. P. (2003). Foreword: The past and future of positive psychology. In C. L. M. Keyes & J. Haidt (Eds.), *Flourishing: Positive psychology and the life well-lived* (pp. XI–XX). Washington, DC: American Psychological Association.

Sroufe, L. A. (2005). Attachment and development: A prospective, longitudinal study from birth to adulthood. *Attachment & Human Development, 7*(4), 349–367.

Stryker, R. (2000). Ethnographic solutions to the problems of Russian adoptees. *Anthropology of East Europe Review, 18*(2), 79–84.

Ungar, M., & Liebenberg, L. (2005). The International Resilience Project: A mixed-methods approach to the study of resilience across cultures. In M. Ungar (Ed.), *Handbook for working with children and youth: Pathways to resilience across cultures and contexts* (pp. 211–226). Thousand Oaks: Sage.

Ungar, M., Liebenberg, L., Boothroyd, R., Kwong, W. M., Lee, T. Y., Leblank, J., . . . Makhnach, A. (2008). The study of youth resilience across cultures: Lessons from a pilot study of measurement development. *Research in Human Development, 5*(3), 166–180.

Werner, E. E. (1993). Risk, resilience, and recovery: Perspectives from the Kauai longitudinal study. *Development and Psychopathology, 5*(4), 503–515.

18

Spirituality and resilience

Explored pathways and unexplored territories

Seema Mehrotra and Ravikesh Tripathi

Spirituality: defining a fundamental phenomenon

Spiritual and religious beliefs and practices are universal phenomena that can be traced in almost all cultures. Spirituality has been defined in multiple ways, which is understandable in view of the complex nature of this phenomenon. Despite a lack of consensus in this regard, most definitions share certain features in common. We confine ourselves to two broad definitions of spirituality that seem to implicitly contain clues regarding its potential connections to well-being and resilience. Hill and Pargament (2008) defined spirituality as a search for that relationship or a process through which person seeks to discover, hold on to and even transform whatever it is that he or she holds sacred. De Jager Meezenbroek et al. (2012) defined spirituality as one's striving for and experience of connection with oneself, connectedness with others and nature and connectedness with the transcendent.

Spirituality–religiosity debate

The scientific literature is replete with debates regarding the conceptualization of the terms religiosity and spirituality. Hinting at the potential connection to religion and yet the distinctiveness of spirituality, Zinnbauer and Pargament (2005) stated that spirituality may be considered as a personal quest for understanding the answers to the ultimate questions about life that may (or may not) lead to or arise from the development of religious rituals and the formation of community. The primary distinctive feature of religiosity, as compared to spirituality, is that the former is said to incorporate those spiritual thoughts, feelings and behaviours that are specifically related to a formally organized and identifiable religion (Zinnbauer & Pargament, 2005). Wuthnow's model (1998) distinguishes between religious 'dwellers' and spiritual 'seekers', but both are seen as seriously engaged in incorporating the sacred in their lives with the basic distinction being in terms of their relationship to religious authority and tradition.

Thus, spirituality and religiosity are viewed as relatively independent constructs representing individual/private and institutional experiences, respectively; these are interrelated as the essential elements in both involve beliefs, emotions and experiences about what is considered as sacred. In addition, several individuals do not distinguish between spirituality and religiosity. Pargament (2013) asserted provocatively that notwithstanding the support for the idea that religion serves psychological, physiological and social functions, the most fundamental function of religion is spiritual. It was argued that spirituality needs to be seen as a basic motivation and process in itself. This process is described in terms of discovery of the sacred, efforts to conserve the relationship with what is perceived as sacred and to transform this relationship as and when necessary.

Adding to the conceptual debate regarding overlaps between spirituality and religiosity is the fact that in the empirical research literature, too, various terminologies, measures and operationalizations have been used, resulting in significant challenges in arriving at a coherent picture through the integration of findings across studies. This is evident in the observation that several reviews and meta-analyses have resorted to use of the phrases such as religion/spirituality or religiousness/spirituality (R/S). This chapter too is not immune from a challenge of this nature, though most attention has been given to understanding the potential links between spirituality and resilience.

Resilience: capturing the essence of the 'ordinary magic' and the spiritual broadway

According to Seaward (2005), the foundations of spirituality in all its forms include four cornerstones, namely, relationships, values, meaning in life and connectedness. Smith, Ortiz, Wiggins, Bernard and Dalen (2012) cited available literature to highlight how each of these may be linked to resilient processes and outcomes in the face of adversities. Coping with adversities through religious and spiritual means can be associated with deriving support from a divine power, from others who follow a similar path/congregation and from meaning making of distressing events resulting in healing and resilience following trauma (Van Dyke, Glenwick, Cecero & Kim, 2009).

In its most generic sense, resilience is a broad construct that refers to "positive adaptation in any kind of dynamic system that comes under challenge or threat" (Masten & Obradovic, 2006). In the behavioural sciences literature, resilience was initially taken up for investigation in the context of children's development (Garmezy, 1974; Rutter, 1999, Werner & Smith, 1992) and then expanded to include the context of potentially traumatic events in adulthood. Rutter (2006) defined resilience as "reduced vulnerability to environmental risk experiences, the overcoming of stress or adversity or a relatively good outcome despite risk experience". Although resilience in response to adversity was often seen initially as an exceptional and rare phenomenon by researchers who focused narrowly on risk factors, subsequent widening of attention tends to repeatedly indicate that resilience is not uncommon. Masten (2001) spoke about the 'ordinary magic' of resilience to refer to the observations that it is not a rare phenomenon limited to the exceptional few and that many children survive major adversities.

Notwithstanding the availability of multiple measures of resilience, it has been seen as a construct that is difficult to operationalize. According to Luthar and Zelazo (2003), resilience is not directly measured but inferred from the presence of two constructs: risk and positive adaptation. Positive adaptation has been examined across studies in multiple ways (e.g. absence of pathology, attainment of developmental tasks and self-reports of well-being etc.). Multiple risk factors may interact with a host of other factors to influence outcomes. Protective factors have been considered as assets or compensatory factors when these are beneficial regardless of exposure to risk/adversity. Marriott, Hamilton-Giachritsis and Harrop (2014) argued that researchers need to rise above debating about a factor being protective (predicting better outcomes under adversity) versus compensatory (beneficial outcomes regardless of risk/adversity). A scan of the available literature indicates that spirituality and religiosity have been examined in the theoretical and empirical literature from both these angles. Studies examining the association of spirituality with well-being and related variables support the assumption that it can serve as an asset and resource that could result in beneficial outcomes regardless of adversity. We have included such studies too in this chapter, guided by the plausibility that some of these beneficial outcomes may in turn promote resilience in the long run.

Readers may observe that we have also included several studies on spirituality that have not explicitly operationalized or assessed resilience as an outcome although these highlight the role of spirituality in positive adaptation and successful coping with various challenges in life. We were prompted to do this in view of two reasons. First is that, surprisingly, studies that have explicitly operationalized and measured resilience in order to examine its links with spirituality are not as many as those which have examined spirituality as a variable shaping the process of coping with challenges and associated outcomes. The second related reason is in line with the assertion that resilience needs to be inferred from the presence of adversity and presence of positive adaptation. We believe that findings of several studies that have not measured resilience directly do seem to imply the operation of resilience processes as gleamed through various health and well-being outcomes.

The following somewhat overlapping sections deal with examples of research studies that provide glimpses of salient findings and proposed mechanisms linking spirituality with well-being and resilience.

Spirituality: well-being, health and other correlates

Using longitudinal data, Wink and Dillon (2003) provided evidence that in late adulthood, religiousness was positively associated with well-being from positive relationships with others, involvement in social and community tasks and generativity. On the other hand, spirituality was linked to well-being from personal growth, involvement in knowledge – building life tasks and wisdom. Lun and Bond (2013) analysed data from World Values Survey of participants from fifty-seven nations and drew attention to the role of macro contexts in understanding variability of relationships of multiple aspects of religion and spirituality with measures of well-being. In national-cultures with emphasis on socialization for religious faith, spiritual practice (frequency of engagement in prayers, meditation etc.) was related positively to subjective well-being.

There is a plethora of studies indicating positive links between spirituality and health in the context of a variety of medical and mental health conditions. In an interesting study, Keefe et al. (2001) found that spirituality and positive aspects of religious and spiritual coping were common part of the experience of living with arthritis pain. Participants with higher spiritual experiences reported higher levels of positive mood, lower levels of negative mood and better social support. Further, participants using religion in coping with pain reported higher levels of instrumental and emotional and social support. Similarly, using a sample of chronically ill patients with sickle cell disease (SCD), Harrison et al. (2005) found that church attendance was significantly associated with measures of pain, after controlling for age, gender and disease severity. Johnstone and Yoon (2009) examined relationships between the religiousness/spirituality and physical and mental health for individuals with chronic disabilities (traumatic brain injury, cerebral vascular accidents and spinal cord injury). Positive spiritual experiences and willingness to forgive were related to better physical health, while negative spiritual experiences were related to worse physical and mental health for individuals with chronic disabilities.

Ironson, Stuetzle and Fletcher (2006) examined spirituality/religiousness after HIV diagnosis. Higher spirituality was significantly related to slower disease progression (better maintenance of CD4 cells). Mouch and Sonnega (2012) reviewed research on spirituality and recovery from cardiac surgery and concluded that a large number of studies support positive association (e.g. fewer complications, superior physical functioning, reduced short-term mortality, lower levels of post-operative depression etc.). However, a few studies with mixed/null findings were also reported. Ginting, Näring, Kwakkenbos and Becker (2015) examined the associations between seven dimensions of spirituality (i.e. meaningfulness, trust, acceptance, caring for others, connectedness with nature, transcendent experiences and spiritual activities) and negative emotions among individuals with Coronary Heart Disease. Spirituality was associated with lower levels of depressive symptoms, anxiety and anger.

A review of studies in the field of mental health conducted between 1990 and 2010 revealed positive association between religious involvement and mental health across several psychiatric conditions in 72% of the studies, with good evidence in the domains of depression, substance abuse and suicide (Bonelli & Koenig, 2013). Koenig (2012), in a landmark review of religion/spirituality (R/S) and indices of physical and mental health, as examined in quantitative peer reviewed empirical studies between 1872 and 2010, lined up evidence for mental health outcomes (positive and negative) and also presented the potential pathways that connect these variables to mental and physical health. R/S influences on mental health were explained through use of religious coping resources, rules and regulations about ways of leading one's life and the prominence given to values such as pro-sociality and compassion. Similarly, the relationship of R/S to physical health was explained through psychological (positive coping and positive emotions); social (supportive social connections, altruism) and health-behaviours pathways. A myriad of mental health issues (depression, suicide, marital instability, delinquency, optimism, hope and well-being) as well as multiple physical health issues (e.g. hypertension, cerebrovascular, cardiac disease, dementia, cancer, physical disability, pain, somatic symptom, immune and endocrine functions, overall mortality) were covered in this review.

Unantenne, Warren, Canaway and Manderson (2013) used ethnographic research to explore the role of spirituality in self-management routines of individuals adapting to a chronic illness such as type 2 diabetes or cardiovascular disease. The data resulted in four lay models of spirituality, namely, the altruistic model (participation in religious community and assisting others), the faith-based model (strong belief in the higher power without an essential focus on religious attendance), the self-belief model (reliance on inner strength and determination) and the naturalistic model (deriving well-being from connecting to nature).

A quantitative review of 147 studies indicated that extrinsic religiosity (motivational orientation that views religion as a means rather than an end) and avoidance of challenges in life through religious activities and blaming God for one's difficulties were associated with higher levels of depression and this was in contrast to the overall results that indicated a modest though reliable negative association of religiousness with depressive symptoms (Smith, McCullough, & Poll, 2003). This review highlighted the need for finer distinctions in the conceptualization and assessment of religiousness. Jordan, Masters, Hooker, Ruiz and Smith (2014) argued that intrapersonal mechanisms of influence have been studied more often than interpersonal mechanisms. Across three studies they reported evidence that different aspects of religiosity/spirituality were associated with contrasting interpersonal variables (e.g. support, warm vs. hostile interpersonal style, loneliness etc.).

A fourteen-year-long longitudinal Canadian study of religious attendance, spirituality and major depression reported a 22% of lower risk of depression for monthly attenders as compared to non-attenders after controlling for a host of variables (such as age, family and personal history of depression, education, perceived support etc.). Self-reported importance of spiritual values and self-identification as a spiritual person were not related to major depression (Balbuena, Baetz, & Bowen, 2013). However, spirituality was not assessed through a standardized measure in this study, which places limits on the nature of conclusion drawn with respect to spirituality.

Aldwin, Park, Jeong and Nath (2014) have utilized a self-regulation framework to propose differential pathways between religiosity, spirituality and physical health. Their model proposes that impact of religiousness (affiliation, service attendance) on health is mediated via self-regulation of health-behaviours/habits. On the other hand, the effect of spirituality is proposed to be mediated by emotional regulation that impacts inflammatory processes in chronic illnesses. They reviewed available literature to conclude that the evidence broadly supports their model. Religiousness was found to be strongly linked to positive health behaviours, including lower smoking, alcohol consumption and greater likelihood of medical screening, but only weakly linked to inflammatory biomarkers. In contrast, spirituality measures were more strongly linked to biomarkers such as blood pressure, cardiac reactivity, immune factors and disease progression.

Spirituality and resilience in the context of interpersonal trauma and other traumatic experiences

In the context of interpersonal trauma, forgiveness has been examined as linked to both spirituality and resilience. In a study on post-traumatic growth following significant interpersonal transgression, Schultz, Tallman and Altmaier (2010) found the positive association between forgiveness and post-traumatic growth to be mediated by the importance of religion and spirituality. In a structured narrative review of resilience following childhood sexual abuse (Marriott et al., 2014), being part of a religious group or a sense of being spiritual was reported to be one of the multiple factors promoting resilience.

Utilizing a high-risk youth sample of individuals exposed to community violence in Brazil, Huculak and McLennan (2010) observed that intrinsic spirituality may mediate the association between institutional activities and certain mental health outcomes.

In an interesting study conducted by Ojeda and Piña-Watson (2013) on Latino day labourers, spirituality and perceived health significantly buffered against the role of perceived discrimination on life satisfaction. Using a meta-analytic review, Davis, Worthington, Hook and Hill (2013) reported that religion/spirituality positively associated with forgiveness, state forgiveness and self-forgiveness. The associations were generally modest and stronger for relationship with trait forgiveness and with reference to certain aspects of spirituality than others. Citing a dearth of significant evidence that religion generally promotes forgiving, Davis, Hook, Van Tongeren, Gartner and Worthington (2012) presented evidence for a model that proposes that how people spiritually interpret a transgression can help or impede forgiveness depending on whether other-oriented (empathy, gratitude, love) or self-focused negative emotions (shame, contempt) are evoked.

Bryant-Davis and Wong (2013), in their selective review of studies to date, highlighted the positive role of positive religious coping and spiritual coping in recovery process in childhood sexual abuse survivors, sexual violence, intimate partner violence, war, refugee trauma and torture trauma. The review summarized results of studies on a variety of interpersonal trauma experiences in multiple socio-cultural contexts across the globe. Aten, O' Grady, Milstein, Boan and Schruba (2014) summarized the role of spiritual and religious variables in the context of dealing with disasters while offering guidelines regarding offering post-disaster care and services that are sensitive to spiritual and religious issues.

Spirituality and positive youth development

Adolescence has been described as a sensitive period for spiritual development as it is characterized by existential search for meaning, enhanced capacity for spiritual experiences and a process of challenging traditional values (Fowler, 1981; Good & Willoughby, 2008). Reviewing existing empirical literature on adolescent spirituality and resilience, Kim and Esquivel (2011) surmised that adolescent spirituality can be seen as a factor that promotes mental health in terms of minimizing externalizing and internalizing problems in youth at risk, promotes well-being, educational performance in certain groups and overall healthy development. The role of environments that can nurture spirituality in family, educational and community contexts was highlighted. An interesting study that uses mixed methods research approach revealed that spiritual well-being and resilience were interrelated, ecologically bound (Smith, Webber, & De Frain, 2013). The researchers argued that spiritual well-being/relationship with their God could enhance family connectedness, social support, experience of positive emotions and healthy behaviours that act as protective factors leading to enhanced resilience. Bryant-Davis et al. (2012) reviewed extant literature on the ways in which children and adolescents applied religion and spirituality in coping with traumatic experiences and its role as a protective factor against substance abuse/initiation of substances, early sexual activity, risky sexual behaviours, deviant peer group involvement etc.

Resilience and spirituality connection: bridge of positive emotions?

Spiritual experiences and practices may directly enhance experience of positive emotions such as joy, love, contentment. In addition, positive reinterpretations of adversities based on one's spiritual framework may generate positive emotions. Smith et al. (2012) summarized the emergent literature, including the links between positive emotions and broad-minded coping. They presented a preliminary model linking healthy spirituality with positive meaning, positive emotions and resilience. While taking into account the evidence regarding reciprocal relationships between spirituality, positive emotions and resilience, they proposed that spirituality is more often the cause rather than an outcome of resilience and positive emotions. Their model indicated that personal meaning may be at least a partial mediator of the relationship between spirituality on one hand and positive emotions and resilience on the other hand. They advocated a need for research on the dimensions of spirituality that are most strongly linked to positive emotions and resilience, the mediators (e.g. personal meaning) of the association and the differential links of high- and low-arousal positive emotions with spirituality in Western and Eastern cultures.

Van Cappellen, Toth-Gauthier, Saroglou and Fredrickson (2014) provided supportive evidence for the role of positive emotions as mediator between the relationship of religiosity/spirituality and well-being. Their line of hypothesizing as well as the study's findings specifically highlighted the role of gratitude, love, awe and peace. These emotions are classified as self-transcendent emotions linked to the interest and welfare of the society as a whole or at least of persons other than the agent (Haidt, 2003). Using ethology and neuroscience, Valliant in a recent paper

(2013) put forth the argument that an amalgam of eight positive emotions, all of which involve human connection (awe, love/attachment, trust/faith, compassion, gratitude, forgiveness, joy and hope) constitutes spirituality. There is some empirical support for the idea that self-transcendent emotions may enhance spirituality through the mediational influence of basic world assumptions (belief in meaningfulness of life and view of others and the world to be benevolent (Van Cappellen, Saroglou, Iweins, Piovesana, & Fredrickson, 2013).

Spirituality–resilience connection: attachment, support and coping pathways

Theorizing and research by Granqvist (1998), Kirkpatrick (1998) and others have resulted in a focus on understanding the relationship individuals have with the divine and thus on the conceptualization of God as an attachment figure. Using an attachment framework, a study of a Baptist community indicated that an insecure attachment to God was related to lower levels of religious spirituality, which in turn was related to higher levels of emotional distress (Freeze & Di Tommaso, 2014).

Spirituality has been associated with traditional personality traits that are recognized to be protective factors (consciousness, agreeableness and low neuroticism) (Simpson, Newman, & Fuqua, 2007). Piedmont (1999) proposed spiritual transcendence as a sixth personality factor based on review of available studies as well as data from two separate studies. Labbe and Fobes (2010) reported a positive autonomic nervous system response in terms of lower respiration rate to laboratory stressors in their young adult participants who had higher ratings on spirituality in addition to higher scores on health protective personality traits.

Hall and Flanagan (2013) noted that the relationship between adolescent spirituality/religiosity and psychosocial adjustment was mediated by coping strategies (e.g. revenge seeking in response to interpersonal offenses). According to the authors, moral teachings and verbal and non-verbal messages about kindness, empathy, compassion, peace and love within religious, family and peer contexts generally discourage revenge seeking by placing a high value on such principles as forgiveness, empathy and grace. Research also indicates association between spirituality and family resilience (Black & Lobo, 2008). Saslow et al. (2013) demonstrated across various studies that spirituality was linked to altruistic behaviours on certain experimental tasks through other-oriented compassion and that the link between religiosity and compassion was no longer significant after controlling for spirituality. The relationship of spirituality with altruism was not explained by personality traits such as extraversion or agreeableness and openness. Daily spiritual experiences have been less frequently examined as compared to religious/spiritual practices/behaviours and spiritual beliefs. Hardy, Zhang, Skalski, Melling and Brinton (2014) conducted a daily level analysis using online surveys to conclude that daily religious activities were linked to daily moral emotions (empathy, forgiveness and gratitude) through daily spiritual experiences. The quality of daily spiritual experiences moderated this link.

According to Koenig's classical model (2008), religiosity/spirituality increases positive outcomes (e.g. meaning, purpose, well-being, connectedness, hope) and decreases negative outcomes (depression, anxiety, addictions). Psychological health thus achieved further affects, psychoneuroimmunological factors that could results in lower the risk of cardiovascular disease, cancer and mortality. In another model (Masters, 2008), spirituality/religiosity influences positive health outcomes through social support, adaptive behaviour and psychological factors (e.g. hope). Levin (1996) put forth a detailed model involving different aspects of religiosity/spirituality, specific pathways and mediators between these aspects and health outcomes. Park's model (2012) highlights three broad influences of R/S on health outcomes. These include general (through health behaviours, support and religious practice); specific beliefs and interpretations (leading to positive, reappraisal, positive affect, access to health promotion resources etc.) and crisis-related (influencing religious meaning, forgiveness, treatment adherence).

The theory of transformative coping (Corry, Lewis, & Mallette, 2014) proposes that positive transformation and personal growth emerge from combined application of creativity and spirituality. The former is said to provide a chance for emotional expression while the latter is expected to increase reflection and self-awareness. Corry, Mallett, Lewis and Abdel-Khalek (2013) generated data that support the proposition that individuals apply creative and spiritual coping in their lives to deal with acute and chronic stress. Using a grounded theory approach, Lancaster and Palframan (2009) found that spirituality supported the process of self-transformation while coping with major negative life events. In their emergent model, openness was seen as a core element in as much as that being open to others and to the transcendent facilitated letting go, enabled acceptance and supported the process of transformation.

Issues of concern: We concur with Bryant-Davis and Wong (2013), who highlighted various concerns in this field of research such as the limited coverage of different religions, racial/ethnic groups and demographic groups and the insufficient attention to problems associated with negative forms of religious coping, bidirectional relationships, as well as dearth of longitudinal studies. The available measures differ in terms of breadth and nature of coverage and overlaps with religiosity, theoretical base and psychometric properties. The available reviews highlight the strengths of these measures as well as raise issues regarding variations in operationalizations, item formulations and confounds with measures of distress and well-being (de Jager Meezenbroek et al., 2012; Kapuscinski & Masters, 2010; Schuumans-Stekhoven, 2010). Novel ways of assessment of spirituality are also being explored (Anderson & Grice, 2014; Hodge, 2013). We wish to add other areas of concern such as inadequate examination of spiritual experiences (in contrast to beliefs and practices), insufficient attention to ecological validity of the measures of spirituality and resilience, individual differences in contents of spiritual beliefs, neural correlates of spirituality–well-being connection and the dynamic nature of spiritually and resilience in the face of adversity. There are a few Indian studies that have highlighted the role of spirituality in coping with adversity (e.g. Mehrotra & Sukumar, 2007; Rammohan, Rao, & Subbakrishna, 2002). Several studies on resilience in the Indian context are reviewed by Mehrotra, Narayanan and Tripathi (in press). A few of these have documented its links with spirituality (e.g. Annalakshmi & Tony, 2011; Narayanan & Mohammed, 2011; Rajkumar, Premkumar, & Tharyan, 2008; Saraf, Singh, & Khurana, 2013), but there is a need for focused research on unravelling the complex relationship between these variables in multiple context within the Indian culture.

Potential links between spirituality and resilience: through the Indian lens

In this section, we attempt to discuss a few constructs in Indian philosophical thought that are likely to be of relevance for researchers who wish to explore the links between spirituality and resilience in the Indian context. Contemporary writings on Indian philosophical thought are ripe with ideas that can be extracted for theory building, hypothesis generation and testing to enrich our understanding of health, well-being and resilience. This section is not meant to provide an exhaustive or in-depth coverage of the same. We merely aim to highlight just a few such constructs and ideas, especially from the Bhagavad Gita, and examine how these may support processes that enable resilience. There has been significant research of theoretical and empirical nature on multiple Indigenous constructs (Kiran Kumar, 2011); however, their relationships with resilience has not been directly/fully examined.

We are tempted to begin this exploration with the concept of karma yoga in the Bhagavad Gita for more than one reason. It is one of the most discussed constructs from Indian philosophical thought in psychology literature. It relates to several other constructs that we wish to subsequently touch upon. Most of all, it is one of those Indian constructs that is common in occurrence in lay dialogues and social discourse in the contemporary India. Karma yoga is described as one of the pathways to self-realization, considered an ultimate aim in life. It is a path that entails two basic ideas (Bhawuk, 2011). First, it promotes the idea that individuals must engage in actions in accordance with their dharma or in other words perform their duties (*svadharma*). This suggests that action is considered as superior to inaction. The second idea is about giving up the attachment to the consequences of one's actions. In other words, *nishkama karma*, or performing of actions without the intention of achieving the fruits of one's actions, is advocated. This conceptualization is closely linked to what has been described as the psychology of desire. According to the process–model of desire (Bhawuk, 2011), one's self interacts with elements of the environment and chooses certain elements, which in turn leads to attachment to these elements. Thinking about such elements/objects and the associated feelings give rise to desire. Desires have an influence on behavioural intention and actual behaviours. Fulfilment of desires lead to pleasant states, but desires are viewed as a fire that is never satiated, with fulfilment of goals leading to further craving and greed and thereby an endless cycle of pursuing desired objects. Non-fulfilment of desire gives rise to frustration and anger. Thus, the Bhagavad Gita advocates conquering of desires in order to attain peace. Desires are seen as obstructions in one's ability to discriminate between right and wrong. All desires are thus seen as source of suffering in the long run, although fulfilment of desires may result in short-lasting experiences of positive effect.

Giving up the attachment to fruits of one's action thus emerges as one of the core teachings of the Bhagavad Gita. This stance has been linked to attainment of a peaceful state of mind that is termed *sthithaprajna*. Here, *sthitha* refers to being steady/firm and *prajna* roughly translates to judgement or wisdom. (Bhawuk, 2011). It is described as a state in which the person experiences a sense of harmony and a state of calm and peace that is independent of external circumstances. As the individual withdraws from sensory attachments, he/she is said to reach a state of equanimity/equipoise wherein he/she is able to transcend or rise above transient positive and negative emotions linked to external events/stimuli. Peace is seen as a natural outcome of conquering desires and following the path of karma yoga. *Nishkama* karma has also been described in terms of *anasakt* action (Pande & Naidu, 2011). *Anasakt* action has been linked to task-excellence as the focus of the actor is completely on the action per se, free from preoccupations, apprehensions or anticipation of the consequences (Pande & Naidu, 2011). Thapa (1983) conducted a theoretical analysis of the construct of *anasakti*, examined its links with motivation and came up with an instrument to measure effort and outcome-orientation as an individual difference variable. Pande and Naidu (2011) dwelt upon several behavioural referents/characteristics of persons high on *anasakti*. These included perception of work as duty, non-attachment to consequences, actions governed by internal rather than external standards and a focus on task-excellence, that is not swayed by the cycles of strong positive and negative emotions or tolerance of pain and discomfort, thereby enhanced ability to exercise ethical judgments in the face of challenges, lack of compulsive engagement in hedonistic pursuits and emotional equipoise. The end state of self-realization can be achieved through practicing performance of *anasakt* actions, but an individual who has attained self-realization is said to become spontaneously *anasakt* (Tart, 1975). In an empirical research study by Pande and Naidu (2011), it was found that *anasakti* scores predicted strain more than stress scores. It was surmised that threat appraisals, emotional instability and ineffective coping were likely to mediate the relationship of low *anasakti* with high levels of strain.

Using a contemporary version of the Bhagavad Gita (Gandhi, 2001) and content analysis of each of the verses, Mulla and Krishnan (2006a) identified the various dimensions of karma yoga. The authors surmised that karma yoga consisted of performing actions without attachment, doing one's duty and being neutral to opposites. Across studies, karma yoga was related to high dutifulness and low achievement striving (Mulla & Krishnan, 2006a), to other-oriented values and moral values (Mulla & Krishnan, 2006b) and to the affective aspects of personality, namely, empathy (Mulla & Krishnan, 2008). Using these strands of findings, the authors proposed the personality profile of a karma-yogi as an individual, who highly values the welfare of others, is empathic, who can understand the feelings and emotions of others without getting personally ruffled and who executes his or her duty without worrying about personal achievements.

The construct of karma is often evoked as an explanation for suffering in various contexts; however, no consistent relationship has been documented between such a causal belief and affective response or psychological recovery following illnesses (Dalal, 2000). In an Indian study utilizing a sample of hundred individuals undergoing treatment for cancer, the utility of Lipowski's framework to understand illness meanings was explored (Tandon, Mehrotra, & Vallikad, 2010). Three out of the five new illness meanings arrived at, namely, "illness as part of life', illness as God's plan and illness as fate", may be viewed as meanings based on spirituality. These meanings, including fate, were associated positively with quality of life and negatively with measures of distress. Folk meanings vary in different socio-cultural contexts. In the fate category, the theory of karma was often invoked, and the present condition was attributed to misdeeds in the present or previous lives. However, the focus was on acceptance of the situation. The authors mention that a although the label 'fate' was loosely assigned to somewhat varying descriptions of illness meanings; what is common to these seems to be an attitude of philosophical acceptance of the current situation and the uncertainty of the final outcome in such a way that it did not detract the participants from doing whatever they thought could be done to improve the situation. The qualitative data of this study suggested that in a majority of cases, the individuals viewing their illness as fate did not 'give up' their attempts at mastery but attached less importance to dwelling on the distressing issue of "Why did it happen to them?" and focused their efforts on actively engaging in treatment while maintaining an uncertain though somewhat hopeful stance regarding outcomes. This seems to be in line with a concept of karma that not only refers to actions in any lifetime influencing present circumstances but also incorporates the notion of a future karma that is constantly being shaped by one's current actions and decisions (Purohit, 2001) and the belief in superiority of action over passivity or inaction as described earlier.

Bhakti yoga in the Bhagavad Gita describes the path of devotion and emphasizes upon surrender and complete trust in God (Bhawuk, 2011). In the Western literature, surrender to God is being researched as a spiritual coping strategy distinct from other religious coping strategies proposed by Pargament et al. (1988). It is described as actively relinquishing one's will and desires to God's will rather than a passive waiting stance (Wong-McDonald & Gorsuch, 2000). Cole and Pargament (1999) conceptualized spiritual surrender to work as a paradoxical pathway to control in the process of coping. However, letting go/surrendering as implied in the Indian philosophical texts exhorts individuals not to erroneously identify their true selves as doers and enjoyers. The Western literature typically emphasizes competence as referring to exercising control over environment often through utilization of environmental resources for one's own good (Sinha, 2011). In contrast, control over senses (*jitendriya*), management of desires and a harmonious relationship with the environment is considered important in the Indian tradition (Sinha, 2011; Srivastava &

Misra, 2003). There is a virtual absence of studies that have explored the experience of surrender and its correlates in the Indian context from a psychological perspective. The path of *Bhakti* yoga is said to involve devotion to God as well as experience of divinity in all that one encounters. The descriptions of a devotee imply frequent experience of emotions such as joy and love. It is plausible that immersion in the path of *bhakti* could enhance resilience through cultivation and maintenance of such positive emotions.

The Indian philosophical tradition with its emphasis on dharma highlights the values that are salient in our culture and the framework of beliefs that may support dealing with adversities in life. Bhangaokar and Kapadia (2009) explored folk interpretations of the concepts of karma and dharma in contemporary urban Indian context through in-depth interviews. The authors concluded that dharma is the larger framework within which individual karma is said to operate. The interpretations of karma were somewhat overlapping and included the following: role-related responsibilities, societal duties, nature of one's deeds & rebirth etc. Ideal fulfilment of dharma was stated by the participants to involve: fulfilment of duties without expectations (familial and societal) goal achievements related (e.g. being self-sufficient, controlling materialistic urges) and conscience related (e.g. coordination between thoughts and feelings, continuing good karma, living in accordance with moral values). Wisdom is another construct of relevance to handling adversities and positive adaptation. Comparison of the conceptualization of wisdom in the Bhagavad Gita with that in modern scientific literature show several similarities, such as rich knowledge about life, emotional regulation, insight and a focus on common good (compassion). Apparent differences include an emphasis on control over desires and renunciation of materialistic pleasures. Importantly, the Bhagavad Gita suggests that at least certain components of wisdom can be taught and learned (Takahashi & Bordia, 2000).

Potential directions of research in the Indian context

The interrelated concepts described earlier are highlighted as examples of constructs whose association with resilience may yield rich observations in the Indian context. The practice of karma yoga is likely to be associated with capacity for resilience due to its inherent emphasis on focus on one's actions and efforts and the renunciation of the consequences of actions. Such a stance could potentially have immense utility in facilitating positive outcomes to adversities through coping that is action-oriented and at the same time devoid of preoccupations with possible consequences and affect laden ruminative cognitions that can reduce one's exercise of discrimination between right and wrong actions. This is in addition to the possibility that the embracing the notion of karma may facilitate meaning making and acceptance of reality in ways that helps in positive adaptation. *Anasakti* as conceptualized earlier, along with the attainment of *sthithpragya* state, can be hypothesized to act as a buffer to the experience of distress and the negative consequences of adversity due to the emphasis on rising above the transient experience of pleasure and pain. An individual's success in transcending of desires and cultivation of an attitude of nonattachment to objects in the external world could also aid in conferring resilience to adversity through changing threat-appraisals and the nature of future expectancies as well as appraisals of outcomes themselves.

On the whole, we propose that the constructs described earlier may aid resilience through activation of the several related processes/mechanisms. These include decreased probability of experience of negative emotions related to stressful situations due to low identification with the material aspects of life, as well as lowered emotional reactivity to adverse circumstances through appraisals that diminish a sense of threat. Salutary coping style with a focus on action-orientation and a sense of spiritual surrender are other factors that could facilitate emergence of resilience.

In addition, an emphasis on other-oriented values (e.g. compassion and selflessness) as well as on a harmonious relationship with the environment may also result in collective actions that help in strengthening resilient capacities of one's socio-cultural context or the environment to face adversities.

The potential linkages mentioned earlier are based upon the assumption of attainment of idealized states as described in religious-philosophical texts. There are significant research gaps to be addressed before a scientific inquiry into such linkages may be undertaken. Some of these gaps and the associated preliminary questions worthy of research are briefly described here.

Extant research and a keen observation of day-to-day discourse in the contemporary Indian context suggests that some of the constructs mentioned earlier (e.g. karma, surrender) are invoked with varying frequency, especially during encounters with challenging situations/adversities. However, there is a dearth of studies that examine the prevalence of these beliefs in the various sections of the general population. More importantly, research indicates that lay meanings attached to these constructs may be highly variable from one individual to another as well as one socio-cultural context to another. It might be a useful exercise to explore the varied meanings of these constructs and to examine whether these meanings can be grouped in different clusters that correlate differentially with coping and well-being. It is essential to capture the meanings ascribed by the individuals themselves in order to examine their psychological influence. The similarities and differences between lay meanings in the contemporary Indian society and the descriptions and interpretations of the sacred texts provided by the experts may also be explored.

Going beyond the lay meanings, it would be useful to explore the salience of these beliefs because salience is a variable that is likely to influence the extent to which individuals attempt to apply these principles/constructs in their day-to-day life as well as in negotiation of major adversities. The efforts made by individuals for whom such principles are salient could be documented through qualitative methods of inquiry. In order to obtain broad coverage of the meanings, practices and actual lived-in experiences, it would be useful to sample a wide range of a population with a special attempt to include individuals who are committed to spiritual paths and who may be considered to be in higher stages of spiritual progress, using pre-defined guidelines for sample selection. Extreme case sampling methods have been used in recent research studies exploring links between spirituality and well-being, for example studies of monks and long-term meditators. This is essential to arrive at a holistic picture about the experiential aspects of practicing such idealized ways of leading life, from the perspective of the common man to that of individuals who have dedicated their efforts to spiritual evolution. In addition, case study methods have also been advocated in similar contexts and may be utilized to obtain some leads as to how saints/spiritual gurus utilize resilient processes (Bhawuk, 2011). Although there is some research available on the construct of spiritual surrender, there is hardly any research in the Indian context as to how it is understood and practiced as well as its similarities or differences to other modes of religious and non-religious coping. Research on the lived experience of surrender may help in understanding the mechanisms through which a surrender style of coping may be salutogenic. Yet another underexplored mechanism that could explain the links between spirituality and resilience in the Indian context is generation and a steady experience of positive emotions such as contentment and peace in individuals leading spiritually oriented lives.

Conclusion

On the whole, it is observed that existing research on the links between spirituality and resilience has highlighted multiple, interacting cognitive, behavioural and affective pathways for further exploration. Also, the interplay between ideas presented in Indian philosophical thought, their lay meanings, extent of internalization, spiritual practice, experiences and their influence on ways of dealing with adversities and adaptational outcomes is an area ripe with challenges and potential breakthroughs for resilience research.

References

Aldwin, C. M., Park, C. L., Jeong, Y. J., & Nath, R. (2014). Differing pathways between religiousness, spirituality, and health: A self-regulation perspective. *Psychology of Religion and Spirituality, 6*(1), 9–21.

Anderson, J. A., & Grice, J. W. (2014). Toward an integrated model of spirituality. *Journal of Psychology and Christianity, 33*(1), 3–21.

Annalakshmi, N., & Tony, P. J. (2011). Spiritual intelligence and resilience among Christian youth in Kerala. *Journal of the Indian Academy of Applied Psychology, 37*(2), 263–268.

Aten, J. D., O'Grady, K. A., Milstein, G., Boan, D., & Schruba, A. (2014). Spiritually oriented disaster psychology. *Spirituality in Clinical Practice, 1*(1), 20–28.

Balbuena, L., Baetz, M., & Bowen, R. (2013). Religious attendance, spirituality, and major depression in Canada: A 14-year follow-up study. *Canadian Journal of Psychiatry, 58*(4), 225–232.

Bhangaokar, R., & Kapadia, S. (2009). At the interface of "Dharma" and "Karma": Interpreting moral discourse in India. *Psychological Studies, 54*(2), 96–108.

Bhawuk, D. P. S. (2011). *Spirituality and Indian psychology: Lessons from the Bhagavad-Gita.* New York: Springer.

Black, K., & Lobo, M. (2008). A conceptual review of family resilience factors. *Journal of Family Nursing, 14*(1), 33–55.

Bonelli, R. M., & Koenig, H. G. (2013). Mental disorders, religion and spirituality 1990 to 2010: A systematic evidence-based review. *Journal of Religion and Health, 52*(2), 657–673.

Bryant-Davis, T., Ellis, M. U., Burke-Maynard, E., Moon, N., Counts, P. A., & Anderson, G. (2012). Religiosity, spirituality, and trauma recovery in the lives of children and adolescents. *Professional Psychology: Research and Practice, 43*(4), 306–314.

Bryant-Davis, T., & Wong, E. C. (2013). Faith to move mountains: Religious coping, spirituality, and interpersonal trauma recovery. *American Psychologist, 68*(8), 675–684.

Cole, B. S., & Pargament, K. I. (1999). Spiritual surrender: A paradoxical path to control. In W. R. Miller (Ed.), *Integrating spirituality into treatment: Resources for practitioners* (pp. 179–198). Washington, DC: American Psychological Association.

Corry, D. A. S., Lewis, C. A., & Mallett, J. (2014). Harnessing the mental health benefits of the creativity–spirituality construct: Introducing the theory of transformative coping. *Journal of Spirituality in Mental Health, 16*(2), 89–110.

Corry, D. A. S., Mallett, J., Lewis, C. A., & Abdel-Khalek, A. M. (2013). The creativity-spirituality construct and its role in transformative coping. *Mental Health, Religion & Culture, 16*(10), 979–990.

Dalal, A. K. (2000). Living with a chronic disease: Healing and psychological adjustment in Indian society. *Psychology and Developing Societies, 12*(1), 67–81.

Davis, D. E., Hook, J. N., Van Tongeren, D. R., Gartner, A. L., & Worthington Jr., E. L. (2012). Can religion promote virtue? A more stringent test of the model of relational spirituality and forgiveness. *International Journal for the Psychology of Religion, 22*(4), 252–266.

Davis, D. E., Worthington Jr., E. L., Hook, J. N., & Hill, P. C. (2013). Research on religion/spirituality and forgiveness: A meta-analytic review. *Psychology of Religion and Spirituality, 5*(4), 233–241.

de Jager Meezenbroek, E., Garssen, B., van den Berg, M., van Dierendonck, D., Visser, A., & Schaufeli, W. B. (2012). Measuring spirituality as a universal human experience: A review of spirituality questionnaires. *Journal of Religion and Health, 51*(2), 336–354.

Freeze, T. A., & Di Tommaso, E. (2014). An examination of attachment, religiousness, spirituality and well-being in a Baptist faith sample. *Mental Health, Religion & Culture, 17*(7), 690–702.

Fowler, J. (1981). *Stages of faith: The psychology of human development and the quest for meaning.* San Francisco, CA: Harper and Row.

Gandhi, M. K. (2001). *The gospel of selfless action.* M. Desai (trans.). Ahmedabad: Navajivan Publishing House. (Original work published in 1946).

Garmezy, N. (1974). The study of competence in children at risk for severe psychopathology. In E. J. Anthony & C. Koupernik (Eds.), The *child in his family: Children at psychiatric risk* (Vol. 3, 3rd ed., pp. 77–97). New York: Wiley.

Ginting, H., Näring, G., Kwakkenbos, L., & Becker, E. S. (2015). Spirituality and negative emotions in individuals with coronary heart disease. *The Journal of Cardiovascular Nursing, 30*(6):537–545.

Granqvist, P. (1998). Religiousness and perceived childhood attachment: On the question of compensation or correspondence. *Journal for the Scientific Study of Religion, 37*(2), 350–367.

Good, M., & Willoughby, T. (2008). Adolescence as a sensitive period for spiritual development. *Child Development Perspectives, 2*(1), 32–37.

Haidt, J. (2003). The moral emotions. In R. J. Davidson, K. R. Scherer, & H. H. Goldsmith (Eds.), *Handbook of affective sciences* (pp. 852–870). Oxford: Oxford University Press.

Hall, S. E., & Flanagan, K. S. (2013). Coping strategies as a mediator between adolescent spirituality/religiosity and psychosocial adjustment. *Journal of Psychology and Christianity, 32*(3), 234–244.

Hardy, S. A., Zhang, Z., Skalski, J. E., Melling, B. S., & Brinton, C. T. (2014). Daily religious involvement, spirituality, and moral emotions. *Psychology of Religion and Spirituality, 6*(4), 338–348.

Harrison, M. O., Edwards, C. L., Koenig, H. G., Bosworth, H. B., Decastro, L., & Wood, M. (2005). Religiosity/spirituality and pain in patients with sickle cell disease. *The Journal of Nervous and Mental Disease, 193*(4), 250–257.

Hill, P. C., & Pargament, K. I. (2008). Advances in the conceptualization and measurement of religion and spirituality: Implications for physical and mental health research. *Psychology of Religion and Spirituality, S*(1), 3–17.

Hodge, D. R. (2013). Implicit spiritual assessment: An alternative approach for assessing client spirituality. *Social Work, 58*(3), 223–230.

Huculak, S., & McLennan, J. D. (2010). "The Lord is my Shepherd": Examining spirituality as a protection against mental health problems in youth exposed to violence in Brazil. *Mental Health, Religion & Culture, 13*(5), 467–484.

Ironson, G., Stuetzle, R., & Fletcher, M. A. (2006). An increase in religiousness/spirituality occurs after HIV diagnosis and predicts slower disease progression over 4 years in people with HIV. *Journal of General Internal Medicine, 21*(S5), S62–S68.

Johnstone, B., & Yoon, D. P. (2009). Relationships between the Brief Multidimensional Measure of Religiousness/Spirituality and health outcomes for a heterogeneous rehabilitation population. *Rehabilitation Psychology, 54*(4), 422–431.

Jordan, K. D., Masters, K. S., Hooker, S. A., Ruiz, J. M., & Smith, T. W. (2014). An interpersonal approach to religiousness and spirituality: Implications for health and well-being. *Journal of Personality, 82*(5), 418–431.

Kapuscinski, A. N., & Masters, K. S. (2010). The current status of measures of spirituality: A critical review of scale development. *Psychology of Religion and Spirituality, 2*(4), 191–205.

Keefe, F. J., Affleck, G., Lefebvre, J., Underwood, L., Caldwell, D. S., Drew, J., . . . Pargament, K. (2001). Living with rheumatoid arthritis: The role of daily spirituality and daily religious and spiritual coping. *The Journal of Pain, 2*(2), 101–110.

Kim, S., & Esquivel, G. B. (2011). Adolescent spirituality and resilience: Theory, research, and educational practices. *Psychology in the Schools, 48*(7), 755–765.

Kiran Kumar, S. K. (2011). Indian indigenous concepts and perspectives: Developments and future possibilities. In G. Misra (Ed.), *Psychology in India, Vol. 4: Theoretical and methodological developments* (ICSSR Survey of Advances in Research) (pp. 93–172). New Delhi: ICSSR.

Kirkpatrick, L. A. (1998). God as substitute attachment figure: A longitudinal study of adult attachment style and religious change in college students. *Personality and Social Psychology Bulletin, 24*(9), 961–973.

Koenig, H. G. (2008). Concerns about measuring "spirituality" in research. *Journal of Nervous and Mental Disease, 196*(5), 349–355.

Koenig, H. G. (2012). Religion, spirituality, and health: The research and clinical implications. *ISRN Psychiatry,* Article ID 278730, 33 pages.

Labbe, E. E., & Fobes, A. (2010). Evaluating the interplay between spirituality, personality and stress. *Applied Psychophysiology and Biofeedback, 35*(2), 141–146.

Lancaster, B. L., & Palframan, J. T. (2009). Coping with major life events: The role of spirituality and self-transformation. *Mental Health, Religion & Culture, 12*(3), 257–276.

Levin, J. S. (1996). How religion influences morbidity and health: Reflections on natural history, salutogenesis and host resistance. *Social Science & Medicine, 43*(5), 849–864.

Lun, V. M. C., & Bond, M. H. (2013). Examining the relation of religion and spirituality to subjective well-being across national cultures. *Psychology of Religion and Spirituality, 5*(4), 304–315.

Luthar, S. S., & Zelazo, L. B. (2003). Research on resilience: An integrative review. In S. S. Luthar (Ed.), *Resilience and vulnerability: Adaptation in the context of childhood adversities* (pp. 510–549). Cambridge: Cambridge University Press.

Marriott, C., Hamilton-Giachritsis, C. H., & Harrop, C. (2014). Factors promoting resilience following childhood sexual abuse: A structured, narrative review of the literature. *Child Abuse Review, 23*(1), 17–34.

Masten, A. S. (2001). Ordinary magic: Resilience processes in development. *American Psychologist, 56*(3), 227–238.

Masten, A. S., & Obradovic, J. (2006). Competence and resilience in development. *Annals of the New York Academy of Sciences, 1094,* 13–27.

Masters, K. S. (2008). Mechanisms in the relation between religion and health with emphasis on cardiovascular reactivity to stress. *Research in the Social Scientific Study of Religion, 19,* 91–116.

Mehrotra, S., Narayanan, A., & Tripathi, R. (in press). Understanding resilience: Global trends and Indian research. In G. Misra (Ed.), *The psycho-social interventions for health and wellbeing.* New Delhi: Springer.

Mehrotra, S., & Sukumar, P. (2007). Sources of strength perceived by females diagnosed with cancer: An exploratory study from India. *Supportive Care in Cancer, 15*(12), 1357–1366.

Mouch, C. A., & Sonnega, A. J. (2012). Spirituality and recovery from cardiac surgery: A review. *Journal of Religion and Health, 51*(4), 1042–1060.

Mulla, Z. R., & Krishnan, V. R. (2006a). Karma Yoga: A conceptualization and validation of the Indian philosophy of work. *Journal of Indian Psychology, 24*(1–2), 26–43.

Mulla, Z. R., & Krishnan, V. R. (2006b, December). *Karma-Yoga: Construct validation using value systems and emotional intelligence.* Paper presented at the First International Conference of Yale-Great Lakes Center for Management Research on Global Mindset–Indian Roots, Chennai, India.

Mulla, Z. R., & Krishnan, V. R. (2008). Karma-Yoga, the Indian work ideal, and its relationship with empathy. *Psychology and Developing Societies, 20*(1), 27–49.

Narayanan, A., & Mohammed, A. (2011). Islamic worldview, religious personality and resilience among Muslim adolescent students in India. *Europe's Journal of Psychology, 7*(4), 716–738.

Ojeda, L., & Piña-Watson, B. (2013). Day laborers' life satisfaction: The role of familismo, spirituality, work, health, and discrimination. *Cultural Diversity and Ethnic Minority Psychology, 19*(3), 270–278.

Pande, N., & Naidu, R. K. (2011). Anasakti and health: An empirical study of anasakti (non-attachment). In A. K Dalal, & G. Misra (Eds.), *New directions in health psychology* (pp. 289–303). New Delhi: Sage Publications.

Pargament, K. I. (2013). Spirituality as an irreducible human motivation and process. *The International Journal for the Psychology of Religion, 23*(4), 271–281.

Pargament, K. I., Kennell, J., Hathaway, W., Grevengood, N., Newman, J., & Jones, W. (1988). Religion and the problem-solving process: Three styles of coping. *Journal for the Scientific Study of Religion, 27*(1), 90–104.

Park, C. L. (2012). Meaning, spirituality, and growth: Protective and resilience factors in health and illness. In A. S. Baum, T. A. Revenson, & J. E. Singer (Eds.), *Handbook of health psychology* (2nd ed., pp. 405–430). New York, NY: Taylor & Francis.

Piedmont, R. L. (1999). Does spirituality represent the sixth factor of personality? Spiritual transcendence and the five-factor model. *Journal of Personality, 67*(6), 985–1013.

Purohit, S. (2001). *Bhagavad Gita: Annotated and explained.* Woodstock, VT: Skylight Paths.

Rajkumar, A. P., Premkumar, T. S., & Tharyan, P. (2008). Coping with the Asian tsunami: Perspectives from Tamil Nadu, India on the determinants of resilience in the face of adversity. *Social Science & Medicine, 67*(5), 844–853.

Rammohan, A., Rao, K., & Subbakrishna, D. K. (2002). Religious coping and psychological wellbeing in carers of relatives with schizophrenia. *Acta Psychiatrica Scandinavica, 105*(5), 356–362.

Rutter, M. (1999). Resilience as the millennium Rorschach: Response to Smith and Gorrell Barnes. *Journal of Family Therapy, 21*(2), 159–160.

Rutter, M. (2006). Implications of resilience concepts for scientific understanding. *Annals of the New York Academy of Sciences, 1094*(Resilience in Children), 1–12.

Saraf, S., Singh, T. B., & Khurana, S. (2013). Cervical cancer survivors: Meaning in life. *Psychological Studies, 58*(2), 144–152.

Saslow, L. R., John, O. P., Piff, P. K., Willer, R., Wong, E., Impett, E. A., . . . Saturn, S. R. (2013). The social significance of spirituality: New perspectives on the compassion – altruism relationship. *Psychology of Religion and Spirituality, 5*(3), 201–218.

Schultz, J. M., Tallman, B. A., & Altmaier, E. M. (2010). Pathways to posttraumatic growth: The contributions of forgiveness and importance of religion and spirituality. *Psychology of Religion and Spirituality, 2*(2), 104–114.

Schuurmans-Stekhoven, J. (2010). "Moved by the spirit": Does spirituality moderate the interrelationships between subjective well-being subscales? *Journal of Clinical Psychology, 66*(7), 709–725.

Seaward, B. L. (2005). *Managing stress* (5th ed.). Boston, MA: Jones & Bartlett.

Simpson, D. B., Newman, J. L., & Fuqua, D. R. (2007). Spirituality and personality: Accumulating evidence. *Journal of Psychology and Christianity, 26*(1), 35–44.

Sinha, D. (2011). Concept of psycho-social well-being: Western and Indian perspectives. In A. K Dalal & G. Misra (Eds.), *New directions in health psychology* (pp. 95–108). New Delhi: Sage Publications.

Smith, B. W., Ortiz, J. A., Wiggins, K. T., Bernard, J. F., & Dalen, J. (2012). Spirituality, resilience, and positive emotions. In L. J. Miller (Ed.), *The Oxford handbook of psychology and spirituality* (pp. 437–454). New York, NY: Oxford University Press.

Smith, L., Webber, R., & De Frain, J. (2013). Spiritual well-being and its relationship to resilience in young people: A mixed methods case study. *SAGE Open, 3*(2), 1–16.

Smith, T. B., McCullough, M. E., & Poll, J. (2003). Religiousness and depression: Evidence for a main effect and the moderating influence of stressful life events. *Psychological Bulletin, 129*(4), 614–636.

Srivastava, A. K., & Misra, G. (2003). Going beyond the model of economic man: An indigenous perspective on happiness. *Journal of Indian Psychology, 21*(2), 12–29.

Takahashi, M., & Bordia, P. (2000). The concept of wisdom: A cross-cultural comparison. *International Journal of Psychology, 35*(1), 1–9.

Tandon, S., Mehrotra, S., & Vallikad, E. (2010). Illness meanings in the context of cancer: An Indian perspective. *Psychological Studies, 55*(3), 230–238.

Tart, C. T. (1975). *Transpersonal psychologies*. New York: Harper & Row.

Thapa, K. (1983). *Effort-consequence orientation as a moderator variable stress-strain relationship* (Post-Doctoral Dissertation). University of Allahabad, Allahabad.

Unantenne, N., Warren, N., Canaway, R., & Manderson, L. (2013). The strength to cope: Spirituality and faith in chronic disease. *Journal of Religion and Health, 52*(4), 1147–1161.

Vaillant, G. E. (2013). Psychiatry, religion, positive emotions and spirituality. *Asian Journal of Psychiatry, 6*(6), 590–594.

Van Cappellen, P., Saroglou, V., Iweins, C., Piovesana, M., & Fredrickson, B., L. (2013). Self-transcendent positive emotions increase spirituality through basic world assumptions. *Cognition and Emotion, 27*, 1378–1394.

Van Cappellen, P., Toth-Gauthier, M., Saroglou, V., & Fredrickson, B. (2014). Religion and well-being: The mediating role of positive emotions. *Journal of Happiness Studies*. Advance online publication. doi: 10.1007/s10902-014-9605-5

Van Dyke, C. J., Glenwick, D. S., Cecero, J. J., & Kim, S. (2009). The relationship of religious coping and spirituality to adjustment and psychological distress in urban early adolescents. *Mental Health, Religion & Culture, 12*(4), 369–383.

Werner, E. E., & Smith, R. S. (1992). *Overcoming the odds: High-risk children from birth to adulthood*. New York: Cornell University Press.

Wink, P., & Dillon, M. (2003). Religiousness, spirituality, and psychosocial functioning in late adulthood: Findings from a longitudinal study. *Psychology of Religion and Spirituality, 18*(4), 916–924.

Wong-McDonald, A., & Gorsuch, R. L. (2000). Surrender to God: An additional coping style? *Journal of Psychology and Theology, 28*(2), 149–161.

Wuthnow, R. (1998). *After heaven: Spirituality in America since the 1950s*. Berkeley: University of California Press.

Zinnbauer, B. J., & Pargament, K. I. (2005). Religiousness and spirituality. In R. F. Paloutzian & C. L. Park (Eds.), *Handbook of the psychology of religion and spirituality* (pp. 21–42). New York: Guilford Press.

19

Posttraumatic growth amongst refugee populations

A systematic review

Katrina Sims and Julie Ann Pooley

Personal growth following adversity is an age-old concept that can be observed in literature drawn from the fields of religion, philosophy and psychology. Fredrick Nietzsche's famous quote "That which does not kill us makes us stronger" is an often cited example of the notion that people can change in beneficial ways following adversity. Scientific interest in growth following adversity commenced in the late 1980s with studies reporting positive changes after traumatic experiences such as combat, cardiac arrest and rape (Joseph & Butler, 2010). Research and interest in this field has grown steadily over the past two decades. Development in posttraumatic growth research has been linked to the expansion of the positive psychology movement. This movement has seen a paradigm shift that has encouraged facilitation of positive emotional states rather than a singular focus on relieving negative symptoms (Joseph & Linley, 2005; Seligman & Csikzentmihalyi, 2000).

Different terms such as benefit finding (Lechner & Weaver, 2009), stress-related growth (Park, 2004) and perceived benefits (McMillen & Fisher, 1998) have been used in literature to refer to similar concepts. Posttraumatic growth (PTG), as proposed by Tedeschi and Calhoun (1996), has become the most commonly used term in current literature to describe positive change following adversity (Joseph & Butler, 2010). Tedeschi and Calhoun (1996) use the term to refer to the experience of positive psychological change following trauma.

It is proposed that after a traumatic event some survivors through their struggle to make sense of their experience perceive psychological development beyond that reported prior to the life-threatening event. Reported positives changes include a greater appreciation of life, enriched intimate relationships, awareness of personal strength, revaluation of priorities and possibilities and positive spiritual change (Tedeschi & Calhoun, 2004). Drawing on the "shattered assumptions" work of Janoff-Bulman (1992), Tedeschi and Calhoun suggest that traumatic events shatter basic world assumptions of benevolence, meaningfulness and self-worth. PTG is assumed to be derived through rebuilding assumptions using processes such as effortful rumination. PTG can therefore be considered a process or an outcome. PTG is not an automatic process that occurs for all people nor is it considered to replace distress. For those who experience PTG, this often occurs alongside ongoing distress.

Within the posttraumatic growth field researchers have reached consensus that PTG occurs following a diverse range of traumatic events and in a range of different populations. PTG has been reported amongst children (Meyerson, Grant, Carter, & Kilmer, 2011), adolescents and adults from different cultures (Splevins, Cohen, Bowley, & Joseph, 2010). Posttraumatic growth has been identified following diverse experiences that include life-threatening illnesses (Hefferon, Grealy, & Mutrie, 2009), survivors of bone marrow transplants (Tallman, Shaw, Schultz, & Altmaier, 2010), bereavement (Cadell & Sullivan, 2006), sexual assault (Frazier, Conlon, & Glaser, 2001), earthquake survivors (Karanci & Acaturk, 2005), terrorist attacks (Peterson & Seligman, 2003) and war (Powell, Rosner, Butollo, Tedeschi, & Calhoun, 2003). A review conducted by Linley and Joseph (2004) indicated that 30–70% of survivors of a range of traumatic events including accidents, medical problems, assaults and natural disasters experienced positive change following a traumatic event. The review found that people who maintained PTG over time were also less distressed. PTG was found to be related to positive well-being and lower rates of depression in a meta-analytic review of seventy-seven studies (Helgeson, Reynolds, & Tomich, 2006). Current research provides evidence to support that posttraumatic growth can occur across different age groups following a diverse range of traumatic events and is related to positive outcomes.

While the body of research into PTG has grown steadily, particularly among Western samples, posttraumatic growth in refugee populations has received much less attention. Given the high incidence of trauma and trauma-related problems reported among many refugee populations and the growing number of refugees settling in Western countries, treatment of refugee trauma-related problems has become an area of importance to health professionals working with refugee populations. The current chapter will review the body of research that has explored posttraumatic growth amongst refugee populations. The United Nations High Commissioner for Refugees (UNHCR, 2012) defines refugees as those who have been forced to relocate for humanitarian reasons including armed conflict, violence, persecution or violation of human rights and natural or manmade disasters. The UNHCR estimate that in 2011 there were 42.5 million refugees globally. Of these, 15.42 million have sought refuge in countries other than their own while 26.4 million were displaced but remain within their own country. Current figures indicate a growth trend in the number of new refugees each year. It was estimated in 2011 there were 800,000 new refugees, the highest number recorded in the past decade. Increase in the number of refugees globally has widespread implications for the displaced individuals and the countries hosting them.

Increase in the number of refugees settling in other countries along with higher incidence mental health problems has stimulated interest in refugee mental health. Estimates of PTSD alone in refugee samples have ranged from 12% to 91% (Johnson & Thompson, 2006). While forced relocation in itself can be considered a traumatic event (Ryff & Essex, 1992), many refugees have been exposed to or have witnessed prolonged and repeated trauma and life-threatening events including starvation, disease, torture, rape, extensive violence and injury or murder of family and friends. Research has identified a link between pre-migration trauma and mental health problems including PTSD, depression, anxiety and substance misuse (Steel, Silove, Phan, & Bauman, 2002). In addition postmigration factors such as loss of identity, acculturation, social isolation, unemployment and discrimination have been found to contribute to the development and maintenance of PTSD (Carlsson, Mortensen, & Kastrup, 2006; Kinzie, 2006).

Recent reviews of interventions to treat refugee mental health have found limited available research but also found some evidence for conventional therapies such as cognitive behaviour therapy and some promising therapies such as narrative exposure therapy (Crumlish & O'Rourke,

2010; Palic & Elklit, 2010). For mental health practitioners in developed countries, there has been a push to respond to refugee mental health in a culturally sensitive manner (Murray, Davidson, & Schweitzer, 2008). While research into effective culturally sensitive therapies to treat refugee populations is limited research into interventions aimed at facilitating posttraumatic growth is in its infancy and has received even less attention (Joseph & Linley, 2006). Nonetheless researchers have begun to explore whether posttraumatic growth can be facilitated through the use of interventions following trauma (Stanton et al., 2002) and through training prior to traumatic events (Tedeschi & McNally, 2011).

A systematic review of the current state of research into posttraumatic growth amongst refugee populations will contribute to the understanding of the phenomenon within this population and identify variables that contribute to posttraumatic growth amongst refugees. This information may in turn inform clinical interventions aimed at promoting psychological growth. To the author's knowledge, a review of this body of research has not been conducted to date.

The following chapter presents the aim of the review, the methodology and results. The results are combined and presented under relevant sub-headings representing common themes in the literature. These include results of measured PTG, the relationship between PTG and posttraumatic stress (PTS), gender and age differences, support for the Tedeschi and Calhoun's (1996) five-factor model and the use of therapy to promote PTG. The chapter concludes with a summary of the findings and the implications for therapists and suggestions for future research. Limitations of the current review and the reviewed studies are discussed.

Aim

The aim of this chapter is to systematically review the PTG literature in relation to refugees who have experienced adversity or trauma. The review will consider whether the phenomenon occurs across different refugee populations, the processes that mediate posttraumatic growth and the use of therapy to promote posttraumatic growth in this population. The review will consider implications for clinical interventions by health practitioners to facilitate posttraumatic growth amongst refugee populations.

Methods

Articles obtained for the review were identified through systematic searches of the electronic databases CINAHL plus Full Text, Proquest, PsychARTICLES, PsychINFO, Scopus and Web of Science. In addition reference lists of the obtained articles were scanned for any missed studies. The key terms "posttraumatic growth", "positive change", "benefit finding", "stress-related growth" and "adversarial growth" were combined with the search terms "refugee", "humanitarian entrant", "asylum seeker" and "displaced person" for the searches. All possible search combinations within the identified databases were conducted.

The articles included in this review are those that contribute to the body of knowledge relating to posttraumatic growth in refugee populations following resettlement. Given that interest in the area of growth following adversity commenced in the 1980s, the search was limited to studies published from 1980 until May 2013. The review is focused on studies that have examined posttraumatic growth in adult refugees. While in most cases samples included adults 18 years and above, one study explored PTG in young people aged 17 to 20 years. Given the majority of participants were adults and the limited number of studies in this area, this study was retained for the review. Participants were those recognised in the study as refugees, humanitarian entrants, asylum seekers or forced migrants from any country. While no limitations were placed on the resettlement country included papers were limited to those published in English. Published, peer-reviewed articles and theses based on quantitative and qualitative research relating to the topic were included.

Once the search process was completed the authors independently screened the generated article titles. Those that did not meet the search criteria were excluded. The abstracts of the retained articles were again independently examined with those meeting the search criteria retained.

Results

The initial search yielded a total of fifty-six studies, thirty-two of these were eliminated during Stages 1 and 2 of the screening process leaving nineteen that met the full inclusion criteria. A further two articles were excluded as they were found to be based on the same research published in different formats. One journal article also appeared as a book chapter (Powell et al., 2003); the other, a thesis, was later published as a journal article (Rodgers, 2012).

Of the seventeen retained articles, fifteen were peer-reviewed journal articles and the remaining two dissertations. While the search criterion was open to studies published after 1980 the retained papers were all published in the last ten years from 2003 with a large number published in the last three years. The majority of the studies were quantitative with a retrospective cross-sectional design, while five of the studies used a qualitative approach. Only one study, Ai, Tice, Whitsett, Ishisaka and Chim (2007), used a longitudinal design. Two studies that tested the use of therapeutic interventions used an experimental approach with one utilising a pretest/posttest design (Gregory & Prana, 2013) and the second a randomised controlled trial (Hijazi, 2012). All studies were reliant on self-report measures to obtain information regarding posttraumatic growth. Table 19.1 presents a brief summary of the review articles. The table includes the authors and date published, the sample size, gender breakdown and the research design for each of the studies. Where reported, ethnicity, religion, resettlement location and time since trauma are included in the table. Also reported is the measurement tool of PTG and the major findings in relation to PTG.

Posttraumatic growth

Each of the reviewed articles reported the existence of PTG within their sample. Fourteen of the studies used a self-report questionnaire as a measure of PTG with eleven of those utilizing Tedeschi and Calhoun's (1996) Posttraumatic Growth Index (PTGI). The remaining three studies used qualitative approaches to analyse interview data.

The PTGI is a twenty-one-item measure using a six-point Likert scale. Scores range from 0 to 126 with higher scores reflecting greater perceived growth (Tedeschi & Calhoun, 1996). Results of the six studies that reported PTGI total mean scores are tabled (Table 19.2). Mean total PTGI scores ranged from 35.82 to 76.68. The highest PTGI mean score resulted from a large sample of Tibetan refugees residing in India (Hussain & Bhushan, 2011). This result may indicate that there is something specific to this group that encourages PTG. A likely explanation is that Tibetans follow a Buddhist philosophy that may support PTG. This idea is discussed in greater detail in the discussion section on cultural factors.

Table 19.1 Summary of review articles

Authors and date	Sample Total, Gender Breakdown	Research Design	Ethnicity	Religion	Location	Time elapsed since relocation	Measure of PTG	PTG Key Findings
Ai, A. L., Tice, T. N., Whitsett, D. D., Ishisaka, T., & Chim, M. (2007)	50, 54% M, 46% F	Longitudinal prospective	Kosovar	96% Muslim	Washington State, USA	Minimum of 10 months	Fifty item Stress Related Growth Scale.	No relationship between PTSD symptoms and PTG. Hope and cognitive coping showed a positive association with PTG
Copping, A., Shakespeare-Finch, J., & Paton, D. (2010).	15, 53% M, 47% F	Qualitative study using grounded theory	Sudanese	100% Christian	Tasmania, Australia	3 months to 5 years		Found values associated to PTG where present prior to trauma and assisted PTG.
Gregory, J.L., & Prana, H. (2013).	49, 41% M, 59% F	Pretest/post test design	Ivorian	No data	Liberia	No data	PTGI	Significant increase in PTG reported following intervention.
Hall, B. J., Hobfoll, S. E., Palmieri, P. A., Canetti-Nisim, D., Shapira, O., Johnson, R. J., & Galea, S. (2008).	190, 44% M, 56% F	Cross sectional	Israeli	70% reported to be religious.	Gaza	Data obtained prior to relocation	6 items of Conservation of Resources Evaluation	PTG related to lower likelihood of probable PTSD but not MDD ($\alpha = .66$) PTG (M = 10.11, SD = 4.62)
Hijazi, A. M. (2012).	53, 49% M, 51% F	Randomized Iraqi controlled trial	Iraqi	75% Chaldean Catholic, 15% Mandean, 9% Muslim Arab	Detroit, Michigan, USA	Mean 2.4 years (SD = 2.4)	PTGI	Significant increase in PTG reported at 2 and 4 months following NET intervention.
Hussain, D., & Bhushan, B. (2011).	226, 50% M, 50% F	Cross sectional design	Tibetan	No data reported; however a Buddhist influence is implied.	Dharmshala, Himachal Pradesh, India	No data	PTGI	Positive correlation between PTS and PTG reported. PTGI total (M = 76.68, SD = 9.39)

Citation	Sample	Design	Population	Religion	Location	Time since trauma	Measure	Findings
Hussain, D., & Bhushan, B. (2013).	12, 67% M, 33% F	Qualitative study using interpretive phenomenological analysis.	Tibetan	No data Buddhism implied	Dharmshala, Himachal Pradesh, India	No data	PTGI	Three themes consistent with PTG theory emerged: change in outlook, personal strength and meaningful relationships.
Jayawickreme, D. E. R. (2011).	237, 69% M, 13% F, 4% U	Cross sectional	Tamil	No data	Sri Lanka	No data	PTGI Short Form	Two factor structure found. Significant gender differences in PTG noted. No relationship was found between PTG and PTSD, depression or functioning.
Kim, H. K., & Lee, O. J. (2009).	5, 60% F, 40% M	Qualitative Phenomenonlogical	North Korean	No data	South Korea	No data		PTG found amongst all participants. Four factors emerged personal, social, religious and mental health.
Kroo, A., & Nagy, H. (2011).	53, 83% M, 17% F	Cross sectional design	Somali	76% reported to be a great deal religious (Muslim)	Hungary	No data	PTGI	PTG reported, PTGI Total (M = 68.92, SD = 16.77). Found a positive relationship between PTG and: hope, religiosity, negative religious coping and perceived social support.
Mattoon, L. (2011).	11, 100% F	Qualitative utilizing the narrative approaches of life story interview and Artistic Inquiry	Uganda and Vietnam	55% Protestant 36% Catholic	California and Uganda	2–27 years since most recent trauma	PTGI	Support for PTG was found. PTG was found to coexist with trauma and to alter religious beliefs. Scores from PTGI range from 66% to 89%.
Nuttman-Shwartz, O., Dekel, R., & Tuval-Mashiach, R. (2011).	269, 37% M, 63% F	Cross sectional	Israeli (from Gaza strip)	84.9% reported being religious	Israel	No data	PTGI	Curvelinear relationship between post traumatic symptoms and growth

(Continued)

Table 19.1 (Continued)

Authors and date	Sample Total, Gender Breakdown	Research Design	Ethnicity	Religion	Location	Time elapsed since relocation	Measure of PTG	PTG Key Findings
Powell, S., Rosner, R., Butollo, W., Tedeschi, R. G., & Calhoun, L. G. (2003).	64, 39% M, 61% F	Cross sectional	Former Yugoslavian	No data	Sarajevo, Bosnia and Herzegovina	3.5 years after war	PTGI Bosnian translation	Low PTGI Total (M = 35.82, SD = 18.09). No relationship was found between PTS and PTG. Support was not found for Tedeschi & Calhoun's 5 factors, a three factor solution was found.
Rodgers, S.T. (2012).	62, 100% F	Cross sectional	Latina (from Colombia 52% El Salvador 21% and Guatemala 11%)	71% Catholic	New York City, NY, USA	6 or more years	PTGI Spanish short form	Reports presence of stress and moderate levels of PTG. Converted PTGI total M = 74.4
Sutton, V., Robbins, I., Senior, V., & Gordon, S. (2006).	8, 12% M, 88% F	Qualitative using Interpretative Phenomenological Analytical Analysis	No data	62% Christian 38% Muslim	United Kingdom	Unclear		Reported varied levels of PTG and co-existence of distress and positive change.
Teodorescu, D. S., Siqveland, J., Heir, T., Hauff, E., Wentzel-Larsen, T., & Lien, L. (2012).	55, 58% M, 42% F	Cross sectional	Eastern Europe 40%, Middle East 26%, Africa 16%, Far East 13%, Latin America 6%	64% Muslim	Norway	Mean 16.7 years	PTGI Short Form	Low PTG reported Converted PTGI M = 47.4 (SD = 10.1). A significant negative association between PTSD symptoms and PTG was found.
Vazquez, C., Cervellon, P., Perez-Sales, P., Vidales, D., & Gaborit, M. (2005).	115, 42% M, 48% F	Naturalistic study	El Salvador	No data	El Salvador	No data	The Community Cohesion Interview.	66% of the sample reported growth or learning

Table 19.2 Summary of PTGI total mean

Authors and date	Sample size and setting	Mean PTGI Score	Standard Deviation
Hijazi (2012)	53 Iraqi refugees settled in USA	49.5 (Control at baseline)	23.9
		43.5 (Control at 4 months)	18.1
		48.5 (Intervention group baseline)	23.8
		58.3 (Intervention group at 4 months)	23.56
Hussain & Bhushan (2011).	266 Tibetan refugees settled in India	76.68	9.39
Kroo & Nagy (2011).	53 Somali refugees living in Hungarian reception centres	68.92	16.77
Powell, et al. (2003).	64 former Yugoslavia refugees living in Sarajevo.	35.82	18.09
Rodgers (2012).	62 Latina women living in New York City	74.4	
Teodorescu, et al. (2012).	55 psychiatric outpatients with a refugee background living in Norway	47.4	10.1

Relationship between posttraumatic stress and posttraumatic growth

While all studies reported the existence of PTG and coexistence of posttraumatic stress symptoms (PTSS), inconsistent results were found between studies that explored the relationship between PTSS and PTG. Three of the studies reported no relationship between PTSS and PTG (Ai, Tice, Whitsett, Ishisaka, & Chim, 2007; Jayawickreme, 2011; Powell et al., 2003) while two reported a negative relationship (Hall et al., 2008; Teodorescu et al., 2012), one study reported a positive association (Hussain & Bhushan, 2011), and one reported a curvilinear relationship (Nuttman-Shwarts, Dekel, & Tuval-Mashiach, 2011). The discrepancy in these results is puzzling and is considered further in the following discussion.

Psychological predictors of posttraumatic growth

Few of the studies explored the role of psychological predictors of PTG among refugee samples. Hope and cognitive coping were found to be positively associated with PTG while avoidance coping was found to have a negative relationship with PTG (Ai et al., 2007). Support was found for the role of hope in the development PTG (Kroo & Nagy, 2011). In addition higher scores on cognitive emotional regulation strategies were found to be associated with higher PTG (Hussain & Bhushan, 2011). Of the nine cognitive coping strategies tested in this study, four (positive refocussing, refocus on planning, putting in perspective and catastrophisizing) were found to partially mediate the relationship between traumatic experience and PTG.

Gender

In general PTG research, females tend to score higher on both stress symptomology and PTG (Linley & Joseph, 2004). Even when exposed to similar traumatic events women tend to experience greater levels of distress. It is theorised that higher levels of distress may be sufficient to shatter previously held assumptions and promote schema change and PTG (Tedeschi & Calhoun,

2004). Among the few studies in the current review that considered gender differences in PTG, two were consistent with findings elsewhere. Hussain and Bhushan (2011) found that females scored higher on PTG along with trauma and PTSS. Jayawickreme (2011) also reported a significant difference in PTG amongst Sri Lankan men and women, with women scoring higher, although their sample included only 13% women.

A third study, however, found no gender difference in PTG among a sample of refugees from the former Yugoslavia following war (Powell et al., 2003). The overall PTGI mean score in this sample was found to be low and thought to be a reflection of high levels of trauma hindering the PTG process. This effect may have impacted both genders equally or perhaps women more so given that women would generally score higher on PTG. Alternatively these results could be a reflection of cultural gender differences.

Age

Age effects were reported in Powell et al. (2003). A significant result was found for the factor changes in self/positive life attitude with the older age group reporting less growth in this area. Rather than age Hussain and Bhushan (2011) examined generational differences in PTG amongst two generations of Tibetan refugees relocated to India. Total PTG difference between the generations was not significant; however, significant differences were found in three of the five sub-factors. First-generation Tibetan refugees scored higher on personal strength and spiritual change while second-generation participants scored higher on new possibilities. First-generation refugees reported greater PTSS.

Use of therapy to facilitate posttraumatic growth

Two studies researched the effect of a specific therapy on PTG in a refugee sample. Compared to a waitlist control group, Hijazi (2012) found that Iraqi refugees provided with three sessions of Narrative Exposure Therapy showed increased PTG at two and four month follow-ups. A trend towards reduced PTSD symptoms was noted but was not found significant at the four-month follow-up. Gregory and Prana (2013) reported a significant increase in PTG as measured by the PTGI following delivery of the Companion Recovery Model to forty-nine Ivorian participants. A third study reported positive effects resulting from the use of a therapeutic interviewing technique (Mattoon, 2011). These initial results show promise for the effectiveness of therapy to facilitate PTG and will be further discussed.

Support for Tedeschi and Calhoun's (1996) five-factor model

To measure PTG, Tedeschi and Calhoun (1996) developed the Posttraumatic Growth Inventory. Five factors or scales emerged from analysis using the PTGI: New Possibilities, Relating to Others, Personal Strength, Spiritual Change and Appreciation of Life. Tedeschi and Calhoun's original five-factor model of PTG was not replicated amongst refugee samples. Jayawickreme (2011) reported a two-factor model while Powell et al. (2003) reported a three-factor solution.

Discussion

The articles reviewed here consistently reported the existence of PTG and the coexistence of PTG and PTSS. The results support that PTG frequently occurs among refugee samples that have experienced often prolonged and complex trauma. The results provide evidence to support that

PTG occurs across many different cultural groups and is likely a universal phenomenon. The co-occurrence of PTG and PTSS found in all studies is consistent with Tedeschi and Calhoun's (2004) PTG model, which purports PTG and PTSS develop from the same events and share similar processes such as rumination.

The importance of PTG to clinicians and health professionals rests in its relationship to mental health outcomes and quality of life. Much research into PTG has attempted to determine whether a relationship between posttraumatic stress symptoms and growth exists and the nature of such a relationship should it exist. Although many studies have explored this relationship, the findings have been inconsistent, and the nature of the relationship remains unclear (Linley & Joseph, 2004). As in other PTG literature, the relationship between posttraumatic stress and growth amongst refugee populations in the current review was found to be inconsistent and confusing with studies reporting null findings, positive, negative and curvilinear relationships.

One hypothesis is that the level of the distress experienced moderates the level of PTG. It is proposed that PTG is highest when the level of posttraumatic stress is moderate and lower when lower or higher doses of trauma are present, thus producing a curvilinear relationship (Butler et al., 2005). Nuttman-Shwartz et al. (2011) reported a curvilinear relationship between psychological distress and PTG in their study of 269 Israeli residents who were forced to relocate from their homes in the Gaza Strip. While causal assumptions cannot be made due to the cross-sectional nature of the study, the authors propose that posttraumatic symptomology at higher levels may be overwhelming and limit PTG and at lower levels may be insufficient to produce the processes that are thought to lead to PTG. Powell et al. (2003) report that their results lend support to the curvilinear hypothesis. While no linear relationship was found in their sample of refugees from the former Yugoslavia exposed to war, high levels of exposure to traumatic events are reported along with relatively low levels of PTG ($M = 35.82$, $SD = 18.09$). It could be assumed that the high levels of trauma produced greater distress, which in turn hindered psychological growth.

Teodorescu et al.'s (2012) finding of a significant negative association between PTSD symptoms and PTG along with relatively low levels of PTG may represent the downward slope of the inverted-U, curvilinear relationship if the sample were to include participants experiencing a high level of distress. This may be the case as the sample was derived from psychiatric outpatients. It would be reasonable to assume that clients seek treatment due to higher levels of symptomology, which may impede their ability to engage in the cognitive processing required for PTG.

Support for a curvilinear relationship between PTSS and PTG has been found elsewhere (Butler et al., 2005) and is reported to be the current dominant explanation for the nature of the relationship (Joseph, Murphy, & Regel, 2012).

The time passed since trauma occurred has also been demonstrated to have an effect on outcomes. Helgeson et al. (2006), in a meta-analysis of general PTG research, considering only Western samples, found greater positive effects on well-being when the time since trauma was greater than two years and conversely that PTG was related to greater distress when the time since trauma was less than two years. Roughly half of the articles presented here did not report time since trauma, and of those that did, the period of time ranged from 3 months to 27 years. Only one of the reviewed articles (Hussain & Bhushan, 2011), considered time since trauma as a factor in their study. These authors considered differences among first-generation and second-generation Tibetan refugees. First-generation refugees were those relocated from their homeland while second-generation refugees were generally born in exile. No difference between the groups was found in traumatic experience or PTG totals; however, first-generation refugees scored higher on PTSS and the PTG factors of personal strength and spiritual change, while second-generation refugees scored higher on new possibilities. These results appear to relate more to generational and age differences than time since trauma.

In addition, trauma that has existed over an extended period of time may have a different impact on PTG. For example in some communities, political unrest or war has occurred over entire lifetimes, and it is possible that exposure to trauma has become part of life. Under these circumstances, assumptions that the world is a safe and benevolent place may not have developed. and assumptions are likely to be very different to the world assumptions of those living in more fortunate circumstances (Copping, Shakespeare-Finch, & Paton, 2010).

Given the differences in samples, level of distress and time since trauma it a possibility that different phases of PTG are being measured. Helgeson et al. (2006) propose the possibility that different studies may be measuring different phases of the PTG process. For example early coping, actual changes and cognitive processes may represent different phases of PTG.

In a study of Israeli's forced to relocate from the Gaza strip, Hall et al. (2008) found that PTG was related to a lower likelihood of probable PTSD but not Major Depressive Disorder (MDD). These authors suggest that the key to PTG amongst this sample may have been actual behavioural change rather than cognitive processes. The participants in the study had chosen to resist instructions to relocate, and in so doing, it was suggested that the participants had actualized their growth cognitions, resulting in a lower likelihood of psychological distress. Refugee groups in other studies appear to have had less control over their situations.

Severity of the trauma reaction may in part explain some of the different findings. Boals, Steward and Schuettler (2010) proposed that, if the impact of trauma did not have a profound effect on core beliefs, study results could be diluted. These authors demonstrated that excluding results from traumatic events that were not central to core beliefs produced greater effect sizes and recommended that future studies exclude data that fail to produce a moderate impact on the participants' core beliefs.

Although many of the studies reported exposure to severe and prolonged traumatic events, the different measures of trauma symptomology ranging from self-report to a clinically administered scale prevent direct comparison. Some studies measured symptoms against PTSD criteria while others measured stress symptomology. It is therefore unclear how the severity of trauma impacted on PTG among refugee samples.

It appears the relationship between PTG and PTSS is complex particularly amongst refugee populations, and current research is still in the early stages of unravelling the nature of the relationship. More stringent research taking into consideration the time since trauma, the level of distress and PTG over time may provide clearer insight into the phenomenon.

Psychological predictors

Few of the studies of PTG in refugee populations explored psychological predictors. Cognitive coping was considered in two studies. Within these, one study considered rumination, which is proposed by Tedeschi and Calhoun (2004) to play a major role in development of PTG. In Hussain and Bhushan's (2011) sample of Tibetan refugees, rumination was not found to be a significant predictor of PTG. No explanation is offered, and it remains unclear whether rumination has a role in development of PTG in other refugee groups.

No studies could be found that considered personality factors, in refugee groups, which are thought to impact PTG. Optimism and hope are discussed in two of the studies. Interestingly hope, but not optimism, was positively related to PTG in both studies (Ai et al., 2007; Kroo & Nagy, 2011). It suggests that hope, compared to optimism, appears more emotional and motivational. Hope offers the perception of ability to effect positive change, which in turn provides motivation to overcome the impacts of trauma (Ai et al., 2007). A possible link between faith and spiritual support with hope is offered. Faith is discussed further under the heading of religious coping.

In their sample of Kosovar war refugees, Ai et al. (2007) found that cognitive coping was positively associated with PTG while a negative relationship was found between avoidance coping and PTG. Hussain and Bhushan (2011) found that higher scores on cognitive emotional regulation strategies were associated with higher PTG. Of the nine cognitive coping strategies tested, four – positive refocussing, refocus on planning, putting in perspective and catastrophisizing – partially mediated the relationship between traumatic experience and PTG. It appears logical that that positive coping strategies such as positive refocusing, refocusing on planning and putting into perspective facilitate growth through positive change in thought patterns; however. the relationship with catastrophisizing appears less clear. It would seem intuitive that catastrophizing would intensify negative thought patterns resulting in less growth; however, the researchers suggest the possibility that catastrophisizing acts as a catalyst for schema change that in turn leads to growth. Tedeschi and Calhoun's (2004) notion that a sufficient level of trauma is required to shatter previous schemas is used to support the hypothesis (Hussain & Bhushan, 2011).

Evidence of psychological factors that promote and hinder PTG is important to the field of clinical psychology. Clinicians can encourage those processes that promote PTG. At this time research into the psychological processes that facilitate growth in refugee populations insufficient to inform clinical practice.

Cultural factors

While some similarities can be drawn between the experiences of refugees from different cultural groups, many cultures have unique beliefs or customs that may impact on their experience as a refugee. These differences may also influence development and experience of PTG. Many cultural practices that may impact on development of PTG were noted throughout the studies. For example Tibetan culture is heavily influenced by Buddhist beliefs such as compassion for others and the "law of karma". A qualitative study of Tibetan refugees revealed that these beliefs aided growth following adversity. Through belief in karma and past deeds, Tibetan's were able to find meaning and acceptance of events that had occurred in their lives (Hussain & Bhushan, 2013). The Tibetans were also found to have pride in their culture and a willingness to make collective efforts to preserve their way of life creating meaning beyond their own survival. The particular beliefs and practices of the Tibetans were found to be conducive to the PTG process, which may explain the high level of PTG reported in a study of a large sample of Tibetans (Hussain & Bhushan, 2011).

Evidence of cultural influence was also found in studies of other cultural groups. Hispanics in the USA were found to believe in divine intervention, which was thought to foster hope among this group (Rodgers, 2012). Collectivism among the Sudanese was found to promote support-seeking behaviour and a sense of shared experience (Copping et al., 2010). A similar collective bond was reported among Tibetans (Hussain & Bhushan, 2013). Evidence that cultural factors influence PTG highlight the value of existing cultural resources and social supports available in some cultural groups. These findings reinforce the need for culturally sensitive practice.

Religious coping

Religious coping was found to be an important factor in PTG across many of the cultures considered in the review. The Sudanese were found to attribute traumatic experience to fate and god (Copping et al., 2010). Faith, prayer and accepting fate were found to be central to posttraumatic growth in Somali refugees in Hungary (Kroo & Nagy, 2011). Of a sample of refugees following an earthquake in El Salvador, 88% report using religion as a means of coping (Vazquez, Cervellon,

Perez-Sales, Vidales, & Gaborit, 2005). Mattoon (2011) found that, not only did religious beliefs influence PTG, but also in many of the participants, PTG was found to have an impact on people's religious beliefs.

The importance of religious coping in the development of PTG across the different cultural groups and religions was one of the most consistent findings across the studies reviewed. This finding has implications for therapists and host countries working with refugees. It is important to note that religious coping among these cultures was often seen as a positive coping strategy. This view may be opposed to that of some Western mental health professionals who often consider religious coping as a form of avoidance (Copping et al., 2010). These results serve as a reminder that mental health professionals working with clients from different cultures should familiarise themselves with the cultural and religious backgrounds of their clients and be careful not to minimise the importance of religious coping on trauma recovery (Mattoon, 2011).

Support for Tedeschi and Calhoun's (1996) five-factor model

Tedeschi and Calhoun's (1996) five-factor model of PTG was not replicated amongst refugee samples. A two- and three-factor model was found in the studies that attempted to explore the factor model. While the results were in line with Tedeschi and Calhoun's model, these results may suggest that the PTGI measures different concepts among different refugee groups. In the studies presented here, the PTGI was often translated to other languages for use with refugee groups. It is possible that meaning was lost between translations. Further research into the relevance of this measure in different cultural groups is required.

Copping et al. (2010) found that PTG outcomes identified by Tedeschi and Calhoun (1996) such as strength, appreciation of life, religious changes and relationships with others were present as coping strategies rather than resulting from traumatic experience, which they explain as a possible artefact of prolonged experience of conflict. Given the cultural differences identified, it is possible that PTG has different meaning and processes among different cultural groups.

The use of therapy to facilitate posttraumatic growth

Only two studies were found to consider the effect of a therapeutic intervention on posttraumatic growth in a refugee population. Gregory and Prana (2013) report that a ten-module (thirty-six-hour) Companion Recovery program delivered to forty-nine Ivorian refugees living in Liberia resulted in significant PTG. The Companion Recovery Model encourages processing of trauma and implementation of positive change through psycho-education, development of counselling skills and selection of a companion to share traumatic experience. PTG was measured using the PTGI before and after the implementation of the program. A significant increase in PTG was identified. The results of this study could have been strengthened through use of a control group to rule out the possibility that a factor other than the intervention contributed to the PTG found among the sample. While PTG is often associated with increases in well-being as discussed previously, it would have been interesting to know what benefits the participants gained alongside PTG and if the gains were maintained over time. The authors suggest that this type of program is a cost-effective means of addressing trauma reactions and empowering refugees to support their peers in refugee centres or camps.

Hijazi (2012) found that Iraqi refugees provided with three 60–90 minute sessions of Narrative Exposure Therapy showed significant increases in PTG at two- and four-month follow-ups as compared to a randomised waitlist control group. A trend towards reduced PTSD symptoms in the intervention group was noted, however, was not found significant at the four-month follow-up. Narrative Exposure Therapy is a manualized short-term intervention drawing on traditional cognitive and behavioural PTSD treatments. The therapy involves processing emotional reactions through repeated telling of the individual's traumatic events and creating a cohesive narrative. The aim is symptom reduction through gradual habituation. Encouraging results were found for this brief therapy.

While not using a psychological intervention, Mattoon (2011) reported anecdotal healing effects from the use of life story interview and artistic inquiry with refugee participants from Vietnam and Africa. Several of the participants from this study found that telling their story was validating and useful in processing events that had occurred in their lives. Some of the participants had never before shared their stories with others. The sharing of life stories was also found to be useful amongst Sudanese refugees in Australia (Copping et al., 2010). These authors identified the value in support groups within Sudanese culture who as a collectivist society are accustomed to seeking support from each other. Refugee groups often share a common experience of suffering regardless of individual difference in stories. Among the Sudanese, reflective counselling was found to be unsatisfactory with a cultural preference for seeking direction and advice noted in this group.

While the results of these studies are encouraging, particularly around the use of narrative therapies amongst certain populations, further research to support the effectiveness is required including whether current treatments for PTSD also produce PTG and what therapies enhance PTG are required to inform clinical practice in this area.

Limitations and conclusions

The overreliance on cross-sectional design is a common criticism of posttraumatic growth research. This criticism is certainly applicable to the research of PTG in refugee populations. Future studies that utilise methodologically sound research designs including longitudinal studies and control groups may help to clarify some of the inconsistencies in current research.

The reliance on self-report questionnaires to measure PTG has also been a major criticism (Coyne & Tennen, 2010). The ability to accurately self-report the extent to which a traumatic event influenced positive change has been described as a difficult and complex task in which people often overestimate past distress. A recent study (Frazier et al., 2009) demonstrated that amongst a sample of college students self-reported growth was not related to actual growth measured pre- and posttrauma. This study does not challenge the existence of PTG but rather the ability of self-report measures to identify actual PTG. More sensitive measures may be required to distinguish perceived growth from illusory growth and actual growth.

A major confounding factor in the study of PTG amongst refugee populations is that the change in environment under some circumstances produces not only relief from threat but actual new opportunities (i.e. housing, job prospects and education) that may not have been possible in the country of origin (Copping et. al., 2010). Refugees relocated to another country have been found to report higher levels of PTG than those internally displaced (Jayawickreme, 2011), and refugees living in temporary housing reported lower levels of growth than did those in independent housing (Nuttman-Shwartz et al., 2011). In order to control for this factor, researchers need to consider the refugees current and previous environmental factors. In the absence of baseline data, researchers could possibly obtain data from a control group from their previous environment.

Limitations of the current review

To the authors' knowledge, all articles that met the inclusion criteria available in the databases searched were obtained for the review. It remains a possibility, however, that some articles were missed. While an effort was made to include unpublished works to avoid a bias toward positive findings, it is probable that unpublished papers have been missed. Non-English-language publications were also excluded. In addition while an effort was made to search reference lists for missed articles, a systematic search for "grey literature" was not conducted and may have been overlooked here. The review therefore is limited to those studies that met the search criteria and may not be a comprehensive overview of all research conducted in this area.

Implications and relevance to clinical psychology

The results obtained here have several implications for clinicians and mental health practitioners. First, it appears clear from the mixed results and rich data from qualitative studies that each culture has different background history, customs and beliefs. It is not news that cultural competence is required when working with different cultural groups. However, it is important that clinicians consider the role that religious coping may play in development of PTG. Second, given that PTG occurs without intervention, it is important to consider the cultural values and practices already present amongst refugee groups and encourage local, traditional coping resources and social support (Kroo & Nagy, 2011). The use of support groups and storytelling may be useful among some cultural groups. Given that hope was found to be a contributing factor to PTG, clinicians have a role in restoring hope and teaching coping strategies (Ai et al., 2007).

It is also important to heed the warning of Tedeschi and Calhoun (2004) that, in the process of encouraging growth care, should be taken not to minimise the very real and damaging impacts of trauma. Until more appropriate culturally sensitive options become available clinicians would be wise to use traditional evidence-based methods to treat PTSD symptoms.

Conclusions and recommendations for future research

This chapter provides a systematic review of research that has explored PTG in adult refugee populations. To date, this area has received limited attention; however, recent interest in the field generated by global growth in refugee populations, combined with interest in positive psychology, has seen sufficient research produced to warrant a review.

Systematic search of electronic databases resulted in seventeen studies matching the search criteria. Differing research methodologies and samples have made direct comparison unfeasible; however, the results taken together provide interesting insight into current knowledge and gaps in PTG research into refugee populations. The results demonstrate that perceived PTG occurs in refugees originating from many different nations and cultural groups. These results support the notion that PTG is a cross-cultural phenomenon.

Research to date has failed to consistently identify the nature of the relationship between PTG and posttraumatic stress symptoms although some support was found for a curvilinear relationship whereby greater PTG is found when moderate levels of stress is present. Some evidence was found to support the use of narrative exposure therapy and the Companion Recovery Program to promote PTG in certain refugee populations; however, much more research is required to establish the effectiveness of these and other interventions in refugee populations.

As research in this area is relatively new, there is much scope for future research. Further research is required to help determine the nature of the relationship between PTG and PTSS and effective use of therapy to promote PTG. Further studies to test the validity of the PTGI in different cultural groups is required. Future research should take into consideration the effects of time since trauma and the severity of trauma responses. New studies would benefit from the consistent use of a measure of trauma symptomology that would allow for comparisons to be made between studies. Research designs that undertake longitudinal and experimental designs where appropriate may produce valuable evidence to add to the growing literature on posttraumatic growth in refugee populations.

References

Ai, A. L., Tice, T. N., Whitsett, D. D., Ishisaka, T., & Chim, M. (2007). Posttraumatic symptoms and growth of Kosovar war refugees: The influence of hope and cognitive coping. *The Journal of Positive Psychology*, 2(1), 55–65.

Boals, A., Steward, J. M., & Schuettler, D. (2010). Advancing our understanding of posttraumatic growth by considering event centrality. *Journal of Loss and Trauma: International Perspectives on Stress & Coping*, 15(6), 518–533.

Butler, L. D., Blasey, C. M., Garlan, R. W., McCaslin, S. E., Azarow, J., Chen, X. H., . . . Spiegel, D. (2005). Posttraumatic growth following the terrorist attacks of September 11, 2001: Cognitive, coping, and trauma symptom predictors in an Internet convenience sample. *Traumatology*, 11(4), 247–267.

Cadell, S., & Sullivan, R. (2006). Posttraumatic growth and HIV bereavement: Where does it start and when does it end? *Traumatology*, 12(1), 45–59.

Carlsson, J. M., Mortensen, E., & Kastrup, M., 2006. Predictors of mental health and quality of life in male tortured refugees. *Nordic Journal of Psychiatry*, 60(1), 51–57.

Copping, A., Shakespeare-Finch, J., & Paton, D. (2010). Towards a culturally appropriate mental health system: Sudanese-Australians' experiences with trauma. *Journal of Pacific Rim Psychology*, 4(1), 53–60.

Coyne, J. C., & Tennen, H. (2010). Positive psychology in cancer care: Bad science, exaggerated claims, and unproven medicine. *Annals of Behavioral Medicine*, 39(1), 16–26.

Crumlish, N., & O'Rourke, K. (2010). A Systematic review of treatments for post-traumatic stress disorder among refuges and asylum-Seekers. *The Journal of Nervous and Mental Disease*, 198(4), 237–251.

Frazier, P., Conlon, A., & Glaser, T. (2001). Positive and negative life changes following sexual assault. *Journal of Consulting and Clinical Psychology*, 69, 1048–1055.

Frazier, P., Tennen, H., Gavian, M., Park, C., Tomich, P., & Tashiro, T. (2009). Does self-reported posttraumatic growth reflect genuine positive change? *Psychological Science*, 20(7), 912–919.

Gregory, J. L., & Prana, H. (2013). Posttraumatic growth in cote d'Ivoire refugees using the companion recovery model. *Traumatology*, 19(3), 232–232.

Hall, B. J., Hobfoll, S. E., Palmieri, P. A., Canetti-Nisim, D., Shapira, O., Johnson, R. J., & Galea, S. (2008). The psychological impact of impending forced settler disengagement in Gaza: Trauma and posttraumatic growth. *Journal of Traumatic Stress*, 21(1), 22–29.

Hefferon, K., Grealy, M., & Mutrie, N. (2009). Post-traumatic growth and life threatening physical illness: A systematic review of the qualitative literature. *British Journal of Health Psychology*, 14(2), 343–378.

Helgeson, V. S., Reynolds, K. A., & Tomich, P. L. (2006). A meta-analytic review of benefit finding and growth. *Journal of Consulting and Clinical Psychology*, 74(5), 797–816.

Hijazi, A. M. (2012). *Narrative exposure therapy to treat traumatic stress in Middle Eastern refugees: A clinical trial* (Doctoral Dissertation). Retrieved from http://ecu.summon.serialssolutions.com

Hussain, D., & Bhushan, B. (2011). Posttraumatic stress and growth among Tibetan refugees: The mediating role of cognitive, emotional regulation strategies. *Journal of Clinical Psychology*, 67(7), 720–735.

Hussain, D., & Bhushan, B. (2013). Posttraumatic growth experiences among Tibetan refugees: A qualitative investigation. *Qualitative Research in Psychology*, 10(2), 204–216.

Janoff-Bulman, R. (1992). *Shattered assumptions: Toward a new psychology of trauma*. New York: Free Press.

Jayawickreme, D. E. R. (2011). *Well-being and war: Competencies and posttraumatic growth among war-affected populations in Sri Lanka* (Doctoral Dissertation). ProQuest Information & Learning, US. (72). Retrieved from http://ezproxy.ecu.edu.au

Johnson, H., & Thompson, A. (2006). The development and maintenance of posttraumatic stress disorder (PTSD) in civilian adult survivors of war trauma and torture: A review. *Clinical Psychology Review*, 28(1), 36–47.

Joseph, S., & Butler, L. D. (2010). Positive changes following adversity. *PTSD Research Quarterly, 21*(3), 1–7.

Joseph, S., & Linley, P. A. (2005). Positive adjustment to threatening events: An organismic valuing theory of growth through adversity. *Review of General Psychology, 9*(3), 262–280.

Joseph, S., & Linley, P. A. (2006). Growth following adversity: Theoretical perspectives and implications for clinical practice. *Clinical Psychology Review, 26*(8), 1041–1053.

Joseph, S., Murphy, D., & Regel, S. (2012). An affective-cognitive processing model of posttraumatic growth. *Clinical Psychology and Psychotherapy, 19*(4), 316–325.

Karanci, A., & Acaturk, C. (2005). Post-traumatic growth among Marmara earthquake survivors involved in disaster preparedness as volunteers. *Traumatology, 11*(4), 307–322.

Kinzie, D. J., 2006. Immigrants and refugees: The psychiatric perspective. *Transcultural Psychiatry, 43*(4), 577–591.

Kroo, A., & Nagy, H. (2011). Posttraumatic growth among traumatized Somali refugees in Hungary. *Journal of Loss and Trauma, 16*(5), 440–458.

Lechner, S., & Weaver, K. (2009). Lessons learned about benefit finding among individuals with cancer or HIV/AIDS. In C. L. Park, S. C. Lechner, M. H. Antoni, & A. L. Stanton (Eds.), *Medical illness and positive life change: Can crisis lead to personal transformation?* (pp. 107–124). Washington, DC: American Psychological Association.

Linley, P., & Joseph, S. (2004). Positive change following trauma and adversity: A review. *Journal of Traumatic Stress, 17*(1), 11–21.

McMillen, J. C., & Fisher, R. H. (1998). The perceived benefit scales: Measuring perceived positive life changes after negative events. *Social Work Research, 22*(3), 173–187.

Mattoon, L. (2011). *The gift of trauma: Stories of posttraumatic growth and spiritual transformation in war survivors from Uganda and Vietnam* (Doctoral Dissertation). ProQuest Information & Learning, US. (71), Retrieved from http://ezproxy.ecu.edu.au

Meyerson, D. A., Grant, K. E., Carter, J. S., & Kilmer, R. P. (2011). Posttraumatic growth among children and adolescents: A systematic review. *Clinical Psychology Review, 31*(6), 949–964.

Murray, K. E., Davidson, G. R., & Schweitzer, J. (2008). *Psychological wellbeing of refugees resettling in Australia: A literature review prepared for the Australian psychological Society*. Melbourne: Australian Psychological Society. Retrieved from www.psychology.org.au/publications/statements/refugees

Nuttman-Shwartz, O., Dekel, R., & Tuval-Mashiach, R. (2011). Post-traumatic stress and growth following forced relocation. *British Journal of Social Work, 41*(3), 486–501.

Palic, S., & Elklit, A. (2010). Psychosocial treatment of posttraumatic stress disorder in adult refugees: A systematic review of prospective treatment outcome studies and a critique. *Journal of Affective Disorders, 131*(1–3), 8–23.

Park, C. L. (2004). The notion of growth following stressful life experiences: Problems and prospects. *Psychological Inquiry, 15*(1), 69–76.

Peterson, C., & Seligman, M. (2003). Character strengths before and after September 11. *Psychological Science, 14*(4), 381–384.

Powell, S., Rosner, R., Butollo, W., Tedeschi, R. G., & Calhoun, L. G. (2003). Posttraumatic growth after war: A study with former refugees and displaced people in Sarajevo. *Journal of Clinical Psychology, 59*(1), 71–83.

Rodgers, S. T. (2012). Exposing the hushed Latina immigration experience: The global reality of refugee-like situations in America. *The Global Studies Journal, 4*(1), 147–159.

Ryff, C. D., & Essex, M. J. (1992). The interpretation of life experience and well being: The sample case of relocation. *Psychology and Aging, 7*(4), 507–517.

Seligman, M., & Csikzentmihalyi, M. (2000). Positive psychology: An introduction. *American Psychologist, 55*(1), 5–14.

Splevins, K., Cohen, K., Bowley, J., & Joseph, J. (2010). Theories of posttraumatic growth: Cross-cultural perspectives. *Journal of Loss and Trauma: International Perspectives on Stress & Coping, 15*(3), 259–277.

Stanton, A. L., Danoff-Burg, S., Sworowski, L. A., Collins, C. A., Branstetter, A., Rodriguez-Hanley., . . . Austenfeld, J. L. (2002). Randomized controlled trial of written emotional expression and benefit finding in breast cancer patients. *Journal of Clinical Oncology, 20*(20), 4160–4168.

Steel, Z., Silove, D., Phan, T., & Bauman, A. (2002). Long-term effect of psychological trauma on the mental health of Vietnamese refugees resettled in Australia: A population-based study. *Lancet, 360*(9339), 1056–1062.

Tallman, B., Shaw, K., Schultz, J., & Altmaier, E. (2010). Well-being and posttraumatic growth in unrelated donor marrow transplant survivors: A nine-year longitudinal study. *Rehabilitation Psychology, 55*(2), 204–210.

Tedeschi, R. G., & Calhoun, L. G. (1996). The post-traumatic growth inventory: Measuring the positive legacy of trauma. *Journal of Traumatic Stress, 9*(3), 455–471.

Tedeschi, R. G., & Calhoun, L. G. (2004). Posttraumatic growth: Conceptual foundations and empirical evidence. *Psychological Inquiry, 15*(1), 1–10.

Tedeschi, R. G., & McNally, R. J. (2011). Can we facilitate posttraumatic growth in combat veterans? *American Psychologist, 66*(1), 19–24.

Teodorescu, D. S., Siqveland, J., Heir, T., Hauff, E., Wentzel-Larsen, T., & Lien, L. (2012). Posttraumatic growth, depressive symptoms, posttraumatic stress symptoms, post-migration stressors and quality of life in multi-traumatized psychiatric outpatients with a refugee background in Norway. *Health and Quality of Life Outcomes, 10*(1), 84–100.

United Nations High Commissioner for Refugees. (2012). *UNHCR Global Trends 2011*. Retrieved from www.unhcr.org

Vazquez, C., Cervellon, P., Perez-Sales, P., Vidales, D., & Gaborit, M. (2005). Positive emotions in earthquake survivors in El Salvador (2001). *Journal of Anxiety Disorders, 19*(3), 313–328.

20

Community-level resiliency intervention in a post-disaster environment

The importance of information

Sandra Prince-Embury

This chapter presents a case illustration of a community-level intervention in a post-disaster environment, mindful of core aspects of resilience. The intervention described is the Three Mile Island (TMI) Health and Environmental Information Series, a community course developed to provide information pertaining to unanswered questions that had remained among TMI community members since the March 28, 1979, nuclear accident at the Three Mile Island Nuclear Generating Facility. This intervention is described within the context of unique post-disaster psychosocial circumstances of the community at that time that contributed to chronic stress. These conditions included lack of clear, understandable information about the accident and its aftermath as well as loss of faith in experts associated with conflicting and incomplete information delivered by officials at the time of the accident. This experience has been referred to as an "information crisis" in the literature.

Also described are the assumptions underlying the design of the intervention: that the delivery of understandable information by credible experts would foster resilience in this community by addressing the "information crisis" created in the aftermath of the accident and that loss of faith in experts might be ameliorated by community participation in the selection of the topics and credible experts to discuss them. The intentions of the community course were the following: (1) to reduce the stressors of risk-related information by delivering the information in a manner designed to minimize emotional reactivity, (2) to restore a sense of mastery by providing understandable information that could be used by community members in processing their experience and making informed decisions, and (3) to restore a sense of relatedness in the community members who attended the course by providing direct personal access to experts who delivered credible information in a way that was understandable to the lay public.

Critical resiliency constructs

Definitions of resiliency have been numerous, and research has operated at different levels of analysis, each with its own language and caveats. Among these definitions of resilience, there are a number of shared features all relating to human strengths, some type of disruption and growth, adaptive coping, and positive outcomes following exposure to adversity (e.g. Bonanno, 2004; Connor & Davidson, 2003; Friborg, Hjemdal, Rosenvinge, & Martinussen, 2003; Masten & Curtis, 2000; Richardson, 2002). Masten and Obradović (2008) suggest the following regarding consideration of resilience in the face of disaster:

> In the event of a flu pandemic, bioterrorism, a natural disaster, or any other large-scale catastrophe, the best surveillance, equipment, communication systems, antiviral supplies, military, and emergency services in the world will not be effective without equal attention to the issues posed by human behavior under conditions of life-threatening danger to children and families. The adaptive systems for positive human adaptation and development, legacies of biological and cultural evolution, must be considered and enjoined to promote resilience.

Towards this end, Masten and Obradović (2008) and others have identified basic, core, adaptive systems that have repeatedly been related to resilience in children and adolescence (Masten & Coatsworth, 1998; Masten & Gewirtz, 2006; Masten & Obradović, 2006; Masten & Powell, 2003; Masten et. al., 2005) and adults (Bonanno, 2004; Charney, 2004). The following is a brief consideration of four of these adaptive systems with comments about how they might relate in the aftermath of technological disaster.

Attachment and sense of relatedness

In a review of resilience studies, Luthar (2006, p. 780) concluded, "Resilience rests, fundamentally, on relationships." Beginning in early development, an attachment figure provides a child with a secure base for reassurance under threat and, when conditions are relaxed, with the confidence to venture out to explore and learn about the world. Separation from attachment figures can cause extreme anxiety to the point of panic, particularly when a threat is perceived, and loss can induce profound grief. Sensitive attachment figures also serve a powerful regulatory function, up- or down-regulating stress and arousal or containing impulses. The presence of a secure-base attachment figure has been shown to moderate stress in threatening situations for infants and toddlers. Disaster may present a threat at the "attachment" level by separating family members, disrupting contact between family members, and obscuring information about the safety among family members. In such circumstances, locator systems and means for communication among family members is critical.

In the vicinity of TMI, findings of loss of faith in experts (Prince-Embury & Rooney, 1987) might be interpreted within this framework, whereby officials and experts who were relied upon to safeguard the community were lost as credible bases of security and replaced by a sudden realization among community members that they were on their own to interpret complex risk information that was beyond their understanding and training. For purposes of discussion, we may distinguish between "attachment", which refers to the psychological process that occurs in early childhood, and "relatedness", which exist in many forms throughout the course of development. At the community level, the aftermath of disaster may disrupt "relatedness" by polarizing community members from each other. For example many of those in the vicinity of the TMI plant worked at the plant and were out of work for as long as the nuclear facility was shut down. For these workers, finding alternative work that paid as well was not likely. On the other hand, members of the community who did not have a family member employed by the nuclear facility were diametrically opposed, wanting the plant to remain shut down. These circumstances contributed to fractures in the community, fewer sources of support, and heightened stress in community members who suddenly found themselves at odds with their neighbors.

Agency, self-efficacy, and the mastery motivation system

As noted by Robert White (1959) in his classic paper on competence and the mastery motivation system, human beings are motivated to adapt to the environment and to experience reward for perceived success. Albert Bandura (1997) elaborated on this system in his empirical work and theory concerning self-efficacy. People with a positive view of their own efficacy will exert more effort to succeed and are more likely to persist in the face of adversity. People who persist are more likely to succeed, which reinforces efforts to adapt. Thus, human individuals who overcome adversity report more positive views of their own effectiveness and self-worth, express more confidence about success, and experience pleasure in doing well. The mastery motivation system can be extinguished by prolonged exposure to unresponsive environments or uncontrollable events, which was noted in learned helplessness experiments (Seligman, 1975). Disaster, presents a threat to human sense of agency, mastery and control on many levels. Disaster by definition is an overwhelming life-threating circumstance that overwhelms one's resources to control outcome. The type of disaster and its aftermath influences the extent of this effect. Prior to the TMI accident, sense of mastery over the safety of community members in the vicinity of Three Mile Island had been deferred to the expertise of the experts and local officials who has assured them that there was little if any chance of an accident. The occurrence of the accident and associated conflicting information disrupted this sense of mastery. If the experts and officials had been wrong, then who was in charge of their safety? Confronted with this dilemma community members were forced to confront the realization that they did not have the expertise to protect themselves or to monitor the level of their safety. Remaining conditions of uncertainty about actual amounts of radiation released during and after the accident and possible health effects further obstructed a sense of mastery over possible consequences. Within this context, many area residents were motivated to seek information for themselves, forming citizens groups, conducting their own informal surveys and studies, and seeking experts who were considered credible. It was within the context of these community efforts that the TMI Public Health and Environmental Information Series was developed.

Central nervous systems for problem solving and information processing

Under conditions of high threat or adversity, the ability to continue thinking and planning effectively is characteristic of resilience; good intellectual skills show protective effects for children and adults dealing with adversity (Luthar, 2006; Masten, 2001). Absence of information or the presence of unclear, ambiguous, or conflicting information in the presence of disaster would impair individuals and the community collectively to process information effectively. It is likely that absence of clear, credible information in the aftermath of the TMI accident obstructed the ability of community members to effectively process information for problem solving. This ability to effectively process information may have been further compromised by chronic arousal and emotional reactivity sustained by conditions of uncertainty in the community.

Regulatory systems for controlling arousal, affect, attention, and action

Overcoming adversity often calls on self-regulation skills to continue functioning effectively under highly stressful or arousing circumstances. Many aspects of voluntary self-control, e.g. voluntary self-restraint and resolving conflicts between competing feelings, thoughts, and behaviors, are associated with higher competence as well as better adaptation during and following adversity and trauma (Masten & Coatsworth, 1998). Fear and anxiety, along with other negative emotions presented by disaster and its aftermath, can influence human self-control systems and the quality of executive functioning including information processing in the aftermath of crisis. High levels of arousal can interfere with decision making, working memory, and other forms of executive functioning. The degree to which one can manage arousal and direct the resources at hand are likely to play a critical role in disaster response and resilience.

In the past, decisions to withhold information from the public in the face of disaster have been justified by the intention of not creating panic. However, this approach has often back-fired when eventually conflicting information is released, resulting in loss of credibility for the information source and loss of faith in experts among the receiving community. Research in the vicinity of TMI following the accident has substantiated the presence of emotional arousal or heightened emotional reactivity (Baum, Gatchel, & Schaeffer, 1983). It is likely that this arousal in addition to incomplete and conflicting information dissemination obstructed information processing.

The nature of disaster

As is the case for defining "resilience," the definition of disaster is not a simple matter. The literature on disaster research and interventions is extensive and beyond the scope of this chapter. Therefore, a brief discussion relevant to this chapter follows. Disasters have been traditionally considered according to the extent of damage done and the extent to which that damage exceeds the ability of the impacted community to cope. Trainer and Bolin (1976) defined disasters as abrupt, unanticipated events that produce severe disruption and a need for relocation. Consideration of resiliency in the face of disaster is informed by consideration of the characteristics of the disaster. Protective factors that facilitate resiliency may differ across type of disaster and whether the intervention is during, immediately after or in the aftermath of the disaster.

Multiple consequences

The more elements of loss, change, lack of control, and uncertainty introduced by the disaster, the more potential psychological difficulty it presents. Disaster impact includes immediate and prolonged danger to self and others, loss of homes and possessions, and relocation in an unpredict-able fashion. The number of negative consequences and the cumulative effect will vary across individuals and their specific circumstances.

Man-made elements

In man-made disasters, there is frequently an assumed element of intentional neglect that is likely to engender more anger and prolonged bitterness. When there is perception that "those in charge or the experts" knew ahead of time and did not prevent or make adequate provi-sions for disaster, this creates another powerful dimension of disaster aftermath: intense anger and blame at those who are perceived to have been negligent or in some way irresponsible. For some this experience is a profound disillusionment or loss of faith that can undermine one's sense of well-being and sense of control. For those who already have lost faith and are skeptical of the intentions of others, such an event serves to confirm the distrust that already exists for them.

Invisible consequences

One characteristic of man-made disasters is that the threat of danger is often posed by invisible consequences such as radiation or other air-borne toxic substances. The lack of ability of community members to see or monitor radiation levels on their own presents ongoing circumstances of uncertainty. This was the case in the aftermath of Three Mile Island, where there had been conflicting reports of how much radiation had been released and continued to be released during clean-up, along with an inability to monitor this. Absence of the ability to see the threat would certainly obstruct effective information processing, thus undermining the community's ability to experience mastery in the situation. The psychological need for visible consequences is illustrated by the persistence of one community member in finding and recording mutated plants in the vicinity of the Three Mile Island facility to document that there had been some effect.

Lack of a clear end point

In circumstances when there is a clear end point, people can begin to recover. When there is no clear end point, it is harder to deal with because conditions of uncertainty are prolonged, closure is prevented, and steps toward recovery are delayed. In the aftermath of the Three Mile Island accident, there was extended clean-up of the damaged Unit 2 reactor (TMI-2) that took many years to complete. Included in this process was the illegal release of 43,000 curies of radioactive Kryton-85 between June and July of 1980. The evaporation of 2.3 million gallons of accident-generated radioactive water that began in December 1990 despite legal objections by a local community organization (TMIA). This evaporation was completed on October 28, 1993, resulting in the release of 658 curies of tritium over a three-year period. Thus, in addition to uncertainty about what radiation levels had been released at the time of the accident, there was continued uncertainty about the levels of radiation being released during clean-up.

Re-traumatization

When disaster conditions are prolonged, or when there is not a clear emergency plan in effect, victims are subject to re-traumatization. As in Katrina, when expected help did not come for some, or perceived promises were not kept, those who felt that they were in the clear may have experienced additional traumatization. In the aftermath of the Three Mile Island accident, residents were confronted with potential sources of re-traumatization. Public statements after the accident suggested that radiation releases and health effects were minimal with the implication that those who thought otherwise were "malcontents." In addition, community members faced restart of Unit 1 (TMI-1), the undamaged reactor, which had been shut down since the time of the accident. It is likely that both of these circumstances may have added stress onto and already stressed community (Prince-Embury, 1992; Prince-Embury & Rooney, 1988).

Three Mile Island nuclear accident

The accident at Unit 2 of the Three Mile Island Nuclear Generating Facility during which there was a partial core meltdown had presented a life crisis for the residents of the neighboring vicinity, the full extent of which had not been completely determined at the time of the conception of this course. At the onset of the accident, which began March 28, 1979, area residents faced threat of a hydrogen explosion and radiation release, were confronted with conflicting information, and, in some instances, were instructed to evacuate their homes (Baum et al., 1983; Bromet,

1980; Dohrenwend, Dohrenwend, Kasl, & Warheit, 1979; Houts, Cleary, & Hu, 1988; Houts & Goldhaber, 1981). TMI-1 had been in operation since September 1974, but TMI-2 had only been online since December 1978, ninety days prior to the accident. Since the accident, conflicting information had remained about the dose estimates of ionizing radiation released at that time, leaving many area residents with uncertainty about the possibility of health and genetic effects that might eventually develop (Lindy & Lindy, 1985).

During the 1979 accident, the nuclear power station at Three Mile Island experienced a pump malfunction, leading to exposure of the core, melting of fuel rods, release of radioactive emissions, and spilling of radioactive water on the reactor building floor. For several days, the release of incomplete, inconsistent, and contradictory information by responsible officials created an information crisis and loss of faith in the credibility of these officials. An example of the information provided at the time of the accident is expressed in the press conference of Lt. Governor William Scranton of Pennsylvania, released on March 28, 1979, 4:30 p.m.:

> This is an update on the incident at Three-Mile Island Nuclear Power plant today. This situation is more complex than the company first led us to believe. We are taking more tests. And at this point, we believe there is still no danger to public health. Metropolitan Edison has given you and us conflicting information. We just concluded a meeting with the company officials and hope this briefing will clear up most of your questions. There has been a release of radioactivity into the environment. The magnitude of this release is still being determined, but there is no evidence yet that it has resulted in the presence of dangerous levels. The company has informed us that from about 11 a.m. until about 1:30 p.m., Three-Mile Island discharged into the air, steam that contained detectable amounts of radiation.

Subsequently, 140,000 residents evacuated when women and children were advised by the governor to do so after earlier reassurances that conditions were safe.

Baum et al. (1983) found chronically elevated levels of stress in TMI area residents as long as six years after the accident and related this to the unique circumstances of man-made disasters including loss of credibility of responsible authorities and remaining conditions of uncertainty. In addition, Davidson and Baum (1986) found that TMI-area residents reported greater feelings of helplessness and less perceived control over their environment than did control subjects and that this appeared to contribute to ongoing stress among TMI residents. Additional studies of Middletown residents revealed a relationship between perceived TMI threat and perceived lack of control and loss of faith in experts among residents in the vicinity after the accident (Prince-Embury & Rooney, 1987). Lack of control was associated with greater perceived threat among area residents consistent with prevailing theory. This finding held primarily for recent arrivers however. Among those present at the time of the accident, loss of faith in experts was more significantly related to lack of perceived control than was threat. Prince-Embury and Rooney (1987) concluded that a profound loss of faith in experts had been a significant psychological impact of the accident for area residents present at the time and that loss of faith had supplanted perceived threat as a psychological concomitant of perception of control.

Additional research by Prince-Embury and Rooney (1987) surveyed a stratified random sample of Middletown residents to determine the extent of interest in information associated with the accident. This survey indicated that 79% were interested in information on cancer detection and treatment, 58% were interested in radiation monitoring, and 56% were interested in information on the epidemiological distribution of cancer in the area. This level of interest in information related to TMI substantiated the need for the Information Series.

Sandra Prince-Embury

The Three Mile Island Public Health and Environmental Information Series

Four years after the TMI accident, the author of this chapter began a collaboration with a small group of community activists representing a number of community organizations, for the purpose of addressing issues remaining in the aftermath of the TMI accident that might have been contributing to continued elevated stress cited earlier. The Three Mile Island Public Health and Environmental Information Series was the result of this collaboration. The intentions of this community course were the following: (1) to reduce the stressors of ambiguous information related to the TMI accident by identifying and delivering relevant information in a manner designed to minimize emotional reactivity, (2) to restore a sense of mastery by providing understandable information to be used by community members in processing their experiences and making informed decisions, and (3) to restore a sense of relatedness in the community members who attended the course by providing direct personal access to experts who delivered credible information in a way that was understandable to the lay public. The proposal was approved by the TMI Public Health Fund, and the course was implemented. Major aspects in the design of the course are presented in the following sections. For a more detailed description, see Prince-Embury (2013).

Underlying assumption regarding understandability, stress, and perceived credibility

The development of the TMI course was based on three of theoretical assumptions. First, access to information related to possible adverse circumstances is sought by impacted community members and can be delivered in a format and manner that increases the experience of understanding of the lay public. Second, intervention in a stressed population should not be avoided because of possible stress reactions but should take this possible effect into account so as to not elevate stress unnecessarily. Such an intervention should address the potential for heightened emotional reactivity and should be designed to minimize the possibility that heightened reactivity will interfere with adequate information processing. Third, an intervention delivered in a stressed population should be sensitive to and address sources of lowered credibility such as perceived and unexplained discrepancies between expert opinions.

Access to information about possible negative circumstances

Whether or not individuals prefer information about possible threat conditions has been a matter of considerable theoretical and empirical interest (Averill, O'Brien, & Dewitt, 1977; Averill & Rosenn, 1972; Berlyne, 1960; Miller & Mangan, 1983; Monat, 1976; Monat, Averill, & Lazarus, 1972). According to the information–seeking model, when faced with uncertainty, people and animals seek information and strive for certainty (Berlyne, 1960). In an earlier study, Prince-Embury and Rooney (1987) had found that 56% to 79% of a stratified random sample of Middletown residents expressed interest in information on radiation epidemiology and cancer five years after the accident. These authors also found that interest in information was significantly correlated with worry about these topics among area residents. Assumptions prevalent at the time of the course were that stressed individuals do not desire information about adverse circumstances particularly if this information does not increase predictability. Miller and Mangan (1983) addressing this issue found that delivery of information that matches the information–seeking style of the individual minimized anxiety while that which does not match increases it. The TMI series was based on the assumption that part of the healing process in the aftermath of

254

technological disaster was the availability of accurate, reliable, and understandable information in a way that allows individuals to pace information intake consistent with their ability to integrate information into a meaningful context. It was recognized, however, that complete healing of a community from the traumatic elements of such an event would not occur from a one-time limited intervention.

Attention to emotional reactivity in stressed populations

Davidson and Baum (1986) identified members of a sample of TMI residents as manifesting symptoms of post-traumatic stress. Researchers have noted that one aspect of post-traumatic stress state is hypervigilance or the ability to continue to respond to stimuli with emotional intensity appropriate only to emergency situations (Kardiner, 1941; Krystal, 1978; Vanderkolk, 1987). McCurdy (1943) identified events that are "near-miss" catastrophes, such as the TMI accident, as critical determinants of hypervigilance. Previous research suggests that hypervigilance interferes with an individual's ability to assess situations calmly as well as the ability to process information appropriately. Specifically, hypervigilance has been described as impairing cognitive functioning by constricting cognition with premature closure, restricting range of attention, narrowing range of perceived alternatives, reduction in immediate memory, and fostering of simplistic ideas (George, 1974; Hamilton, 1975; Janis, 1971; Janis & Leventhal, 1968; Janis & Mann, 1977). Thus, residents at TMI who might remain hypervigilant were seen as possibly less capable of processing information accurately and completely. Among the factors most frequently implicated as antecedents of hypervigilant reactions are lack of perceived control over dangerous events and lack of preparatory information about what is to be expected (Epstein, 1973; Janis, 1971; Monat et al., 1972). The TMI course was designed mindful of potential interference by hypervigilance in the information processing by course participants.

Attention to potentially perceived discrepancies

Reports of incidents during and following the TMI accident suggest that the situation had lent itself to cognitive contradiction in that area residents were given contradictory messages during and after the accident: local radio stations had reported safe conditions, cable stations at a distance were reporting warnings, and officials were offering reassuring messages to be followed by emergency evacuation instructions (Lindy & Lindy, 1985; Walsh, 1988). The origin of theoretical concern about congruence of reality and expectation is found in the theory of cognitive dissonance offered by Festinger (1957). According to Festinger, dissonance refers to cognitive contradiction, which is associated with discomfort and drive toward consistency. It was hypothesized that sensitivity to information inconsistency remained in the post-accident environment and might be relevant to the delivery of new information. The TMI course design took into account the possible negative effects of perceived contradiction and inconsistency among course presenters.

Providing access to understandable information

A primary goal of the information series was providing information that was understandable. Increased potential for individual understanding of information was addressed in preliminary instruction to scientist presenters to express concepts in lay language. Increased potential for individual understanding was also addressed in the format of each session, which provided the second hour for dialogue and individual's questions to the speaker. This format was implemented to address the specific questions of individuals so that they might integrate the information into a context that was understandable to them. It was also believed that information received in an interactive fashion could be more readily adjusted to the unique needs of the individuals.

Structure for managing emotional reactivity to lessen the possibility of increased stress as an obstacle to understanding

The series was based on the assumption that communication of information in an environment of intense polarization on different sides of the nuclear power debate (Walsh, 1988) must in some way address the possibility of intense emotionality among course participants. Ground rules were developed by this author to maximize the likelihood of information flow and comprehension by minimizing or controlling emotional reactivity. The specific ground rules were read to participants at the beginning of each session and were presented in the form of a mutually agreed upon verbal contract for participation in the sessions. Additional mechanisms for managing emotional reactivity included the following: break times between the first and second half of each session and following each session allowed informal debriefing to occur. The opportunity to express questions and comments to the speaker in a formal way during the second half of each session served also as a tension release. The coordinator of the series, a psychologist, and two psychology graduate students were available to individuals who wanted to express concerns individually.

Structure for managing uncertainty and perceived discrepancy in expert opinion as sources of lowered credibility

Informal observation and community collaboration revealed that, at the time of the accident and afterwards, members of the Three Mile Island community were confronted with discrepancies between reports of experts and between official statements. This was associated with a significant loss of credibility attributed to official statements. This lack of perceived credibility of information was associated with a significant loss of faith in experts and demoralization (Dohrenwend et al., 1979; Prince-Embury & Rooney, 1987). Lack of credibility was addressed in the choice of credible scientist presenters and in designing the structure of sessions. The choice of scientist experts included national experts in their areas of expertise, who were knowledgeable about areas of uncertainty and disagreement in their field and could discuss this openly. Furthermore, many of these individuals were identified by a panel of scientists commissioned by the Three Mile Island Public Health Fund, as politically neutral on potentially controversial issues relevant to their areas of expertise. In addition, dialogue periods in each session allowed attendees to ask questions. For more specific information about the structure of the community course and participant responses, see Prince-Embury (1991, 1992, 2013).

General conclusions

Overall, this description provides a case example of the dissemination of information in an environmentally impacted polarized community. Also illustrated is how a community intervention may be designed based on unique needs and remaining stressors in the aftermath of technological disaster informed by an understanding of core aspects of community resilience. It is recognized, however, that the Three Mile Public Health and Environmental Information Series occurred twenty-six years ago and much has changed since that time. For example access to information has been greatly increased by prevalent access to the internet in the homes of technologically developed societies. However, the possibility of technological disaster is ever present as evidenced by the disaster in the Japanese nuclear reactor at Fukushima. In addition, threat of terrorist attacks has increased the environment of uncertainty world-wide. For this reason, consideration of information dissemination as a means of fostering resiliency in the aftermath of technological disaster or under pervasive conditions of uncertainty remains a valid pursuit.

This importance of communicating accurately about risks was persuasively expressed by Baruch Fischhoff in a special issue of the *American Psychologist*, entitled "9/11: Ten Years Later" (Fischhoff, 2011): "Psychological Research has essential roles to play in identifying the public's information needs, designing responsive communications and evaluating their success. Fulfilling these roles requires policies that treat two-way communication as central" (p. 520). Fischhoff warns against obstacles to this pursuit such as underestimating the public's ability to learn and make decisions, a tendency seen in the myth of panic and popular accounts of human frailty. In this article, Fischhoff identifies steps to be taken in creating communications about risks of terror (or anything else). Some of these steps may be summarized as follows: identifying the information most relevant to helping audience members make decisions; identifying subject matter experts, who can ensure fidelity to the best available technological knowledge; drafting communications in precise and comprehensive form; and assuring the maintenance of respectful, two-way communications channels. To the extent that the Three Mile Island Health and Environmental Information Series followed these steps in 1985, it provided an early model for threat-related communication.

References

Averill, J. R., O'Brien, L., & DeWitt, G. W. (1977). The influence of response effectiveness on the preference for warning and on physiological stress reactions. *Journal of Personality, 45*(3), 396–418.

Averill, J. R., & Rosenn, M. (1972). Vigilant and non-vigilant coping strategies and psych-physiological stress reactions during the anticipation of an electric shock. *Journal of Personality and Social Psychology, 23*(1), 128–141.

Bandura, A. (1997). Self-efficacy: The exercise of control. New York, NY, USA: Freeman.

Baum, A., Gatchel, R. J., & Schaeffer, M. A. (1983). Emotional, behavioral and physiological effects of chronic stress at Three Mile Island. *Journal of Consulting and Clinical Psychology, 51*(4), 565–572.

Berlyne, D. E. (1960). *Conflict arousal and curiosity.* New York: McGraw Hill.

Bonanno, G. A. (2004). Have we underestimated the human capacity to thrive after extremely aversive events? *American Psychologist, 59*(1), 20–28.

Bromet, E. (1980). *Three Mile Island: Mental health findings.* Pittsburgh: Western Psychiatric Institute and Clinic and the University of Pittsburgh.

Charney, D. (2004). Psychobiological mechanisms of resilience and vulnerability: Implications for successful adaptation to extreme stress. *American Journal of Psychiatry, 161*(2), 195–216.

Connor, K. M., & Davidson, J. R. T. (2003). Development of a new resilience scale: The Connor-Davidson resilience scale (CD-RISC). *Depression and Anxiety, 18*(2), 76–82.

Davidson, L., & Baum, A. (1986). Chronic stress and post-traumatic stress disorders. *Journal of Consulting and Clinical Psychology, 54*(3), 303–308.

Dohrenwend, B. P., Dohrenwend, B. S., Kasl, S. V., & Warheit, G. J. (1979). *Report of the Task Force on Behavioral Effects of the President's Commission on the accident at Three Mile Island.* Washington, DC.

Epstein, S. (1973). Expectancy and magnitude of reaction to a noxious. *Psychophysiology, 10*(1), 100–107.

Festinger, L. (1957). *A theory of cognitive dissonance.* Stanford, CA: Stanford University Press.

Fischhoff, B. (2011). Communicating about the risks of terrorism (or anything else). *American Psychologist, 66*(6), 520–531.

Friborg, O., Hjemdal, O., Rosenvinge, J. H., & Martinussen, M. (2003). A new rating scale for adult resilience: What are the central protective resources behind healthy adjustment? *International Journal of Methods in Psychiatric Research, 12*(2), 65–76.

George, A. (1974). Adaptation to stress in political decision making: The individual, small group and organizational content. In G. V. Coelho, D. A. Hamberg, & R. J. E. Adams (Eds.), *Coping and adaptation* (pp. 176–245). New York: Basic Books.

Hamilton, V. (1975). Socialization and information processing: A capacity model of anxiety-induced performance deficits. In I. G. Sarason & C. D. Speilberger (Eds.), *Stress & anxiety* (Vol. 2, pp. 45–68). Washington, DC: Hemisphere.

Houts, P. S., Cleary, P. O., & Hu, Teh-Wei (1988). *The Three Mile Island crisis: Psychological, social and economic impacts on the surrounding population.* University Park and London: The Pennsylvania State University Press.

Houts, P. S., & Goldhaber, N. K. (1981). Psychological and social effects on the population surrounding Three Mile Island after the nuclear accident. In S. Majumdar (Ed.), *Energy, environment and the economy* (pp. 151–164). PA: Pennsylvania Academy of Science.

Janis, I. L. (1971). *Stress & frustration.* New York: Harcourt.

Janis, I. L., & Leventhal, H. (1968). Human reactions to stress. In E. Borgatta & W. Lambert (Eds.), *Handbook of personality theory and research* (pp. 167–224). Chicago: Rand McNally.

Janis, I. L., & Mann, L. (1977). *Decision making.* New York: The Free Press.

Kardiner, A. (1941). *The Traumatic Neuroses of War.* New York: P. Hoeber.

Krystal, H. (1978). Trauma and affects. *Psychoanalytical Study of the Child, 33,* 81–116.

Lindy, J. D., & Lindy, J. G. (1985). Observation in the media and disaster recovery period. In J. Laube & S. A. Murphy (Eds.), *Perspectives on disaster recovery* (pp. 295–303). Norwalk, CT, US: Appleton-Century-Crofts.

Luthar, S. S. (2006). Resilience in development: A synthesis of research across five decades. In D. Cicchetti & D. J. Cohen (Eds.), *Developmental psychopathology. Volume 3: Risk, disorder, and adaptation* (2nd ed., pp. 739–795). New York, NY: Wiley.

McCurdy, J. (1943). *The structure of morale.* New York: Macmillan.

Masten, A. S. (2001). Ordinary magic: Resilience processes in development. *American Psychologist, 56*(3), 227–238.

Masten, A. S., & Coatsworth, J. D. (1998). The development of competence in favorable and unfavorable environments: Lessons from research on successful children. *American Psychologist, 53*(2), 205–220.

Masten, A. S., & Curtis, W. J. (2000). Integrating competence and psychopathology: Pathways toward a comprehensive science of adaptation in development [Special issue]. *Development & Psychopathology, 12*(3), 529–550.

Masten, A. S., & Gewirtz, A. H. (2006). Vulnerability and resilience in early child development. In K. McCartney & D. A. Phillips (Eds.), *Handbook of early childhood Development* (pp. 22–43). Malden, MA, USA: Blackwell.

Masten, A. S., & Obradovic, J. (2006). Competence and resilience in development. *Annals of the New York Academy of Science, 1094*(1), 13–27.

Masten, A. S., & Obradović, J. (2008). Disaster preparation and recovery: Lessons from research on resilience in human development. *Ecology and Society, 13*(1), 9.

Masten, A. S., & Powell, J. L. (2003). A resilience framework for research, policy, and practice. In S. S. Luthar (Ed.), *Resilience and vulnerability: Adaptation in the context of childhood adversities* (pp. 1–25). New York, NY: Cambridge University Press.

Masten, A., S., Roisman, G. I., Long, J. D., Burt, K. B., Obradovic, J., Riley, J. R., . . . Tellegen, A. (2005). Developmental cascades: Linking academic achievement and externalizing and internalizing symptoms over 20 years. *Developmental Psychology, 41*(5), 733–746.

Miller, I. M., & Mangan, C. E. (1983). Interacting effects of information and coping style in adaptation to gynecology and stress: Should the doctor tell all? *Journal of Personality and Social Psychology, 45*(1), 223–236.

Monat, A. (1976). Temporal uncertainty, anticipation time, and cognitive coping under threat. *Journal of Trauma Stress, 2*(2), 32–43.

Monat, A., Averill, J. R., & Lazarus, R. S. (1972). Anticipatory stress and coping reactions under various conditions of uncertainty. *Journal of Personality and Social Psychology, 24*(2), 237–252.

Prince-Embury, S. (1991). Information seekers in the aftermath of technological disaster. *Journal of Applied Social Psychology, 21*(7), 569–584.

Prince-Embury, S. (1992). Information attributes as related to psychological symptoms and perceived control among information seekers in the aftermath of technological disaster. *Journal of Applied Social Psychology, 22*(14), 1148–1159.

Prince-Embury, S. (2013). Community-level resiliency intervention in a post-disaster environment: The Three Mile Island health and environmental information series: Theoretical assumptions, implementation and participant response. In S. Prince-Embury & D. Saklofske (Eds.), *Resilience in children, adolescents and adults: Translating research for practice* (pp. 227–237). New York: Springer.

Prince-Embury, S., & Rooney, R. (1987). Perception of control and faith in experts among residents in the vicinity of Three Mile Island. *Journal of Applied Social Psychology, 17*(11), 953–968.

Prince-Embury, S., & Rooney, J. (1988). Psychological symptoms of residents in the aftermath of the Three Mile Island nuclear accident and restart. *Journal of Social Psychology, 128*(6), 779–790.

Richardson, G. E. (2002). The metatheory of resilience and resiliency. *Journal of Clinical Psychology, 58*(3), 307–321.

Seligman, M. E. P. (1975). *Helplessness: On depression, development, and death.* San Francisco: W. H. Freeman.

Trainer, P., & Bolin, R. (1976). Persistent effects of disasters on daily activities: A cross-cultural comparison. *Mass Emergencies, 1,* 279–290.

Vanderkolk, K. (1987). *Psychological trauma.* Washington: American Psychiatric Press.

Walsh, E. (1988). *Democracy in the shadows.* New York: Greenwood Press.

White, R. W. (1959). Motivation reconsidered: The concept of competence. *Psychological Review, 66,* 297–333.

21

United States Special Operations Command

Reducing risk by fostering resiliency

Lori Holleran, Kate Maslowski,
Harry L. McCleary, Captain Gordon Hanson,
Captain Thomas Chaby, Karen J.
Friday and Bruce Bongar

Throughout the past decade, the prevalence of suicide fatalities among special operators and general military populations has exceeded rates observed during the 1900s, suggesting a modern epidemic of soldiers taking their own lives (Nock et al., 2013). Suicide rates among military service members have historically been lower than those witnessed amongst their civilian counterparts. However, between 2005 and 2008, suicide fatalities within the Army nearly doubled and surpassed the civilian population rates for the first time in history (Black, Gallaway, Bell, & Ritchie, 2011).

In the past, suicide interventions implemented by the United States military have been targeted towards prevention and detection systems. While the United States government and its respective military branches have implemented several interventions in response to the increased suicidal ideation and behaviors of its service members over the past decade, suicide rates have not significantly decreased (Black et al., 2011). This ineffectiveness in managing risk for suicide is encouraging subsets of the military to develop their own intervention programs in an effort to face the problem from a more localized framework.

One group in particular, the United States Special Operations Command (SOCOM), is taking a different approach towards suicide prevention. SOCOM is addressing risk by removing the focus from suicide prevention programs, and emphasizing the physical, psychological, social, and spiritual well-being, or overall resiliency, of its elite war fighters (United States Special Operations Command, 2013). The following examines the interventions employed by the Department of Defense (DOD) and the military over the last decade to help mitigate suicidal behaviors amongst the general military population as well as special operations forces (SOF). Specifically, information-gathering and interpersonal strategies utilized over the past decade will be reviewed. The success, or lack thereof, of these interventions and the ways in which they informed SOCOM's innovative strategy to foster resiliency will be considered. Finally, we will examine the core components of this vanguard strategy and highlight potential implications for future military and SOF.

Information gathering strategies

Department of Defense Suicide Event Report

In recent years, the DOD has implemented the Department of Defense Suicide Event Report (DoDSER) to track suicide-related fatalities (Alexander, Reger, Smolenski, & Fullerton, 2014). When a service member's death has been ruled a suicide by the Armed Forces Medical Examiner System, the command is required to make a record in the DoDSER regarding the service members death and history. The DoDSER is informed by an epidemiological data collection system used to analyze the circumstances of completed suicides amongst military service members (Alexander et al., 2014).

The DoDSER examines both protective and suspected risk factors and can be utilized to identify possible intervention points for healthcare providers and military leaders (Bush et al., 2013). However, it only collects data on individuals who have completed suicide (Alexander et al., 2014). The system could be used to predict suicidal behaviors within the general military population if the DoDSER gathered reported experiences of suicidal ideation and suicide attempts that did not result in a fatality, and therefore it could be increasingly effective. Additionally, inconsistency and lack of standardization in reporting limit the DoDSER's effectiveness and further complicates the reported suicide data (Stein & Ursano, 2013).

Army Study to Assess Risk and Resilience in Service Members (Army STARRS)

In 2008 the Army implemented the Army STARRS program in response to the Army's increasing suicide rates. The Army STARRS is a database that is jointly funded and supported by the Army and the National Institute of Mental Health. The program is aimed at further investigating suicidal behavior and ideation amongst active duty service members in an attempt to inform how the military understands modifiable risk factors (Stein & Ursano, 2013). This data can then be utilized to inform policy makers and high-ranking military advisors when making policy adjustments to mitigate suicide risk.

In terms of size, the Army STARRS is incomparable to most other suicide databases and has the potential for significant data analysis within the general military population (Jobes, 2013). However, the inconsistency of reporting can be problematic with the Army STARRS, as it is with DoDSER (Stein & Ursano, 2013), yet both yield a large amount of data regarding risk. For example it is generally accepted that one of the most significant risks for suicide is a history of suicide attempts (Weiner, Richmond, Conigliaro, & Wiebe, 2011). This type of information is vital in creating future preventative interventions. Several studies have already been conducted examining the relationship between suicidal behavior and numerous factors, including demographics (Ursano et al., 2015), gender (Street et al., 2015), combat experience (Jobes, 2013), and recent recruitment into the Army (Kessler et al., 2013) using data from the Army STARRS. The STARRS program represents a substantial effort on the part of the Army to engage in preventative actions to reduce suicidal behavior.

Mental health assessments

There are several mental health factors that influence suicidal behaviors and ideation, such as depression, post-traumatic stress disorder (PTSD), and traumatic brain injury (TBI) (Bliese, Wright, Adler, Thomas, & Hoge, 2007). The United States and several other countries are now implementing Post Deployment Health Assessments (PDHA) in order to guide and facilitate mental health treatment referrals. Depression, alcohol use, PTSD, and relationship and sleep problems are some of the potential suicide risk factors screened for in these post-deployment assessments (Hughes, Wagner, Willkomm, & Smykala, 2004). PDHAs were integrated into standard practice by each of the armed services in April 2003. Moreover, The Post Deployment Health Reassessment (PDHRA) was mandated in March 2005.

Both the PDHA and the PDHRA are required health assessments for all armed servicemen returning from deployment. The PDHA must be completed within 30 days, and the PDHRA, within 90 to 180 days post-deployment (Sharkey & Rennix, 2011). These assessments examine potential risk factors for suicide and mental health issues in order to address symptomology as soon as possible (Bliese et al., 2007). These assessments inform commanders, physicians, and mental health providers of potential developing or current mental health issues that may influence risk for suicide and overall performance.

Interpersonal approaches

Social support

Interpersonal support is a well-accepted protective factor for suicide, demonstrating an inverse relationship with suicidal ideation and behaviors (Bryan & Hernandez, 2013). While some debate remains regarding the function of social support and whether it directly or indirectly mitigates suicidal risk, it is widely agreed upon that social support diminishes risk of suicide (Bryan & Hernandez, 2013). This is witnessed amongst active duty United States Air Force personnel, with greater levels of perceived social support correlating with lower levels of suicidal ideation. This finding supports previous research, examining risk witnessed in the special operations community prior to 2010, demonstrating that the lower suicide prevalence was related to the smaller unit populations, and subsequently increased cohesion amongst its members (Hanwella & Silva, 2012). However, within the last three years, a greater prevalence of suicide has been reported within SOCOM than within the general Army population (Shanker & Oppel, 2014; Ursano et al., 2015).

Military chaplain services

Chaplains serve as individuals that special operators can consult with while in theater, in daily life, and throughout one's service regarding spiritual and emotional issues. Chaplains have a unique role when considering that they have the power to maintain confidentiality even when service members report dangerous behavior, while mental health professionals and other service members do not hold this right. Military chaplains have served a role in the armed forces since General George Washington established the Chaplain Corps in 1775 (Trotter, 2014). Since then, they have served a large role in the intervention processes in multiple facets.

Military mental health providers train military chaplains to evaluate who is "at risk" for suicide and to provide referrals to those identified (Budd, 1999). This training is mandatory for military chaplains, in an attempt to offer chaplains and mental health providers an opportunity to work as a team to aid in reducing risk. This collaboration is important due to stereotypes and biases regarding mental health within the military, potentially leading service members to feel more comfortable voicing their issues and concerns to a chaplain.

Command involvement

SOCOM and the general military are entities that possess a heavily structured ranking system. The highest-ranking officer within a unit or battalion has the power to implement programs that will reach each individual special forces operator (Theriault, 2015). Moreover, they have the capability to mandate trainings and services. This command involvement sets a tone conveying what is a priority and what is of secondary importance within any given environment. Command support involves the monitoring and implementation of orders or policy that help to reduce suicidal behaviors (Warner et al., 2011).

One form of command support involves the creation of Suicide Risk Management Teams (SRMT). These teams consist of representatives from a command in the areas of mental health, medical, and the chaplain corps. The SRMT encourages junior officers and non-commissioned officers (NCOs) to take the lead in suicide prevention practices. It is then the job of these officers and NCOs to promote help-seeking behavior regarding mental health issues (Warner et al., 2011). Through advising the commanding officer regarding what strategies can and should be implemented, SRMT ultimately influence suicide risk approaches within a unit or battalion.

Education and awareness programs

Education and awareness programs are implemented regarding numerous situations and issues that apply directly to service members, with the goal of providing information, increasing knowledge, and encouraging responsiveness to various topics relevant to soldiers, marines, sailors, and airmen. Within military culture, there exists a stigmatization regarding seeking mental health services (Vogt, 2011). This broad issue, and specifically concerns related to suicide risk, are addressed through mandatory suicide awareness programs.

One specific suicide-related program is the Army Suicide Intervention Skills Training Program. This is a program that the Army and other services have adopted that aims to teach military populations about the possible warning signs of suicide and how to seek help if and when they need it (Reyes & Hicklin, 2005). This program has demonstrated utility within the general military; however, special operators belong to a small elite community where reputation is, not only a social aspect of life, but also a factor that influences occupational advancement (Shanker & Oppel, 2014). Maintaining this professional reputation amongst others factors may make it more difficult for a special operator to seek mental health treatment or refer a peer to mental health treatment despite knowledge of a possible hazardous situation.

Moving forward

Afghanistan, Iraq, and other theaters of war create austere combat environments. Extreme weather, rigid operational tempo, unknown length of deployments, and challenging terrain further complicate the war zone experience of special operators (Reyes & Hicklin, 2005).

However, while combat places unique physical and psychological stressors on military individuals, combat experience has not been found to directly influence suicidal behaviors (Jobes, 2013). This is not to imply that combat exposure does not influence risk for suicide. The stressors of these operators, often related to combat, can be complicated by substance abuse, historical developmental concerns, and psychiatric illness (Reyes & Hicklin, 2005). Furthermore, traumatic experiences that involve loss, separation, and changes in self-esteem may exacerbate their stress levels. The heavy burden of these potential combinations of factors can trigger suicidal behaviors.

Despite all of these interventions for suicide prevention, which represent just some of the components that the military has put into place in order to address the issue of risk, the frequency of both suicide attempts and suicide completions have not declined significantly within either the special operations community or the general military population (Black et al., 2011). Instead, these strategies have resulted in the creation of large databases regarding possible risk factors and stressors related to suicide. Unfortunately, to date, more attention has been placed on identifying risks factors related to suicide, which have not been found to significantly impact the current suicide epidemic, rather than protective factors (Bryan & Hernandez, 2013).

The next foreseeable step is to utilize the expanding cache of research findings to implement policies and measures, which promote lifestyle and occupational changes to effectively address suicidal ideation and behavior. Currently, SOCOM is attempting to do just that. SOCOM has committed itself to advancing its resources and interventions in order to confront this issue in an innovative way. In order to effectively address this occurrence, SOCOM has adapted its response to the presence of risk, striving to be more proactive than reactive in its approach. Completed suicides and suicidal behaviors among elite war fighters in the special operations community quickly resonate within this exclusive and small community. Thus, suicides under the SOCOM umbrella do not go unnoticed.

Building resilience through four domains

The life of a US Special Forces operator is demanding and unique and involves not only the service member but also their family. The demands that this prestigious career requires can be overwhelming at times for both the operator and his family. More recently, the demands of this career have seemingly been too much to bear for forty-nine special operators, all of whom committed suicide since 2011 (Shanker & Oppel, 2014). In response to the unprecedented suicide rate witnessed amongst these elite combat soldiers, Congress has shifted millions of dollars into therapies for PTSD, TBI, and building resiliency within the SOF. To build resiliency and improve readiness for the amplified operational expectations that are associated with the job, SOCOM has focused on four specific domains within each service member's life (United States Special Operations Command, 2013). These four domains emphasize the physical, psychological, social, and spiritual well-being of each SOF operator.

Physical performance

Physical standards are a priority in the military. Within the SOF, physical health can make the difference between a successful or failed mission (Miles, 2013). The importance of physical exercise and conditioning and its impact on mental health has become common knowledge within the general public, including the improved mood and enhanced cognitive functioning that cardio-respiratory fitness provides (Hötting & Röder, 2013). The great importance placed on physical health and fitness has caused SOCOM to take action in order to reduce injuries while training for missions. Taking this type of initiative will lead to the reduced likelihood of operators experiencing debilitating injuries or death while in the field (United States Special Operations Command, 2013). To help establish this domain, SOCOM has developed a Human Performance Program that incorporates strength and conditioning, nutrition, and physical therapy to help develop a physically well-rounded, yet extraordinary operator.

Operators train like high-performance athletes. As with performance athletes, a physical injury can be debilitating or the end of a career. Physical injury within elite athletes has been found to have a strong negative effect on social functioning, vitality, and mental health (McAllister, Motamedi, Hame, Shapiro, & Dorey, 2001). Furthermore, physical injury has been associated with post-traumatic stress reactions and poorer general mental health (Dyster-Aas et al., 2012). To reduce the amount of physical injuries sustained during training, which in turn reduces stress for operators (Miles, 2013), SOCOM has enlisted the expertise of strength and conditioning coaches that develop specific workout plans and monitor operators as they work out. Moreover, they also utilize the services of physical therapists to attend to physical injuries as they occur and to monitor the recovery progress over time (Miles, 2013). However, more goes into physical fitness than training.

The nutrition of an operator can greatly affect muscle performance, body composition, and cognitive performance (Ford & Glymour, 2014). Although the average SOF operator is 29 to 34 years old, married, and often has children (United States Special Operations Command, 2013), his knowledge of proper nutrition is inadequate when considering the physical performance levels that he is expected to maintain. When asked to identify the proper use of proteins, supplements, and role of vitamins in their diet, over half of operators were unable to correctly do so (Bovill, Tharion, & Lieberman, 2003).

To address these weaknesses, SOCOM has brought in nutritionists to help educate operators and their families on the proper nutrition during training periods and in daily life (Miles, 2013). By educating operators on topics like proper nutrition and providing them with healthier food options while training and in the field, there is evidence that better nutrition can improve both their physical and cognitive performance and enhance resiliency (Ford & Glymour, 2014). By enlisting the help and knowledge of trained professionals to attend to the performance-related training, physical injuries, and nutrition of these SOF operators, SOCOM is hoping to reduce the physical injuries sustained by operators and improve their physical preparedness, subsequently enhancing performance and resiliency.

Psychological performance

The DOD, specifically SOCOM, is committed to eliminating the stigma surrounding seeking psychological help in the military (Miggantz, 2014; Quartana et al., 2014; Shanker & Oppel, 2014). Throughout the previous decade, mental health utilization in the military has risen, but stigma is still an omnipresent problem (Quartana et al., 2014). In the past, fear of being found unfit for duty or losing the trust and confidence of fellow teammates likely deterred operators from seeking mental health treatment (Brown, Creel, Engel, Herrell, & Hoge, 2011; Clark-Hitt, Smith, & Broderick, 2012). One way to effectively help reduce stigma is to have high-ranking military leaders who have been exposed to combat themselves support, utilize, and speak openly about seeking mental health treatment (Britt, Wright, & Moore, 2012; Clark-Hitt et al., 2012).

To help fully utilize mental health services, SOF units have embedded mental health professionals within each unit to accommodate unpredictable training and deployment schedules (Miles, 2013). Furthermore, having a mental health professional specifically trained in the needs of the special operations community assists in improving therapeutic rapport and increases treatment adherence. It is hoped that having mental health providers readily available, combined with leadership supporting help-seeking behavior, will lead to an increase in operators seeking mental health services (Miggantz, 2014). This may have exponential influence based on findings indicating that once an operator receives mental health treatment, they are more likely to seek help again in the future (Brown et al., 2011). This finding illustrates the importance of creating an environment, which encourages operators to make those initial contacts with mental health services. Further, in recognition that many operators who need supportive services remain hesitant to reach out, SOCOM currently conducts post-deployment PDHAs and periodic assessments on operators' mental health as previously examined in this document (Miggantz, 2014). Beyond providing mental health information, this process also exposes operators to the assessment process, which may normalize this interaction potentially influencing future help-seeking behaviors.

Psycho-education also plays a large role in the mental health status of the operators and their families. Mental health professionals are teaching operators dedicated stress-inoculation strategies to help improve performance in the field and at home (United States Special Operations Command, 2013). Stress Inoculation Training (SIT) is an individually tailored form of cognitive behavioral therapy that is employed in a three-phase intervention to eventually teach coping skills tailored to specific stressors operators may face (Meichenbaum, 1996). When operators are in the field, some dedicated stress inoculation strategies used could involve problem solving, cognitive restructuring, or self-soothing techniques to appropriately deal with the stressors within a mission. While at home, operators may use emotional self-regulation, communication skills, utilization of social support systems, and fostering meaning-related activities to deal with the stresses of reintegration into the family unit (Meichenbaum, 1996).

Social performance

Positive social support is a cornerstone to good mental health. This is particularly important within the military, especially SOCOM, because of the unique stressors that may arise in the life of an SOF operator due to unpredictable deployment and training cycles. SOF requires stability and reliability in all aspect of operators' lives including family cohesion and social networks (United States Special Operations Command, 2013). The ability to not only establish meaningful relationships but to maintain them throughout training and deployment is important in an operator's life. The lack of social support has been found to exacerbate suicide symptoms, therefore increasing the overall risk of suicide, while developing social supports promotes resiliency (Griffith, 2012). The unique requirements of an operator's career makes having a baseline of normality to return to when the mission is complete increasingly valuable (United States Special Operations Command, 2013).

The average SOF operator is married with two children (United States Special Operations Command, 2013). Thus, the toll associated with the unique demands that a SOF career requires, such as unpredictable deployments, must take into consideration numerous individuals. This includes the impact on operators' respective partners and children and the global effect on family dynamics. The strain that unaccompanied deployments can have on families includes increased rates of marital conflict, domestic violence, and spousal depression and anxiety (Saltzman, 2011). Specifically, marital conflict is an important factor to emphasize in terms of building resiliency, because divorce and separation has been identified as risk factors for suicide (Hyman, Ireland, Frost, & Cottrell, 2012).

To address these interpersonal issues, SOCOM hopes to build trust and interpersonal effectiveness between the operator, their family, and the command. A way of improving effectiveness between an operator and his family is achieved through the provision of psycho-education regarding underlying causes of behavior amongst returning operators and learning to open lines of communication within a family unit (Saltzman, 2011). Failures in family communication among spouses and between parents with their children can adversely affect family functioning (Saltzman, 2011). Impaired communication while a parent or spouse is away for long periods of time can lead to feelings of estrangement and exclusivity, weakened attachment, and role confusion. Teaching both the operator and their family member's proper ways to stay connected while the loved one is away, and how to reconnect once they return home, can dramatically increase family cohesion.

One way of improving the relationship between the family and the command relies on the leadership within the command and members of individual teams to embrace family members as part of the team. Including families in the deployment process and scheduling and keeping open lines of communications between the leadership, operators, and their families allows for a better understanding about what the operators are doing (Palmer, 2008; Saltzman, 2011). Further, these interactions provide additional information to the family related to the sacrifices they are making. Obtaining acceptance and support of the mission from an operator's family is strongly predictive of effective future coping and adaptation among their children (Palmer, 2008). Additionally, when an operator's home life and social support is stable, it diminishes outside stressors like worrying about marital problems or an issue with a child and allows the operator to fully focus on the mission (Hosek, Miller, Kavanagh, & Rand, 2006).

Spiritual performance

Religiosity, or the degree to which a person adheres to religious values or beliefs, and spirituality, an internal, personal, subjective and private experience, are seen as effective resiliency resources (Reutter & Bigatti, 2014). Within this context, spiritualty does not require subscription to a specific religion or belief in a certain god. Here, spirituality is defined as one's core spiritual beliefs, values, awareness, relationships, and experiences (United States Special Operations Command, 2013). Spiritual performance is designed to enhance these ideals.

Spiritual attachments have been recognized as worthwhile resources for dealing with stress, with self-reported higher spirituality associated with lower perceived stress levels (Reutter & Bigatti, 2014). The improvement of spiritual performance is accomplished through chaplain-led or chaplain-supported programs for both operators and their families. Chaplains often focus on building a faith community and a sense of belongingness within their command (Doty & Spencer-Thomas, 2009). By holding discussion groups, educational programs and developing peer support groups for operators and their families, chaplains look to build that sense of community. For those who do not identify with a particular religion, inter-faith forums are held where leaders from multiple faiths come together to discuss religion and faith in hopes to educate and develop a sense of spirituality (Doty & Spencer-Thomas, 2009).

Spirituality ultimately affects operators' mission performance and ability to deal with challenges within SOF by strengthening their core beliefs and values, which assist in better decision making and dealing with stress (Miles, 2013). Studies suggest that spiritualty may relate to more positive appraisals of life stressors and less psychological distress (Reutter & Bigatti, 2014). Chaplains base their programs off the notion that religiously committed people tend to report greater subjective well-being and life satisfaction (Richards & Bergin, 2000). By developing or strengthening the spirituality of operators and their families, SOCOM looks to increase resiliency in a high-stress environment that is indicative of an SOF career (Miles, 2013).

Conclusion

SOCOM, its operators, and their families are essential to the defense mission of the United States. However, because of these operators' stoic appearance and disciplined behavior, their physical, mental, social, and spiritual needs are often overlooked. Unfortunately, not responding to these aspects of well-being amongst operators in the past led to a greater prevalence of suicide within this group. While many strategies have been developed and implemented in an attempt to address this increased suicidality, these previous approaches have been largely unsuccessful. While there are various potential reasons why these strategies have not ultimately experienced success, one prominent weakness is that they have focused primarily on identifying risks factors related to suicide, rather than factors serving protective functions.

SOCOM has developed a multi-dimensional method to address the comprehensive needs of an operator proactively. Based on initial response, this approach seems preferable to allowing mental health issues to evolve overtime potentially developing into readiness and risk issues. Attending to the unique stressors these operators encounter with a holistic preventative approach develops resilience amongst this population, reducing risk of suicide and further preparing them to face the many challenges associated with their specialized role.

References

Alexander, C. L., Reger, M. A., Smolenski, D. J., & Fullerton, N. R. (2014). Comparing US army suicide cases to a control sample: Initial data and methodological lessons. *Military Medicine, 179*(10), 1062–1066.

Black, S. A., Gallaway, M. S., Bell, M. R., & Ritchie, E. C. (2011). Prevalence and risk factors associated with suicides of army soldiers 2001–2009. *Military Psychology, 23*(4), 433–451.

Bliese, P. D., Wright, K. M., Adler, A. B., Thomas, J. L., & Hoge, C. W. (2007). Timing of postcombat mental health assessments. *Psychological Services, 4*(3), 141–148.

Bovill, M. E., Tharion, W. J., & Lieberman, H. R. (2003). Nutrition knowledge and supplement use among elite US army soldiers. *Military Medicine, 168*(12), 997–1000.

Britt, T. W., Wright, K. M., & Moore, D. (2012). Leadership as a predictor of stigma and practical barriers toward receiving mental health treatment: A multilevel approach. *Psychological Services, 9*(1), 26–37.

Brown, M. C., Creel, A. H., Engel, C. C., Herrell, R. K., & Hoge, C. W. (2011). Factors associated with interest in receiving help for mental health problems in combat veterans returning from deployment to Iraq. *Journal of Nervous and Mental Disease, 199*(10), 797–801.

Bryan, C. J., & Hernandez, A. M. (2013). The functions of social support as protective factors for suicidal ideation in a sample of air force personnel. *Suicide & Life-Threatening Behavior, 43*(5), 562–573.

Budd, F. C. (1999). An air force model of psychologist-chaplain collaboration. *Professional Psychology: Research & Practice, 30*(6), 552–556.

Bush, N. E., Reger, M. A., Luxton, D. D., Skopp, N. A., Kinn, J., Smolenski, D., & Gahm, G. A. (2013). Suicides and suicide attempts in the US military, 2008–2010. *Suicide & Life-Threatening Behavior, 43*(3), 262–273.

Clark-Hitt, R., Smith, S. W., & Broderick, J. S. (2012). Help a buddy take a knee: Creating persuasive messages for military service members to encourage others to seek mental health help. *Health Communication, 27*(5), 429–438.

Doty, T. D., & Spencer-Thomas, S. (2009). *The role of faith communities in suicide prevention: A guidebook for faith leaders.* Golden, CO: Carson J Spencer Foundation.

Dyster-Aas, J., Arnberg, F. K., Lindam, A., Johannesson, K. B., Lundin, T., & Michel, P. (2012). Impact of physical injury on mental health after the 2004 Southeast Asia tsunami. *Nordic Journal of Psychiatry, 66*(3), 203–208.

Ford, K., & Glymour, C. (2014). The enhanced warfighter. *Bulletin of the Atomic Scientists, 70*(1), 43–53.

Griffith, J. (2012). Suicide and war: The mediating effects of negative mood, posttraumatic stress disorder symptoms, and social support among army national guard soldiers. *Suicide & Life-Threatening Behavior, 42*(4), 453–469.

Hanwella, R., & Silva, V. (2012). Mental health of special forces personnel deployed in battle. *Social Psychiatry & Psychiatric Epidemiology, 47*(8), 1343–1351.

Hosek, J. R., Miller, L. L., Kavanagh, J., & Rand, C. (2006). *How deployments affect service members.* Santa Monica, CA: RAND.

Hötting, K., & Röder, B. (2013). Beneficial effects of physical exercise on neuroplasticity and cognition. *Neuroscience and Biobehavioral Reviews, 37*(9, Part B), 2243–2257.

Hughes, J. G., Wagner, A., Willkomm, B., & Smykala, P. (2004). *NATO research task group 20, stress and psychological support in modern military operations: Clinical sub-group initial report.* RTO-TR-HFM-081, Brussels, Belgium.

Hyman, J., Ireland, R., Frost, L., & Cottrell, L. (2012). Suicide incidence and risk factors in an active duty US military population. *American Journal of Public Health, 102*(S1), S138–S146.

Jobes, D. A. (2013). Reflections on suicide among soldiers. *Psychiatry, 76*(2), 126–131.

Kessler, R. C., Colpe, L. J., Fullerton, C. S., Gebler, N., Naifeh, J. A., Nock, M. K., . . . Heeringa, S. G. (2013). Design of the army study to assess risk and resilience in service members (Army STARRS). *International Journal of Methods in Psychiatric Research, 22*(4), 267–275.

McAllister, D. R., Motamedi, A. R., Hame, S. L., Shapiro, M. S., & Dorey, F. J. (2001). Quality of life assessment in elite collegiate athletes. *The American Journal of Sports Medicine, 29*(6), 806–810.

Meichenbaum, D. (1996). Stress inoculation training for coping with stressors. *The Clinical Psychologist, 49,* 4–7. Miggantz, E. L. (2014). Stigma of mental health care in the military. Naval Center for Combat & Operational Stress Control. Retrieved from: www.med.navy.mil/sites/nmcsd/nccosc/healthProfessionalsV2/reports/Documents/Stigma%20White%20Paper.pdf

Miles, D. (2013, June 14). SOCOM strives to boost operators' resilience, readiness. *American Forces Press Services.* Retrieved from http://archive.defense.gov/news/newsarticle.aspx?id=120289

Nock, M. K., Deming, C. A., Fullerton, C. S., Gilman, S. E., Goldenberg, M., Kessler, R. C., . . . Ursano, R. J. (2013). Suicide among soldiers: A review of psychosocial risk and protective factors. *Psychiatry: Interpersonal and Biological Processes, 76*(2), 97–125.

Palmer, C. (2008). A theory of risk and resilience factors in military families. *Military Psychology, 20*(3), 205–217.

Quartana, P. J., Wilk, J. E., Thomas, J. L., Bray, R. M., Rae Olmsted, K. L., Brown, J. M., . . . Hoge, C. W. (2014). Trends in mental health services utilization and stigma in US soldiers from 2002 to 2011. *American Journal of Public Health, 104*(9), 1671–1679.

Reutter, K. K., & Bigatti, S. M. (2014). Religiosity and spirituality as resiliency resources: Moderation, mediation, or moderated mediation? *Journal for the Scientific Study of Religion, 53*(1), 56–72.

Reyes, V. A., & Hicklin, T. A. (2005). Anger in the combat zone. *Military Medicine, 170*(6), 483–487.

Richards, P. S., & Bergin, A. E. (2000). *Handbook of psychotherapy and religious diversity.* Washington, DC, US: American Psychological Association.

Saltzman, W. W. (2011). Mechanisms of risk and resilience in military families: Theoretical and empirical basis of a family-focused resilience enhancement program. *Clinical Child & Family Psychology Review, 14*(3), 213–230.

Shanker, T., & Oppel Jr., R. A. (2014, June 6). War's elite tough guys, hesitant to seek healing. (Cover story). *New York Times,* pp. A1–A16.

Sharkey, J. M., & Rennix, C. P. (2011). Assessment of changes in mental health conditions among sailors and marines during post deployment phase. *Military Medicine, 176*(8), 915–921.

Stein, M. B., & Ursano, R. J. (2013). Suicide among United States military personnel: determining the root causes. *Depression & Anxiety, 30*(10), 896–897.

Street, A. E., Gilman, S. E., Rosellini, A. J., Stein, M. B., Bromet, E. J., Cox, K. L., . . . Kessler, R. C. (2015). Understanding the elevated suicide risk of female soldiers during deployments. *Psychological Medicine, 45*(4), 717–726.

Theriault, E. (2015). Empowered Commanders. *Air & Space Power Journal, 29*(1), 99–111.

Trotter, S. (2014). The combined arms support command chaplain capabilities developer. *Army Sustainment, 46*(6), 22–25.

United States Special Operations Command. (2013). *Preservation of the force and family* [Brochure]. Tampa, FL: Author.

Ursano, R. J., Heeringa, S. G., Stein, M. B., Jain, S., Raman, R., Sun, X., . . . Kessler, R. C. (2015). Prevalence and correlates of suicidal behavior among new soldiers in the US army: Results from the army study to assess risk and resilience in service members (Army STARRS). *Depression and Anxiety, 32*(1), 3–12.

Vogt, D. (2011). Mental health–related beliefs a barrier to service use for military personnel and veterans: A review. *Psychiatric Services, 62*(2), 135–142.

Warner, C. H., Appenzeller, G. N., Parker, J. R., Warner, C., Diebold, C. J., & Grieger, T. (2011). Suicide prevention in a deployed military unit. *Psychiatry: Interpersonal & Biological Processes, 74*(2), 127–141.

Weiner, J., Richmond, T. S., Conigliaro, J., & Wiebe, D. J. (2011). Military veteran mortality following a survived suicide attempt. *BMC Public Health, 11*, 374.

22

Experience of terrorist threat among urban populations in Russia[1]

PTSD and resilience

Nadezhda V. Tarabrina and Julia V. Bykhovets

In the last few decades, millions of people from the multinational civil population of Russia do live in the environment of increased danger of terrorist activity. The terrorism that has existed during all history of mankind now has changed qualitatively: first, it became almost permanent (rare are the newscasts without reports of an act of terrorism happening somewhere); second, it became international: it is now difficult to name a country where acts of terrorism do not happen. The heads of governments consider the fight against terrorism to be a priority state task. It is possible to assert that there is a war going on in the world that is directed towards the destabilization of peaceful coexistence of countries. The number of acts of terrorism grows continuously, and most experts do not forecast any decline in the foreseeable future. Therefore, studying influence of acts of terrorism on the psyche (psychological traumatization of population) is one of the most urgent medical-social problems.

Empirical study of presentations and perception of the terrorist threat has been executed in the Laboratory of Psychology of Posttraumatic Stress of the Institute of Psychology, Russian Academy of Sciences (Bykhovets, 2008; Bykhovets & Tarabrina, 2010a; Tarabrina & Bykhovets, 2006, 2009). We researched how a regular person who was not victimized personally from the act of terrorism perceives terroristic acts. How does such an event influence his ideas, feelings, and behavior? The results of this study show a correlation between the level of sensitivity to a terrorist threat and PTSD. The data obtained in our work manifests that a high level of terrorist threat is a stressor for vulnerable parts of a population. The levels of terrorist threat sensitivity were compared in different regions of the Russian Federation. It is necessary to note that research of psychological consequences of acts of terrorism has been conducted at a new level in recent years: while earlier research had a descriptive character of types of psychical reactions to this stressor, now more issues present scientific interest for specialists, such as the hierarchy of PTSD symptoms in clinical and nonclinical groups, the role of mass-media in forming of characterizations of enemy (in relation to members of terrorist organizations), and the vulnerability and resistance of populations to traumatic influence. This development suggests that psychological science has begun to determine a wider scope of research on the psychological consequences of acts of terrorism.

Emphasis on those areas of knowledge will help to forewarn of the threatening influence of acts of terrorism on a population's psyche. It is obvious to psychologists that participation in terrorist organizations and in terrorist acts is influenced by different and compound psychological complexes and by internal and external reasons that explain such behavior. We should note some modern research that attempts to consider the problems of terrorism from the "other" side. For example A. Speckard studied that issue for more than a decade, at times using difficult and dangerous methods of conducting interviews with terrorists, their friends, and their relatives in different countries. During those years, she recorded more than 400 interviews in different parts of the world, setting before itself the task to understand the inner world of terrorist, motivation of acts of terrorism. The results of this original research were expounded in a professional and accessible way in her book *Conversation with a Terrorist* (Speckhard, 2012); in the conclusion, she writes that nobody is born a terrorist: something or someone sends a man to the terrorist trajectory. And the global task of politicians and scientists is to search and find the ways to return these people from that dangerous voyage.

Acts of terrorism have become an integral part of modern public life; therefore, the members of social help professions (doctors, psychologists, social workers) must realize the necessity of working with the hidden consequences of acts of terrorism. For example psychiatrists found that people are afraid, not only of terrorists, but also of their victims. An idea exists in the majority consciousness that a victim of an act of terrorism is also dangerous, that the mood of such a person after stress changes to the worse, and that the victim acquires the negative charge of energy, of conflict. Such watchful attitude toward witnesses and victims of acts of terrorism is observed not only in Russia but also other countries. Thus, the study of psychological influence of "waves of information" about the acts of terrorism on citizenry has a high socially relevant value.

Categories of the persons injured from acts of terrorism are defined differently in different sources. For example V. S. Yastrebov distinguished four groups of victims: 1) "first line" victims, victims of acts of terrorism who appear in its epicentre; 2) rescuers, professionals executing rescues or other workers directly involved in the terrorism response and also in other actions within the framework of counterterrorism activity; 3) victims of the "second line", witnesses of acts of terrorism, inhabitants of neighbouring territories; and 4) the population indirectly connected to the acts of terrorism through administrative agencies, mass-media, etc. (Yastrebov, 2004).

Rudovski, Voloshina, and Aksenova (2004) distinguished the following categories of victims: 1) direct participants of events; 2) relatives of those lost and injured as a result of an act of terrorism; 3) eyewitnesses of dramatic events; and 4) persons with the emotional trauma, induced by the stories of eyewitnesses, mass-media, anxiety, and searches for information about friends and relatives. Some authors consider that, among the victims of acts of terrorism, it is possible to distinguish primary and secondary victims. Primary victims are the directly injured from the act of terrorism. However, there has been no attention given to "secondary victims". Other authors consider that secondary victims are, foremost, friends and relatives of victims (Kohanov, Krasnov, & Kekelidze, 2000), while another suggests that secondary victims were not victims or witnesses but had neurotic reactions (anxiety, phobia, depression) developed as a result of information about the event (Pisarenko, 1986).

We believe that it is necessary to distinguish direct and indirect victims of acts among victims of terrorism (Enikolopov, Lebedev, & Bobosov, 2004). Direct victims of acts of terrorism are directly injured, their relatives, and their close acquaintances. Indirect victims are those who became witnesses of acts of terrorism by means of mass-media and other sources of communication.

Complex analysis of psychological consequences of acts of terrorism for indirect victims is constrained by development of a theoretical model studying the consequences of the psychological influence of terrorist threat, which is the special form of injuring influence, a complex emotional-personality concept – the perception of terrorist threat.

The goal of this research is a study of the perception of terrorist threat by indirect victims (witnesses of acts of terrorism by means of mass-media) in different regions of Russia and its correlation with PTSD. To this purpose, the following tasks have been identified: 1) to compare regional groups on the level of intensity of terroristic sensitivity, 2) to divide the sample into three subgroups based on expression of PTSD, 3) to compare the distinguished subgroups on the level of terroristic sensitivity, and 4) to estimate the connection between terroristic sensitivity and PTSD in the groups of respondents with the different levels of PTSD.

Terroristic threat and resilience

The concept of resilience implies adaptability and a certain ability to be restored after a collision with a stressor. "Terrorist threat" differs from other stressors. First, experienced threat to life is related to one's future, as a rule, formed after a person has been a victim or a witness (either direct or indirect) of a terrorist act and its consequences (Tarabrina & Bykhovets, 2007). Analysis and forecasting of the probability of becoming a victim of terrorism turned into the basis for the development of emotional-cognitive structures that contain assumptions about terrorist threat. Individuals that directly or indirectly experienced an act of terrorism may develop expectations and assumptions of undesirable consequences of terrorist acts that they are not capable of preventing. This personal and subjective assessment may be expressed either through increased anxiety, through complete indifference to the frightening perspective, or through other forms of attitudes to the actuality of threat. Distinctions in objectivity of the assessment of "terrorist threat" after an actual terrorist act may be considered as a result of experiencing that event. Afterward, even if it there is not an objective basis to feel the threat of the terrorist act, some individuals will anyway anticipate such ominous prospects (Tarabrina & Bykhovets, 2007). Thus, terroristic sensitivity is examined by us as a subjective estimation of risk of becoming a victim of act of terrorism.

The second notion is the complexity of forecasting terrorism, meaning that it is impossible to predict the time, place, or type of terror acts. Unpredictability itself renders oppressing effects on the mentality of an individual. H. Selye in his research demonstrated that unpredictable and unmanageable events are more dangerous than expected and controllable ones (Selye, 1992). The third factor is the uncompromising character of terrorist acts, i.e. the individual realize that he/she does not have informational opportunities to prevent the threat hanging above him. And, fourth, an individual starts to realize his/her own personal vulnerability in the face of terrorist acts. There is a comprehension that a terrorist act is capable of disrupting anyone's life. Fifth, description is an activity that places terrorist actions outside the norm of usual actions and states.

In this study, we refer to authors studying society's emotional stability versus terrorism. D. Simeon, Greenberg, Knutelska, Schmeidler, and Hollander (2003) has shown that, for indirect victims, acts of terrorism educed: decline in the level of perceiving life's safety; fear of death; enhanced aggression; enhanced levels of emotional reaction; high levels of peritraumatic dissociation; loss of life prospects and ability to cope with vital difficulties; anxiety; and increased of consumption of alcohol, cigarettes, and drugs.

Reflections about potential of becoming a victim of act of terrorism assisted development of signs of stress (Dixon, Rehling, & Shiwach, 1993). The psychological influence of information about September 11 was perceived in Italy (Apolone, Mosconi, & La Vecchia, 2002) and in India (Roetzer & Walch, 2004). American expatriates in Belgium sharply experienced these events

(Speckhard, 2002, 2003). Many similar researchers have examined mass-media, especially TV influences, as an important predictor of stress or traumatic symptoms.

The influence of mass-media can operate as an injuring reminder and lead to the permanent symptoms today. Information about the acts of terrorism in mass-media and other communication media can be considered as a traumatic stressor that leads to the development of signs of PTSD in the indirect victims.

The concept of resilience is defined as a dynamic variable, influenced by many co-variates (defined in the following) and existing in a continuum of adaptability (Saltzman, Pynoos, Layne, Steinberg, & Aisenberg, 2001). According to this definition, an individual who is resilient to high-threat security environment must retain, or in the best-case scenario even show, gains, flexibility, adaptability, functionality, and empathy. Loss of resilience likewise is indicated by the appearance of pathological symptoms interfering with normal functioning including symptoms of posttraumatic stress (including flashbacks, high arousal states, loss of concentration, irritability, etc.); dissociation (a separation of normal cognitive functions, emotional numbing, inability to think, etc.); anxiety; depression; and panic, all of which interfere with and create a loss of normal functioning. Likewise a gain in xenophobia (hatred of outsiders such as Muslims or Arabs in this case) is also assessed in this model as contributing to a loss of resilience (Speckhard, Verleye, & Jacuch, 2012).

Method

The following questionnaires have been used to attain the purpose and goals of the research: a questionnaire of terroristic sensitivity (QTT-50; Bykhovets & Tarabrina, 2010b); the Mississippi Scale (MS; Vreven, Gudanowski, & King, 1995); and the Symptom Check List-90-Revised (SCL-90-R; Derogatis, Rickels, & Rock, 1976).

A special questionnaire was designed for this purpose – the Questionnaire of the Terrorist Threat (QTT; Tarabrina & Bykhovets, 2006). This instrument is based on the notion that the perception of terrorist threat can be analyzed from the point of view of its three components, dissimilar in their psychological content: cognitive, emotional, and behavioral. The QTT is intended to evaluate the content and the structure of an individual's awareness of both objective and subjective stressful factors experienced after actual terrorist attacks. The basic psychometric properties and the factor structure of the QTT are reported in a sample of 494 subjects. The results indicate that the QTT possesses strong reliability and validity. A Cronbach's alpha coefficient was .93, the equal-length Spearman-Brown coefficient was .91, the Guttmann Split-Half coefficient was .91, and item-total score correlations ranged from .18 to .71.

Samples

Four hundred and ninety-four respondents have taken part in the research. All participants were volunteers and participated in the research study during April–August 2006. The sample is represented by three groups: the Moscow group ($n = 288$), respondents of Chechen Republic (ChR) ($n = 73$), and Chita (West Siberia, Russia) ($n = 133$). The choice of research groups is not random. Intensity of influence of information about the acts of terrorism (identical in different regions) is different depending on their frequency in a region and degree of closeness to the epicentre of events: in ChR, battle actions and acts of terrorism have taken place everywhere since 1994; in Moscow, thirteen acts of terrorism happened from 1999 to 2006; and Chita is relatively quiet in terms of terrorist threat. The Moscow group included people from 16 to 60 years old. (Dates are presented in Table 22.1.)

Table 22.1 Descriptive statistics of Moscow respondents' age

	Age				
	Mean	*Median*	*Range*	*Std.Dev.*	*N*
Students, female from 16 to 20 years	18.53	19.00	3.00	1.06	92
Students, male from 16 to 21 years	19.38	19.00	5.00	1.11	39
Young adults, female from 21 to 35 years	24.97	24.00	14.000	3.82	71
Young adults, male from 22 to 35 years	26.58	24.50	13.00	4.51	24
Middle aged adults, female from 36 to 55 years	46.6	50.000	19.00	5.99	43
Middle aged adults, male from 36 to 60 years	50.05	51.00	23.000	7.28	19

Table 22.2 Descriptive statistics of ChR respondents' age

	Age				
	Mean	*Median*	*Range*	*Std.Dev.*	*n*
Students, female from 16 to 20 years	18.27	18.000	4.000	1.16	22
Students, male from 16 to 21 years	18.24	18.000	5.000	1.72	29
Young adults, female from 21 to 35 years	22.71	22.000	5.000	1.19	21
Middle aged adults, female from 36 to 55 years	–	–	–	–	1

Table 22.3 Descriptive statistics of Chita respondents' age

	Age				
	Mean	*Median*	*Range*	*Std.Dev.*	*n*
Students, female from 16 to 20 years	18.36	18.000	3.000	.99	104
Students, male from 16 to 21 years	18.88	19.000	3.000	.93	9
Young adults, female from 21 to 35 years	22.16	22.000	4.000	1.07	19
Young adults, male from 22 to 35 years	–	–	–	–	1

Second group consists from the respondents of Chechen Republic cities (Grozyi, Gydermes, Nozay-Urt). Battle actions and acts of terrorism have occurred everywhere in this territory since 1994. The population of ChR continuously lives in the situation of threat to their own life and life of their acquaintances. Thus, acts of terrorism have become for them a chronic stressor. Its cumulative influence maybe considerably traumatic. The ChR group included people from 16 to 55 years old. (Dates are presented in Table 22.2.)

The third group included of the respondents from Chita (West Siberia, Russia). They live on territory of relative quiet as far as terrorist threat is concerned. They are subject to messages of acts of terrorism far away from the epicentre of events. Information about acts of terrorism from mass-media and other communication media creates the threat of the personal safety to a lesser degree as compared to other regional groups. The Chita group included people from 16 to 35 years old. (Data is presented in Table 22.3.)

Results

Our study shows the connection between terroristic sensitivity and region of residence. Randomization of the regional groups was conducted. Persons not of student age eliminated from analysis. Thus, only persons of student age were entered for research: first, Moscow, $N = 130$; second, ChR. $N = 73$; and third, Chita, $N = 133$.

We suppose that the levels of distress, terroristic sensitivity, and PTSD must be higher in the group of respondents of ChR than in the groups of Moscow and Chita, connected to military operations on territories of ChR. The frequency of acts of terrorism and closeness of residence to the places of battle actions can be factors in development of signs of PTSD, signs of psychopathology, and intensive terroristic sensitivity. Further, in accordance with the logic of our reasoning, expressions of the examined indexes must be higher in the group of Moscow respondents as compared to the group of Chita. For verification of this hypothesis, we made a comparison of the regional groups on the level of expressed indexes of two test batteries: MS and QTT-50. Results are represented in Table 22.4.

Our hypothesis was confirmed partially. Residents of Chechen Republic experience terrorist threat and PTSD symptoms with the highest intensity. Residents of the city of Chita (West Siberia, Russia) experience threat of terrorism in a greater degree, than Muscovites. However, the groups of Moscow and Chita differ on expression of PTSD.

The residents of ChR are subject to traumatic influence of acts of terrorism in a greater degree. They watch what is going on, acts of terrorism, mainly on television and live in this reality. They suffer from PTSD and experience the threat of acts of terrorism in a greater degree than Muscovites and residents of Chita. Moscow is a large megalopolis. The stressors are more various than in small cities. People that live in a megalopolis possess greater vitality and resilience. They were tempered under influence of surrounding stressors. The residents of Chita live in a large remoteness far from large megalopolises. In spite of the fact that acts of terrorism occur more often in Moscow, it rather formed resilience for the citizens of Moscow, compared to the residents of Chita.

Rubin et al. (2007) write about the specific psychological stability of a population of a megalopolis to traumatic influence of acts of terrorism, commenting on the psychological consequences of explosions in July 2005 in London. We got data that the residents of Chita experienced the threat of terrorism to a greater degree than Muscovites. On its face, this result conflicts with the logic that the closeness of residence to the acts of terrorism stimulates higher intensity of terroristic sensitivity.

However, in our work, we got data about the semantic analysis of ideas about acts of terrorism in the three regional groups. This data allows us to explain the low value of terroristic sensitivity

Table 22.4 Values of Mann–Whitney U-test

	Group 1	Median	Mode	Range	Dispersion	Group 2	Median	Mode	Range	Dispersion	U	p
MS	Moscow	81	Mult	69	196.547	ChR	103	Mult	68	500.213	2939	.000
	ChR	103	Mult	68	500.213	Chita	79	79	70	212.348	3062.5	.000
	Chita	79	79	70	212.348	Moscow	81	Mult	69	196.547	8612	.96
QTT-50	Moscow	129	120	152	715.64	ChR	148	148	112	359.266	2803.5	.000
	ChR	148	148	112	359.266	Chita	138	130	108	513.727	4022	.041
	Chita	138	130	108	513.727	Chita	129	120	152	715.64	6595.5	.000

Table 22.5 Values of Mann–Whitney U-test

Symptom Check List-90-Revised (SCL-90-R) Scales	Group 1	Median	Mode	Range	Dispersion	Group 2	Median	Mode	Range	Dispersion	U	p
Somatization (SOM)	Moscow	.37	0	2	.198	CHR	1.5	Mult	2.67	.658	2002	.000
	ChR	1.5	Mult	2.67	.658	Chita	.58	.25	2	.228	2394	.000
	Chita	.58	.25	2	.228	Moscow	.37	0	2	.198	7415	.071
Obsessive-Compulsive (O-C)	Moscow	.7	9	2.9	.28	ChR	1.4	1.4	3.6	.612	2836	.000
	ChR	1.4	1.4	3.6	.612	Chita	.6	.4	2.4	.305	2776.5	.000
	Chita	.6	.4	2.4	.305	Moscow	.7	9	2.9	.28	7789.5	.24
Interpersonal Sensitivity (INT)	Moscow	.765	1	3.25	.409	ChR	1.44	1.22	3.56	.678	2787.5	.000
	ChR	1.44	1.22	3.56	.678	Chita	.78	Mult	3.11	.371	2776	.000
	Chita	.78	Mult	3.11	.371	Moscow	.765	1	3.25	.409	8202.5	.61
Depression (DEP)	Moscow	.538	0	3.231	.354	ChR	1.23	2	2.85	.7	2698	.000
	ChR	1.23	2	2.85	.7	Chita	.54	.23	2.69	.321	2838.5	.000
	Chita	.54	.23	2.69	.321	Moscow	.538	0	3.231	.354	8331.5	.77
Anxiety (ANX)	Moscow	.3	0	2.1	.228	ChR	1.4	Mult	2.8	.661	2228.5	.000
	ChR	1.4	Mult	2.8	.661	Chita	.4	.2	2.3	.199	2481	.000
	Chita	.4	.2	2.3	.199	Moscow	.3	0	2.1	.228	7821	.26
Hostility (HOS)	Moscow	.5	5	2.5	.276	ChR	1.33	Mult	3.33	.72	2834.5	.000
	ChR	1.33	Mult	3.33	.72	Chita	.5	.33	2.5	.281	2603	.000
	Chita	.5	.33	2.5	.281	Moscow	.5	5	2.5	.276	7443.5	.08
Phobic Anxiety (PHOB)	Moscow	.14	0	7	.485	ChR	1	0	2.86	.748	2009	.000
	ChR	1	0	2.86	.748	Chita	.14	0	2.14	.15	2333	.000
	Chita	.14	0	2.14	.15	Moscow	.14	0	7	.485	7638	.15
Paranoid Ideation (PAR)	Moscow	.668	1	2.33	.334	ChR	1.5	2.17	3.5	.754	2641	.000
	ChR	1.5	2.17	3.5	.754	Chita	.67	.33	2.5	.307	2525.5	.000
	Chita	.67	.33	2.5	.307	Moscow	.668	1	2.33	.334	7861	.29

(Continued)

Table 22.5 (Continued)

Symptom Check List-90-Revised (SCL-90-R) Scales	Group 1	Median	Mode	Range	Dispersion	Group 2	Median	Mode	Range	Dispersion	U	p
Psychoticism (PSY)	Moscow	.4	0	1.9	.172	ChR	1.5	2.2	2.7	.798	2588	.000
	ChR	1.5	2.2	2.7	.798	Chita	.3	0	2.3	.228	2539	.000
	Chita	.3	0	2.3	.228	Moscow	.4	0	1.9	.172	7852.5	.28
Additional Items (ADD)	Moscow	.43	0	15	5.184	ChR	1.86	0	2.2	37.9	2604	.000
	ChR	1.86	0	2.2	37.9	Chita	.43	0	2.57	.229	2191.5	.000
	Chita	.43	0	2.57	.229	Moscow	.43	0	15	5.184	7552	.12
Global Severity Index (GSI)	Moscow	.523	.3	2.32	.185	ChR	1.73	Mult	2.7	.567	2425	.000
	ChR	1.73	Mult	2.7	.567	Chita	.53	Mult	3.11	.224	2445	.000
	Chita	.53	Mult	3.11	.224	Moscow	.523	.3	2.32	.185	8393.5	.92
Positive Symptom Total (PST)	Moscow	36	37	82	308.2	ChR	70	Mult	84	65.2	2280	.000
	ChR	70	Mult	84	65.2	Chita	36.5	30	89	373.87	2559	.000
	Chita	36.5	30	89	373.87	Moscow	36	37	82	308.2	8065	.53
Positive Symptom Distress Index (PSDI)	Moscow	1.375	1	3.058	.159	ChR	2.09	Mult	2.96	.374	2620	.000
	ChR	2.09	Mult	2.96	.374	Chita	1.295	1	2.68	.176	2427.5	.000
	Chita	1.295	1	2.68	.176	Moscow	1.375	1	3.058	.159	7409.5	.09

in Muscovites. The high value of terroristic sensitivity in the respondents of ChR is conditioned by constant involvement in the situation of terrorist threat. Muscovites are plugged into this situation from time to time. Fear is in implicit conceptions of act of terrorism in the Moscow group, but data from the QTT-50 show that they do not fear terrorism.

It is possible to suppose that protective reactions work for them: "I do not want to show that I am afraid". Probably the high values of terroristic sensitivity in the group from Chita are conditioned by that the source of the stress is specific of social life in a province: absence of existential confidence in economic prosperity and low quality of life. Undoubtedly, information about acts of terrorism in mass–media and other communication media force the general situation of anxiety, but residents of Chita are remote from the places of acts of terrorism: they never had the real experience of this stressor. We got data that their implicit conceptions about acts of terrorism were not ordered.

The data from SCL-90-R represented that levels of distress were higher in the respondents from ChR than in the Moscow and Chita groups (see Table 22.5).

Study of correlation of terroristic sensitivity with PTSD

Information about acts of terrorism in mass–media and other communication media can be considered a traumatic stressor. We have singled out three subgroups to verify this assumption: first the subgroup named "PTSD" (their MS index corresponds with clinical PTSD) and, second, the "Not PTSD" subgroup (their MS index is low). The bottom quartile of distribution MS included estimations: from 48 to 68 points ($M = 62.512$; $SD = 4.575$); top quartile – rom 90 to 131 ($M = 102.597$; $SD = 10.988$). The respondents who have scored on MS from 68 to 90 points ($M = 79.35$; $SD = 5.838$) have entered a group of "Partial PTSD".

The sample of respondents has been divided into three subgroups:

1   "PTSD" ($n = 123$)
2   "Partial PTSD" ($n = 237$)
3   "Not PTSD" ($n = 134$)

The mean values using the QTT-50 index were compared in these distinguished groups: "PTSD", "Partial PTSD", and "Not PTSD" (see Table 22.6).

We have obtained the following data: intensity of terroristic sensitivity is higher in the subgroup "PTSD" than in any other subgroup. This result is confirmed by data of correlation analysis between the MS and QTT-50 indexes in the distinguished groups (see Table 22.7).

Table 22.6 Values of Mann–Whitney U-test

	"PTSD"[a]		"Partial PTSD"[b]		"Not PTSD"[c]	
	U	P	U	P	U	p
"PTSD"	–	–				
"Partial PTSD"	15522	.000	–	–		
"Not PTSD"	5454	.000	13209	.000	–	–

a Median = 100; mode = 90; range = 4; dispersion = 120.75.
b Median = 79; mode = Multiple R; range = 20; dispersion = 34.08.
c Median = 64; mode = Multiple R; range = 20; dispersion = 20.94.

Table 22.7 Correlation between the MS and QTT-50 indexes

	"PTSD"	"Partial PTSD"	"Not PTSD"
Rs	.21	.29	.11
p	.015	.000	.238

Table 22.7 presents data about the statistically meaningful correlations between the level of terroristic sensitivity and signs of PTSD, which were only in groups of respondents in the high and middle level of the MS.

Thus, two contrasting groups can be distinguished. They differentiate on the level of expressed of the MS and by the level of terroristic sensitivity. The subgroups "PTSD" can be certain as unsteady to influence of information about acts of terrorism. The subgroup "Not PTSD" consists of persons with expressed of resilience, i.e. the psyche of these people appeared less susceptible to traumatic influence of pictures of acts of terrorism in mass-media. This type of traumatic event was effectively processed and included in the register of stressors. Adaptation of a person to the terms of life is based on the mutual change of personality and his/her surroundings (Kharlamenkova & Nikitin, 2000).

Respondents of subgroup "PTSD" intensely experience any type of information related to acts of terrorism. They are in a state of suspicion, hyperarousal, anxiety, and emotional lability. Respondents with a high intensity of symptoms of PTSD acutely experience the potential threat of acts of terrorism, i.e. terroristic sensitivity contributes to the development of PTSD. The one factor analysis of variance of ANOVA was conducted for verification of this hypothesis. The result of the analysis is presented in Tables 22.8, 22.9, and 22.10. We have singled out

Table 22.8 Descriptive statistics for MS

	N	Mean	Std. Deviation	Std. Error
First subgroup	124	76.081	14.359	1.294
Second subgroup	245	80.453	15.846	1.012
Third subgroup	125	89.104	16.503	1.4782
Total	494	81.54	16.332	.736

Table 22.9 Leven Statistic

Leven Statistic	df1	df2	Sig.
.598	2	491	.551

Table 22.10 ANOVA

	Sum of squares	Df	Mean square	F	Sig.
Between groups	11050.653	2	5525.32	22.53	.000
Within groups	119925.5	491	245.246		
Total	130976.2	493			

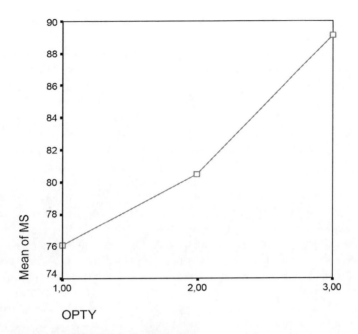

Chart 22.1 Mean of the QTT-50 and MS indexes

three subgroups by terroristic sensitivity level. The first subgroup is presented by respondents whose QTT-50 index value is lower than 121 points ($M = 103.22$; $SD = 15.09$); the second, by respondents whose QTT-50 index value is more than or equal to 121 but below 153 points ($M = 137$; $SD = 9.3$); the third, by respondents whose QTT-50 index value is more than or equal to 153 points ($M = 166.08$; $SD = 12.08$). A calculation of top and lower quartiles was used to divide the sample.

The Leven Statistic shows that statistically reliable distinctions were not discovered (Sig. > .05) between dispersions. Consequently, application of ANOVA is possible.

Results confirm the hypothesis that expressed terroristic sensitivity is statistically related to expression of signs of PTSD (Chart 22.1).

The MS value monotonously increase with the increase of values in the QTT-50 index, as apparent in the table. Posttraumatic stress disorder arises as a result of effect of the traumatic events related to death or serious wounds of people or with the possible threat of such death or wounds. Thus, a man surviving similar traumatic events can witness both and be the victim of what is going on in the suffering of other persons. Results of our study allow us to assert that perception of terrorist threat, which is formed as a result of the influence of information about acts of terrorism in mass-media and other communication media, is connected with high levels of signs of PTSD. This connection allows us to include the phenomenon of terrorist threats in the number of traumatic stressors.

Conclusion

The present research is a study of the psychological consequences of stress from the influence of information messages about acts of terrorism in mass-media and other sources of communication. The data about the correlation of PTSD and terroristic sensitivity, which arises after perceiving horrific pictures of death and wounds of direct victims of acts of terrorism in a body and in broadcasting, publications in mass–media, and other sources of communication, suggests inclusion of these type of stressors in the list of traumatic situations.

The thesis about the need to include the subject in any observation is evident. Visual images that appear in electronic or printed mass–media possess powerful effects on the psyche of the population. From here, the effects of "participation" follow appropriate senses of fear, guilt, etc. It is necessary to note that, by virtue of the all-embracing character of modern electronic mass–media, victims of every act of terrorism are practically seen by all populations. The origin of signs of PTSD is assisted by not only experiencing of actual act of terrorism but also by the idea about a "terrorist threat" and the expectation formed after the anticipation of acts of terrorism.

The results of most studies show that one of primary purposes of an act of terrorism is intimidation of population and evocation of feelings of fear. Data from our previous research shows that "fear" is the most often used in association with acts of terrorism for respondents from the different regions of Russia (Bykhovets, 2008; Tarabrina, Vorona, & Bykhovets, 2007). Thus, fear of witnesses, i.e. those who heard about them from mass–media, in opinion of some authors, exceeds the horror of direct victims who succeeded to pull through. Fear and later horror of direct victims carries concrete character. The fear of those who became a witness is more general and abstract. For direct victims, fear is always related to the repetitive experiencing of a traumatic situation. For those who were a witness, there is no such concrete remembrance. They are tormented by a fear that they do not simply know yet nor know how to behave in such cases. Direct victims over the course of time have horror from the disbelief that they suc-ceeded to pull through. For witnesses, fear appears from ignorance, that it is sometimes possible to pull through.

It is possible to assert on the basis of data from this study that, as a result of information mes-sages about acts of terrorism, the perception of terrorist threat does not depend on the sex or age of subjects (Bykhovets, 2008; Tarabrina & Bykhovets, 2006) and is formed in mass–media and other sources of communication. Both among men and among women, the group of people sub-ject to the influence of this type of traumatic stressor can be distinguished across different ages.

In our work, perception of terrorist threat is examined as a subjective estimation of risk to fall a victim of act of terrorism. Acting from mass–media and other sources of communication, information about acts of terrorism and supposed consequences (number of victims, features of damages, etc.) and, similarly, internal information in the form of remembrances about past terrorist events and their consequences are starting mechanisms, contingent on increases in the subjective risk estimate that one will fall prey to a future act of terrorism. The possible predictors of the terroristic sensitivity are emotional instability and unsteady individuals from data of our additional research (Bykhovets, 2008; Tarabrina & Bykhovets, 2006).

Terroristic sensitivity is related to a high level of signs of PTSD; this allows us to include the phenomenon of terrorist threat into the number of traumatic stressors. The specificity of answers from peaceful populations of different regions Russia regarding terrorist threats testifies to the low tolerance for this type of stressor. It is shown that residing in a region with a high frequency of acts of terrorism (ChR) increases the risk of terroristic sensitivity and posttraumatic reactions. Remoteness far from the locations of acts of terrorism (Chita) reduces intensity of terroristic sensitivity. In our view, it can be related to the fact that terroristic sensitivity actualizes a necessity to be out of harm's way, for defense, as one of the basic, dominant necessities for a person. Aspir-ing for organization, stability, legality, and order adds to the predictability of events and frees one from such threatening factors as illness, fear, or chaos.

Probably, there is some dissonance between information from mass–media and other sources of communication about the inevitability of acts of terrorism and information on the organization of protective measures for their prevention. This data indicates an expedient need for a more detailed study of the psychological consequences of the influence of acts of terrorism on the population. The necessity to develop complex models of psychological stability to the traumatic influences of acts of terrorism is obvious, and it should include socially demographic and personal characteristics that are able to influence processes of coping with a traumatic event.

Continuation of research in this direction is, not only interesting, but also necessary. Knowledge about similar psychological aspects of the problem of terrorism and about mechanisms of its effects on a population has not only scientific but also practical importance.

Note

The study was supported by State task FANO RF No .0159-2015-0010.

References

Apolone, G., Mosconi, P., & La Vecchia, C. (2002). Post traumatic stress disorder (letter). *New England Journal of Medicine, 346*, 1495–1496.

Bykhovets, J. V. (2008). *Ideas about acts of terrorism and perception of the terrorist threat by population of the different regions of Russian federation.* Ph.D. Thesis. Moscow (Bykhovets, J. V. (2008). Predstavlenie o terroristicheskom acte I perezivanie terroristicheskoi ygrozi zitelyami raznih regionov RF. Dissertazia kandidata psyhologicheskih nauk. Moscow] (in Russian).

Bykhovets, J. V., & Tarabrina, N. V. (2010a). *Dependence between level of terroristic threat and parameters of psychological well-being at schoolchildren.* In School and health for the 21st century. Health education: International experiences (pp. 433–441). Brno.

Bykhovets, J. V., & Tarabrina, N. V. (2010b). *Psychological estimation of perception of the terrorist threat: Guidance.* Moscow: Institute of Psychology RAN. [Bykhovets, J. V., & Tarabrina, N. V. (2010). Psichologicheskaya ozenka perezivaniya terroristicheskoi ygrozi: Rukovodstvo. Moscow: IP RAN] (in Russian).

Derogatis, L. R., Rickels, K., & Rock, A. (1976). The SCL-90 and the MMPI: A step in the validation of a new self-report scale. *British Journal of Psychiatry, 128*(3), 280–289.

Dixon, P., Rehling, G., & Shiwach, R. (1993). Peripheral victims of the Herald of free enterprise disaster. *British Journal of Medical Psychology, 66*(2), 193–202.

Enikolopov, S. N., Lebedev, S. V., & Bobosov, E. A. (2004). Influence of extreme events on indirect victims. *Psikhologicheskiy zhurnal, 25*(6), 73–76. [Enikolopov, S. N., Lebedev, S. V., & Bobosov, E. A. (2004). Vliyanie ekstremalnih sobiti na kosvennih zerts. *Psikhologicheskiy zhurnal, 25*(6), 73–76] (in Russian).

Kharlamenkova, N. E., & Nikitin, E. P. (2000). *Phenomenon of human self-affirmation.* St. Peterburg: Alteya. [Kharlamenkova, N. E., & Nikitin, E. P. (2000). Fenomen chelovecheskogo samoutverzdenia. St. Peterburg: Alteya] (in Russian).

Kohanov, V. P., Krasnov, V. N., & Kekelidze, Z. I. (2000). Psychological and psychiatric aspects of a medical and preventive and rehabilitation help in emergencies. *Zhurnal Medicina katastrof, 1*(29), 61–63. [Kohanov, V. P., Krasnov, V. N., & Kekelidze, Z. I. (2000). Psihologo-psihiatricheskie aspect v lechebno-profilacticheskoi i reabilitazionnoi pomoshi v chrezvichainih situaziyah. Zhurnal Medicina katastrof, 1*(29), 61–63] (in Russian).

Pisarenko, V. M. (1986). A role of psyche is providing of emotional stability of man. *Psikhologicheskiy zhurnal, 7*(1), 62–72. [Pisarenko, V. M. (1986). Rol psihiki v obespechenii emozionalnoi ustoichivosti cheloveka. Psikhologicheskiy zhurnal, 7*(1), 62–72] (in Russian).

Roetzer, L. M., & Walch, S. E. (2004). *Undergraduate reactions to terrorism: A phenomenological analysis.* In The International Society for Traumatic Stress Studies 20th Annual Meeting. Final Program and Proceedings (pp. 34–36). War as a Universal Trauma, New Orleans, LA.

Rubin, G. J., Brewin, C. R., Greenberg, N., Hughes, J. H., Simpson, J., & Wessely, S. (2007). Enduring consequences of terrorism: 7-month follow-up survey of reactions to the bombings in London on 7 July 2005. *British Journal of Psychiatry, 190*(4), 350–356.

Rudovski, A. A., Voloshina, I. A., & Aksenova, I. V. (2004). Department of urgent psychological help of MSPP and his participating in liquidation of consequences of the dramatic February events 2004 in Moscow. In M. M. Reshetnikov (Ed.), *Psihologiya I psihopatologiya terrorizma. Gumanitarnie strategii antiterrora* (pp. 238–248). St. Peterburg: Vostochno-Evropeiski Institut Psihoanaliza. |Rudovski, A. A., Voloshina, I. A., & Aksenova, I. V. (2004). Otdel ecstrennoy psyhologicheskoi pomoshi MSPP I ego uchastie v likvidazii posledstvii dramaticheskih fevralskih sobitii 2004 goda v Moskve. In M. M. Reshetnikov (Eds.) *Psihologiya I psihopatologiya terrorizma. Gumanitarnie strategii antiterrora* (pp. 238–248). St. Peterburg: Vostochno-Evropeiski Institut Psihoanaliza| (in Russian).

Saltzman, W. R., Pynoos, R. S., Layne, C. M., Steinberg, A. M., & Aisenberg E. (2001). Trauma and grief focused intervention for adolescents exposed to community violence: Results of a schoolbased screening and group treatment protocol. *Group Dynamics: Theory, Research and Practice, 5*(4), 291–303.

Selye, H. (1992). *When stress does not bring grief.* Moscow: Misl. |Selye, H.(1992). Kogda stress ne prinosit gorya. Moscow: Misl| (in Russian).

Simeon, D., Greenberg, J., Knutelska, M., Schmeidler, J., & Hollander, E. (2003). Peritraumatic reactions associated with the World Trade Center disaster. *American Journal of Psychiatry, 160*(9), 1702–1705.

Speckhard, A. (2002). Inoculating resilience to terrorism: Acute and posttraumatic stress responses in US military, foreign & civilian serving overseas after September 11th. *Traumatology, 8*(2), 105–122.

Speckhard, A. (2003). Acute stress disorder in diplomats, military and civilian Americans living abroad following the September 11th terrorist attacks on America. *Professional Psychology: Research & Practice, 34*(2), 151–158.

Speckhard, A. (2012). *Talking to terrorists: Understanding the psycho-social motivations of militant Jihadi terrorists, mass hostage takers, suicide bombers & martyrs.* McLean, VA: Advances Press.

Speckhard, A., Verleye, G., & Jacuch, B. (2012). Assessing psycho-social resilience in diplomatic, civilian & military personnel serving in a high-threat security environment during counter insurgency and counter-terrorism operations in Iraq. *Perspectives on Terrorism, 6*(3), 23–44.

Tarabrina, N. V., & Bykhovets, J. V. (2006). The empirical study of the terrorist treat. In J. Victorov (Eds.), *NATO security through science series: Human and societal dynamics. Tangled roots: Social and psychological factors in the genesis of terrorism* (Vol. 11, pp. 242–258). USA: IOS Press, University of Southern California Keck School of Medicine. Oxford.

Tarabrina, N. V., & Bykhovets, J. V. (2007). Perception of the terrorist threat by habitants of Moscow. In A. L. Zuravlev, A. I. Lyashenko, & V. E. Inozemzeva (Eds.), *Tezisi pervoi mezdunarodnoi nauchno-prakticheskoi konferenzii «Psihologicheskie problem sem'i i lichnosti v megapolise"* (pp. 119–123). Moscow: Institut Psyhologii RAN. |Tarabrina, N. V., & Bykhovets, J. V. (2007). Perezivanie terroristicheskoi ygrozi zitelyami Moskvi: empiricheskoe issledovanie. In A. L. Zuravlev, A. I. Lyashenko, & V. E. Inozemzeva (Eds.), *Tezisi pervoi mezdunarodnoi nauchno-prakticheskoi konferenzii «Psihologicheskie problem sem'I I lichnosti v megapolise"* (pp. 119–123). Moscow: Institut Psyhologii RAN| (in Russian).

Tarabrina, N. V., & Bykhovets, J. V. (2009). *Relationship between level of terrorist threat experience and PTSD.* Final Program and Proceedings. Traumatic Stress Disorders: Toward DSM-V and ICD-11. ISTSS 25th Annual Meeting. P.221.

Tarabrina, N. V., Vorona, O. A., & Bykhovets, J. V. (2007). Ideas about acts of terrorism by population of the different regions of Russian Federation. *Psikhologicheskiy zhurnal, 28*(6), 40–50. |Tarabrina, N. V., Vorona, O. A., & Bykhovets, J. V. (2007). Predstavleniya o teracte u naseleniya razlichnih regionov Rossii. Psikhologicheskiy zhurnal, 28(6), 40–50| (in Russian).

Vreven, D. L., Gudanowski, D. M., & King, L. A. (1995). The civilian version of the Mississippi PTSD scale: A psychometric evaluation. *Journal of Traumatic Stress, 8*(1), 91–109.

Yastrebov, V. S. (2004). Terrorism and psychical health (scale of problems, tolerance of population, organization of help). *Zhurnal nevrologii i psihiatrii, 6,* 4–8. |Yastrebov, V. S. (2004). Terrorism i psihicheskoe zdorov'e (macshtab problem, tolerantnost' naseleniya, organizaziya pomoshi). *Zhurnal nevrologii i psihiatrii, 6,* 4–8| (in Russian).

23

Martyrdom as a result of psychosocial resilience

The case of Palestinian suicide terrorists

Jonathan Matusitz

This paper examines the development of Palestinian martyrs (i.e. suicide terrorists) by applying key tenets of psychosocial resilience. Psychosocial resilience refers to a person's ability to adapt to stress and adversity. Examples of psychosocial stress and adversity include family problems, workplace hardships, and cultural and societal predicaments (Rutter, 1985, 1987). Martyrdom is a particular type of suicide terrorism. It refers to heroic death, usually in "holy war," sanctified by a deity. Death in battle leads to a new life (i.e. immortality), and the deceased is lionized as a martyr (Matusitz, 2014). In the Palestinian territories, martyrs-to-be are sometimes interviewed before embarking on their last missions. Some have actually been interviewed in Israeli jails after being caught. A recurrent theme, across many narratives, is that they express a desire to escape such "cultural and societal predicaments." Their abhorrence of living on earth stems, in part, from their abject economic miseries and stressful living situations. According to the World Bank (2001), over one-third of the Palestinian population – roughly one million people – live below the poverty line of $2.10 per day.

Past studies (e.g. Luthar, Cicchetti, & Becker, 2000; Reissman, Klomp, Kent, & Pfefferbaum, 2004; Zimmerman & Arunkur, 1994) have shown that a great deal of research has concentrated on the person, mostly ignoring social affiliations or contextual factors. In this paper, this shortcoming is overhauled through the examination of Palestinian martyrs' psychological development within their social milieu, context, and personal experiences. Research on resilient youths suggests that adaptational approaches are strongly correlated to, not only their milieu and context, but their competence and determination as well -- based on their experiences and interpretations of the world (Masten & Coatsworth, 1998; Nettles & Mason, 2004). Such approaches involve (1) attachment to people, a highly motivational system that creates and sustains relationships with mentors and "guides" (i.e. the individual can surmount difficulties in a social environment) and (2) self-efficacy, the belief in one's ability to accomplish objectives in a given situation (i.e. martyrdom itself) by being able to "pull through" and "go elsewhere." The first approach will be explained through the structuralist perspective; the second one will be explained through the phenomenological perspective. This chapter ends with a discussion that also offers suggestions for future research.

Psychosocial resilience

Psychosocial resilience refers to as a person's ability to overcome stress and adversity by taking certain actions (whether short or long term) to improve themselves. Examples of stress and adversity are personal problems (e.g. psychological, health related, etc.), family or relationship strains, and job-related and financial stressors, among others (Rutter, 1985, 1987). Resilient individuals can successfully adapt to daily life and easily steer their way around crises and rely on effective methods of coping (Werner & Smith, 1992). Resilience should be regarded as a process, instead of a trait to be had (Masten, Best, & Garmezy, 1990). Stressful experiences can affect not only the developmental process of children and adolescents, but the health and welfare of adults as well (Compas, 1987; Dubow & Tisak, 1989). This topic is of utmost importance here because a certain number of Palestinian suicide terrorists are still in their teens (Child Soldiers International, 2004; Myre, 2004). The number of developmental and behavioral changes occurring in teenage years is unusually high, as compared with that of other age groups. Adolescence marks a period of precipitous mental, social, emotional, and physical change (Forman, 1993).

Protective factors

Protective factors are particular competencies required for the process of resilience to take place. Generally, competencies are healthy skills and capacities that a person can access and may happen within both the individual and group (i.e. interpersonal or family) environment (Dyer & McGuinness, 1996). Individual factors that protect people from risks include, but are not limited to, self-esteem and internal locus of control (the belief that one can control one's life) (Garmezy, 1983, 1987; Werner & Smith, 1982). Group factors consist of family cohesion and a healthy relationship with at least one relative or close friend/mentor (Campbell, 1987; Rutter, 1979). As one can see, protective factors are greatly influenced by supportive elements in the larger environment. They function at different levels and through various mechanisms – individual, family, collective, institutional, and so forth – and often relate to and complement one another (Boyden & Mann, 2005). Now, psychosocial resilience is not a novel concept. It has been established by psychological and human development theories (Stewart, Reid, & Mangham, 1997). Two of these approaches are the structuralist perspective and the phenomenological perspective.

Structuralist perspective

The structuralist perspective (or structuralism *tout court*) rests on the premise that the main objects of knowledge are formed by the relationships between behaviors and the events that constitute the life of individuals or groups (Lacharité, 2005). Put another way, although practically anyone is capable of resilience, it is the interplay between the person and his or her broader environment that accounts for the level of resilience (Egeland, Carlson, & Sroufe, 1993; Tusaie & Dyer, 2004). According to structuralism, the mélange of interaction skills, relationships, and achievements facilitates resilience because it has a positive impact on relationships with others. Such mélange can be created through participation in community life, talents or accomplishments valued by oneself or esteemed by others, access to and utilization of protective processes, adaptive coping mechanisms appropriate to the situation and the individual, and maturing out of negative experiences (Williams & Drury, 2009).

From this vantage point, psychosocial resilience possesses dynamic, interactional, and systemic traits; personal factors intermingle with experience and fluctuating circumstances. In many cases, the quality of our family, peer, school, and workplace relationships; the events we go through in life; and the type of attachments we have are crucial formative elements (Williams & Drury, 2009). The structuralist perspective of resilience assumes transactional stimuli between individual and other systems. People and their peers, families, teachers, and many other folks with whom they communicate on a daily basis reciprocally shape each other (Sameroff & MacKenzie, 2003). At the macro-level of interaction, individuals (particularly youths) in modern society can influence cultural traditions (e.g. style of dress, culinary practices, movies, music) that are produced and how they are marketed (Masten, 2004). At the same time, observance of cultural traditions through constant learning and implementing one's local and/or global cultural practices, values, and beliefs eventually shapes those practices, values, and beliefs. As we will see with the macro-level environmental factors that shape would-be Palestinian suicide terrorists, cultural traditions that seem to address the needs and concerns of youths are actually fulfilling the needs of a specific culture or society at large.

Phenomenological perspective

Phenomenology examines the structures of experience and consciousness. A person becomes who he or she is through his or her life experiences, judgments, and perceptions of the world (Zahavi, 2003). Therefore, the phenomenological perspective rests on the premise that life is seen as an occurrence experienced by the person. In the context of resilience, it entails taking a "subjectifying" look that focuses on the person's experience in circumstances of vulnerability. It also concentrates on the relationship with self and others that risk creates in such circumstances. Thus, the phenomenological approach improves our understanding of the "horizons" of actions and identity of people when they experience vulnerability (Lacharité, 2005).

In phenomenological resilience, the individual is in the position to face up to the situation of hardship. Now, such individual can realize and create a "thick description" of his or her own history, path through life, and the means he or she has used to take action. This type of experience enables the conversion (instead of just mobilization) of resources: a revitalization of suppressed or untapped resources, a restoration of resources that were not honored, and an actualization of future resources (e.g. through terrorist training) so that they acquire new meanings in new contexts. Unlike the structuralist perspective, this phenomenological process of resilience is mostly identity based (Soulet, 2003).

Martyrdom as suicide terrorism

Suicide terrorism refers to a violent attack on a target in which a terrorist aims at killing others, while being cognizant that he or she will die in the attack itself (Pedahzur, 2006). Unlike other terrorist or militant tactics, in suicide terrorism, the achievement of a suicide attack hinges exclusively on the destruction of the perpetrator(s) – e.g. via a massive explosion – who uses him- or herself as a weapon against individuals and/or material objects (Baloch, 2010). Using one's body as a terrorist weapon is called "biopolitics"; the body is turned into a destructive weapon (the shattered body parts are now devastating projectiles) (Hardt & Negri, 2005). Schweitzer, Levin, and Yogev (2014) found that, in 2014, close to 600 suicide bombings occurred, which is a 94% increase over 2013.

Martyrdom

In the jihadist context, martyrdom is a specific kind of suicide terrorism. It refers to heroic death, often in holy war, that is hallowed by a deity or Supreme Being. Death in battle leads to eternal life, and the "hero" is lionized as a martyr (Matusitz, 2014). Islamist martyrdom is often group-assisted mass destruction by way of suicide bombings. Martyrdom is nurtured through a group-held fantasy of annihilating infidels (Jews, Christians, pagans, and sometimes even fellow Muslims perceived as unfaithful Muslims). In Islamism, a martyrdom operation (i.e. what we call a suicide mission or suicide attack in the West) is justifiable; it is an acceptable way to die at the hands of the enemy and a legitimate approach to please Allah. Some Islamist leaders even claim that it is Allah, not the martyr-to-be, who determines whether the latter will die and whether innocent people will die alongside the martyr (Kobrin, 2010). The essence of this section can be encapsulated in one concept: *istishhad*. In Arabic, *istishhad* means martyrdom, a martyr's death, or an heroic death. When translated word for word, it actually signifies "self-chosen martyrdom" (Juergensmeyer, 2000). The Arabic label for the martyr him- or herself is *shahid* (*shuhada* in the plural) (Gruber, 2012).

Palestinian martyrdom

In the Palestinian territories, terrorist organizations like Hamas recruit, indoctrinate, and coach their martyrs-to-be. Hence, the martyr is frequently a product of his or her social environment. He or she depends, in large part, on the ideology of the society/community and other central catalysts as well. There is a growing inclination to consider martyrdom an emblem of resistance and terrorism (Barlow, 2007). Hamas is a Palestinian organization that has been labeled as a terrorist organization by countries such as Australia, Canada, Israel, Japan, and the United States. Hamas is very active in the Gaza Strip (Hilsenrath & Singh, 2007). Hamas terrorism has much to do with *istishhad* in the Palestinian territories. In Palestinian society, the *shahid* can gain high social status – even after his or death – if the suicide mission is accomplished successfully (Juergensmeyer, 2000). The Israel Ministry of Foreign Affairs (2008) reported that, between 2000 and 2007, no fewer than 140 Hamas-linked suicide terrorist attacks took place in Israel and the Palestinian territories, which killed over 540 people.

Palestinian martyrdom as a result of psychosocial resilience

The psychological development of Palestinian suicide terrorists must first be considered within their social milieu and context. Extreme violence as a resilient method was introduced by Elsass (1992) in his field studies with South American Indians and African Americans. Survival and resilience were successfully accomplished because the community capitalized on "good violence." "Good violence" was akin to legitimate and necessary brutality that had to be seen and heard (Hunter & Chandler, 1999). In this regard, psychosocial resilience induces the promise of something good out of misfortune, misery, or adversity (Dyer & McGuinness, 1996). A common assumption is that stressful life events cause individuals to become more vulnerable to psychological, behavioral, or somatic problems (Compas, 1987; Cowan, Cowan, & Schulz, 1996; Garmezy, 1983; Hetherington & Blechman, 1996). By definition, vulnerability is a human condition that increases the probability (i.e. à propos incidence, severity, or duration) of a person or group to develop a particular problem when facing a given risk. It is an issue that interacts with the risk and exacerbates the impact of that risk on the person or group (Lacharité, 2005).

Resilience is particularly salient during times of transition, when stresses reach their highest levels. Examples of such transitions are school entry and dissociation from family and friends (Luthar & Zigler, 1992). Research on resilient youths suggests that survival of stressful life events and adaptation to a new life are associated with competence and practice (Masten & Coatsworth, 1998). Competence and practice include emotional attachment to like-minded others; a high degree of relationships with caregivers and mentors; self-regulation (being able to modulate emotion); and self-efficacy (a strong belief in oneself, so as to achieve the goals required in certain circumstances) (Nettles & Mason, 2004). All these traits suggest that individuals learn how to "work against" tough situations through strategies that avoid bending or backing down in the face of misfortune, misery, or adversity. As we will see, these traits bestow the necessary underpinnings that guide many Palestinian suicide terrorists.

Structuralist perspective

Psychosocial resilience can be determined by a vigorous interaction between the person, the family environment, and the larger social context (Werner & Johnson, 1999). In fact, the influence of just one older mentor can yield a tremendous impact on a person's resilience (Werner & Smith, 1992). Family members and close friends can play a big part in helping individuals understand, process, and overcome difficult times. Even peer mentors can become role models for problem solving, inspiration, and other coping skills (Punamaki, 1987; Turton, Straker, & Mooza, 1990). Dyer and McGuinness (1996) refer to this whole idea as "prosocial attitude," a sociable, benign attitude that promotes attachment to those who need the development of resilience.

In the Palestinian territories, there is "no child left behind." He or she often enjoys social protection through such prosocial attitude: by being welcome, nurtured, and taken care of by local communities until mature enough to start his or her own family (Burgoon, 2006). The problem is that seemingly innocuous social welfare programs are sometimes designed to turn disaffected youths into suicide killing machines. Furthermore, becoming a martyr for the cause actually means to die for Allah, a status symbol that attracts many of these disaffected youths. For many Palestinians, *istishhad* is the ultimate performance of sacrifice: by removing any infidel off the earth, *shahids* perform a ritual in which they raise their status and prove themselves indomitable over their targets (Matusitz, 2014). Through such sanctimonious acts, their Palestinian brethren emphathize with them. When interviewed on their last journey (before exploding their grenades or suicide vests), martyrs-to-be usually wish their wives and children would do the same in the future. After all, martyrdom is a form of communal healing, and it is the greatest honor for a martyr's family (Hareven, 1983).

Communal routines and rituals can help youths surmount the effects of stress in their lives. Simple routines like collective meals, storytelling, and sports can be important sources to achieve a sense of order and structure (Gilligan, 2000). They can help preserve or restore predictability in a person's life. Predictability is of utmost importance for martyrdom training; the young recruit needs to be extremely focused to complete his or her suicide mission successfully. Therefore, the recruit needs to be constantly nurtured so as to reach a steady mental state and behavior, which allows terrorist leaders to know in advance what to expect from the recruit (Berko, 2009). Frequent celebrations and rituals can also assume great symbolic significance. According to Sandler, Miller, Short, and Wolchik (1989), "rituals have symbolic significance in that they signify collective identity and continuity" (p. 279). They can give a young recruit a sense of order in a life that was previously ruled by disorder.

Being in a cult as ritual is important when understanding the motives of Palestinians to engage in martyrdom (Matusitz, 2012). When a recruit agrees and abides by the rules of the cult, it is called "positive cult." The positive cult imposes the norms for collective and normative behavior. It consists of a series of rituals that unite group members around the sacred. One of those sacred rites is a mystical rite called the "last night." The "last night" is a poem or a bunch of verses that martyrs-to-be recite before embarking on their ultimate mission. Metaphorically speaking, the "last night" means that true Muslims are those who risk or sacrifice their lives against the enemies (whereas coward ones recoil in shame behind closed doors or on the back rows) (Cook, 2002). Such a positive cult is a ritual through which humans "have always believed that they upheld positive and bilateral relations with religious forces" (Durkheim, 1915, p. 326). The positive cult serves two purposes: to reinforce recruits' commitment to collective values and to evoke the power of religious/cultural symbols over the recruits' consciousness (Brow, 1981).

Interpersonal connections give youths an arena of support where they can cultivate certain skills and attitudes and learn to take care of one another. Nevertheless, within certain districts of the Palestinian territories, even those groups that have such positive peer-to-peer support may intentionally get confined to isolated environments. If new recruits agree to live within such positive cults, they will be more likely to give up their associations with certain previous groups – this is analogous to a replacement of relationships. A positive cult may contribute enormously to an individual's psychosocial resilience, but it also creates a "milieu control" based on the reasoning that previous group identities would encumber the unconditional commitment required by the martyrdom training team (Singer & Lalich, 1995). Such circumstances give rise to the concept of herd behavior, whereby people discard their sense of self, become whipped into a larger group experience, and are no longer restricted by sentiments of morality or humanity. This is how martyrs-to-be subdue their own identity to the collective identity of the group; now, what serves the group cause is the only thing that matters (Orléan, 1995; Post, 2010).

In both the Western and non-Western worlds, institutions such as non-profit organizations and organized community groups can boost disaffected people's self-esteem by providing them with a supportive context. When both local neighborhoods and the powers-that-be act as the welfare state, people tend to improve their psychosocial resilience. As such, assisting people through a series of interventions, including food aid, housing, collective insurance, and specialized institutions of childhood (e.g. child care and leisure centers) can be a great addition to traditional family support (Boyden & Mann, 2005). In fact, in times of predicament, they may be a substitute for family altogether. In case the state does not intervene to help disaffected people, the latter can improve their resilience when relying on the mobilization efforts of civil society and community organizations. These are informal protective processes that may even include joint labor on community developments, therapies proposed by traditional healers, and spiritual guidance by religious leaders (Boyden & Mann, 2005).

In academic jargon, civic duties and community developments implemented by organizations are sometimes referred to as "corporate citizenship." Corporate citizenship describes the activities carried out by organizations to fulfill their social responsibilities (Smith, 1996). Even though the concept of corporate citizenship originates from the business world (Miller, 1996), it is also practiced in the terrorist world. Hamas has gained widespread support among the Palestinians, partly because it has done a great deal of social work for the Palestinian people: it runs state-of-the-art and affordable clinics in areas of need; it provides assistance to locals in mosques and schools. Already in the mid-1980s, Hamas operated 40% of the mosques in the Gaza Strip. It also controls the IUG (Islamic University of Gaza) (Gunderson, 2003). Hence, the peaceful side of Hamas tends to be more visible to local Palestinians, many of whom also enjoy Hamas-supported food aid programs (Juergensmeyer, 2000).

In line with these contentions, Hamas tends to the martyr's family by covering their financial needs. In the beginning of the First Intifada (1987–1993), the cost of a Palestinian *shahid* was approximately $2,000. More exactly, those who agreed to become suicide bombers were promised that their entire families would obtain $2,000 when mission accomplished – an astronomical amount of money in that society (Saad, 2001). According to Hassan (2001), after a successful martyrdom operation, Hamas may even give the martyr's family between $2,800 and $5,000 (based on the actual damage caused by the operation). College scholarships for siblings and compensation for their families' resettlement – if their homes were destroyed by the Israel Defense Forces (IDF) – are guaranteed as well (Kelly, 1994).

Phenomenological perspective

When a person believes that he or she has new direction in life, this may help combat his or her sense of failure in other spheres of life as well. In this situation, success is not necessarily based on competition, but it is based on a person's interpretations of experience and consciousness (Rutter, 1990). Phenomenology, in and of itself, investigates the interpretations of experience and consciousness. An individual views him- or herself through his or her life experiences, beliefs, and outlooks on the world (Zahavi, 2003). This process can be so essential to the experience of resilience that individuals navigating through difficult times can eventually come to terms with their own needs. This allows them to develop both their own selves and personal goals so as to overcome their adversity. For Lacharité (2005), two types of goals are possible in phenomenological approaches of resilience: "pulling through" and "going elsewhere."

1   "Pulling through": a goal that is part of the actual circumstance of vulnerability. It does not rise above the situation but involves the individual getting past the difficult situation by ascribing it a new meaning. "Pulling through" is similar to "facing up to"; it denotes a commitment to become involved in a process so essential to the experience of resilience. The individual can give a new meaning to his or her situation by developing a new narrative about the predicament that he or she is experiencing (Soulet, 2003).
2   "Going elsewhere": This goal depends on the individual rising above the actual circumstance of vulnerability. Generally, the individual has a new project in life (Lacharité, 2005). For Palestinian martyrs-to-be, the new project is the achievement of eternal life in *janna* (Arabic for Paradise or the Heavenly Garden).

In academic terms, "pulling through" and "going elsewhere" would be associated with self-efficacy. Self-efficacy is the extent to which one believes in one's ability to complete tasks and reach goals (Bandura, 1982). A crisis can be a massive motivator for youths to develop new ideas. In the Palestinian territories, scores of martyrs-to-be have been questioned before embarking on their ultimate mission. Those who were caught by Israeli authorities are willing to answer key questions. A shared belief, in the Islamists' narratives, is that they express high uncertainty about living on earth. This, in part, relates to their miserable economic situations and resultant stressful lives (Matusitz, 2014). The World Bank (2001) reports that over a third of Palestinians, about 1 million of them, make less than $2.10 a day. Consequently, Palestinian youths can "pull through" by committing themselves to train as future martyrs and "go elsewhere" by experiencing eternal life in Paradise. To this point, martyrs-to-be are persuaded that, by exploding their bodies (and infidels in the process), the safest place in Paradise is awaiting them. They like to follow certain Quranic verses, such as Qur'an 4:74: "He who fights in the cause of Allah and is killed or achieves victory, we will bestow upon him the greatest reward." It is the martyrs' assumption that a true

Muslim is one who sacrifices him- or herself for Allah. Only then will they be bestowed an authentic and dignified life.

Generally, individuals who maintain lofty hopes about the future are more adaptable, have better problem-solving skills, and are actively attempting to control their own lives. By the same token, they are less likely to be vulnerable to their own adversity (Punamaki, 1987). For suicide terrorists, there is arguably no better self-gratification than the conviction that they will reap the highest rewards that Allah grants his favorite people: *janna* (Zeidan, 2001). Described in the Qur'an, it alludes to the Garden of Paradise for pious Muslims – i.e. true believers who have achieved martyrdom (Holtmann, 2009). In Islamist discourse, *janna* is a profound notion. It evokes a paradisiac world of lush greenery, beautiful waterfalls, and *huris* (black-eyed virgins) (Moghadam, 2003).

Discussion and future directions

What this paper has demonstrated is that both the structuralist and phenomenological approaches can bestow the theoretical foundations for the rationales that guide many Palestinian suicide terrorists. In both cases, psychosocial resilience can determine how Palestinian martyrs-to-be are able to overcome adversity. Resilience should be identified as an assemblage of traits. As we have seen, these traits include the adaptability to stress, the development of interpersonal relationships in a social environment, motivation, self-efficacy, the focus on new projects, and so forth. Resilience, then, is contingent upon stress-resistant personal qualities – in spite of ill-starred life experiences (Markstrom, Marshall, & Tryon, 2000). Comprehending youths' unsuccessful pathways is fundamental to the body of knowledge concerned with the development of Palestinian martyrs. From a structuralist perspective, social support from mentors, guides, or even peers can significantly enhance a person's resilience. In the Palestinian territories, examples of social support are social protection (e.g. prosocial attitude), as in reflected in the "no child left behind" philosophy, and Hamas's corporate citizenship by feeding and assisting the disaffected ones. From a phenomenological perspective, the Palestinian recruits' belief in their ability to achieve eternal life in *janna* (i.e. martyrdom itself) rests on two pillars: "pull through" and "go elsewhere."

An important conclusion is that, in the context of Palestinian martyrdom, the ideal type of psychological resilience is both structuralist and phenomenological. The two types are of equal relevance in surmounting difficulties and boosting self-esteem: on the one hand, through secure and harmonious relationships in the social and larger environment and, on the other hand, through a strong belief in the success of reaching objectives by assigning new meanings to their situations (i.e. Palestinian recruits develop new narratives about both their former predicaments and future "lives").

For future research, it would be interesting to continue investigating the effects of psychosocial resilience on Palestinian martyrs-to-be by addressing the following questions. Are there other strategies that martyrdom-oriented Palestinian communities have used (or could use) to reduce stress and adversity for their future "heroes"? If that would be the case, would there be gender differences between male and female Palestinian recruits? Lastly, many individuals seem to have enough regulatory abilities to live through difficult times. However, even in the Western world, psychosocial resilience may be misdirected for negative purposes or even misused by ill-intentioned adults. This may engender depraved communities of immigrants, who will harbor feelings of oppression or discrimination toward the West. Could this depravity account for the psychosocial development of the Kouachi brothers (i.e. the ones responsible for the Charlie Hebdo terrorist attacks in Paris) or the jihadists in the July 7, 2005, London bombings?

References

Baloch, Q. B. (2010). Suicide missions: Power of the powerless and powerlessness of the powerful. *The Dialogue, 2*(2), 45–66.

Bandura, A. (1982). Self-efficacy mechanism in human agency. *American Psychologist, 37*(2), 122–147.

Barlow, H. (2007). *Dead for good.* New York: Paradigm Publishers.

Berko, A. (2009). *The path to paradise: The inner world of suicide bombers and their dispatchers.* Dulles, VA: Potomac Books.

Boyden, J., & Mann, G. (2005). Children's risk, resilience and coping in extreme situations. In M. Ungar (Ed.), *Handbook for working with children and youth: Pathways to resilience across cultures and contexts* (pp. 3–25). Thousand Oaks, CA: Sage.

Brow, J. (1981). Class formation and ideological practice: A case from Sri Lanka. *The Journal of Asian Studies, 40*(4), 703–718.

Burgoon, B. (2006). On welfare and terror: Social welfare policies and political–economic roots of terrorism. *Journal of Conflict Resolution, 50*(2), 176–203.

Campbell, A. (1987). Self-reported delinquency and home life: Evidence from a sample of British girls. *Journal of Youth Adolescence, 16*(2), 167–177.

Child Soldiers International. (2004). *Global report 2004.* London: Child Soldiers International.

Compas, B. E. (1987). Stress and life events during childhood and adolescence. *Clinical Psychology Review, 7*(3), 275–302.

Cook, D. (2002). Suicide attacks or martyrdom operations. *Contemporary Jihad Literature, 3,* 17–19.

Cowan, P. A., Cowan, C. P., & Schulz, M. S. (1996). Thinking about risk and resilience in families. In E. M. Hetherington & E. A. Blechman (Eds.), *Stress, coping, and resiliency in children and families* (pp. 1–38). Mahwah, NJ: Lawrence Erlbaum.

Dubow, E. F., & Tisak, J. (1989). The relation between stressful life events and adjustment in elementary school children: The role of social support and social problem-solving skills. *Child Development, 60*(6), 1412–1423.

Durkheim, E. (1915). *The elementary forms of religious life.* New York: Free Press.

Dyer, J. G., & McGuinness, T. M. (1996). Resilience: Analysis of the concept. *Archives of Psychiatric Nursing, 10*(5), 276–282.

Egeland, B., Carlson, E., & Sroufe, L. A. (1993). Resilience as a process. *Development and Psychopathology, 5*(4), 517–528.

Elsass, P. (1992). *Strategies for survival: The psychology of cultural resilience in ethnic minorities.* New York: University Press.

Forman, S. G. (1993). *Coping skills intervention during childhood and adolescence.* San Francisco: Jossey-Bass.

Garmezy, N. (1983). Stressors in childhood. In N. Garmezy & M. Rutter (Eds.), *Stress, coping, and development in children* (pp. 43–84). New York: McGraw-Hill.

Garmezy, N. (1987). Stress, competence, and development: Continuities in the study of schizophrenic adults, children vulnerable to psychopathology, and the search for stress-resistant children. *American Journal of Orthopsychiatry, 57*(2), 159–174.

Gilligan, R. (2000). Adversity, resilience and young people: The protective value of positive school and spare time experiences. *Children & Society, 14*(1), 37–47.

Gruber, C. (2012). The martyrs' museum in Tehran: Visualizing memory in post-revolutionary Iran. *Visual Anthropology, 25*(1), 68–97.

Gunderson, C. G. (2003). *Terrorist groups.* Edina, MN: ABDO Publishing Company.

Hardt, M., & Negri, A. (2005). *Multitude: War and democracy in the age of empire.* London: Hamish Hamilton.

Hareven, A. (1983). Victimization: Some comments by an Israeli. *Political Psychology, 4*(1), 145–155.

Hassan, N. (2001, November 19). An arsenal of believers: Talking to the "human bombs." *The New Yorker,* pp. 36–41.

Hetherington, E. M., & Blechman, E. A. (1996). *Stress, coping, and resiliency in children and families.* Mahwah, NJ: Lawrence Erlbaum.

Hilsenrath, P. E., & Singh, K. P. (2007). Palestinian health institutions: Finding a way forward after the Second Intifada. *Peace Economics, Peace Science and Public Policy, 13*(1), 1–15.

Holtmann, P. (2009). *Martyrdom, not suicide: The legality of Hamas' bombings in the mid-1990s in modern Islamic jurisprudence.* Munich: GRIN Publishing.

Hunter, A. J., & Chandler, G. E. (1999). Adolescent resilience. *Image: The Journal of Nursing Scholarship, 31*(3), 243–247.

Israel Ministry of Foreign Affairs. (2008). *Suicide and other bombing attacks in Israel since the declaration of principles (Sept 1993).* Jerusalem: Israel Ministry of Foreign Affairs.

Juergensmeyer, M. (2000). *Terror in the mind of god: The global rise of religious violence.* Berkeley: University of California Press.

Kelly, M. (1994, November 29). In Gaza, peace meets pathology. *The New York Times*, p. 56.

Kobrin, N. H. (2010). *The banality of suicide terrorism: The naked truth about the psychology of Islamic suicide bombing.* Dulles, VA: Potomac Books.

Lacharité, C. (2005). From risk to psychosocial resilience: Conceptual models and avenues for family intervention. *Texto Contexto Enferm, 14*(spe.), 71–77.

Luthar, S. S., Cicchetti, D., & Becker, B. (2000). The construct of resilience: A critical evaluation and guidelines for future work. *Child Development, 71*(3), 543–562.

Luthar, S. S., & Zigler, E. (1992). Intelligence and social competence among high-risk adolescents. *Development and Psychopathology, 4*(2), 287–299.

Markstrom, C. A., Marshall, S. K., & Tryon, R. J. (2000). Resiliency, social support, and coping in rural low-income Appalachian adolescents from two racial groups. *Journal of Adolescence, 23*(6), 693–703.

Masten, A. S. (2004). Regulatory processes, risk, and resilience in adolescent development. *Annals of the New York Academy of Sciences, 1021*, 310–319.

Masten, A. S., Best, K. M., & Garmezy, N. (1990). Resilience and development: Contributions from the study of children who overcome adversity. *Development and Psychopathology, 2*(4), 425–444.

Masten, A. S., & Coatsworth, J. D. (1998). The development of competence in favorable and unfavorable environments: Lessons from research on successful children. *American Psychologist, 53*(2), 205–220.

Matusitz, J. (2012). *Terrorism & communication: A critical introduction.* Thousand Oaks, CA: Sage.

Matusitz, J. (2014). *Symbolism in terrorism: Motivation, communication, and behavior.* Lanham, MD: Rowman & Littlefield.

Miller, W. H. (1996). Citizenship that's hard to ignore. *Industry Week, 245*(16), 21–24.

Moghadam, A. (2003). Palestinian suicide terrorism in the second intifada: Motivations and organizational aspects. *Studies in Conflict & Terrorism, 26*(2), 65–92.

Myre, G. (2004, March 25). Israeli soldiers thwart a boy's suicide bombing attempt. *The New York Times*, p. A1.

Nettles, S. M., & Mason, M. J. (2004). Zones of narrative safety: Promoting psychosocial resilience in young people. *Journal of Primary Prevention, 25*(3), 359–373.

Orléan, A. (1995). Bayesian interactions and collective dynamics of opinion: Herd behavior and mimetic contagion. *Journal of Economic Behavior & Organization, 28*(2), 257–274.

Pedahzur, A. (2006). *Root causes of suicide terrorism: The globalization of martyrdom.* New York: Routledge.

Post, J. M. (2010). "When hatred is bred in the bone:" The social psychology of terrorism. *Annals of the New York Academy of Sciences, 1208*, 15–23.

Punamaki, R. L. (1987). Content of and factors affecting coping modes among Palestinian children. *Scandinavian Journal of Development Alternatives, 6*(1), 86–98.

Reissman, D. B., Klomp, R. W., Kent, A. T., & Pfefferbaum, B. (2004). Exploring psychological resilience in the face of terrorism. *Psychiatric Annals, 33*(8), 627–632.

Rutter, M. (1979). Maternal deprivation, 1972–1978: New findings, new concepts, new approaches. *Child Development, 50*(2), 283–305.

Rutter, M. (1985). Resilience in the face of adversity: Protective factors and resistance to psychiatric disorder. *British Journal of Psychiatry, 147*(6), 598–611.

Rutter, M. (1987). Psychosocial resilience and protective mechanisms. *American Journal of Orthopsychiatry, 57*(3), 316–331.

Rutter, M. (1990). Psychosocial resilience and protective mechanisms. In J. Rolf, A. S. Masten, D. Cicchetti, K. H. Nüchterlein, & S. Weintraub (Eds.), *Risk and protective factors in the development of psychopathology* (pp. 181–214). Cambridge: Cambridge University Press.

Saad, R. (2001). Weapons of the weak. *Al-Ahram Weekly*, p. A1.

Sameroff, A. J., & MacKenzie, M. J. (2003). Research strategies for capturing transactional models of development: The limits of the possible. *Development and Psychopathology, 15*(3), 613–640.

Sandler, I. N., Miller, P., Short, J., & Wolchik, A. A. (1989). Social support as a protective factor for children in stress. In D. Belle (Ed.), *Children's social networks and social supports* (pp. 277–307). New York: John Wiley.

Schweitzer, Y., Levin, A., & Yogev, E. (2014). *Suicide attacks in 2014: The global picture.* Tel Aviv: Institute for National Security Studies (INSS).

Singer, M. T., & Lalich, J. (1995). *Cults in our midst: The hidden menace in our everyday lives*. San Francisco: Jossey-Bass.

Smith, C. (1996, September 8). Corporate citizens and their critics. *The New York Times*, p. A11.

Soulet, M. H. (2003). Faire face et s'en sortir: vers une théorie de l'agir faible. In V. Châtel & M. H. Soulet (Eds.), *Agir en situation de vulnérabilité* (pp. 67–99). Québec: Presses de l'Université Laval.

Stewart, M., Reid, G., & Mangham, C. (1997). Fostering children's resilience. *Journal of Pediatric Nursing*, *12*(1), 21–31.

Turton, R., Straker, G., & Mooza, F. (1990). The experiences of violence in the lives of township youth in "unrest" and "normal" conditions. *South African Journal of Psychology*, *21*(2), 77–84.

Tusaie, K., & Dyer, J. (2004). Resilience: A historical review of the construct. *Holistic Nursing Practice*, *18*(1), 3–10.

Werner, E., & Johnson, J. L. (1999). Can we apply resilience? In M. D. Glantz & J. L. Johnson (Eds.), *Resilience and development: Positive life adaptations* (pp. 259–268). New York: Academic/Plenum Publishers.

Werner, E., & Smith, R. S. (1982). *Vulnerable but invincible: A study of resilient children*. New York: McGraw-Hill.

Werner, E., & Smith, R. S. (1992). *Overcoming the odds: High risk children from birth to adulthood*. Ithaca, NY: Cornell University Press.

Williams, R., & Drury, J. (2009). Psychosocial resilience and its influence on managing mass emergencies and disasters. *Psychiatry*, *8*(8), 293–296.

World Bank. (2001). *Poverty in the West Bank and Gaza*. Washington, DC: West Bank.

Zahavi, D. (2003). *Husserl's phenomenology*. Stanford: Stanford University Press.

Zeidan, D. (2001). The Islamic fundamentalist view of life as a perennial battle. *Middle East Review of International Affairs*, *5*(4), 26–53.

Zimmerman, M. A., & Arunkur, R. (1994). Resiliency research: Implications for schools and policy. *Society for Research in Child Development*, *8*(4), 1–19.

24

The impact of resilience on our ability to survive, adapt and thrive

Reuven Bar-On

In that the author emphasizes the close connection between resilience and adaptability throughout this chapter, what follows is how he defines adaptability, which will hopefully facilitate a better understanding of the relationship between them:

> Adaptability means being aware of the immediate environment as well as realistically and flexibly attempting to understand and address challenges when they arise. This, in turn, facilitates the ability to manage and adapt to an ever-changing human existence. One's level of adaptability moreover, determines how successful one will be in coping with change. People who have a high level of adaptability are generally effective in understanding problematic situations as well as finding suitable solutions to them, as well as constructive ways of dealing with setbacks and resiliently recovering from them.

Adaptability is one the five meta-factors of the author's conceptual and psychometric model of "emotional and social intelligence" (Bar-On, 1997), which has been considerably influenced by Darwin's concept of *survival* and *adaptation*, which is thought to be one of the driving forces behind human existence, behavior and performance (Darwin, 1872/1965). As such and because of the close relationship between adaptability and resilience, the author will frequently focus on findings generated by the adaptability composite scale of the Emotional Quotient Inventory (*EQ-i*) as well as the three sub-scales of this composite scale (flexibility, problem solving and reality testing) in order to gain a better understanding of resilience. It will also be shown that the four other meta-factors of the Bar-On conceptualization of emotional intelligence, which are measured with the *EQ-i*, shed light on the nature of resilience as well. The following are the four other meta-factors that will also be referred to in this chapter: intra-personal strength, inter-personal compatibility, stress management and general mood (Bar-On, 1997, 2000, 2004, 2006b). As will be seen, all of these meta-factors interact with resilience in varying degrees, individually and jointly to contribute to one's ability to be resilient. It is also logical that one can be more resilient if one possesses intra-personal strength, can rely on support from significant others, copes well with stress and is able to remain positive and optimistic when facing difficulties and setbacks in addition to being adaptable (i.e. capable of realistically understand the immediate challenge and flexibly coming up with effective solutions to deal with it).

1 The impact of resilience on cognitive functioning

This first section of the chapter examines the impact of flexibility, adaptability and other factors that are closely associated with resilience on problem solving, decision making and other important aspects of cognitive functioning.

In that problem solving is thought to represent a key component of cognitive intelligence (Gardner, 1983), it is important to begin this section by examining the impact of resilience on problem solving, decision making and other aspects of cognitive functioning. This will be done by presenting findings from four studies that the author has been involved with.

The EQ-i study

When the *EQ-i* was normed in the United States and Canada between 1996 and 1997 (Bar-On, 1997), an interesting finding emerged that has relevance for the present discussion on resilience. In analyzing the data generated by the normative sample ($n = 3,831$), a significant correlation of .47 ($p < .001$) was observed between the *EQ-i*'s flexibility and problem-solving scales. Very similar correlations were observed between these two scales in the United Kingdom (.43), Israel (.46) and many other countries (Bar-On, 1997, 2000, 2004). These findings indicate that flexibility, which is a key component of adaptability and resilience, is significantly associated with the problem-solving aspect of cognitive intelligence and functioning. This also shows that there is a significant overlap between these two sub-components of the adaptability meta-factor within the factorial structure of Bar-On's conceptualization of emotional intelligence, which was further demonstrated by the fact that the flexibility, problem-solving and reality-testing factors load high on the adaptability meta-factor statistically justifying the *existence* of this meta-factor (Bar-On, 1997).

The IDF study

When the *EQ-i* was normed and validated in Israel, much of this work was conducted in the Israeli Defense Forces (IDF) in that it represents a cross-section of the local population, in spite of the narrow age range due to 2–3 years of compulsory military service for both females and males upon completing secondary school. When examining the construct validity of this instrument in Israel on a sample of 2,014, a correlation of .33 ($p < .001$) was obtained between *EQ-i*'s problem-solving scale and the *Standard Progressive Matrices* (Raven, 1958), demonstrating that the *EQ-i* problem-solving scale is, at least to some extent, assessing the problem-solving aspect of cognitive functioning. More importantly for the present discussion, the correlation between *EQ-i*'s adaptability scale and the *Standard Progressive Matrices* proved to be significant ($p < .001$) although low to moderate in magnitude as well (.30). In spite of this relatively low correlation, the results suggest that adaptability, which is associated with resilience, has an impact on cognitive functioning. It is also interesting to note that Kobasa's conceptual and psychometric model of *hardiness* (Kobasa, 1979), which is considered to be an important component of resilience (Bartone & Hystad, 2010; Bonanno, 2004), correlated significantly ($R = .36, p < .00$) with the *Standard Progressive Matrices*. These findings indicate that adaptability and hardiness are associated with the cognitive functioning. This validity study was described in detail in Fund (2001) and referred to elsewhere in Bar-On, Handley and Fund (2006).

The CCL study

In 2001, the author examined results obtained from a sample 300 adults who participated in a leadership development program at the Center for Created Leadership (CCL) in the US (Bar-On, 2006a, 2006b). The participants completed the *EQ-i*, and shortly before the program began, their performance was rated using the *Benchmarks* rating format by an average of seven to eight supervisors, peers and direct-reports. The *EQ-i* adaptability scale scores for this sample were found to be significantly correlated ($R = .32, p = .006$) with the *Benchmarks* "resourcefulness" ratings (the ability to think strategically, to flexibly solve problems and make good decisions), which is thought to assess problem solving. Their "resourcefulness" ratings were then compared with the "change and adaptation" ratings (the ability to resiliently cope with change and learn from mistakes), which essentially assesses resilience as described here. This rendered a significant and moderately high correlation ($R = .49, p < .001$), which indicates that resilience significantly impacts the problem-solving and decision-making aspects of cognitive functioning.

The IL-i study

When norming the *Inspiring Leadership Inventory* (IL-i), on 1,101 adults in the United Kingdom as was described by Travers in 2014, it was found that its "resilience" scale correlates significantly and highly ($R = .68, p < .001$) with its "general intelligence" scale. A correlation of .68 suggests that more than 45% of cognitive intelligence and functioning is based on resilience.

In an effort to briefly expand the discussion after demonstrating that adaptability impacts cognitive functioning based on these four studies, the author would like to present additional findings indicating that flexibility, adaptability, resilience, creative problem solving and the desire to do one's best are inter-related.

A number of researchers have presented findings showing that creativity and innovative thinking lead to a heightened level of problem analysis, problem solving and decision making, which is examined in the following. Before discussing these findings, however, it is important to first clarify the relationship between giftedness, creativity and innovative problem solving.

While giftedness and creativity have traditionally been associated with elevated cognitive intelligence, Peterson (1997) rightfully cautions against confusing giftedness and the capacity for creative thinking with simply possessing a significantly high IQ. He stresses that it is important to point out that many gifted students are not high achievers at school, and many high performers at school are not necessarily creative. Thompson and Rudolph (1992) stress, moreover, that a key characteristic of gifted individuals is that they are not only more effective problem-solvers than their peers but they appear to have a keen *desire* to solve problems. Additionally, they are thought to be more *flexible* and tend to apply more innovative and creative methods in attempting to find solutions to problems (Parker, 1997).

Maree and Ebersohn (Ebersohn & Maree, 2006; Maree, 2006) have presented research findings that support their hypothesis that creativity and innovative thinking play a critical role in *survival*. Their findings demonstrate that being *flexible* and *resilient* increases the ability to survive and adapt. These findings emerged from their study of copying mechanisms among a sample of South African children whose parents suffered from AIDS. The findings showed that the more cognitively, emotionally and socially gifted children coped significantly better than the less gifted in their sample. They were also found to be more *flexible*, *adaptive* and *resilient* than the others. These findings were based on test results they received from administering the youth version of the *EQ-i* (*EQ-i:YV*). They found that those children who coped better with having to run the household after their parents became ill, incapacitated and died demonstrated higher levels of

(1) self-awareness, (2) independence, (3) stress tolerance, (4) optimism and (5) flexibility. They concluded that *flexibility* and *resilience* represent the two most important contributors to survival and adaptation (Ebersohn & Maree, 2006).

It is important to emphasize that enhanced cognitive functioning and elevated levels of resilience are insufficient, in and of themselves, to effectively cope with difficulties and setbacks if one is insufficiently motivated to do so. People must be motivated to come up with potentially effective solutions and effectively apply them. Being *motivated* depends on being *engaged* and *driven to do one's best*. In that the desire and drive to do one's best is assessed by the *EQ-i* "self-actualization" scale (Bar-On, 1997, 2001), it is interesting to note that the there is a significant and moderately high correlation ($R = .53, p < .001$) between this scale and the *EQ-i*'s "problem-solving" scale (Bar-On, 1997).

Summary: The key findings presented in this section indicate that adaptability and resilience play a significant role in cognitive functioning. Moreover, the findings support the assumption that flexibility, adaptability and hardiness are all important aspects of resilience. Additionally, being motivated, engaged and driven to do one's best most likely interact with resilience in order to enhance one's ability to survive, adapt and effectively navigate through life.

2   The impact of resilience on academic performance

In that the previous section shows that resilience plays a significant role in cognitive functioning, it is logical to assume that it also plays an important role in academic performance. This assumption is not only logical according to the way cognitive intelligence is defined but is also based on the need for originally developing cognitive intelligence assessment at the end of the nineteenth century: in order to justify the placement of a learner in a specific class based on his or her *academic potential*.

For many years, the emphasis in education has been placed on strengthening cognitive skills such as (1) acquiring and applying knowledge; (2) exercising logical thinking and good judgement; and (3) combining knowledge, experience and good judgment to solve problems and make good decisions. The capacity for applying these skills is assessed with "intelligence tests" that render an "IQ" score. The more adept one is at performing these specific skills, the higher one's IQ is expected to be as well as his or her academic performance; and the higher one's IQ is, the greater are the chances that individuals will perform these cognitive skills better as well as receive higher grades (Wagner, 1997). All of this is important for succeeding at school in addition to being successful at work later on. However, being cognitively intelligent, in and of itself, is insufficient to succeed at school. In addition to being cognitively intelligent, there are other important factors that are needed in order to perform well academically. In addition to IQ, a few of the most important predictors of successful academic performance are finding meaning and purpose in what one studies, being adequately self-motivated and engaged as well as being sufficiently *resilient* to effectively cope with difficulties and failures as well as learn from them.

This section focuses primarily on the impact of adaptability and resilience on academic performance. Research findings are presented that are thought to empirically confirm this important relationship, based on four major studies conducted in Canada, South Africa, England and the United States.

The British study

In the study described here (Bar-On, 2003, 2007a, 2007b), 197 students at a secondary school for the musically gifted in England completed the youth version of the *EQ-i* (*EQ-i:YV*). This sample comprised 96 males and 101 females whose average age was 14.4 at the time they completed the *EQ-i:YV*. A multiple regression analysis examined the ability of Bar-On's five meta-factors of emotional intelligence to predict performance at school, which was rated by teachers on a five-point scale ranging from "very poorly" (1) to "very well" (5). This analysis generated a four-factor regression model with an overall correlation of .50 ($F = 12.91, p < .001$), indicating that emotional intelligence has a very significant impact on school performance. The adaptability meta-factor emerged as the strongest contributor to academic performance ($\beta = .428, t = 5.61$, $p < .001$) followed by intra-personal strength ($\beta = .187, t = 2.61, p = .010$), stress management ($\beta = .168, t = 2.26, p = .025$) and inter-personal compatibility ($\beta = .162, t = 2.16, p = .032$).

The Canadian study

In this study, a path analysis was conducted by Parker and his colleagues on 667 Canadian high school students (2004). The overall degree of correlation between emotional intelligence, assessed with the *EQ-i*, and academic performance, evaluated by grades, was found to be .41 indicating a moderate yet statistically significant relationship between emotional intelligence and academic performance. Although this is a moderate correlation, the adaptability component of this path analysis proved to be the most robust contributor to the predictive model, with an inner-path correlation of .67, when compared with the other four meta-factors of Bar-On model of emotional intelligence.

The South African study

This study was conducted on 448 South African university students (Bar-On, 1997; Swart, 1996), and clearly demonstrated that there are significant differences in emotional intelligence between more successful and less successful students. Swart (1996) examined the ability of *EQ-i* scores to differentiate between more successful and less successful students (based on one standard deviation above and below their grade point average calculated at the end of their first academic year). When compared with the other four composite scales, the adaptability scale demonstrated the most robust ability to distinguish between successful and less successful students ($t = 2.87$, $p = .010$); and this scale was closely followed by the stress management composite scale ($t = 2.64$, $p = .010$).

The American study

In this study, which was first described by Bar-On in 1997, 1,125 individuals who were admitted to the US Naval Academy at Annapolis completed the *EQ-i*. After completing their first academic year, the degree of correlation between the *EQ-i* adaptability scores and the grade point average for 821 students was examined. While multiple regression analysis generated a relatively low correlation of .26, it was nevertheless highly significant ($F = 23.03, p < .001$), showing that adaptability plays a role in academic performance at least to some extent.

Summary: In addition to showing that adaptability is significantly associated with academic performance, based on the studies described here, it was also demonstrated that adaptability is capable of significantly distinguishing between more successful and less successful students.

After showing that the adaptability significantly impacts academic performance, it is reasonable to ask if adaptability can be enhanced in order to improve success at school. In an edited book on educating people to be more emotionally and socially intelligent (Bar-On, Maree, & Elias 2007), many of the contributing authors have presented detailed approaches to how this can be done as well as the results from developing such educational programs.

3 The impact of resilience on general occupational performance, leadership and organizational profitability

In that the findings presented in the previous section demonstrate that resilience plays an important role in academic performance, it is logical to assume that it also impacts occupational performance. This section presents empirical findings that support this assumption, based on the following five studies.

The IL-i study

When the *Inspiring Leadership Inventory* (*IL-i*) was normed in the UK (Travers, 2014), one of the initial findings suggested that resilience plays an important role in occupational performance. This was based on obtaining a significant bivariate correlation of .42 ($p < .001$) between scores on the *IL-i* resilience scale for 1,101 adults and their responses to a question regarding their current performance at work. A second finding, based on criterion-group nomination, confirmed these initial results (Travers, 2014). After creating a sample of 87 individuals who were identified by colleagues as "inspiring leaders" (the designated criterion group of high performers), an analysis of variance was applied by the author to examine the ability of *IL-i* scales to distinguish between them and a randomly selected group of individuals from the normative sample. The results clearly indicated that resilience emerged as one of the most robust predictors of high occupational performance and capable of distinguishing between average performance and "inspiring" performance ($F = 12.43, p < .001$).

The USAF study

In the US Air Force (USAF) study, the role played by resilience in occupational performance was examined with a criterion-based approach (Bar-On, 1997, 2006b; Bar-On, Handley, & Fund, 2006; Handley, 1997). In this study, the *EQ-i* scores of 1,171 military recruiters were compared with their ability to meet annual recruitment quotas. High performance was defined by the USAF as meeting or exceeding 100% of their annual recruitment quotas, while low performance was defined as meeting less than 80% of their quotas. This was considered a robust measure of their occupational performance (i.e. what they do on a daily basis). After equally matching the number of female recruiters with their male counterparts, a multiple regression analysis of the three factorial components of the adaptability meta-factor revealed a correlation of .33 ($F = 13.08, p < .001$) indicating that adaptability plays a significant role in occupational performance based on the sample studied and the method applied to assess performance. Two of the three factorial components of adaptability entered the regression model that emerged; and the stronger of the two was the problem-solving component ($\beta = .204, t = 2.79, p = .006$) followed by flexibility ($\beta = .171, t = 2.34, p = 020$). Logistic regression analysis was also applied to the results, in order to examine the full range of emotional intelligence factors that were thought to impact the occupational performance of the military recruiters who participated in this study. This rendered an overall predictive coefficient of .53, demonstrating that the predictive model that emerged was able to accurately predict the recruiters' ability to meet their quotas. These results demonstrate a moderately high relationship between emotional intelligence and occupational performance. In addition to (1) the ability to *flexibly understand problems, generate effective solutions and make wise decisions*, the following are most powerful predictors of performance based on the model that emerged for this sample: (2) the ability to manage stress and work effectively in stressful situations; (3) the ability to be aware of others' feelings and work well with them; (4) the ability to constructively assert oneself; and (5) the ability to be sufficiently energized, motivated and fully engaged. After one year of comparing the *EQ-i,* scores of new candidates with this predictive model in order to make better selection decisions, the USAF increased its ability to select successful recruiters by nearly threefold decreasing first-year attrition due to costly mismatches and reducing financial losses by 92% saving the military approximately $3 million in the first year.

Based on the USAF's success with selecting more effective military recruiters described in the previous paragraph, they discussed a number of additional projects with the author of this chapter in 2007. They began to explore the potential use the *EQ-i* to predict performance in training programs for pilots, air traffic controllers and para-rescue jumpers ("PJs"). The USAF's "PJ Project" was considered top priority, at the time, and the first of these projects to be implemented (Consortium for Research on Emotional Intelligence in Organizations, 2010). The PJ course takes two years to complete and includes numerous hours of combat training, parachuting, diving, para-medical instruction as well as extensive air rescue and evacuation preparation. The total cost of completing the training was estimated at $250,000 per trainee when this study began. The USAF's aim was to explore possibilities of using the *EQ-i* to identify those candidates for the PJ course, early on, who have the best chance of successfully completing this highly specialized and expensive course. All of the 200 PJ trainees who began the 2008 course completed the *EQ-i,* and the results of those who successfully completed the program in 2010 were compared with those who did not complete it. A discriminant function analysis was applied to examine the results, which generated an overall predictive coefficient of .45 demonstrating that some of the factors assessed by the *EQ-i* have a significant impact on performance among PJ trainees and are capable of predicting who will successfully complete this course and who will most likely not complete the course. Additionally, the accuracy level of this model was considered 75% accurate based on the results of the analysis. In addition to (1) *the ability to multitask and resiliently adapt in order to effectively address new situations,* the following are the most powerful predictors of performance based on the predictive model that emerged: (2) the ability to work effectively under pressure and in stressful situations; (3) the ability to maintain composure and control of one's emotions in difficult situations; (4) the ability to be keenly aware of one's surroundings and to quickly size up the immediate situation; and (5) the ability to be energized, motivated and fully engaged in what one does. It is also interesting and important to note that the *flexibility* scale score was the highest score (113) for those who successfully completed the course when compared with those who did not complete the course (108), and it also represented the highest significant difference in scores between the two groups. By applying the model, the USAF calculated that it would save them approximately $190 million over a five-year period by significantly reducing costly mismatches and by helping the Air Force make better selection decisions. These results further confirm the important role played by resilience in performance, including performance under pressure and in potentially life-threatening situations, as well as its impact on organizational profitability.

The IDF study

In this study (Bar-On et al., 2006; Fund, 2001), leadership potential was examined by applying a criterion-group approach. This method was used, once again, to examine the potential impact of resilience on leadership performance.

Similar to the USAF's desire to make more cost-effective selection decisions, the Israeli Defense Forces (IDF) expressed an interest in seeing if emotional intelligence assessment could help identify leadership potential and better predict leadership performance. This analysis was done by comparing the *EQ-i* scale scores for 470 officer trainees (the criterion group) with a randomly selected group of 470 soldiers (the control group). This approach was thought to represent a very robust and realistic approach to identifying key leadership characteristics, because it was based on comparing a group of individuals who were actually enrolled in officer training with a group of soldiers who did not meet the requirements for officer training, did not pass the psychological screening required and/or did not express a desire to be officers. Both groups were composed of males with a mean age of 19.0 at the time they completed the *EQ-i*. The results of applying an analysis of variance revealed very significant differences between the two groups. In addition to highly significant differences ($F = 59.42, p < .001$) between the Total EQ scores obtained by the criterion group ($EQ = 107.7$) and those obtained by the control group ($EQ = 101.0$), there were significant differences between the two groups on all of the scale scores. What is particularly interesting for the present discussion is that there were large and significant differences between the criterion group ($EQ = 107.3$) and the control group ($EQ = 101.0$) on the adaptability scale ($F = 62.36, p < .001$). When examining the three sub-scale scores that contribute to adaptability, moreover, it was found that the strongest contributor to adaptability was the ability to solve problems and make decisions ($F = 87.02, p < .001$) followed by the ability to flexibly ($F = 40.97, p < .001$) size up the immediate situation ($F = 18.95, p < .001$).

These findings support the results from the previous studies presented in this section, regarding the significant impact of adaptability and resilience on leadership in general. Additionally, the findings suggest that adaptability can significantly distinguish between average soldiers and officers ("officer material"). This would also justify its use in screening, together with other key predictors of military leadership. Based on these results, moreover, a recommendation was made to High Command to use this approach as part of the existing admission procedures used in selecting officer trainees (Fund, 2001).

The CCL study

In this study (Bar-On, 2006a), the Center for Creative Leadership (CCL) used a $360°$ multi-rating system to evaluate leadership performance. This study was conducted on 300 individuals who were admitted to the CCL leadership development program. Before the course began, the participants' leadership performance was rated by an average of seven to eight supervisors, co-workers and direct-reports based on the *Benchmarks* rating format that rates 21 different predictors of effective and successful leadership. All of these individuals completed the *EQ-i* shortly after beginning the leadership program they were attending. Their averaged leadership performance, based on averaging the ratings for the twenty-one predictors of successful leadership, was then compared with their *EQ-i* scale scores including adaptability. Four of the five composite scores entered into the regression model rendering an overall regression correlation of .95 ($F = 241.18, p < .001$) in the following order of their predictive ability: adaptability ($\beta = .392, t = 8.91, p < .001$); inter-personal compatibility ($\beta = .352, t = 7.23, p < .001$); stress management ($\beta = .300, t = 7.12, p < .001$); and intra-personal strength ($\beta = .113, t = 2.28, p = .025$). This demonstrates that resilience is very closely associated with leadership performance and is the strongest predictor of this type of performance, based on the sample studied and the way resilience and performance were assessed. More succinctly and based on the way Bar-On has described these meta-factors of emotional and intelligence (1997, 2000, 2006b), those leaders who are more adaptable and resilient, adept at constructively interacting with others and capable of working well under pressure are expected to be the more successful leaders.

The Langhorn study

In the last study described in this section, the author would like to stress, once again, that adaptability and resilience are not only important for leadership performance, but they have an impact organizational profitability as well (i.e. "the bottom line"). This was also demonstrated in the USAF studies previously described. A doctoral student in the UK, Steven Langhorn, examined the relationship between (1) the emotional intelligence of 161 managers in one of Whitbread Corporation's largest restaurant chains and (2) the profitability of the restaurants they managed (Langhorn, 2004). He assessed emotional and social intelligence with the *EQ-i* and measured profitability in terms of the annual profit growth of the restaurants they managed over a one-year period. An initial examination of the data revealed a bivariate correlation of .31 (p =.014) between the *EQ-i* adaptability composite scale scores and annual profit growth, which was the second highest correlation that emerged between the five composite scales and annual profit growth. In a more powerful multivariate examination of this relationship, a multiple regression analysis produced an overall regression correlation of .47 between the regression model that emerged and annual profit growth. Among those factors that proved to be the strongest predictors of annual profit growth, the adaptability meta-factor surfaced as a significant and robust predictor. Additionally, Langhorn found that restaurants managed by managers with higher emotional intelligence, including higher levels of adaptability, showed an annual profit growth of 22% (7% above the anticipated 15% growth for the same year) representing an increase of approximately £110 million in the organization's revenues during the same period (Langhorn, 2004).

Summary: The results from these five studies clearly indicate a significant relationship between emotional intelligence and occupational performance. Within this general relationship moreover, adaptability appears to be significantly associated with occupational performance, leadership and organizational profitability. This means that adaptability and resilience can also predict performance in the workplace. Additionally, *the ability to adapt and manage change as well as to resiliently cope with challenges* can distinguish between high and low performers as well as between more inspiring and less inspiring leaders. These findings appear to justify the need to evaluate adaptability and resilience, together with the other important predictors of performance that emerged from these studies, when hiring and promoting employees for leadership positions. After hiring the best people for the position, these important predictors of performance need to be strengthened further through group training and executive coaching in order to enhance individual performance and organizational profitability.

For some time, the types of predictive models presented here have provided *roadmaps* for organizations to make better selection and development decisions that have significantly reduced costly mismatches and helped them hire more effective and productive employees who have contributed to the organization's overall productivity and profitability (see, for example Bar-On et al., 2007).

4   The relationship between resilience and physical health, with implications for coping with and recovering from serious medical conditions

This section examines the relationship between resilience and physical health as well as its potential impact on the ability to cope with serious medical conditions and life-threatening situations.

To better understand the relationship between resilience and physical health, the results from five studies are presented in the following sections. In presenting and discussing these results, an attempt will be made to address the following question: "Are people who are more resilient healthier than those who are less resilient?"

The North American study

In order to explore the general relationship between adaptability and physical health, the first study presented here examined the degree of correlation between the two (Bar-On, 2012b). This was done by conducting a multivariate correlation between the *EQ-i* adaptability scale scores and responses to a question regarding the respondents' physical health. In the North American sample upon which the *EQ-i* was originally piloted and normed (Bar-On, 1997), which included 1,867 males and 1,945 females with an average age of 34.2 years, an additional question was asked about their physical health: "I feel good about my health in general." Although this is a subjective and potentially biased estimate of one's health, such self-assessed health estimates appear to correlate significantly with medical examinations conducted by healthcare providers (Shadbolt, Barresi, & Craft, 2002) justifying its use here as an indication of physical health. The correlation that emerged from this multiple regression analysis of the data was .35 ($F = 174.97$, $p < .001$), suggesting that adaptability is significantly associated with physical health. In the three-factor regression model that emerged, the strongest contributor to adaptability was reality testing ($\beta = .181, t = 8.95, p < .001$) followed by flexibility ($\beta = .141, t = 7.47, p < .001$) and problem solving ($\beta = .102, t = 5.26, p < .001$). These results suggest that the ability to realistically and flexibly cope with challenges, which also means putting things in correct perspective, have an impact on one's health.

The British study

The second study described here more directly studied the relationship between resilience and physical health, by examining the degree of correlation between the "resilience" and "health" scales of the *IL-i* (Travers, 2014). This was carried out on a British sample of 1,101 adults. After matching for gender, a significant correlation of .36 ($p < .001$) was obtained. This appears to support the results of the previous study described here. Although correlations of this magnitude are considered moderate, these results are statistically significant and suggest the existence of a meaningful relationship.

The Annapolis study

In this study, a more rigorous and accurate evaluation of the subjects' physical health was applied by using medical ratings made by physicians. This sample comprised a total of 1,125 who were accepted to the US Naval Academy in Annapolis, which is described in greater detail by Bar-On (1997). Upon re-examining the original data, 821 individuals were identified who completed the *EQ-i* and also possessed complete medical records describing their health at the time they were accepted to the Naval Academy. A multiple regression analysis examined the degree of correlation between the individuals' *EQ-i* adaptability scores and their five-point physical health ratings. This revealed a significant regression correlation of .35 ($F = 28.75, p < .001$). Within the adaptability regression model that emerged, flexibility was the most important contributor to adaptability ($\beta = .190, t = 4.19, p < .001$) followed by problem solving ($\beta = .168, t = 3.69.$, $p < .001$) and reality testing ($\beta = .072, t = 1.88, p = .060$). This tends to confirm the findings from the two previous studies, indicating that adaptability does indeed have a significant impact on physical health.

In order to examine the ability of adaptability to distinguish between healthier and less healthy individuals, a factorial analysis of variance was applied to the data after dividing the sample into high and low levels of adaptability (based on .5 standard deviations above and below the mean adaptability score respectively). After designating gender as the covariate, the differences in medically assessed physical health between the two groups were examined. This revealed a significant difference ($F = 25.58, p < .001$) between the two groups, 4.8 and 3.2, respectively, based on the previously mentioned five-point rating scale, empirically demonstrating the important impact adaptability has on physical health.

The IDF study

This study was conducted in the Israeli Defense Forces (IDF) and compared the EQ-i scale scores of 941 new conscripts with the medical profiles they received at the Office of Mobilization (Bar-On, 2012b; Fund, 2001). Similar to the previously described study at the US Naval Academy in Annapolis, physical health was very rigorously and extensively assessed by physicians who also had access to past medical records. Medical profiles given in the IDF are composed of five digits. The first four digits describe the type medical problems that may have been diagnosed, and the fifth digit describes their severity. A multiple regression analysis was applied to compare their medically rated physical health with EQ-i scores. This rendered a regression correlation of .37 indicating a low-moderate yet significant relationship between emotional intelligence and physical health. The problem-solving component of the adaptability meta-factor contributed significantly to this regression model ($\beta = .104, t = 2.22, p = .027$).

In addition to the significant relationship between adaptability and physical health demonstrated in this study (Bar-On, 2012b), an analysis of variance examined the ability of emotional intelligence to distinguish between healthier individuals ($n = 587$) and less healthy individuals ($n = 354$). The results indicated that the flexibility component of the adaptability meta-factor was more robust than the others in significantly distinguishing between these two groups ($F = 16.91, p < .001$).

As with the previous studies described here, this study shows that adaptability and the various other factors closely associated with resilience are capable of both predicting physical health as well as distinguish between healthier and less healthy individuals.

The cancer survivorship study

The fifth and last study to be described in this section examined differences in emotional intelligence between thirty-five cancer survivors and a matched control group (Bar-On, 2012b; Krivoy, Weyl Ben-Arush, & Bar-On, 2000). This study was conducted in the Pediatric Oncology Department at Rambam Hospital in Israel. A group of eighteen females and seventeen males, who were classified as "cancer survivors" (i.e. symptom free for at least five years), were randomly selected from the hospital's records. The individuals in this group were initially diagnosed with various types of cancer in childhood or during early adolescence. In one of their follow-up examinations, they completed the EQ-i. Their EQ-i scores were then used to compare them with a control group comprising 35 randomly selected individuals from the local normative population sample matched for gender and age. While the adaptability meta-factor rendered a low correlation of .25, which was not significant at the .05 level of probability, its problem-solving component was the most robust among the three components of this meta-factor ($\beta = .266$, $t = 2.02, p = .047$). It is important to point out the most of the EQ-i scores were higher for the cancer survivors. Although the ability of the adaptability scale to predict cancer survivorship is questionable at this stage based on the results presented here, these preliminary results suggest that adaptability and resilience might still play a role in the ability to survive cancer. As such, it is recommended that future research should apply a variety of different measures of resilience on larger and more homogeneous clinical samples whilst focusing on a range of different types of cancer diagnosed at different age levels.

Summary: The results produced by the studies reviewed in this section suggest that adaptability and other aspects of resilience play a role in physical health.

5   The impact of resilience on emotional health and on overall well-being

This section describes findings from four studies that demonstrate the impact of adaptability and resilience on psychological health and overall well-being.

The EQ-i normative study

During the norming and validation of the *EQ-i* (Bar-On, 1997), this instrument was concomitantly administered with a wide variety of different measures of psychopathology including the following: (1) the Beck Depression Inventory; (2) the Eysenck Personality Questionnaire; (3) the Minnesota Multiphasic Personality Inventory; (4) the Ninety Symptom Check List; (5) the Personality Assessment Inventor; (6) and the Zung Self-Rating Depression Scale. Based on applying these and other psycho–diagnostic procedures in six major studies conducted on 765 individuals in Canada, South Africa and the United States, the results indicate that deficiencies in flexibility, adaptability and resilience are associated with the following symptoms of psychopathology based on the correlation coefficients appearing in the brackets: (1) anxiety (ranging from .35 to .58 in two studies); (2) phobias (ranging from .29 to .41 in two studies); (3) somatization (.63 in one study); (4) obsessive-compulsive traits (.71 in one study); (5) depressive mood (ranging from .31 to .69 in five studies); (6) suicidal thoughts (.55 in one study); (7) borderline personality trends (ranging from .50 to .66 in two studies); (8) paranoid tendencies (.70 in one study); and (9) psychotic ideation (.66 in one study). These results indicate that flexibility and adaptability impact psychological health (Bar-On, 2012a).

The inpatient and outpatient study

In addition to showing that deficiencies in flexibility, adaptability and other aspects of resilience are associated with a variety of psycho–pathology as was shown in the previous section, it is important to also summarize a number of actual clinical studies that demonstrate that factors closely associated with resilience are capable of significantly distinguishing between individuals diagnosed with various psychiatric disorders and non-clinical control groups. In one of the first clinical studies that directly studied this relationship, the *EQ-i* scores of 418 psychiatric patients were compared with matched control groups in Argentina, Israel, South Africa and the United States (Bar-On, 1997). The clinical samples in the United States and South Africa were obtained from psychiatric outpatient facilities, and the Israeli clinical sample comprised patients being treated in an inpatient facility, while the Argentinean clinical sample included both outpatients and inpatients. In addition to significant differences in a number of the *EQ-i* scale scores between the clinical and control groups in these samples, the findings revealed significant differences on the adaptability scale scores. The average differences, in EQ points, between the outpatient samples and controls in both the United States and South Africa were 8.4, and the difference in EQ points between the inpatient sample and the control group in Israel was 18.4 EQ points, while the difference for the mixed outpatient and inpatient sample and the control group in Argentina was 15.1 EQ points. All differences in adaptability between the clinical and control groups were significant at a probability level smaller than .01 (Bar-On, 1997, 2012a), meaning that the differences observed were highly significant. It is interesting to note that the difference in adaptability is more severe with inpatients than with outpatients, which was expected and is logical (i.e. individuals suffering from more severe psychopathology usually require treatment in inpatient rather than outpatient facilities).

The IDF mental health study

In another study (Bar-On, 2006b, 2012a; Fund, 2001), which included a sample of 2,514 males who completed the EQ-i at the time of their induction into the Israeli Defense Forces (IDF), the author identified 152 new recruits who were eventually discharged for psychiatric reasons. He then randomly selected an additional group of 152 soldiers who were diagnosed with less severe psychiatric disturbances that allowed them to continue their tour of duty with relatively few limitations. The EQ-i scores of these two groups were compared with a randomly selected group of 152 recruits, within the same population sample ($n = 2,514$), who did not receive a psychiatric profile during the entire period of their military service. This created three groups representing three different levels of psychological health: (1) individuals who were so severely disturbed that they were incapable of serving a full tour of duty, (2) individuals who received less severe psychiatric profiles that allowed them to continue active military service until completion and (3) individuals who completed their military service without having received a psychiatric profile. It was found that the adaptability scale of the EQ-i revealed a significant multivariate correlation of .39 with these three different levels of psychological health. In addition to correlating with psychological health, the adaptability scale proved to be the most robust factor that distinguishes between the groups ($F = 51.67, p < .001$). The results indicate that adaptability, flexibility and other closely associated aspects of resilience can distinguish between individuals diagnosed with psychiatric problems from others who were never diagnosed with such problems. These findings suggest, moreover, that adaptability has a significant impact on psychological health and is capable of significantly distinguishing between different levels of psychological health as well as the severity of psychiatric problems (Bar-On, 2012a).

The well-being study

In addition to having an impact on psychological health and psychopathology, as was demonstrated in the previous three studies, there is also compelling evidence indicating that adaptability and resilience have a significant impact on overall subjective well-being (i.e. how well people feel about themselves, their interpersonal relationships, their work and about life in general). A study conducted by the author in 2005 examined this relationship in detail (Bar-On, 2005). The primary focus of that study was the development of a three-factor measure of subjective well-being, based on a North American sample comprising 3,831 adults who completed the EQ-i as well as 19 additional items thought to cover various aspects of life satisfaction and overall well-being. A factor analysis of the responses revealed three distinct factors related the following areas of well-being: (1) satisfaction with one's health and oneself in general, (2) satisfaction with one's close interpersonal relationships and (3) satisfaction with one's work and source of livelihood. Bar-On argued that this particular factorial structure comprises most of the reoccurring themes traditionally used to describe subjective well-being in the literature (see, for example Diener, 2000; Helliwell & Putnam, 2004; Oswald, 1997; Ryff, 1989). In re-examining the data from this earlier study (Bar-On, 2005),the author re-ran bivariate correlations between the EQ-i adaptability scale and responses to the well-being measure that was developed. This revealed a significant and relatively high degree of correlation between adaptability and subjective well-being (R =.58, p < .001). He next applied an analysis of variance to specifically examine the ability of the EQ-i adaptability scale to distinguish between individuals with higher and lower levels of subjective well-being (one standard deviation above and below the mean for overall well-being, respectively). Among the five EQ-i composite scales, the adaptability scale emerged as the third strongest in distinguishing between these two groups (F = 1056.56, p < .001). The two other stronger composite scales were general mood (F = 1954.00, p < .001) followed by inter-personal compatibility (F = 1611.19, p < .001). These findings may indicate that healthy adaptability impacts one's overall sense of well-being by interacting with satisfying inter-personal relationships and maintaining positive mood. The directionality of (1) effective adaptability and resilience, (b) mutually satisfying inter-personal relationships and (2) positive mood needs to be further addressed by future research, in order to determine the direction of the vectors involved (i.e. what impacts what, how and to what degree).

Summary: The findings presented in this section demonstrate that adaptability significantly impacts psychological health and overall subjective well-being. Based on these findings, more-over, it appears that individuals who are adaptable and resilient typically have better psychological health and a higher sense of overall well-being than those who are less adaptable and resilient. As such, it can be said that the findings presented justify the need to focus more on adaptability and resilience in psycho-assessment, psycho-diagnostics and psycho-therapeutic intervention. In another publication, moreover (Bar-On, 2012a), the author describes in detail how this can be done.

Concluding comments

The results provided by the twenty-two studies reviewed in this chapter indicate that resilience plays a significant role in (1) cognitive functioning, (2) academic performance, (3) occupational performance, (4) physical health and (5) psychological health and overall subjective well-being.

In order to gain greater insight into what was presented and discussed here, future research in this area will need to apply a wider array of assessment methods on larger and more diverse population samples. In light of the fact that the studies presented here were cross-sectional in design, future studies should attempt to examine how resilience develops over time.

It is the author's hope that the findings discussed in this chapter, and those presented by the other contributors to this volume, will add to the literature by demonstrating the importance of resilience for performance, health and well-being. Hopefully these findings will also inspire other researchers to learn more about resilience and eventually inspire parents, educators and practitioners to apply this growing body of knowledge, in order to not only help people *survive* but to *thrive*.

References

Bar-On, R. (1997). *The Bar-On Emotional Quotient Inventory (EQ-i): Technical manual*. Toronto, Canada: Multi-Health Systems.

Bar-On, R. (2000). Emotional and social intelligence: Insights from the Emotional Quotient Inventory (EQ-i). In R. Bar-On & J. D. A. Parker (Eds.), *Handbook of emotional intelligence: Theory, development, assessment and application at home, school and in the workplace* (pp. 363–388). San Francisco: Jossey-Bass.

Bar-On, R. (2001). Emotional intelligence and self-actualization. In J. Ciarrochi, J. Forgas, & J. D. Mayer (Eds.), *Emotional intelligence in everyday life: A scientific inquiry* (pp. 82–97). New York: Psychology Press.

Bar-On, R. (2003). How important is it to educate people to be emotionally and socially intelligent, and can it be done? *Perspectives in Education, 21*(4), 3–13.

Bar-On, R. (2004). The Bar-On Emotional Quotient Inventory (EQ-i): Rationale, description, and summary of psychometric properties. In G. Geher (Ed.), *Measuring emotional intelligence: Common ground and controversy* (pp. 111–142). Hauppauge, NY: Nova Science Publishers.

Bar-On, R. (2005). The impact of emotional intelligence on subjective well-being. *Perspectives in Education, 23*(2), 41–61.

Bar-On, R. (2006a). *The EQ-i leadership user's guide.* Toronto, Canada: Multi-Health Systems.

Bar-On, R. (2006b). The Bar-On model of emotional-social intelligence. *Psicothema, 18,* 13–25.

Bar-On, R. (2007a). How important is it to educate people to be emotionally intelligent, and can it be done? In R. Bar-On, J. G. Maree, & M. Elias (Eds.), *Educating people to be emotionally intelligent* (pp. 1–14). Westport, CT: Praeger.

Bar-On, R. (2007b). The impact of emotional intelligence on giftedness. *Gifted Education International, 22*(1), 122–137.

Bar-On, R. (2012a). Applying emotional intelligence in clinical psychology. In A. Di Fabio (Ed.), *The psychology of counseling* (pp. 109–124). Hauppauge, NY: Nova Science Publishers.

Bar-On, R. (2012b). The impact of emotional intelligence on health and wellbeing. In A. Di Fabio (Ed.), *Emotional intelligence: New perspectives and applications* (pp. 29–50). Rijeka, Croatia: InTech.

Bar-On, R., Handley, R., & Fund, S. (2006). The impact of emotional and social intelligence on performance. In V. Druskat, F. Sala, & G. Mount (Eds.), *Linking emotional intelligence and performance at work: Current research evidence* (pp. 3–19). Mahwah, NJ: Lawrence Erlbaum.

Bar-On, R., Maree, J. G., & Elias, M. J. (2007). *Educating people to be emotionally intelligent.* Westport, CT: Praeger.

Bartone, P. T., & Hystad, S. W. (2010). Increasing mental hardiness for stress resilience in operational settings. In P. T. Bartone, B. H. Johnsen, J. Eid, J. M. Violanti, & J. C. Laberg (Eds.), *Enhancing human performance in security operations: International and law enforcement perspective* (pp. 257–272). Springfield, IL: Charles C. Thomas.

Bonanno, G. A. (2004). Loss, trauma, and human resilience: Have we underestimated the human capacity to thrive after extremely aversive events? *American Psychologist, 59*(1), 20–28.

Consortium for Research on Emotional Intelligence in Organizations. (2010). Retrieved from *www.eiconsortium.org/pdf/USAFPeliminaryPJStudy--Revised-b.pdf*

Darwin, C. (1872/1965). *The expression of the emotions in man and animals.* Chicago: University of Chicago Press.

Diener, E. (2000). Subjective well-being: The science of happiness and a proposal for a national index. *American Psychologist, 55*(1), 34–43.

Ebersohn, L. E., & Maree, J. G. (2006). Demonstrating resilience in an HIV & AIDS context: An emotional intelligence perspective. *Gifted Education International, 21*(2), 14–30.

Fund, S. (2001). *The emotional intelligence study.* Tel-Aviv: IDF Department of Human Resources.

Gardner, H. (1983). *Frames of mind: The theory of multiple intelligences.* New York: Basic Books.

Handley, R. (1997, April). AFRS rates emotional intelligence. *Air Force Recruiter News, 28,* 797–812.

Helliwell, J. F., & Putnam, R. D. (2004). The social context of well-being. *Philosophical Transactions of the Royal Society of London: Biological Sciences, 359*(1449), 1435–1446.

Kobasa, S. C. (1979). Stressful life events, personality, and health: Inquiry into hardiness. *Journal of Personality and Social Psychology, 37*(1), 1–11.

Krivoy, E., Weyl Ben-Arush, M., & Bar-On, R. (2000). Comparing the emotional intelligence of adolescent cancer survivors with a matched sample from the normative population. *Medical & Pediatric Oncology, 35*(3), 382.

Langhorn, S. (2004). How emotional intelligence can improve management performance. *International Journal of Hospitality Management, 16*(4), 220–230.

Maree, J. G. (2006). A fairer deal for the gifted disadvantaged in rural areas in South Africa. In B. Wallace & G. Erikson (Eds.), *Diversity in gifted education: International perspectives on the global issues* (pp. 136–141). London: Routledge.

Oswald, A. J. (1997). Happiness and economic performance. *The Economic Journal, 107*(445), 1815–1831.

Parker, J. D. A., Creque, R. E., Barnhart, D. L., Harris, J. I., Majeski, S. A., Wood, L. M., . . . Hogan, M. J. (2004). Academic achievement in high school: Does emotional intelligence matter? *Personality and Individual Differences, 37*(7), 1321–1330.

Parker, J. R. (1997). Who are the gifted? *Gifted Education International, 12*(2), 85–90.

Peterson, J. S. (1997). Bright, tough, and resilient–and not in a gifted program. *Journal of Secondary Gifted Education, 9*7(8), 121–137.

Raven, J. C. (1958). *Standard progressive matrices.* London: H. K. Lewis & Co. Ltd.

Ryff, C. D. (1989). Happiness is everything, or is it? Explorations on the meaning of psychological well-being. *Journal of Personality and Social Psychology, 5*7(6), 1069–1081.

Shadbolt, B., Barresi, J., & Craft, P. (2002). Self-rated health as a predictor of survival among patients with advanced cancer. *Journal of Clinical Oncology, 2*0(10), 2514–2519.

Swart, A. (1996). The relationship between well-being and academic performance. Unpublished master's thesis, University of Pretoria, South Africa.

Thompson, C. L., & Rudolph, L. B. (1992). *Counseling children.* Pacific Grove, California: Brooks/Cole Publishing Company.

Travers, L. (2014). *Inspiring women leaders.* Pool-in-Wharfedale, England: Fisher King Publishing.

Wagner, R. K. (1997). Intelligence, training, and employment. *American Psychologist, 5*2(10), 1059–1069.

Section IV

Proposed implications and resilience building

25

Resilience and vulnerability in coping with stress and terrorism

Zvi Zemishlany

The world-wide increase in terrorist activities poses new challenges to health professionals, clinicians and policy makers who need to confront the impact of terror-related trauma on individuals and communities. Many communities across the world are chronically exposed to extreme violence. Exposure to a potentially traumatic event, like a terror attack, disrupts the homeostatic state, triggering a series of responses intended to enable the organism to adjust to the altered condition. These responses are generally adaptive in the short run but can lead to a state of chronic dysregulation and psycho-physiologic imbalance. Studies of the impact of war, political violence and terrorism around the world have revealed a range of detrimental mental consequences, including heightened anxiety and depression; reduced sense of safety; increased use of tobacco, alcohol, drugs and psychotropic medications; and post-traumatic stress symptoms. On the community level, the resulting damage to the community infrastructure has an impact on the economy, displaces populations and lowers community morale and well-being.

The immediate mental health effects of the notorious terrorist attack of September 11, 2001, in the United States were assessed using a nationally representative sample of American adults who were asked about their reactions to the terrorist attack and their perceptions of it. Three to five days following the attack, 44% of this cohort reported that they experienced at least one of five substantial stress symptoms. Although the people who were in or close to New York City had the highest rate of substantial stress reactions, others throughout the country, in large and small communities, also suffered from them. Five to nine weeks after the attack, 7.5% of adults living south of 110th Street in Manhattan reported symptoms consistent with post-traumatic stress disorder (PTSD), and 9.7% reported symptoms consistent with current major depression. Additionally, those living closest to the World Trade Center site were nearly three times as likely to develop PTSD as those living farther away. The people who experienced the attack directly as well as those who experienced it indirectly, through the media, showed elevated levels of distress, a lowered sense of security and subsequent pathological reactions such as PTSD and depression (Galea et al., 2002). In their severe form, these stress reactions can lead to acute stress disorder (ASD) and chronic PTSD in keeping with the time-span they occupy.

Lawyers et al. (2006) characterized peri-traumatic reactions of residents of New York City during and immediately following the September 11th terrorist attack, identified predictors of those reactions and identified predictors of PTSD four months later. Three related, but distinct, peri-traumatic response patterns were revealed: dissociation, emotional reactions, and panic/physiological arousal. These results support a growing literature concerning the predictive value of peri-traumatic reactions in relation to PTSD. Understanding the early phase of emotional disturbances may shed some light on the development of the early stages of chronic stress reaction that result from repeated terrorist attacks.

Amital and colleagues (Amital, Amital, Shohat, Soffer, & Bar-Dayan, 2012) reported on the short-term emotional effects and disturbances in daily life two days after a suicide bomber's attack in the southern Israeli city of Dimona. A higher prevalence of stress and fear and a lower prevalence of joy were reported in the population of Dimona compared with the general population in Israel. Subjects who reported being less resilient had a higher prevalence of stress and fear, disturbances in daily life activities and changes in leisure activities than subjects who reported being more resilient.

The immediate response to the traumatic event in individuals who may develop ASD or PTSD involves intense fear, helplessness or horror. ASD is experienced during or immediately after the trauma, lasts for at least two days, and either resolves within four weeks or the diagnosis has to be adjusted. A diagnosis of PTSD may be appropriate provided the full criteria for PTSD are met (American Psychiatric Association, 2013). Of the individuals who respond to the trauma with intense fear or horror, 15–35% develop eventually a significant degree of dysfunction and distress (Fairbank, Ebert, & Costello, 2000), namely PTSD, lasting a considerable length of time. The PTSD symptoms can be grouped into four main clusters. The first is persistent re-experience of the traumatic event, such as recurrent dreams and flashbacks. The second is persistent avoidance of internal or external cues associated with the trauma. The third consists of negative alterations in cognitions or mood. These negative alterations can be expressed in exaggerated negative beliefs and expectations about oneself, others or the world; feelings of fear, anger, shame, guilt or detachment; and diminished interest and inability to experience positive emotions. The fourth is increased arousal, which is manifested in difficulty in concentrating, hypervigilance and exaggerated startle response (American Psychiatric Association, 2013). PTSD is a devastating disorder chronically disrupting the lives of the sufferer and his family, while imposing a burden on society.

Resilience and vulnerability

The marked discrepancy between the proportion of the general population exposed to traumatic events and the proportion that ultimately fulfill the criteria for PTSD is a challenging aspect of the study of stress-related disorders. Identification of factors that increase vulnerability of individuals and factors that increase resilience may have important implications in public health.

Recent studies have addressed the characteristics of resilience, defined by Bonanno (2004) as "the ability . . . to maintain a relatively stable, healthy level of psychological and physical functioning in the face of highly disruptive events." This concept is particularly important in view of the findings that following a range of traumatic events, a large percentages of people (40–78.2%) exposed to these events are either entirely or almost entirely symptom free (Bonanno, Rennicke, & Dekel, 2005; Bryant, Harvey, Guthrie, & Moulds, 2000; Galea et al., 2002).

Moscardino, Scrimin, Capello, and Altoe (2010) investigated the influence of socio-contextual variables on depressive symptoms in 158 adolescent survivors of the 2004 terrorist attack in Balsan, Russia. Over 1,300 children and adults were taken hostage by a group of 32 terrorists at the traditional celebration for the opening school day. Hundreds of young children spent fifty-seven hours sitting in an overcrowded gymnasium wired with explosives. They witnessed the beating and murder of family members, friends and teachers. On the third day, the hostage crisis ended in extreme violence that caused the deaths of 329 persons and the injury of many hundreds. The survivors were assessed eighteen months after the traumatic event for depressive symptoms, social support, sense of community and collectivism. The findings suggest that social support and community connectedness may serve as protective resources and were associated with lower rates of depressive symptoms.

Kaplan, Matar, Kamin, Sadan and Cohen (2005) investigated stress-related responses after three years of exposure to terror from Gaza Strip (2003–2005) in three different types of population centers in Israel: a suburb of Tel Aviv, a settlement in the West Bank (Kiryat Arba) and the Gush Katif settlement cluster around the Gaza Strip. Symptoms of acute stress and chronic (post-traumatic) stress as well as symptoms of general psychopathology and distress were assessed. The inhabitants of Gush Katif, in spite of first-hand daily exposure to violent attacks, reported the fewest and least severe symptoms of stress-related complaints, the least sense of personal threat and the highest level of functioning of all three samples. The most severely symptomatic and functionally compromised were the inhabitants of the Tel Aviv suburb, who were the least affected by exposure to violent attacks both in terms of frequency and of directness. Due to the Gush Katif population tending to be particularly religious, the data were reassessed according to religiousness. The religious inhabitants of Kiryat Arba had almost the same symptom profile as the Gush Katif population, whereas secular inhabitants of Kiryat Arba reported faring worse than any of the other populations. The authors conclude that religiousness combined with common ideological convictions and social cohesion is associated with substantially higher resilience as compared to the secular metropolitan urban populations.

In another Israeli study by Dekel and Nuttman-Shwartz (2009) the findings are similar. Their study assessed a sample of 134 residents, 67 of whom were residents from two kibbutzim and the other 67 were inhabitants from the city of Sderot. Both groups have been the target of Qassam rocket attacks. The city residents reported more post-traumatic symptoms. It was suggested that the kibbutz ideology, solidarity and communal lifestyle provide a measure of protection against stress.

Similar findings were shown recently by Gelkopf, Berger, Bleich, and Silver (2012) who compared the responses to seven years of continuous rocket fire of residents from the urban community of Sderot, with the rural communities bordering the Gaza Strip, and with non-exposed rural and urban populations as comparison groups. As expected, the residents bordering the Gaza Strip evidenced little symptomatology. In contrast, PTS, distress, functional impairment and health care utilization were substantially higher in the highly exposed urban community of Sderot than in the other three communities. The authors explain the low level of vulnerability in the rural community that was exposed to chronic rocket attacks by their reporting on higher levels of community commitment and feeling that they were an integral part of their community. They reported having a strong social network for both instrumental and social support and having greater confidence in the army and in the national leadership of the country, which seemed to be protective against the chronic stress. In addition, each rural community had a local officer who was responsible for the security of the inhabitants and served as the liaison with the army and an elected committee handling community issues. These officers were responsible for the state of the local shelters, which was in contrast to the situation in the cities, where shelters were not always clean, lacked water and electricity, and lacked liaison personnel for less mobile populations. These emphasize the role of the logistic preparations and the creation of "culture of safety" in the development of resilient communities.

When combining all these findings, "sense of belonging" appears to be an important characteristic of resilience. "Sense of belonging" refers to people feeling part of a collective, be it the neighborhood, the immediate community, the nation or any other group or place. It is characterized by mutual concern, connection, community loyalty and trust that one's personal needs will be fulfilled by means of commitment to the group as a whole. Within the same line, it was found that during the 1973 war in Israel, there were lower rates of combat stress in army units that had high levels of solidarity and cohesion than in those in which the soldiers' sense of belonging was lower (Steiner & Neumann, 1978).

Even residents of communities that are indirectly exposed to political violence and terrorism show psychological effects (Bleich, Gelkopf, Melamed, & Solomon, 2006; Gelkopf, Solomon, Berger, & Bleich, 2008), but here, too, variability in response across communities is evident (Gelkopf et al., 2008). This is likely a function of differences in ethnic, economic, ideological and social composition across communities, with different resources and risk factors. Thus, the impact of exposure to political violence may depend on the wider social context in which it occurs. This context can be defined by proximity to the disaster as well as by social factors (Kawachi & Subramanian, 2006). Indeed, Nakagawa and Shaw (2004) observed that, within the same cities, neighborhoods recovered at different rates depending upon the available social capital, and Kawachi and Berkman (2001) have discussed the importance of availability of social connections as a buffer against the impact of disasters. Residents of poorer communities (Ahern & Galea, 2006) and communities with a narrow range of economic resources (Cutter et al., 2006) appear more vulnerable to stressful conditions. Furthermore, war and political violence can cause or worsen local stressful social and material condition such as poverty, social marginalization, isolation, inadequate housing and changes in family structure and functioning (Miller & Rasmussen, 2010), which can exacerbate mental health problems.

The central role of the contextual and community risk factors can be illustrated in the case of minorities. Minority ethnic groups share a common heritage and cultural values that differ from the mainstream population. Identification as a member of an ethnic minority may affect the individual's interaction with the social network. The actual and perceived low social support can lead to different traumatic exposure rates and increased vulnerability to develop PTSD (Gelkopf et al., 2012; Perilla, Norris, & Lavizzo, 2002). Discriminated minority groups often have disparities in access to economic and social resources like healthcare, education and income, leading to increased risk of psychosocial distress when further resources are threatened. Furthermore, the perception of discrimination may prevent the individual from seeking support and using available social resources and may intensify feelings of decreased self-worth. Moreover, the degree of integration and acculturation affects PTSD development. In a study of the Taiwanese aboriginal population, it was found that those with a lower degree of acculturation were twice as likely to develop PTSD as their higher acculturated counterparts (Lee et al., 2009). Individuals with low acculturation tend to be less integrated and have less support from social networks. Similar to the mainstream population, political and ideological convictions have been shown to be a protective factor. Servan-Schreiber, Le Lin and Birmaher (1998) found increased resilience in Tibetan refugee children with a strong sense of participating in their nation's struggle against an oppressor.

Children and adolescents often exhibit higher levels of psychological distress to disasters than adults despite seeming to perform normally on a superficial level. While rates vary greatly depending on the type of trauma and the population exposed, level of PTSD often reach or exceed 50% (Attanayake et al., 2009; Yule et al., 2000). Protective factors described in children include personal characteristics like optimism, high self-esteem, good temperament, strong self-efficacy and positive coping (Benight & Bandura, 2004; Boscarino & Adams, 2009). A supportive family (Thabet, Ibraheem, Shivram, Winter, & Vostanis, 2009) and strong social networks are key predictors of resilience (Moore & Varela, 2010).

Lack of resources was associated with increased vulnerability among urban residents. Individual risk factors for increased vulnerability to adverse psychological effects of terror found across studies included being female, older age, minority or an immigrant; having lower education, direct exposure or prior experience of highly stressful events; suffering economic loss; proximity to the disaster; ongoing sense of threat; lack of optimism and lack of social support (Bleich, Gelkopf, & Solomon, 2003; Bleich et al., 2006; Gelkopf et al., 2012). In children, lower age, poor parental response and inadequate family cohesion are additional factors that contribute to their increased vulnerability (Hobfoll et al., 2009; Moore & Varela, 2010).

Preventive interventions

Mental health interventions are meant to increase resilience in adults and children exposed to a disaster or terrorism. However, during disaster situations, traditional mental health resources are overwhelmed. Therefore, a public health ecological approach targeting the whole community should be adopted. According to Norris and Stevens (2007), community resilience emerges from four primary sets of adaptive capacities: economic development, information and communication, community competence and social capital. Social capital is defined as mutual trust and social networking among individuals and groups, as they willingly partake in mutually beneficial collective action (Putnam, 2000).

A panel of international experts (Hobfoll et al., 2007) identified and gained consensus on five empirically supported intervention principles that should be used at the early and mid-term stages of a mass trauma. These are promoting 1) a sense of safety, 2) calming, 3) a sense of self and community efficacy, 4) social connectedness and 5) hope. They emphasize that, for children, the restoration of the school community is an essential step in re-establishing a sense of self-efficacy.

Several studies described preventive interventions in accordance with these principles in order to increase resilience, mainly in children, during a continuing situation of stress and political violence. School-based interventions are effective, especially when delivered to small groups. In a randomized controlled trial of a ten-session small-group intervention delivered by school clinicians, students reported fewer symptoms, and parents reported less psychosocial dysfunction among their children in comparison to a waitlist group (Stein et al., 2003). In disaster situations, the limited number of professionals is insufficient to reach all the children in need. Therefore, Wolmer et al., 2013) proposed to empower teachers to serve as clinical mediators in order to assist the children with their psychological distress.

Wolmer, Hamiel and Laor (2011) conducted a study that consisted of 1,488 children studying in fourth and fifth grades in the south of Israel and thus vulnerable to being exposed to periods of continuous rocket attacks (in 2008–2009). A teacher-led intervention was implemented 3 months prior to the traumatic exposure ($n = 748$). The control group included 740 children matched by age and exposure characteristics, who did not receive the preventive intervention. The intervention protocol consisted of 14 weekly 45-minute sessions presenting a didactic module. The intervention protocol focused on resilience building rather than directly addressing trauma symptoms. By providing training in effective coping skills prior to exposure, the intervention was based on a stress inoculation training (SIT) approach aimed at preparing individuals for coping more favorably with stressful events while enhancing performance. The intervention group displayed significantly lower levels of post-traumatic stress symptoms, lower rates of PTSD and lower rates on a scale assessing stress, mood and anxiety than the control group ($p < .001$). Among the children in the control group, there were 57% more detected cases of PTSD than among the children in the intervention training group. The difference was significantly more pronounced among boys (10.2% vs. 4.4%) than among girls (12.5% vs. 10.1%).

Another study by Wolmer et al. (2013) investigated the influence of exposure to rockets attacks during the 2006 Lebanon war on a group of Jewish and two groups of Arab Israeli children studying in the fourth and fifth grade in schools located in northern Israel. Children from both ethnic groups ($n = 1372$) were assessed for stressful life events, symptoms and parental concern regarding adaptation before a 16-week program and after its completion. It focused on strengthening adaptive coping mechanisms and socio-emotional competences. Topics included processing positive and negative experiences, managing stress, dealing with emotions, correcting negative cognitions and implementing adaptive coping mechanisms. Teachers completed a twenty-hour training program and were supervised weekly by school counselors. As expected, Arab children, being a minority in Israel, reported more severe symptoms before the program. The three groups showed a significant decrease to the same level after the program. The authors conclude that the results suggest that school-based programs with teachers as clinical mediators could be a valuable, cost-effective cross-cultural model of intervention after mass trauma, moderating vulnerabilities of ethnic minorities.

Hamiel, Wolmer, Spirman and Laor (2013) described a comprehensive urban resilience program aimed to reinforcing the more vulnerable urban civilian resilience and to prepare the population to cope with the consequences of disasters. The program was implemented first in Tel Aviv and since 2010 in eighteen Israeli cities. The model operates in areas at risk by forming coordinated networks of multi-disciplinary and multi-systemic teams with clear lines of command and control. It includes four components: training health and mental health professionals, providing an effective flow of information by the city's emergency system, delivering basic needs of the population and development of resilience-focused, preventive, teacher-delivered interventions from preschool through high school. Expertise is developed throughout the entire system by municipal sub-units responsible for organizing the response to disaster. A similar integrated model for building resilience in communities exposed to ongoing missiles attacks has been suggested by Pat-Horenczyk et al. (2012). In the clinical level, distressed parents and children were identified and engaged in a dyadic therapy adjusted for peri-traumatic and post-traumatic circumstances. In the community level, resilience-building interventions by workshops for parents and teachers were initiated, as well as training of local professional staff, specializing in treatment of young children. In these programs, the participants learned to identify their own coping mechanisms and those of the young children and acquire the capability to enrich and to vary the ways of coping. The mutual dialog between parents, teachers and staff created circles of mutual support that increased the sense of belonging to the community. Follow-up studies on the teacher-delivered intervention approach have shown a significant and immediate decrease in symptoms and increased hope, in comparison to a waitlist group (Berger & Gelkopf, 2009; Berger, Pat-Horencyzk, & Gelkopf, 2007; Wolmer, Laor, Dedeoglu, Siev, & Yazgan, 2005). The positive effect persisted over a course of three years (Wolmer et al., 2005).

Specifically for children, one of the most vulnerable populations, such a comprehensive framework offers the opportunity to strengthen their capacity to handle severe events through the preparatory enhancement of personal and familiar coping strategies. It augments the social capital of urban institutions, communities and families and may serve as an effective holding environment in times of disaster and its aftermath. It creates a unified, coordinated continuity of preparedness and care among child services such as schools, medical providers and community resources.

It is of note that two recent Israeli studies emphasized the possible prevention of PTSD through early treatment of the exposed person. Cognitive psychotherapy and prolonged exposure therapy, but not the antidepressant medication escitalopram, effectively prevented chronic PTSD in recent survivors (Shalev et al., 2012). A high dose of hydrocortisone (100–140 mg), a glucocorticoid associated with stress, administered immediately after trauma may also alter the trajectory of PTSD (Zohar et al., 2011).

In summary, a preventive approach towards terror-exposed communities should focus on helping vulnerable groups such as disadvantaged city populations lacking economic and social support. Special care should be given to populations with high proportion of children, minorities and immigrants. Resiliency can be enhanced by preparedness of professionals and key figures in the community, delivering the basic needs by the local authorities, as well as strengthening community solidarity and confidence in the local and national leadership competence. Common ideology, religion and social connectedness are significant protective factors against the devastating consequences of exposure to the trauma of terrorism, war and political violence.

References

Ahern, J., & Galea, S. (2006). Social context and depression after a disaster: The role of income inequality. *Journal of Epidemiology and Community Health, 60*(9), 766–770.

American Psychiatric Association. (2013). *Trauma-and stressor-related disorders:* Diagnostic and statistical manual of mental disorders: DSM-5. Washington, DC: American Psychiatric Association.

Amital, D., Amital, H., Shohat, G., Soffer, Y., & Bar-Dayan, Y. (2012). Resilience emotions and acute stress reactions in the population of Dimona and the general population of Israel two days after the first suicide bombing attack in Dimona. *Israel Medical Association Journal, 14*(5), 281–285.

Attanayake, V., McKay, R., Joffers, M., Singh, S., Burkle, F. Jr., & Mills, E. (2009). Prevalence of mental disorders among children exposed to war: A systematic review of 7920 children. *Medicine, Conflict and Survival, 25*(1), 4–19.

Benight, C. C., & Bandura, A. (2004). Social cognitive theory of posttraumatic recovery: The role of perceived self-efficacy. *Behaviour Research and Therapy, 42*(10), 1129–1148.

Berger, R., & Gelkopf, M. (2009). School-based intervention for the treatment of tsunami-related distress in children: A quasi-randomized controlled trial. *Psycotherapy and Psychosomatics, 78*(6), 364–371.

Berger, R., Pat-Horencyzk, R., & Gelkopf, M. (2007). School-based intervention for prevention and treatment of elementary-student's terror related distress in Israel: A quasi-randomized controlled trial. *Journal of Traumatic Stress, 20*(4), 541–551.

Bleich, A., Gelkopf, M., Melamed, Y., & Solomon, Z. (2006). Mental health and resiliency following 44 months of terrorism: A survey of an Israeli national representative sample. *BMC Medicine, 4*, 21–32.

Bleich, A., Gelkopf, M., & Solomon, Z. (2003). Exposure to terrorism, stress–related mental health symptoms, and coping behaviors among a nationally representative sample in Israel. *JAMA, 290*(5), 612–620.

Bonanno, G. A. (2004). Loss, trauma, and human resilience: Have we underestimated the human capacity to thrive after extremely aversive events? *American Psychologist, 59*(1), 20–28.

Bonanno, G. A., Rennicke, C., & Dekel, S. (2005). Self-enhancement among high-exposure survivors of the September 11th terrorist attack: Resilience or social maladjustment? *Journal of Personality and Social Psychology, 88*(6), 984–998.

Boscarino, J. A., & Adams, R. E. (2009). PTSD onset and course following the world trade center disaster: Findings and implications for future research. *Social Psychiatry and Psychiatric Epidemiology, 44*(10), 887–898.

Bryant, R. A., Harvey, A. G., Guthrie, R. M., & Moulds, M. L. (2000). A prospective study of psychophysiological arousal, acute stress disorder, and posttraumatic stress disorder. *The Journal of Abnormal Psychology, 109*(2), 341–344.

Cutter, S. L., Emrich, C. T., Mitchell, J. T., Boruff, B. J., Gall, M., Schmidtlein, M. C., . . . Melton, G. (2006). The long road home: Race, class, and recovery from Hurricane Katrina. *Environment, 48*(2), 8–20.

Dekel, R., & Nuttman-Shwartz, O. (2009). Posttraumatic stress and growth: The contribution of cognitive appraisal and sense of belonging to the country. *Health and Social Work, 34*(2), 87–96.

Fairbank, J., Ebert, L., & Costello, E. (2000). Epidemiology of traumatic events and post-traumatic stress disorder. In D. Nutt, J. Davidson, & J. Zohar (Eds.), *Post-traumatic stress disorder: Diagnosis, management and treatment* (pp. 17–27). London, UK: Martin Dunitz Publishers.

Galea, S., Ahern, J., Resnick, H., Kilpatrick, D., Bucuvalas, M., Gold, J., & Vlahov, D. (2002). Psychological sequelae of the September 11 terrorist attacks in New York city. *New England Journal of Medicine, 346*(13), 982–987.

Gelkopf, M., Berger, R., Bleich, A., & Silver, R. C. (2012). Protective factors and predictors of vulnerability to chronic stress: A comparative study of 4 communities after 7 years of continuous rocket fire. *Social Science & Medicine, 74*(5), 757–766.

Gelkopf, M., Solomon, Z., Berger, R., & Bleich, A. (2008). The mental health impact of terrrorism in Israel: A repeat cross-sectional study of Arabs and Jews. *Acta Psychiatria Scandinavica, 117*(5), 269–380.

Hamiel, D., Wolmer, L., Spirman, S., & Laor, N. (2013). Comprehensive child-oriented preventive resilience program in Israel based on lessons learned from communities exposed to war, terrorism and disaster. *Child and Youth Care Forum, 42*(4), 261–274.

Hobfoll, S. E., Palmieri, P. A., Johnson, R. I., Canetti-Nisim, D., Hall, B. J., & Galea, S. (2009). Trajectories of resilience, resistance, and distress during ongoing terrorism: The case of Jews and Arabs in Israel. *The Journal of Consulting and Clinical Psychology, 77*(1), 138–148.

Hobfoll, S. E., Watson, P., Bell, C. C., Bryant, R. A., Brymer, M. J., Friedman, M. J., . . . Ursano, R. J. (2007). Five essential elements of immediate and mid-term mass trauma intervention: Empirical evidence. *Psychiatry, 70*(4), 283–315.

Kaplan, Z., Matar, M. A., Kamin, R., Sadan, T., & Cohen, H. (2005). Stress-related responses after 3 years of exposure to terror in Israel: Are ideological-religious factors associated with resilience? *The Journal of Clinical Psychiatry, 66*(9), 1146–1154.

Kawachi, I., & Berkman, L. F. (2001). Social ties and mental health. *Journal of Urban Health, 78*(3), 458–467.

Kawachi, I., & Subramanian, S. V. (2006). Measuring and modeling the social and geographic context of trauma: A multilevel modeling approach. *Journal of Traumatic Stress, 19*(2), 195–203.

Lawyer, S. R., Resnick, H. S., Galea, S., Ahern, J., Kilpatrick, D. G., & Vlahov, D. (2006). Predictors of peritraumatic reactions and PTSD following the September 11th terrorist attacks. *Psychiatry, 69*(2), 130–141.

Lee, C. S., Chang, J. C., Liu, C. Y., Chang, C. J., Chen, T. H. H., Chen, C. H., & Cheng, A. T. (2009). Acculturation, psychiatric comorbidity and posttraumatic stress disorder in a Taiwanese aboriginal population. *Social Psychiatry and Psychiatric Epidemiology, 44*(1), 55–62.

Miller, K. E., & Rasmussen, A. (2010). War exposure, daily stressors, and mental health in conflict and post-conflict settings: Bridging the divide between trauma-focused and psychosocial frameworks. *Social Science and Medicine, 70*(1), 7–16.

Moore, K. W., & Varela, R. E. (2010). Correlates of long-term posttraumatic stress symptoms in children following Hurricane Katrina. *Child Psychiatry & Human Development, 41*(2), 239–250.

Moscardino, U., Scrimin, S., Capello, F., & Altoe, G. (2010). Social support, sense of community, collectivistic values, and depressive symptoms in adolescent survivors of the 2004 Beslan terrorist attack. *Social Science & Medicine, 70*(1), 27–34.

Nakagawa, Y., & Shaw, R. (2004). Social capital: A missing link to disaster recovery. *International Journal of Mass Emergencies and Disasters, 22*(1), 5–34.

Norris, F., & Stevens, S. (2007). Community resilience and the principles of mass trauma intervention. *Psychiatry, 70*(4), 320–328.

Pat-Horencyzk, R., Achituv, M., Kagan-Rubenstein, A., Khodabakhsh, A., Brom, D., & Chemtob, C. (2012). Growing up under fire: Building resilience in young children and parents exposed to ongoing missile attacks. *Journal of Child & Adolescent Trauma, 5*(4), 303–314.

Perilla, J. L., Norris, F. H., & Lavizzo, E. A. (2002). Ethnicity, culture and disaster response: Identifying and explaining ethnic differences in PTSD six months after hurricane Andrew. *Journal of Social and Clinical Psychology, 21*(1), 20–45.

Putnam, R. (2000). Bowling alone: The collapse and revival of American community. New York, NY: Simon & Schuster.

Servan-Schreiber, D., Le Lin, B., & Birmaher, B. (1998). Prevalence of posttraumatic stress disorder and major depressive disorder in Tibetan refugee children. *Journal of the American Academy of Child Psychiatry, 37*(8), 874–879.

Shalev, A. Y., Ankri, Y., Israeli-Shalev, Y., Peleg, T., Adessky, R., & Freedman, S. (2012). Prevention of posttraumatic stress disorder by early treatment: Results from the Jerusalem trauma outreach and prevention study. *Archives of General Psychiatry, 69*(2), 166–176.

Stein, B. D., Jaycox, L. H., Kataoka, S. H., Wong, M., Tu, W., Elliot, M. N., & Fink, A. (2003). A mental health intervention for school children exposed to violence: A randomized controlled trial. *JAMA, 290*(5), 603–611.

Steiner, M., & Neumann, M. (1978). Traumatic neurosis and social support in the Yom Kippur war returnees. *Military Medicine, 143*(12), 866–868.

Thabet, A. A., Ibraheem, A. N., Shivram, R., Winter, E. A., & Vostanis, P. (2009). Parenting support and PTSD in children of a war zone. *International Journal of Social Psychiatry, 55*(3), 226–237.

Wolmer, L., Hamiel, D., & Laor, N. (2011). Preventing children's posttraumatic stress after disaster with teacher-based intervention: A controlled study. *Journal of the American Academy of Child & Adolescent Psychiatry, 50*(4), 340–348.

Wolmer, L., Hamiel, D., Slone, M., Faians, M., Picker, M., Adiv, T., & Laor, N. (2013). Post-traumatic reaction of Israeli Jewish and Arab children exposed to rocket attacks before and after teacher-delivered intervention. *Israel Journal of Psychiatry and Related Sciences, 50*(3), 165–173.

Wolmer, L., Laor, N., Dedeoglu, C., Siev, J., & Yazgan, Y. (2005). Teacher-mediated intervention after disaster: A controlled three-year follow-up of children's functioning. *Journal of Child Psychology and Psychiatry, 46*(11), 1161–1168.

Yule, W., Bolton, D., Udwin, O., Boyle, S., O'Ryan, D., & Nurrish, J. (2000). The long-term psychological effects of a disaster experienced in adolescence: I: The incidence and course of PTSD. *Journal of Child Psychology and Psychiatry, 41*(4), 503–511.

Zohar, J., Yahalom, H., Kozlovsky, N., Cwikel-Hamzany, S., Matar, M. A., Kaplan, Z., . . . Cohen, H. (2011). High dose hydrocortisone immediately after trauma may alter the trajectory of PTSD: Interplay between clinical and animal studies. *Eur Neuropsychopharmacol, 21*(11), 796–809.

26

Posttraumatic growth
A pathway to resilience

Richard G. Tedeschi and Cara L. Blevins

The experience of suffering is ubiquitous. While the parameters of what constitutes a traumatic experience are broad, reviews of large-scale, population-based studies consistently indicate that most, if not all, individuals will experience at least one tragedy, significant loss, or catastrophe in their lifetime (Bonanno, Westphal, & Mancini, 2012; Calhoun & Tedeschi, 1999). These events may be severe enough to meet criteria from the *Diagnostic and Statistical Manual of Mental Disorders, Fifth Edition* (American Psychological Association, 2013) for a psychological trauma (e.g. an event that threatens or causes serious personal harm, injury, or death), or they may be sufficiently upsetting without meeting clinical thresholds of official diagnoses. Regardless, highly stressful events or major life tragedies have the potential to result in a variety of negative outcomes including posttraumatic stress disorder (PTSD), depression, anxiety, isolation, and an increased risk of chronic disease and illness (Ramos & Leal, 2013; Tedeschi & Calhoun, 2004).

The fields of psychology and psychiatry have historically focused on "fixing" those problems or deficits associated with exposure to traumatic circumstances. However, over the course of the past decade, the field of psychology has begun to depart from these traditional disease or deficit-focused models of mental health to incorporate a positive psychological perspective (Seligman & Csikszentmihalyi, 2000; Tedeschi & Calhoun, 1995; Tedeschi & Kilmer, 2005). The notion that one might grow as a result of trauma has existed throughout history, and themes of growth and transformation following adversity are central components of religious and philosophical traditions (Calhoun & Tedeschi, 1999; Calhoun & Tedeschi, 2013). These lineages have inspired the contemporary empirical investigation into the experiences of individuals who, not only recover from trauma, but use their experiences as a stepping stone to further growth, development, and resilience (Tedeschi, Park, & Calhoun, 1998).

Whereas some confuse the concept of posttraumatic growth (PTG) with resilience or traumatic recovery (Bonanno, 2004; Bonanno et al., 2012), we suggest that the concepts are quite distinct. Resilience represents a dynamic process that encompasses positive adaptation despite significant adversity or sources of stress (Aldwin, Park, & Spiro, 2007; Bonanno, 2004; Luthar, Cicchetti, & Becker, 2000; Zerach, Soloman, Cohen, & Ein-Dor, 2013). Resilience has been conceptualized as an inherent personal trait or attribute and as a component of developmental processes (Aldwin et al., 2007); however, resilience is defined as a return to baseline levels of functioning that existed before encounters with adverse circumstances.

PTG represents more than just a return to baseline and reflects development beyond previous levels of functioning. In other words, individuals who display resilience following a highly stressful or traumatic experience have adjusted successfully despite adversity, whereas persons who experience PTG are *transformed by their struggles with adversity* (Calhoun & Tedeschi, 2013; Tedeschi & Kilmer, 2005). Interestingly, individuals with higher degrees of pre-trauma resilience may be less likely to report outcomes of PTG (Tedeschi & Calhoun, 1995). For these more resilient individuals, the traumatic event may not disrupt the assumptive world to the extent necessary to cognitively restructure or rebuild the core belief system. As we will describe in this chapter, it is not the trauma itself that produces PTG but rather the processes of cognitive and emotional struggle in the aftermath of trauma that prompt outcomes of positive change, transformation, and growth. Therefore, we conceptualize PTG as both a process and an outcome with distinct cognitive and emotional components that have the potential to result in behavioral changes and transformation (Tedeschi & Calhoun, 1996, 2004). Yet, while the experience of PTG is distinct from resilience, we believe that PTG has the potential to provide new pathways or baselines for resilience and recovery. Therefore, this chapter will attempt to provide readers with (1) a review of the origins and principles of the theory of PTG, (2) a description of selected characteristics and contexts that may help facilitate PTG, (3) a review of the tools used to quantify and assess outcomes of growth, and (4) an understanding of how PTG may represent a pathway in the development of resilience following trauma.

Origins of posttraumatic growth (PTG)

References to the transformative potential of suffering can be found in the writings of both ancient and contemporary religious, philosophical, and psychological lineages (Calhoun & Tedeschi, 2013). Buddhism is believed to have originated from Siddhartha's attempts to understand and navigate the inevitability of human suffering, Hindu mythology speaks of Kali, the goddess of change, power, and destruction from which re-creation stems, and Christianity is centered around the belief that Jesus's suffering and death on the cross was in the service of the forgiveness and rebirth of humanity (Tedeschi & Calhoun, 2004). Further, the transformative potential of suffering is a central theme to seminal works in philosophy (e.g. Nietzsche's "what does not kill me makes me stronger"), literature, drama, and poetry.

Pioneers of twentieth-century psychological theory also detailed ways in which trauma and suffering could initiate processes of positive transformation. Frankl (1963) described processes relating to the search for meaning following experiences in World War II concentration camps, Bugental (1965) wrote of the search for authenticity and existential inquiry as fundamental to human nature, Maslow (1970) sought to examine predictors of positive human functioning, and Caplan (1964) wrote of the potential for healthy development following effective coping in the aftermath of trauma (Tedeschi & Calhoun, 2004).

Processes and basic principles of PTG

These influences led to the empirical investigation of PTG and the development of a theoretical model of PTG that has undergone several revisions (Calhoun, Cann, & Tedeschi, 2010; Calhoun & Tedeschi, 2006; Tedeschi & Calhoun, 1995, 2004).

PTG is a process and an outcome, stemming from an individual's engagement with complex cognitive, emotional, and social variables that have the potential to contribute to a greater sense of well-being and life satisfaction post-trauma. PTG highlights the capacity for people to respond well to adverse situations and refers to positive changes, which may occur following the process of attempting to make sense of a disrupted world. Those experiencing PTG do not return to the same baseline that existed prior to trauma but rather emerge transformed with a benchmark for future resilience trajectories (Tedeschi & Kilmer, 2005). Further, individuals may not experience a cessation of distressing symptoms and still recognize that they have experienced some benefit as a result of their experience. Continued distress may operate to produce the cognitive processing and deliberate rumination necessary to prompt PTG (Calhoun & Tedeschi, 2013; Maercker & Zoellner, 2004; Tedeschi & Kilmer, 2005).

The assumptive world

To effectively navigate daily existence, humans function on the basis of assumptive world views comprised of personal theories, attributions, and schemas. The assumptive world enables humans to bring a sense of order and understanding to an otherwise chaotic world and is comprised of core belief structures that allow one to plan, (re)organize, and act effectively within a framework that comprises normal, day-to-day living (Epstein, 1980; Janoff-Bulman, 1992; Parkes, 1971). In general, these core beliefs are held at a preconscious level (Janoff-Bulman, 1992). However, at certain times in our lives, we are exposed to highly impactful circumstances or events that bring these basic assumptions and belief structures to a more conscious level, requiring us to reorganize, re-conceptualize, and perhaps redefine the nature of our assumptive world and system of core beliefs (Calhoun & Tedeschi, 2013; Janoff-Bulman, 2006).

Seismic events

Central to the model of PTG is the seismic nature of traumatic or highly adverse circumstances. We have used a metaphor of earthquakes to describe this process (Tedeschi & Calhoun, 1995, 2004). Similar to how an earthquake disrupts the physical environment, traumatic events have the capacity to disrupt, challenge, or even shatter an individual's assumptions or way of understanding the world (Janoff-Bulman, 1992). Therefore, the severity of a traumatic experience can be understood as the degree to which one's assumptive world is challenged. The more "seismic" an experience is, the more an individual is caused to question and to develop their fundamental assumptions regarding safety, predictability, identity, and meaning (Tedeschi & Calhoun, 2004). Disruptions to assumptive worlds are generally accompanied by a significant degree of psychological distress (Tedeschi & Calhoun, 2004), which initiates cognitive processes by which one attempts to understand the event and rebuild the assumptive world/core belief structure (Cann et al., 2011). These cognitive processes, or ruminations, have the potential to result in outcomes of posttraumatic growth.

Rumination: intrusive and deliberate

The term rumination has historically had a negative connotation, due largely to its association with clinical literature. In these contexts, rumination has referred to excessive worry or self-focused negative thinking with related diagnoses of depression and PTSD (Calhoun & Tedeschi, 2013; Cann et al., 2011). We suggest that rumination may be better understood in accordance with its general definition as the tendency to think in-depth or engage in repetitive thoughts with relation to psychological topics (Cann et al., 2011). In understanding how PTG might emerge from ruminative thinking, we distinguish between two styles of ruminative thought: intrusive rumination and deliberate rumination. Intrusive ruminations are thoughts relating to events or experiences that appear in one's consciousness unexpectedly, without invitation or conscious intent. Deliberate ruminations are event-related thoughts that an individual invites, welcomes, and engages in purposefully, often with the intent of trying to understand or make sense of events and their implications (Cann et al., 2011). Intrusive thoughts following a traumatic event are not abnormal; rather, they are to be an expected outcome of trauma and may represent an individual's attempt to make sense of their changing life circumstances.

The model of PTG suggests that following a disruption to one's core belief structure, both intrusive and deliberate rumination play distinct roles in the growth process. Evidence suggests that intrusive ruminations relating to traumatic events are positively associated with distress and a failure to cope (Cann et al., 2011). Deliberate or purposeful ruminations relating to traumatic events have been positively associated with PTG (Lindstrom, Cann, Calhoun, & Tedeschi, 2013). Higher levels of intrusive rumination are also believed to predict higher levels of deliberate rumination as a way to better understand and bring meaning to a traumatic experience (Calhoun et al., 2010; Cann et al., 2011). For many people who have experienced a highly stressful or traumatic event, the process of deliberate rumination directly relates to outcomes of growth and helps facilitate well-being in the aftermath of trauma (Cann et al., 2011).

Self-disclosure, social resources, and responsiveness

While cognitive processing is inherent to outcomes of PTG, evidence suggests that self-disclosure is also a key component. Self-disclosure, or processes of verbal or written communication whereby one reveals aspects of their identity or experience to another, is essential in cultivating and maintaining relationships and alleviating distressing thoughts and emotions (Taku, Cann, Tedeschi, & Calhoun, 2009). Self-disclosure has been identified as an important component of cognitive processing and coping in the aftermath of trauma and has been associated with a variety of positive outcomes, including lower levels of distress, enhanced physical functioning, a resilient self-concept, and outcomes of PTG (Calhoun & Tedeschi, 2013; Pennebaker, 2003; Taku et al., 2009). In accordance with the model of PTG, disclosing distressing emotions or thoughts relating to traumatic experiences may be an essential component to a trauma survivor's ability to understand and make sense or meaning of their experiences, thereby initiating the process of re-configuring the assumptive world following seismic disruption (Calhoun & Tedeschi, 2013). Self-disclosure may also help alleviate the frequency of intrusive thoughts relating to the traumatic experience and contribute to processes of deliberate rumination that are an important precursor to experiences of PTG.

Recounting and disclosing traumatic experiences requires a large degree of courage and can be a difficult process for survivors to engage in. The very nature of disclosure requires that the survivor make him or herself vulnerable to another, with no guarantee that others will understand, empathize, or maintain a sense of confidentiality relating to the shared experiences (Calhoun & Tedeschi, 2013). It is a risk, but identifying a person whom it is safe to disclose emotional topics to may help survivors begin to make sense of their experience and result in a deepened sense of relational intimacy and closeness (Calhoun & Tedeschi, 2013; Lindstrom et al., 2013; Taku et al., 2009). Benefits stem from both verbal and written disclosure, and studies indicate that the frequency and complexity of disclosure may help facilitate PTG (Pennebaker & Chung, 2007; Taku et al., 2009).

The perceived reactions of the recipient of self-disclosure are also important to outcomes of PTG and those survivors who perceive recipients as being empathic, having a matched understanding of the traumatic experience, and providing a sense of validation to the survivor of the trauma report greater of outcomes of PTG (Calhoun & Tedeschi, 2004; Taku et al., 2009). Research has also indicated that perceiving disclosure as a mutual process or having the perception that one is working through the process with another helps alleviate symptoms of distress and facilitates PTG (Cann et al., 2011; Taku et al., 2009).

The five domains of PTG

Trauma survivors tend to report PTG across five domains: a greater appreciation for one's life, a greater sense of personal strength, improvements in relationships, recognition of new life possibilities, and spiritual development. These domains emerged empirically in the development of a quantitative measure of PTG (Tedeschi & Calhoun, 1996).

Many individuals report experiencing an increased appreciation for life following trauma. They may begin to take pleasure in "the small things life has to offer", such as seeing a child smile, feeling the breeze against one's skin, or taking pleasure in the beauty of the setting sun at the end of the day (Tedeschi & Calhoun, 2004). Survivors may indicate that, as a result of their trauma, they feel "lucky" and may feel as if they were given a second chance. They may report viewing life with "a new set of eyes", experiencing an increased sense of meaning, beauty, and importance in things that may have formerly been taken for granted or seemed trivial (Calhoun & Tedeschi, 2013). Survivors may also indicate that they recognize and/or possess a sense of increased personal strength as a result of traumatic experience. They may experience increased psychological flexibility, such that they feel better able to handle difficult life situations or that "things that used to be big deals aren't big deals anymore" (Tedeschi & Calhoun, 2004, p. 6). They may recognize or celebrate positive attributes and personal character strengths and feel better able to perform certain skillful actions, such as the ability to listen empathically. Paradoxically, an increased sense of personal strength is often reported simultaneously with an increased sense of vulnerability. Survivors report having a heightened recognition that much of life is uncontrollable and that bad things can and do happen; however, they also report feeling stronger, such that, if they were able to get through this experience, they could handle anything (Janoff-Bulman, 1992; Tedeschi & Kilmer, 2005).

Trauma survivors may report deeper and more meaningful relationships as an outcome of PTG and an increased sense of compassion, empathy, and connection to others experiencing similar circumstances (Calhoun & Tedeschi, 2013; Taku et al., 2009; Tedeschi & McNally, 2011). Further, the loss of some relationships as a result of tragedy has the potential to increase appreciation or deepen the intimacy of other relationships. Trauma survivors may also acknowledge the presence of new possibilities and/or opportunities based on a revaluation of priorities. Finally, struggles with highly seismic or traumatic circumstances may prompt the initiation or deepening of engagement with existential questions about the fundamental nature or meaning of life (Tedeschi & Calhoun, 2004). This can apply to religious and nonreligious or atheistic persons, and survivors may report a deepened sense of faith, belief in God or a higher power, or general spiritual and existential development.

There is often a paradoxical nature that often accompanies growth experienced in each of these five domains. PTG represents the actualization of the proverbial "from loss comes gain", and outcomes of growth in certain areas would not be possible without a loss in others (Calhoun & Tedeschi, 2013). For example traumatic exposure makes an individual vulnerable in many ways but also presents the potential for an enhanced sense of personal strength. Loss in one aspect of life may present the potential for new opportunities or possibilities in another aspect, and spiritual or existential doubt presents the potential for deepened, reinvigorated, or re-conceptualized faith (Tedeschi & Calhoun, 2004). Helping survivors recognize and appreciate these paradoxes is similar to helping clients think dialectically, or consider two extremes in tandem, in therapy. We suggest that it is from this dialectical thought and appreciation of paradox that the potential for growth, wisdom, life satisfaction, and new resilience trajectories emerge (Calhoun & Tedeschi, 2013; Triplett, Tedeschi, Cann, Calhoun, & Reeve, 2012).

Measurement tools for PTG processes and outcomes

A critical step in deepening our understanding of the positive changes that may result from exposure to highly adverse or traumatic experiences was the development of empirical instruments to help quantify the phenomenon of PTG (Cann et al., 2009). The PTGI (Tedeschi & Calhoun, 1996) is the most widely used and well-known tool used to assess the experience of PTG. The PTGI developed as a result of years of clinical experience, extensive literature searches and interviews with survivors of traumatic experiences. The final items of the twenty-one-item scale have been subjected to numerous evaluations of its factor structure, validity, and reliability, and the scale consistently demonstrates excellent internal consistency and reliability (Cann et al., 2009; Tedeschi & Calhoun, 1996). Convergent validity has been demonstrated in the corroboration of PTGI responses by close others (Shakespeare-Finch & Enders, 2008), and discriminant validity has been illustrated in the distinction of PTGI scores from measures of social desirability (Cann et al., 2009). PTG may be assessed globally, as a total score, or across subscales representing the five domains of growth previously detailed. To capture the potential for growth depreciation and assess possible negative consequences that may result from exposure to traumatic circumstances, researchers developed the PTGI-42, which allows respondents to report on outcomes of both PTG and posttraumatic depreciation (PTD; Cann, Calhoun, Tedeschi, & Solomon, 2010).

Several variations of the PTGI have been published, including the PTGI-C, a twenty-one-item inventory suitable to assess growth in children (Cryder, Kilmer, Tedeschi & Calhoun, 2006); the PTGI-C-R, a shortened ten-item inventory of the original PTGI-C (Kilmer et al., 2009); and the PTGI-SF, a shortened ten-item measure of the full twenty-one-item PTGI (Cann et al., 2009). Shortened forms of the PTGI and PTGI-C have demonstrated excellent convergent validity for the assessment of growth both globally and across subscales. However, it is recommended that researchers use the full inventories should they be interested in exploring PTG domains in depth.

The core belief and event-related rumination inventories

As described earlier, the disruption of core beliefs and resultant cognitive processing are essential components to the experience of PTG. To quantify and assess this process, we developed the Core Beliefs Inventory (CBI; Cann et al., 2010). The CBI has been shown to reliably measure the degree to which an individual's assumptive world and core belief structure are challenged following traumatic experience, and higher scores have been positively associated with the five PTG domains in a wide variety of samples (Cann et al., 2010).

The model of PTG also posits that deliberate rumination is an important precursor to outcomes of PTG (Cann et al., 2011; Tedeschi & Calhoun, 2004), and we developed the Event Related Rumination Inventory (ERRI; Cann et al., 2011) as an assessment tool for this hypothesis. The ERRI is a valid and reliable measure consisting of two 10-item Likert scales reflecting event-related intrusive and deliberate ruminations. Initial work suggests that scores on this measure support the theoretical model of PTG such that intrusive rumination has been positively associated to PTD and deliberate rumination has been positively associated with PTG (Cann et al., 2011; Lindstrom et al., 2013).

Prosocial and altruistic behavior in the aftermath of PTG

Studies using the CBI, ERRI, and PTGI have supported the association of PTG with a variety of positive outcomes including the recognition of personal strengths, new possibilities, and an enhanced sense of well-being and life satisfaction. In addition, it is not uncommon for trauma survivors report prosocial or altruistic behavior as an outcome of PTG (Frazier et al., 2013; Staub & Vollhardt, 2008). Prosocial and altruistic behaviors are associated with outcomes of resilience and well-being in the fields of developmental and social psychology (Staub, 2004) and serve to decrease posttrauma distress, enhance one's ability to maintain social relationships, and increase one's overall sense of self (Vollhardt, 2009). Additionally, prosocial value orientations, or concerns for other humans and a perceived responsibility for their general well-being, have been associated with secure attachment styles and an increased sense of connection and belonging with others (Eisenberg, 2010; Twenge, Baumeister, DeWall, Ciarocco, & Bartels, 2007). These factors have been associated with resilience and both cognitive and affective well-being in both children and adults (Vollhardt, 2009).

Increased altruistic behavior is often associated with the occurrence of natural disasters (e.g. hurricanes, earthquakes, tornados) or personally experienced tragedy (e.g. war, loss, and chronic illness; Frazier et al., 2013), and victims of these events tend to display greater altruistic behaviors than nonvictims (Kaniasty & Norris, 1995). A tendency towards altruistic behavior, not only despite traumatic experience but precisely because of it, has been associated with PTG in a variety of studies (Frazier et al., 2013; Staub, 2004). Individuals reporting PTG may engage in altruistic behavior in an attempt alleviate distress and negative affect (Vollhardt, 2009); however, research suggests that these behaviors are more likely attributed to increases in empathy and compassion for others that often accompany growth in relational PTGI domains following trauma (Calhoun & Tedeschi, 2013; Frazier et al., 2013). As individuals reporting PTG frequently report altruistic behaviors, and as research has established relationships between altruistic behavior and resilience, it is possible that PTG may represent a pathway to resilience following traumatic experiences through the increase of altruistic action.

Expert companionship

We have spent the majority of this chapter defining the concept of PTG and describing the proposed mechanisms by which PTG may occur, how it may be measured, and several outcomes of PTG. We now turn our discussion to ways in which an experience of PTG may be facilitated. PTG involves, to a large extent, intentional or unanticipated change that evolves from survivors' coping strategies, ways of thinking about and reconstructing their shattered belief systems, and as a result of disclosure and interaction with the social environment (Calhoun & Tedeschi, 2013; Zoellner & Maercker, 2006). PTG may also be facilitated by the presence of an expert companion, or one who "consistency displays compassion, humility, and respect for a survivors' narrative and perspective while highlighting the potential for strength and change" (Tedeschi & McNally, 2011, p. 21).

The term expert companion implies that a degree of professional competency and human companionship are critical to the processes of healing and growth in survivors (Calhoun & Tedeschi, 2013). Effective expert companions display an open and nonjudgmental presence that echoes Rogers' (1957) necessary and sufficient conditions for therapeutic change (i.e. empathy, genuineness, and unconditional positive regard) and listen to the subtle underlying meanings behind a trauma survivor's disclosure (Calhoun & Tedeschi, 2013; Kelly, 1969). Expert companions should be open, not just to learning about trauma survivors, but to learning *from* them

(Calhoun & Tedeschi, 2013). By allowing ourselves to "learn the language of trauma survivors, empathize with their worldviews, and tolerate not only hearing about but feeling some of the impact of the story of their suffering, we create circumstances where the best trauma treatment can be accomplished" and where the potential for PTG is most likely (Calhoun & Tedeschi, 2013, pp. 25–26). An effective expert companion seeks to do more than just administer evidence-based trauma treatments to remove distress symptomology. Rather, they seek to appreciate the experience of the survivor such that the person can feel safe to explore the situation emotionally and cognitively. It is important to note that not all survivors of trauma will experience PTG. We therefore emphasize that seeking to initiate change should not be the goal of providing expert companionship. Rather, we suggest that embodying the characteristics described earlier and acting an expert companion to survivors of trauma may help to initiate processes of deliberate rumination and facilitate the re-conceptualization of core belief structures that have the potential to contribute to outcomes of PTG. Ways to incorporate expert companionship into a model of PTG intervention have been described elsewhere in the literature (Calhoun & Tedeschi, 1999, 2013; Tedeschi & McNally, 2011).

Conclusions

In this chapter, we have sought to familiarize readers with the origins and principles of the theory of PTG. We have described a selection of characteristics and contexts, such as self-disclosure and expert companionship, believed to facilitate outcomes of PTG. We have also sought to explain how PTG is distinguished from resilience, yet may represent a pathway to new degrees of resilience and resilience trajectories in the aftermath of trauma. These overarching themes of growth and resilience have been well documented and further exploration of how these distinct, yet related, processes complement each other is warranted. Future longitudinal studies should seek to trace varied trajectories of the PTG process in a similar fashion to the latent growth mixture models frequently employed in studies of resilience (Bonanno, Brewin, Kaniasty, & La Greca, 2010) to assess for mechanistic similarities and differences between the two processes. Researchers should also continue to examine the way in which self-disclosure, the presence of supportive others, and expert companions may help to facilitate an experience of PTG. Additionally, investigation of the outcomes of PTG, including altruistic and prosocial behaviors as well as other biopsychosocial outcomes, should continue in a thoughtful and systematic manner. The development of interventions that might serve to foster outcomes of PTG is intriguing, yet, we implore researchers to adequately familiarize themselves with the origins and theoretical principles of PTG and clearly articulate the goals and consequences of these interventions before implementation. We also encourage researchers to take a more nuanced and incremental approach to intervention design, and to appreciate the importance of expert companionship in facilitating outcomes of PTG.

References

Aldwin, C. M., Park, C. L., & Spiro, A. (2007). *Handbook of health psychology and aging.* New York: Guilford Press.
American Psychiatric Association. (2013). *Diagnostic and statistical manual of mental disorders, fifth edition, text.* Washington, DC: Author.
Bonanno, G. A. (2004). Loss, trauma, and human resilience: Have we underestimated the human capacity to thrive after extremely aversive events? *American Psychologist, 59*(1), 20–28.
Bonanno, G. A., Brewin, C. R., Kaniasty, K., & La Greca, A. M. (2010). Weighing the costs of disaster consequences, risks, and resilience in individuals, families, and communities. *Psychological Science in the Public Interest, 11*(1), 1–49.

Bonanno, G. A., Westphal, M., & Mancini, A. D. (2012). Loss, trauma, and resilience in adulthood. *Annual Review of Gerontology & Geriatrics, 32*(1), 189–210.

Bugental, J. F. T. (1965). *The search for authenticity: An existential-analytic approach to psychotherapy.* New York: Holt, Rinehart & Winston, Inc.

Calhoun, L. G., Cann, A., & Tedeschi, R. G. (2010). The posttraumatic growth model: Sociocultural considerations. In T. Weiss & R. Berger (Eds.), *Posttraumatic growth and culturally competent practice* (p. 114). Hoboken, NJ: Wiley.

Calhoun, L. G., & Tedeschi, R. G. (1999). *Facilitating posttraumatic growth: A clinician's guide.* Mahwah, NJ: Erlbaum.

Calhoun, L. G., & Tedeschi, R. G. (2004). The foundations of posttraumatic growth: New considerations. *Psychological Inquiry, 15*(1), 93–102.

Calhoun, L. G., & Tedeschi, R. G. (2006). *Handbook of posttraumatic growth: Research and practice.* Mahwah, NJ: Erlbaum.

Calhoun, L. G., & Tedeschi, R. G. (2013). *Posttraumatic growth in clinical practice.* New York: Routledge.

Cann, A., Calhoun, L. G., Tedeschi, R. G., Kilmer, R. P., Gil-Rivas, V., Vishnevsky, T., & Danhauer, S. C. (2009). The core beliefs inventory: A brief measure of disruption in the assumptive world. *Anxiety, Stress, & Coping, 23*(1), 19–34.

Cann, A., Calhoun, L. G., Tedeschi, R. G., & Solomon, D. T. (2010). Posttraumatic growth and depreciation as independent predictors of well-being. *Journal of Loss and Trauma, 15*(3), 151–166.

Cann, A., Calhoun, L. G., Tedeschi, R. G., Triplett, K. N., Vishnevsky, T., & Lindstrom, C. M. (2011). Assessing posttraumatic cognitive processes: The event related rumination inventory. *Anxiety, Stress, and Coping, 24*(2), 137–156.

Caplan, G. (1964). *Principles of preventive psychiatry.* New York: Basic Books.

Cryder, C., Kilmer, R., Tedeschi, R., & Calhoun, L. (2006). An exploratory study of posttraumatic growth in children following a natural disaster. *American Journal of Orthopsychiatry, 76*(1), 65–69.

Eisenberg, N. (2010). Empathy-related responding: Links with self-regulation, moral judgment, and moral behavior. In M. Mikulincer & P. R. Shaver (Eds.), *Prosocial motives, emotions, and behavior: The better angels of our nature* (pp. 129–148). Washington, DC: American Psychological Association.

Epstein, S. (1980). The self-concept: A review of the proposal of an integrated theory of personality. In E. Staub (Ed.), *Personality: Basic issues and current research.* Englewood Cliffs, NJ: Prentice-Hall.

Frankl, V. E. (1963). *Man's search for meaning.* New York: Pocket Books.

Frazier, P., Greer, C., Gabrielsen, S., Tennen, H., Park, C., & Tomich, P. (2013). The relation between trauma exposure and prosocial behavior. *Psychological Trauma: Theory, Research, Practice, and Policy, 5*(3), 286–294.

Janoff-Bulman, R. (1992). *Shattered assumptions.* New York: The Free Press.

Janoff-Bulman, R. (2006). Schema-change perspectives on posttraumatic growth. In L. G. Calhoun & R. G. Tedeschi (Eds.), *Handbook of posttraumatic growth: Research & Practice* (pp. 81–99). Mahwah, NJ: Erlbaum.

Kaniasty, K., & Norris, F. (1995). Mobilization and deterioration of social support following natural disasters. *Current Directions in Psychological Science, 4*(3), 94–98.

Kelly, G. (1969). Personal construct theory and the psychotherapeutic interview. In B. Maher (Ed.), *Clinical psychology and personality: The selected papers of George Kelly* (pp. 224–264). New York: Wiley.

Kilmer, R., Gil-Rivas, V., Tedeschi, R., Cann, A., Calhoun, L., Buchanan, T., & Taku, K. (2009). Use of the revised posttraumatic growth inventory for children. *Journal of Traumatic Stress, 22*(3), 248–253.

Lindstrom, C. M., Cann, A., Calhoun, L. G., & Tedeschi, R. G. (2013). The relationship pf core belief challenge, rumination, disclosure, and socio-cultural elements to posttraumatic growth. *Psychological Trauma: Theory, Research, Practice, and Policy, 5*(1), 50–55.

Luthar, S. S., Cicchetti, D., & Becker, B. (2000). The construct of resilience: A critical evaluation and guidelines for future work. *Child Development, 71*(3), 543–562.

Maercker, A., & Zoellner, T. (2004). The Janus face of self-perceived growth: Toward a two component model of posttraumatic growth. *Psychological Inquiry, 15*(1), 41–48.

Maslow, A. H. (1970). *Motivation and personality.* New York: Harper.

Parkes, C. M. (1971). Psycho-social transitions: A field for study. *Social Science and Medicine, 5*(2), 101–115.

Pennebaker, J. W. (2003). Writing about emotional experiences as a therapeutic process. In P. Salovey & A. J. Rothman (Eds.), *Social psychology of health* (pp. 362–368). New York: Psychology Press.

Pennebaker, J. W., & Chung, C. K. (2007). Expressive writing, emotional upheavals, and health. In H. Friedman & R. Silver (Eds.), *Handbook of health psychology* (pp. 263–284). New York: Oxford University Press.

Ramos, C., & Leal, I. (2013). Posttraumatic growth in the aftermath of trauma: A literature review about related factors and application contexts. *Psychology, Community, and Health, 2*(1), 43–54.

Rogers, C. R. (1957). The necessary and sufficient conditions of therapeutic personality change. *Journal of Consulting Psychology, 21*(2), 95–103.

Seligman, M.E.P., & Csikszentmihalyi, M. (2000). Positive psychology: An introduction. *American Psychologist, 55*(1), 5–14.

Shakespeare-Finch, J., & Enders, T. (2008). Corroborating evidence of posttraumatic growth. *Journal of Traumatic Stress, 21*(4), 421–424.

Staub, E. (2004). Basic human needs, altruism, and aggression. In A. G. Miller (Ed.), *The social psychology of good and evil* (pp. 51–84). New York: Guilford.

Staub, E., & Vollhardt, J. (2008). Altruism born of suffering: The roots of caring and helping after victimization and other trauma. *American Journal of Orthopsychiatry, 78*(3), 267–280.

Taku, K., Cann, A., Tedeschi, R. G., & Calhoun, L. G. (2009). Intrusive versus deliberate rumination in post-traumatic growth across US and Japanese samples. *Anxiety, Stress, & Coping, 22*(2), 129–136.

Tedeschi, R. G., & Calhoun, L. G. (1995). *Trauma & transformation: Growing in the aftermath of suffering.* Thousand Oaks, CA: Sage.

Tedeschi, R. G., & Calhoun, L. G. (1996). The posttraumatic growth inventory: Measuring the positive legacy of trauma. *Journal of Traumatic Stress, 9*(3), 455–471.

Tedeschi, R. G., & Calhoun, L. G. (2004). Target article: "Posttraumatic growth: Conceptual foundations and empirical evidence". *Psychological Inquiry, 15*(1), 1–18.

Tedeschi, R. G., & Kilmer, R. P. (2005). Assessing strengths, resilience, and growth to guide clinical interventions. *Professional Psychology: Research and Practice, 36*(3), 230–237.

Tedeschi, R. G., & McNally, R. J. (2011). Can we facilitate posttraumatic growth in combat veterans? *American Psychologist, 66*(1), 19–24.

Tedeschi, R. G., Park, C., & Calhoun, L. G. (1998). *Posttraumatic growth: Positive changes in the aftermath of crisis.* Mahwah: Lawrence Erlbaum.

Triplett, K. N., Tedeschi, R. G., Cann, A., Calhoun, L. G., & Reeve, C. L. (2012). Posttraumatic growth, meaning in life, and life satisfaction in response to trauma. *Psychological Trauma: Theory, Research, Practice, and Policy, 4*(4), 400–410.

Twenge, J. M., Baumeister, R. F., DeWall, N., Ciarocco, N. J., & Bartels, J. M. (2007). Social exclusion decreases prosocial behavior. *Journal of Personality and Social Psychology, 92*(1), 56–66.

Vollhardt, J. R. (2009). Altruism born of suffering and prosocial behavior following adverse life events: A review and conceptualization. *Social Justice Research, 22*(1), 53–97.

Zerach, G., Soloman, Z., Cohen, A., & Ein-Dor, T. (2013). PTSD, resilience, and posttraumatic growth among ex-prisoners of war and combat veterans. *Israeli Journal of Psychiatry Related Science, 50*(2), 91–99.

Zoellner, T., & Maercker, A. (2006). Posttraumatic growth in clinical psychology-a critical review and introduction of a two component model. *Clinical Psychology Review, 26*(5), 626–653.

27

Spirituality, culture and resilience

A virtue-informed approach to well-being

Chandra Bhal Dwivedi

Resilience is generally thought of as a positive adaptation after a prolonged stressful or adverse situation. It is an ability to gear up one's resources and bounce back from a negative or threatening experience. Resilience is not only about overcoming a deeply devastating situation but also coming out of it with a renewed energy and competent functioning. Resilience makes an individual to rebound from adversity as a strengthened and more resourceful person. No matter how threatening the stressor is, resilience empowers an individual to adapt and prosper.

What is resilience?

The term resilience is derived from the Latin root *resiliere* which means "to spring back". According to the *Oxford English Dictionary*, this word means "being able to withstand or recover quickly from difficult conditions". In essence, resilience stands for the ability to bounce back from negative emotional experiences and flexibly adapt to changing demands of stressful experiences. Uses of this term in psychology share a common core of meaning, focusing on good outcomes following significant life challenges. Ann Masten (2001) has defined resilience as "a class of phenomenon characterized by *good outcomes in spite of serious threats to adaptation or development*" (p. 228, italics in original).

More specifically, Ryff and Singer (2003) have defined resilience as "*maintenance, recovery, or improvement in mental or physical health following challenge*" (p. 20, italics in original). Windle (2010) conducted an extensive review of over 270 research articles on resilience and based on that review suggested the following operational definition of resilience:

> Resilience is the process of negotiating, managing and adapting to significant sources of stress or trauma. Assets and resources within the individual, their life and environment facilitate this capacity for adaptation and 'bouncing back' in the face of adversity. Across the life course, the experience of resilience will vary.

It has been shown that two factors are involved for a judgment of resilience to be made. First, a person must face a "significant" threat or risk that has the potential to produce negative outcomes. There are a variety of factors that may threaten normal development. Studies have shown that children who grow up in physically abusive homes, who have parents suffering from mental illness or alcoholism, or who are raised in utter poverty are at a significant risk for a variety of problems (see Masten, 2001; Ryff & Singer, 2003, for a review of studies). Steve Baumgardner and Marie Crothers (2009) argue that a judgment of resilience requires that the person has faced a significant risk or threat to well-being. Without a demonstrated risk there is no resilience. Second, a judgment of favourable or good outcome is required for resilience. The standards for judging outcomes may be defined by the normative expectations of society for the age and situation of the individual. Finally, it must be noted that resilience is not an absence of problem behaviours or psychopathology following adversity; resilient responses to adversity are common across the life span. We all encounter a variety of challenges as we journey through life. This is a process that Masten (2001) calls "ordinary magic", consistent with which researchers have emphasized the normal and everyday bases of resilience.

Numerous factors contribute cumulatively to a person's resilience. The single most important factor that helps in handling both ordinary and extraordinary levels of stress is having positive relationships inside or outside one's family. These positive relationships that aid in bolstering a person's resilience include traits such as mutual, reciprocal support and caring. Besides positive relationships, there are many other factors that help in developing and sustaining a person's resilience, such as the ability to make realistic plans and the capability of taking necessary steps to follow through with them, a positive self-concept and confidence in one's strengths and abilities, communication and problem-solving skills, and the ability to manage strong impulses and feelings.

Three definitional approaches to resilience

In the past decade, researchers have conducted many theoretical and empirical studies on resilience (e.g. Cohn, Fredrickson, Brown, Mikels, & Conway, 2009; Davydov, Stewart, Ritchie, & Chaudieu, 2010; Karairmak, 2010; Karreman & Vingerhoets, 2012; Liu, Wang, & Li, 2012). Individuals demonstrate resilience when they face difficult experiences and rise above them with ease. Resilience is found in almost every individual, and it can be learned and developed by virtually anyone. However, there is a lack of a uniform definition for resilience and a corresponding methodology for studying it. Current definitional approaches to resilience include trait, outcome and process orientations.

The trait approach to resilience suggests that resilience is a personal trait that helps individuals cope with adversity and achieve good adjustment. This approach views resilience as a personality trait that presumably inoculates persons against the impact of adversity or traumatic events (Conor & Davidson, 2003; Ong, Bergeman, Bisconti, & Wallace, 2006). An outcome-oriented approach to resilience regards this phenomenon as a function or behavioural outcome that can conquer and help individuals in recovering from adversity or traumatic events in life (Harvey & Delfabbro, 2004; Masten, 2001). The process approach to resilience considers resilience as a dynamic process that helps individuals adapt to and recover rapidly from adversities in life (Rutter, 2008). It becomes intuitively clear that, like state and trait aspects of anxiety, resilience should also be considered in totality with traits working as a predisposing factor while process provides a precipitating role toward the outcome.

Positive emotions and resilience

There is significant amount of research that supports the view that resilience and positive emotions are related. It has been demonstrated in a number of studies that maintaining positive emotions while facing adversity promotes flexibility in thinking and problem solving.

Maintaining a positive emotionality not only increases personal well-being, it also helps in counteracting the physiological effects of negative emotions. Inasmuch as feeling positive emotions during stressful experiences enhances adaptive benefits in the coping process of the individual, they have been described as critical to trait resilience (Tugade & Fredrickson, 2004). Ong et al. (2006) have shown that individuals who have a propensity for coping strategies that concretely elicit positive emotions, such as benefit-finding and cognitive reappraisal, humour, optimism, and goal-directed problem-focused coping, appear to strengthen their resistance to stress.

Low positive affect has been implicated as a distinguishing characteristic of depression. Contrarily, frequent positive affect, along with infrequent negative affect, has been characterized as both a necessary and sufficient condition to produce a state of happiness or affective well-being (Diener, Sandvik, & Pavot, 1991). High positive affect has been shown to indicate as well as promote optimal well-being or flourishing. Positive emotions not only have physical outcomes, but they also have physiological ones. It has been demonstrated that some physiological outcomes caused by humour include improvements in immune system functioning and increment in levels of salivary immunoglobin A, a vital system antibody that serves as the body's first line of defence in respiratory illnesses. Tugade and Fredrickson (2004) studied positive emotions in trait-resilient individuals and their cardiovascular recovery rate following negative emotions. The results showed that trait-resilient individuals experiencing positive emotions demonstrated acceleration in the speed in rebounding from cardiovascular activation initially generated by negative emotional arousal.

Hu, Zhang, and Wang (2015) used 60 published studies and 111 effect sizes in their meta-analysis and reported that trait resilience was negatively correlated with negative indicators of mental health and positively correlated with positive indicators of mental health. Age was found to moderate the relationship between trait resilience and negative indicators of mental health but not the positive indicators of mental health, with adults showing stronger effects than did children and adolescents. Besides this, gender also moderated the relationship between trait resilience and mental health. Another fact that was evident was that the effect sizes were significantly stronger for people in adversity than those not in adversity. These results support the contentions of Baumgardner and Crothers (2009) that resilient individuals seem to use positive emotions, knowingly or unknowingly, to offset negative emotions.

Culture

The current American psychological thinking, despite being local, culture-specific and indigenous, has assumed a global representation and claims itself to be treated as "universal" with a so-called pan-human level legitimacy. As a result of this American hegemony, the mainstream psychology has maintained a unicultural stance at the cost of ignoring other substantive possibilities from disparate cultural traditions. It tries to study every conceivable area of human behaviour – perception, cognition, motivation, intelligence, personality, memory, child development, psychopathology, social behaviours, prejudice, diagnosis and treatment of mental disorders – from the said unicultural and so-called scientific perspective.

The underlying belief in such an attempt is the hope that by so doing it might be possible that the value systems of diverse cultures, particularly those in the third world, would become homogenized over the years. In all probability, this is also guided by a desire that the impact of science and technology combined with large-scale multinational financial aid and investments would foster the growth of material affluence and economic prosperity, which would transform the values of the third world countries and bring them in line with those of the West. It has been thought by those scholars that, as a result of this type of globalization, all the developing countries would eventually imbibe the so called "gold standard" of Western values of *individualism, humanism, empiricism, secularism* and *scientism* and thus would become indistinguishable from other Western countries.

The idea underlying such a broad-based homogenization, as Parekh (2000) has pointed out, is based on the belief that "there is only one correct, true or normal way to understand and structure the relevant areas of life" (p. 1), which indeed is nothing but Euro-American. The impression one gets out of all this is a deep rooted belief in the Western psychologists that the world is only that much as they see it. They also believe that the rest of the people in the world see the world as they see it – through Western spectacles. What they have been proposing is referred to as "absolutist position" by Berry, Poortinga, Segall and Dasen (1997), which assumes that "human phenomena are basically the same (qualitatively) in all cultures: honesty is honesty, and depression is depression, no matter where one observes it" (p. 1103). However, the world as construed by an American scholar cannot be accepted as universally true for all cultures for all time to come. Therefore, doubts concerning the all-pervading power of American psychology began to spread among psychologists all around the world. Psychologists in other cultures found that many of the problems and issues that the Americans paid great attention to were of little or no concern to their own cultural needs.

Culture and psychological processes

Psychologists working across the globe have observed that the psychological processes are rooted in historically variable and culturally mediated activities. Human behaviour does not take place in a vacuum; every human being is part of a cultural system. It can be easily observed that culture and cognitive processes are interlocked and that human beings are both creatures as well as creators of culture. The cultural practices or folk psychology is nothing but "a culture's account of what makes a human being tick" (see Bruner, 1990). It is in terms of folk psychological categories that our experience of ourselves and others is structured. Our participation in culture is essentially indispensable, and indeed, no psychology can be imagined on the basis of individual alone; participation in culture makes meaning public. According to Misra and Mohanty (2002),

> People construct multiple socio-historically grounded realities and apprehending reality from an observer-independent perspective is virtually impossible. Cultural psychological studies underscore the constitutive role of the context of activities. We as human beings operate within socially constituted worlds. This defies the assumptions of a lawful universe and absolute objects with context-free properties.
>
> *(p. 16)*

Diverse cultures provide differing world-views embedded in the practices that sustain them. These world-views inform the way people characteristically look outward upon the universe; it includes ideas about "ought" that influence patterns of thought and affective aspects of things. It teaches them whether "to identify themselves closely with the rest of the cosmos or to see themselves distinct from 'what is out there'" (Redfield, 1953, p. 84). Self actually works as the axis of our world-view; if the self is taught that the human being is unique, to be set apart, the crowning achievement of creation, then that self must tend to relate to the world differently than that of another culture that teaches that the self is only a variation on a single theme, an element whose identity is known by its participation in the whole. In view of this, Western psychological theories and concepts can hardly be treated as universal inasmuch as they are the

337

products of a specific set of social, structural and historical circumstances and accompanying assumptions.

Our self-construals provide an interpretive framework that shapes the way a given socio-cultural group engages in thinking, feeling and acting. Markus and Kitiyama (1991) have shown how interdependent and independent modes of self-construals demonstrate diverse implications for defining and shaping psychological processes. They have also shown that such self-construal simultaneously constrains and affords a range of psychological processes that the members of a given culture might have developed through socialization in order to conduct themselves. Being unique as well as interdependent provides cultural imperatives in their respective cultures. Diverse self-construal encourages different sets of customs, practices, artifacts, norms and institutions in the society. Some of them remain explicit while others remain less conspicuous. Thus, they constrain and afford differing options for human actions. It is this sense that psyche and culture jointly make each other (Shweder, 1990, 1991). Laungani (2004/2010) has also pointed out that

> from a psychological point of view it needs to be stressed that although all human beings share a variety of common biological, physical, and psychological characteristics and behaviours, they have uniquely different, diverse and idiosyncratic ways of responding to their environment and to their own world. Human behaviour is neither static nor a "finished" product. It evolves. It reconstitutes itself culturally. Human behaviour is self-reflective and diversified. Human beings, regardless of their cultural origins, have the ability to share certain common values and agree to common commitments.
>
> *(p. 213)*

It does not, therefore, follow that such consensual agreements will necessarily lead to a corrosion of their traditional values or cultural identity. Laungani (2004/2010) has also contended that "human beings, like chameleons, have the distinct ability to adapt and incorporate the changes within their cultural identity, without wrecking their ancient structure" (p. 213).

The realization that culture plays an important role in psychopathology was realized in the *Diagnostic and Statistical Classification of Mental Disorders, Fourth Edition* (DSM-IV). There is a controversy about the indicators of good psychological and social development when resilience is studied across different cultures (see, for a review, Castro & Murray, 2010). The American Psychological Association's Task Force on Resilience and Strength in Black Children and Adolescents (2008), took note of the fact that there could be some special skills that Black children and youth along with their families have that help them cope with all sorts of disadvantages and trauma, including ability to resist racial prejudice against them.

Researchers have shown that the indigenous factors like culture, history, community values and geographical settings have considerable impact on resilience in indigenous communities. Ungar (2004) has contended that persons who cope with distress or trauma may also show "hidden resilience" when they don't conform to society's expectations. Most of the contemporary research on resilience has demonstrated almost unequivocally that resilience is the result of individual's ability to interact with his/her environment and the processes that either promote well-being or protect them against the overwhelming influence of risk factors.

Spirituality and resilience

Until recently spirituality was regarded as a discipline belonging exclusively to the domain of religion and in so doing the use of the term "religion" was confined to the realm of faith. In such an event, spirituality formed only a side stream that was known as mysticism. However, in recent years, that mysticism has been demystified, and spirituality is now the subject of independent study. Spirituality these days is making headway in all walks of life including psychotherapy (see Miller, 2012; Pargament, 2011), though one cannot fail to notice that there are many different views on what it means to be spiritual.

In modern usage, it includes such a wide range of human experience – traditional religious practices, personal mystical experiences, ecstatic meditational experiences and the quest for meaning in life – that researchers have not been able to agree on a universal definition.

Spirituality appears to be a multidimensional construct in which a few core constructs repeatedly emerge. Spirituality implies that there is a deeper dimension to human life, an inner world of the soul. It assumes that humans are fundamentally spiritual in their pure consciousness. K Ramakrishna Rao (2011, pp. 14–15) has contended that

> Spirituality and consciousness are at the extreme end of ambiguity. Even the notion of science with its intrinsic implication of objectivity has gone through a bewildering array of disputations. To further compound the confusion, the concepts of science and spirituality are conceived in the Western tradition as polar opposites that are hermetically sealed in the tightly compartmentalized behavioural loops. However, in the classical Indian tradition, the dichotomies such as science and spirituality are less sharp permitting their possible coexistence in a holistic conception of human nature.

While attempting a psychological analysis of the concepts of the Bhagavadgīta, Dharam Bhawuk (2011) also noted,

> A major difference between philosophy and spirituality, or for that matter religion and spirituality, is that spirituality, as practiced in India, has an action bias over and above cognitive (thinking or thoughts) or value (considering something important) concerns. Spirituality has been valued in the Indian culture from time immemorial, and it is no surprise that many innovations in the field of spirituality originated in India.
>
> *(p. 25)*

The word "spirituality" is more frequently described in a variety of ways than defined operationally. The word derives from the Latin *spirare*, which means, to breathe. Koenig, McCullough, and Larson (2001) have defined spirituality as "the personal quest for understanding answers to ultimate questions about life, about meaning and about relationship to the sacred or transcendent" (p. 18). According to Peter Hill and Kenneth Pargament (2003),

> [T]he sacred, which includes the divine and the transcendent, is the common denominator of religious and spiritual life. Spirituality is a search for the sacred, a process through which people seek to discover, hold on to, and, when necessary, transform whatever they hold sacred in their lives.
>
> *(p. 65)*

It would be clear that in the West, spirituality is considered as a concept of an immaterial reality. It is considered as an inner path enabling a person to discover the essence of one's being or the deepest values and meanings by which people live. As such spiritual practices including prayer, meditation and contemplation are intended to develop an individual's inner life (Husain, Beg,

& Dwivedi, 2013). Akbar Husain (2011, pp. 24–43) attempted to describe and operationalize spiritual knowledge and practice.

On the other hand, a spiritual aspiration has been the governing force or the core of thought and ruling passion of Hinduism. Every Hindu follows *sanātana dharma* (which may be roughly translated as the Eternal Code). It had made spirituality its highest aim of life, and it tried to turn the whole of life towards spirituality. It is seen in the importance attached by the Hindus to the four *puruṣārthas,* namely, *dharma, artha, kāma,* and *mokṣa.* The first three *puruṣārthas* are only meant for preparing oneself toward the last *puruṣārtha* of *mokṣa,* or deliverance from the cycle of birth, which shows the inherent spirituality in the Hindu mindset. The fact that *mokṣa* was considered as the most important *puruṣārtha* becomes apparent when we see the four *aśramas,* that were proposed for attaining each of these *puruṣārthas* in an orderly sequence, namely, the *Brahmacarya, Gārhasthya, Vānaprastha,* and *Sannyāsa.*

Spirituality, positive emotions and resilience contribute to personal meaning in life

Spirituality, positive emotions and resilience engender personal meaning and purposefulness in a person's life. Personal meaning has been defined as "the cognizance of order, a sense of coherence, the purpose and attainment of worthwhile goals and an accompanying sense of fulfillment" (Smith, Ortiz, Wiggins, Bernard, & Dalen, 2012, p. 439). A person with a remarkably high degree of personal meaning has a clear conceptualization of purposefulness in life, a sense of directedness, a sense of fulfillment in life, a determination to make one's future also quite meaningful and a striving for self-actualizing sort of goal orientation as is visible in the *mokṣa,* the ultimate goal of life of every ardent Hindu. Thus, personal meaning is very much rooted in an individual's culture and is relatively stable (see Smith, et al., 2012).

Another construct that is relevant in the context of resilience is posttraumatic growth that is used more specifically to refer to what occurs in the context of traumatic or stressful events. Posttraumatic growth is also referred to as "stress-related growth" (Park, Cohen, & Murch, 1996) or "benefit finding" (Affleck & Tennen, 1996). Posttraumatic growth involves positive changes such as improved relationships, changes in the values ascribed to one's life, changes in priorities, viewing oneself as a stronger or better person, and finally in spiritual growth. It is the spiritual growth that is most clearly visible in the aftermath of stressful events. Posttraumatic growth always involves attributing something positive after having undergone a highly stressful event in life.

Spirituality increases resilience by affecting relationships and life values

Spirituality emphasizes ethical conduct in relationships with other people. It promotes viewing oneness in all living creatures, and Hinduism includes satiating the entire universe during daily observance of *sandhyopāsana* and *tarpana* (Dwivedi, 2014). Values of love, acceptance, mutual respect, nonviolence, truth and the like are present in almost all religious faiths of the world. It is through spirituality that people start the service of all human beings. This effort also generates social support, which is regarded as a key factor in resilience and coping with stress.

In every form of religion and spirituality, there are "do's and don'ts" or ethical codes for healthy living. These ethical codes may be viewed as either external mandates or as functioning to cultivate internal value system in the individual. Many of these take the shape of formal principles or structured guidelines, such as daily Hindu rituals, meditation and reading of scriptures among others that may prevent or reduce stress. On the other hand, there are certain virtues, such as humility, charity, kindness and veracity that everyone ought to strive for in order to be humane.

The *Yogasutra* of Patanjali has enlisted certain *yamas* or restraints and *niyamas* or observances that are prescribed to be inculcated as the first two steps (from among the eight) in order to become a *yogin* (Dwivedi, in press). "Additionally, religion often explicitly fosters forgiveness and reconciliation as virtues. In fact some form of forgiveness is espoused in the religious doctrines of Judaism, Christianity, Islam, Buddhism, and Hinduism" (Smith et al., 2012, p. 441). The process of forgiveness involves an inner process of making peace by means of positive emotional and cognitive processing that support meaning making and acceptance.

Besides, religiousness and spirituality are intimately related to a personal quest for understanding the questions about travails of life, one's existence, reality, meaning and what is perceived as sacred. In a study of Black families of South Africa, Greeff and Lobuser (2008) asked open-ended questions about strengths that had recently helped their families. They found that people strongly identified spirituality as an important coping resource. It would thus appear that spirituality, positive emotions and resilience have reciprocal relationship and that each of them fosters others and together they help develop a personal meaning for life.

Character strengths and the virtue-informed approach

One of the central themes of positive psychology concerns describing the features of a life well-lived, and inasmuch as the meaning of a good person and good life are intimately connected to virtue, positive psychology has given prominence to virtue-informed approach as well. This has been visible in the Values in Action Project (Peterson & Seligman, 2004), which had the very lofty goal of developing a classification of character strengths and virtues that would parallel the *Diagnostic and Statistical Classification of Mental Disorders* (DSM), developed by the American Psychiatric Association.

Developing a classification of character strengths is indeed a very daunting task. Peterson and Seligman (2004) began by finalizing a set of criteria that was to be applied for selecting character strengths. To be included in the final classification, a character strength had to meet all or nearly all criteria. Half of the strengths selected met the entire set of criteria; the other half did not. Taken as a whole, the final classification of virtues and character strengths "hangs together" as a reasonably coherent effort. The final classification included wisdom and knowledge, courage, humanity, justice, temperance and transcendence.

In a critique of this classification system, Ciarrocchi (2012) questioned "the assumptions and organizational structure behind character strengths and virtues" (p. 427). It stands to reason also that practical wisdom is not just one of the six virtues; it guides a person in choosing which specific action is good in a particular situation. According to Ciarrocchi, "a corollary of this is that virtues need to be integrated and in some sense are hierarchical. That is some virtues such as practical wisdom count more" (p. 427).

Flourishing, in the view of the positive psychology, works on a linear model where more of a virtue is thought to be better. To cite an example, too much or too little optimism is counterproductive, and a person ought to have an optimal balance between too little and too much optimism. A virtue-informed approach to well-being maintains virtue as a mean between two extremes. Ciarrocchi (2012) has suggested,

From a methodological standpoint, positive psychology can determine the linear or curvilinear aspects of a measured virtue, thereby testing whether a measurable virtue is indeed a

341

mean between extremes. Most work on character strengths continues to support the linear hypothesis that more is better. Perhaps more research looking for moderation effects of character strengths will bring to life the nuances virtue ethics suggest.

(p. 427)

Religion and spirituality are only one type of character strength comprising the virtue of transcendence – a virtue that forges "connections to the larger universe and provides meaning" (Peterson & Seligman, 2004, p. 30). Defining character strengths in this cluster include appreciation of beauty and excellence, gratitude, hope and humour. To transcend means to go beyond or rise above the ordinary and the everyday. Transcendence keeps things in proper perspective and keeps us from worrying about or striving for things that don't really matter. Religion and spirituality involve a belief in a higher and abiding power and a far greater purpose for life. Transcendent beliefs connect the individual to a more encompassing and deeper meaning of life. The Indian view of spirituality provides us a connectedness to the entire universe, and Hindu daily practices highlight that aspect quite explicitly.

A virtue-informed approach to well-being caters to those aspects of flourishing that are about meaning making in life. Obviously meaning making and spirituality in their ultimate contexts is not one asset among many but are integral to all remaining virtues put together. Spirituality is undoubtedly a form of meaning making that prescribes the whole point of a good virtuous life. As discussed elsewhere (Dwivedi, 2014), spirituality is about a life that takes care in satiating the entire universe with a firm belief that a human being owes even his existence to Mother Nature. This view is apropos to Martin (2007) who has suggested that it is more comprehensible to place transcendence "as an axis that cuts across all the virtues when they are linked to spirituality" (p. 97).

Is spirituality the master virtue?

In this regard, it is equally important to consider which is the master virtue from among the six virtues proposed by Peterson and Seligman (2004). The master virtue for most of Indians would presumably revolve around practical wisdom with spirituality. Virtue ethics views flourishing as what one ultimately desires and practical wisdom with spirituality helps one to achieve it. Obviously flourishing is not an aggregate of a select number or even all the virtues and character strengths; it is how we take it for our own sake. It is with that respect that spirituality becomes important.

Practical wisdom with prudence judges what the right amount of self-control is adequate for the person in a particular situation. The virtue-informed approach formulates a spiritual or philosophical virtue to inculcate practical wisdom. In all major world religions and most forms of spirituality, there is an emphasis on ethical conduct in relationships with other people. This point has been expanded in Hinduism to include all entities of the universe in its fold regarding developing relationships. In daily rituals, Hindus satiate everything in the universe, and that includes rivers, mountains, seas, oceans, trees and all creatures however small or big they might be, for that matter. At their most basic level in other forms of faith too, religion promotes human kindness through civil conduct and dedication to community. All sacred scriptures advise one to treat others equally on values such as love, acceptance and mutual respect. Can there be strife if one believes in one's heart of hearts that we all are kinsmen? Is there a better way to well-being than to emulate the principle of universal brotherhood?

Summary and future directions

In summarizing the relationship between spirituality, culture and resilience, we notice the close linkages between them, and it becomes amply clear from the brief review of studies cited in the present chapter that they may lead to increases in each other over time. Positive emotions are beneficial in the process of coping with stress in those individuals who are more resilient tend to utilize cultural beliefs and spirituality in coping strategies that elicit positive emotions. Smith et al. (2012) have reviewed studies that show that positive emotions may serve as protective factors that are helpful in promoting both short-term coping and long-term health benefits.

Studies have shown that positive emotions, resilience, and spirituality are linked to one another. Thus, trait-positive emotion may broaden and build resources for resilience and spirituality, and vice versa. Ultimately people who are high in resilience may not only cultivate positive emotions and spirituality in them but also be adept in eliciting positive emotions in others with whom they have close relationships. The main limitation for research examining the relationship between spirituality, resilience, culture and positive emotions is that each of these constructs has been defined and measured in so many different ways. It is important for researchers to operationally define these constructs so that a model showing the interrelationships between them could be worked out.

References

Affleck, G., & Tennen, H. (1996). Construing benefits from adversity: Adaptational significance and dispositional underpinnings. *Journal of Personality, 64*(4), 899–922.

American Psychological Association's Task Force on Resilience and Strength in Black Children and Adolescents. (2008). *Resilience in African American children and adolescents: A vision for optimal development.* Washington, DC: Author.

Baumgardner, S. R., & Crothers, M. K. (2009). *Positive psychology.* New Delhi: Pearson Education, Inc.

Berry, J. W., Poortinga, Y. H., Segall, M., & Dasen, P. R. (1997). *Cross-cultural psychology: Research and applications.* Cambridge, UK: Cambridge University Press.

Bhawuk, D. P. S. (2011). *Spirituality and Indian psychology: Lessons from the Bhagavad-Gita.* New York: Springer.

Bruner, J. (1990). *Acts of meaning.* Cambridge, MA: Harvard University Press.

Castro, F. G., & Murray, K. E. (2010). Cultural adaptation and resilience: Controversies, issues and emerging models. In J. W. Reich, A. J. Zautra, & J. S. Hall (Eds.), *Handbook of adult resilience* (pp. 375–403). New York: Guilford Press.

Ciarrocchi, J. W. (2012). Positive psychology and spirituality: A virtue-informed approach to well-being. In L. J. Miller (Ed.), *The Oxford handbook of psychology and spirituality* (pp. 425–436). New York: Oxford University Press.

Cohn, M. A., Fredrickson, B. L., Brown, S. L., Mikels, J. A., & Conway, A. M. (2009). Happiness unpacked: Positive emotions increase life satisfaction by building resilience. *Emotion, 9*(3), 361–368.

Conor, K. M., & Davidson, J. R. T. (2003). Development of a new resilience scale: The Conor-Davidson Resilience Scale (CD-RISC). *Depression and Anxiety, 18*(2), 76–82.

Davydov, D. M., Stewart, R., Ritchie, K., & Chaudieu, I. (2010). Resilience and mental health. *Clinical Psychology Review, 30*(5), 479–495.

Diener, E., Sandvik, E., & Pavot, W. (1991). Happiness is the frequency, not the intensity, of positive versus negative affect. *Subjective Well-Being: An Interdisciplinary Perspective, 21,* 119–139.

Dwivedi, C. B. (2014). Hindu daily rituals as indigenous culture-centered means of counseling. In S. Banerjee & A. Mukhopadhyaya (Eds.), *Guidance and counseling: An over-view* (pp. 1–28). Varanasi: Green Leaf Publication.

Dwivedi, C. B. (in press). Self-restraints (*yamas*) and self-observances (*niyamas*) as aids in inculcating spirituality in Hinduism. In A. Husain (Ed.), *Spiritual psychology: Recent trends in research, theory, practice and training.* New Delhi: Research India Press.

Greeff, A., & Lobuser, K. (2008). Spirituality as a resiliency quality in Xhosa-speaking families in South Africa. *Journal of Religion and Health, 47*(3), 288–301.

Harvey, J., & Delfabbro, P. H. (2004). Psychological resilience in disadvantaged youth: A critical overview. *Australian Psychologist, 39*(1), 3–13.

Hill, P. C., & Pargament, K. I. (2003). Advances in the conceptualization and measurement of religion and spirituality: Implications for physical and mental health research. *American Psychologist, 58*(1), 64–74.

Hu, T., Zhang, D., & Wang, J. (2015). A meta-analysis of the trait resilience and mental health. *Personality and Individual Differences, 76,* 18–27.

Husain, A. (2011). *Spirituality and holistic health: A psychological perspective.* Delhi: Prasad Psycho Corporation.

Husain, A., Beg, M. A., & Dwivedi, C. B. (2013). *Psychology of humanity and spirituality.* New Delhi: Research India Press.

Karairmak, O. (2010). Establishing the psychometric qualities of the Conor-Davidson Resilience Scale (CD-RISC) using exploratory and confirmatory factor analysis in a trauma survivor sample. *Psychiatry Research, 179*(3), 350–356.

Karreman, A., & Vingerhoets, A. (2012). Attachment and well-being: The mediating role of emotion regulation and resilience. *Personality and Individual Differences, 53*(7), 821–826.

Koenig, H. G., McCullough, M. E., & Larson, D. B. (2001). *Handbook of religion and health.* Oxford, UK: Oxford University Press.

Laungani, P. (2004/2010). Counselling and therapy in a multicultural setting. In R. Moodley, A. Rai & W. Alladin (Eds.), *Bridging East-West psychology and counselling: Exploring the work of Pittu Laungani* (pp. 205–219). New Delhi: Sage Publications.

Liu, Y., Wang, Z. H., & Li, Z. G. (2012). Affective mediators of the influence of neuroticism and resilience on life satisfaction. *Personality and Individual Differences, 52*(7), 833–838.

Markus, H. R., & Kitiyama, S. (1991). Culture and the self: Implications for cognition, emotion, and motivation. *Psychological Review, 98*(2), 224–253.

Martin, M. W. (2007). Happiness and virtue in positive psychology. *Journal for the Theory of Social Behavior, 37*(1), 89–103.

Masten, A. S. (2001). Ordinary magic: Resilience processes in development. *American Psychologist, 56*(3), 227–238.

Miller, L. J. (2012). *The Oxford handbook of psychology and spirituality.* New York: Oxford University Press.

Misra, G., & Mohanty, A. K. (2002). Introduction. In G. Misra & A. K. Mohanty (Eds.), *Perspectives on indigenous psychology* (pp. 13–33). New Delhi: Concept Publishing Company.

Ong, A. D., Bergeman, C. S., Bisconti, T. L., & Wallace, K. A. (2006). Psychological resilience, positive emotions, and successful adaptation to stress in later life. *Journal of Personality and Social Psychology, 91*(4), 730–749.

Parekh, B. (2000). *Rethinking multiculturalism: Cultural diversity and political theory.* New York: Palgrave.

Pargament, K. I. (2011). *Spiritually integrated psychotherapy: Understanding and addressing the sacred.* New York: Guilford Press.

Park, C. L., Cohen, L. H., & Murch, R. L. (1996). Assessment and prediction of stress-related growth. *Journal of Personality, 64*(1), 71–105.

Peterson, C., & Seligman, M. E. P. (2004). *Character strengths and virtues: A handbook of classification.* Washington, DC: American Psychological Association/New York: Oxford University Press.

Rao, K. R. (2011). *Cognitive anomalies, consciousness and yoga.* New Delhi: Matrix Publishers.

Redfield, R. (1953). *The primitive world and its transformation.* Ithaca: Cornell University Press.

Rutter, M. (2008). Developing concepts in developmental psychopathology. In J. J. Hudziak (Ed.), *Developmental psychopathology and wellness: Genetic and environmental influences* (pp. 3–22). Washington, DC: American Psychiatric Publishing.

Ryff, C. D., & Singer, B. (2003). Flourishing under fire: Resilience as a prototype of challenged thriving. In C. L. M. Keyes & J. Haidt (Eds.), *Flourishing: Positive psychology and the life well-lived* (pp. 15–36). Washington, DC: American Psychological Association.

Shweder, R. A. (1990). Cultural psychology-what is it? In W. Stigler, R. A. Shweder, & G. Herdt (Eds.), *Cultural psychology: Essays on comparative development* (pp. 1–43). Cambridge: Cambridge University Press.

Shweder, R. A. (1991). *Thinking through cultures: Expeditions in indigenous psychologies.* Cambridge, MA: Harvard University Press.

Smith, B. W., Ortiz, J. A., Wiggins, K. T., Bernard, J. F., & Dalen, J. (2012). Spirituality, positive emotions and resilience. In L. J. Miller (Ed.), *The Oxford handbook of psychology and spirituality* (pp. 434–454). New York: Oxford University Press.

Tugade, M. M., & Fredrickson, B. L. (2004). Resilient individuals use positive emotions to bounce back from negative emotional experiences. *Journal of Personality and Social Psychology, 86*(2), 320–333.

Ungar, M. (2004). *Nurturing hidden resilience in troubled youth.* Toronto: University of Toronto Press.

Windle, G. (2010). The resilience network: What is resilience? A systematic review and concept analysis. *Reviews in Clinical Gerontology, 21,* 1–18.

28

Building resilience by teaching and supporting the development of social emotional skills and wellness in vulnerable children

Todd I. Herrenkohl and Logan A. Favia

Resilience, as conceptualized in this chapter, is a life course process that characterizes successful adaptation to adverse childhood experiences (Herrenkohl, 2011). Adverse childhood experiences, which include abuse and neglect, are known risk factors for a range of developmental and functional impairments in children, as well as later-occurring problems, such as drug and alcohol abuse, violence, and mental illness. Research also shows a link to physical health, the onset of disease, and premature death in adults. However, adverse childhood experiences do not always lead to negative outcomes, nor do they consistently limit what any individual can achieve in her or his lifetime. Those who rebound from adversity and avoid at least some of the associated negative consequences are considered resilient (Herrenkohl, 2011; Klika & Herrenkohl, 2013).

Theory underscores the finding that resilience is not a stable pattern of behavior, nor is it a reflection of an individual's fixed traits or dispositions, although it is a reflection of an individual's capacity to overcome trauma and cope under stress (Luthar, 2006; Luthar, Cicchetti, & Becker, 2000). According to scholars like Luthar (2006) and Masten (1994, 2001) and others before them, resilience is a reflection of how an individual responds over time to unfolding life circumstances, some of which are within an individual's control and others of which are not. Generally, when an individual's surroundings are conducive to health and recovery (e.g. there is adequate social support, safety, and opportunity for growth and nurturance), functioning will improve or be sustained at a high level. When surroundings are not conducive to health and recovery, as when abuse is ongoing or an individual is repeatedly threatened with violence from within or outside the family, individual functioning will deteriorate or remain at a low level. Thus, researchers often talk about resilience in relation to environmental risk or stress (Leadbeater, Schellenbach, Maton, & Dodge, 2004). In Figure 28.1, Leadbeater et al. (2004) illustrate how individual functioning changes in response to stress and protection in the environment. In Figure 28.1, they refer to individual "competence" in relation to changes over time in stress and protective influences. The same general logic applies to resilience, a closely related concept.

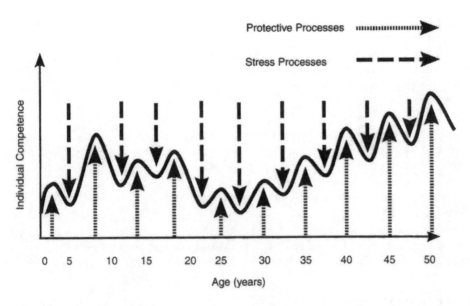

Figure 28.1 Interaction of risk and protective processes related to individual competence
Source: Leadbeater et al. (2004).

Studies on the protective processes and the building blocks of resilience in vulnerable children point to the importance of early interventions to lessen conflict within families and to restore functioning in relationships (adding protection) to a point that children feel safe and nurtured (Herrenkohl, 2011). Various models of primary and secondary prevention programs for families at risk for abuse have been tested, and some show success in preventing family violence and improving the lives of children. These include parenting programs that focus on helping young mothers acquire support and skills to parent successfully. A well-published and often cited example is the Nurse-Family Partnership model (www.nursefamilypartnership.org/). Nurse-Family Partnership (NFP) is a home-visiting program that focuses on helping young, first-time mothers who have limited resources. The intent of the program is to improve prenatal care by assisting mothers to obtain necessary services and to ready mothers for the tasks of parenting young children. Tested in several trials, the program has shown promise for reducing several risk factors for child maltreatment and also lessening developmental problems in children as they age. Mothers, too, appear to benefit from the program in showing better prenatal health and improved functioning, as well as more positive interactions with their children (Blueprints for Healthy Youth Development, www.blueprintsprograms.com/programResults.php).

Triple P is another example of an evidence-based program that has shown promise for reducing risk factors and the consequences of child maltreatment and for promoting health and wellness in parents and their children (www.triplep.net/glo-en/home/). Like NFP, Triple P focuses on improving parenting practices and lessening behaviors in parents and children that can impede child development. Both programs, NFP and Triple P, have been evaluated using cost–benefit methods and are shown to produce a positive return on initial investments made (www.blueprintsprograms.com/programResults.php).

Other programs outside of the home focus on providing children with opportunities to develop skills that allow them to perform well in school and interact successfully with others (Trickett, Kurtz, & Pizzigati, 2004). Many programs of this type are based in schools because schools provide the best access to children from all backgrounds, including those who have experienced adversity.

Programs delivered in schools are often oriented to reducing risk factors (e.g. poor academic achievement, disengagement from school, negative peer modeling) and preventing problems, like aggression and bullying (Herrenkohl, Chung, & Catalano, 2004; Walker & Shinn, 2002). Certain programs in prevention teach skills to enhance healthy social interaction and promote positive youth development by empowering children to take initiative in their education, learning life skills, etc. These include universal programs in social emotional learning (SEL). Universal SEL programs seek to equip all children with skills and competencies that will help them succeed not only in school but also in other aspects and domains of their lives (Brackett & Rivers, 2014; Brackett, Rivers, Reyes, & Salovey, 2012). They provide opportunities for children to learn how to solve problems and negotiate conflict, persevere in the face of difficulties, manage stress, and share emotions (Durlak, Weissberg, Dymnicki, Taylor, & Schellinger, 2011). In the section that follows, we focus on research about SEL and explore the intersection between SEL programs, integrated models of care, and resilience in vulnerable populations. Specifically, we explain how SEL programs can help position children of all backgrounds to succeed in school and to build resilience.

Social emotional learning (SEL)

A widely accepted definition of social emotional learning was posited by Zins and Elias (2006). They define social emotional learning, or SEL, as "the process of acquiring and effectively applying the knowledge, attitudes, and skills necessary to recognize and manage emotions; developing caring and concern for others; making responsible decisions; establishing positive relationships; and handling challenging situations capably" (p. 1). The Collaborative for Academic, Social, and Emotional Learning (CASEL), a nationally recognized organization dedicated to promoting the use of evidence-based programs in SEL, uses this definition to support its emphasis of five core competencies. These competencies include self-awareness, self-management, social awareness, relationship skills, and responsible decision making (www.casel.org/). Developmental studies of SEL programs show that mastery of these competencies is associated with greater well-being and general improvement in student conduct (Durlak et al., 2011). Specifically, students who are socially and emotionally skilled are more able to develop strong relationships that nurture good habits and promote self-confidence. They also feel generally more connected to school and are motivated to learn and do well academically (US Department of Health and Human Services, 2009). Moreover, research shows that mastery of the five CASEL competencies is linked to success much later in life in the domains of employment (e.g. securing and maintaining a well-paying job); relationships (e.g. forming adult relationships, starting a family, etc.); and participating as a productive citizen in one's community.

Although no one skill or competency affords more opportunity for growth and development than another, the core competency of self-management is highly valued because it allows a young person to cope and even thrive under stress. Likewise, the core competency of decision making is critical because responsible decision making leads to good life choices that promote health and wellness (Bradshaw, O'Brennan, & McNeely, 2008).

School-based SEL programs

When SEL is not prioritized, children have fewer opportunities to meet the five CASEL competencies, and there is evidence that deficits in one or more of these areas can increase a child's risk for underachieving (Ruby & Doolittle, 2010). Unfortunately, exposure to childhood adversities, such as abuse and neglect, increases the likelihood that a child will not develop the skills reflected in the five competency areas before entering school (Webster-Stratton, Reid, & Stoolmiller, 2008). Children from stressful, highly problematic home environments where violence is a common occurrence are least likely to enter school with skills that allow them to focus and do well on tasks or to interact with others in ways that strengthen social connections and build self-confidence (Frick, Cornell, Barry, Bodin, & Dane, 2003). Instead, children who are repeatedly exposed to violence in their homes come to school having learned behaviors (e.g. being hostile and controlling to others, showing disregard for others' well-being, and being disruptive) that further diminish their chances of succeeding in that context. Thus, special programming efforts often are required to allow these children opportunities to re-learn and re-tool so that their social interactions and orientation to school is positive and productive. In the sections that follow, we comment on universal and more targeted approaches to helping these and other children succeed.

Universal SEL programs

Whole-school and classroom-based models of SEL can take the form of universal programs (i.e. those that focus on increasing skills and competencies in an entire population of students), or they can be more tailored to the needs of particular subgroups of students (Goncy, Sutherland, Farrell, Sullivan, & Doyl, 2015). Classroom-based, universal SEL programs often include explicit skill instruction and possibly group-based activities that are guided by a structured skills curriculum. There are a variety of examples, some of which have been reviewed and vetted by organizations like CASEL. More information on programs recommended by CASEL can be found on their website (http://casel.org/).

Evidence to date of the promise of universal SEL programs for reducing risk factors and promoting protective factors that lead to resilience is generally favorable (Durlak et al., 2011). In fact, reviews of research on these SEL programs show they can reduce disruptive behaviors among elementary school children *and* increase students' academic performance. Durlak et al.'s (2011) meta-analytic review of 213 school-based SEL programs found consistent gains in students' academic performance, with an average effect size above .20 across the different intervention formats. In addition, they found positive and significant effects from SEL programs on students' skills, attitudes, and behaviors. Students who received SEL instruction exhibited fewer conduct problems and less emotional distress on average than did students who did not receive SEL instruction. Of note, however, the quality of program implementation and instructional practices in SEL mattered, such that better quality programs led to more student success. More specifically, programs that followed four highly recommended procedures to teach SEL skills (e.g. followed steps for sequencing activities and making expectations clear and explicit) yielded better results than did programs that did not follow these procedures.

The CASEL Guide, published online, provides a rating system for evaluating the quality of SEL programs and offers guidance to schools and districts that are considering SEL for their students. The guide is organized to allow readers quick access to information that can help them decide which program(s) is/are best suited to the needs of their students. CASEL's rating system is useful because it provides school and district staff with a set of criteria on which to evaluate the strengths and merits of programs using common or even disparate approaches. The strongest programs in the rating system typically are those that have been studied using rigorous methods. Among the review criteria are the "contexts" in which SEL is taught (e.g. schools) and whether the programs generalize to other settings (e.g. community). Although many programs teach skills applicable to a range of settings and contexts, not all include community outreach components

– an important consideration when reviewing and adopting an intervention for children from diverse backgrounds. Particularly for children who enter school without early skills-training, building capacity for SEL that extends beyond the school setting is critically important because it allows them to focus on applying skills in those other settings.

Integrated school-based programs

To build resilience among children who experience the most serious and chronic forms of adversity, such as extreme violence and chronic disruption, universal programs in SEL are critical but insufficient. Research has begun to show that system-level reforms focused on changing schools on behalf of vulnerable children can have profound effects on their learning and resilience. In a well-written and comprehensive case study of her work in an urban charter high school, Mulloy (2014) examined the concept of resilience as it applies to the school environment. Consistent with the public health model, Mulloy describes the advantages of school-level changes designed to make the environment more conducive to learning for children who have experienced adversity. This approach involves understanding and applying what is known about resilience and protective factors to the school setting by providing targeted academic supports and intensive skills training. The model described by Mulloy has some of the same elements as a full-service community school approach, where an emphasis is placed on the whole child (Dryfoos, 1994).

The community school model is related to other models of integrated services (Walker & Shinn, 2002), where schools become a hub for activities designed to meet the multiple needs of children. Services in these settings can include physical and mental health services, as well as after-school recreation programs and family support. The goal is to develop and implement a holistic model of learning and support that revolves around student success in the broadest sense of the term. In community schools, the basic needs of children and families are addressed by bringing mental and physical health services into the school building and by relying on community organizations to help mentor students around academic goals. It is understood by proponents of this model that learning is maximized when they and their families have basic needs met and that bringing schools, families, and community providers together promotes collective ownership of children's schooling and life successes. In addition, collaborations build political strength to press for more resources in typically underresourced schools. Further, community-based organizations bring the culture of the community into the school and, in doing so, help to create an environment in which children from diverse ethnic and cultural backgrounds feel welcomed and included (Warren, 2005).

Children who enter school having experienced adversity can exhibit symptoms of some of the more common childhood mental health problems, including attention deficit hyperactivity disorder (ADHD), oppositional defiant disorder, conduct disorder, and depression. To address the needs of children with mental health problems, specialized mental health services are often required. Such services can include individual- and group-therapy models that help children identify and appropriately respond to feelings of distress; to develop coping skills, and to routinize strategies of help-seeking when negative emotions become overwhelming (Rones & Hoagwood, 2000). Several school-based, cognitive-behavioral therapy interventions have been shown to reduce symptoms of posttraumatic stress disorder (PTSD) and depression. These include the Cognitive Behavioral Intervention for Trauma in Schools (CBITS) and Trauma-Focused Coping in Schools (TFC).

CBITS is a group-based, trauma intervention delivered in the school setting by school-based clinicians with training in the implementation of trauma-related services. In about 10 sessions (as well as one to three individual sessions, two parent sessions, and one teacher session), children and adolescents from the ages of 10 to 15 learn cognitive-behavioral techniques, including coping (e.g. relaxation) and social problem-solving strategies in order to relieve symptoms of PTSD. Several clinical and randomized control trials of the CBITS model have shown positive outcomes for children with clinically significant levels of PTSD after reported exposure to violence. In one trial, sixth grade students attending large middle schools in Los Angeles experienced significant improvement in PTSD and depressive symptoms after participating in a ten-session CBITS intervention (Stein et al., 2003). Additionally, those who support this approach suggest it can be flexibly implemented to in order to integrate culturally relevant strategies and examples (NCTSN, 2012).

TFC is similar to CBITS in that it is a group-based, skills-focused, cognitive-behavioral intervention for children and adolescents. TFC is designed for children and adolescents from the ages of 6 to 18 who have experienced a single incidence of trauma. In about fourteen to eighteen sessions, youth learn to manage anxiety, anger, and grief and process the memory and story of their trauma, individually and with their peers (NCTSN, 2012). In clinical trials, this program has demonstrated beneficial effects of treatment for reducing symptoms of PTSD, depression, anxiety, and anger immediately after participation in the intervention and six months after participation (March, Amaya-Jackson, Murray, & Schulte, 1998).

The CBITS and TFC models of embedded supports are characteristic of an integrated framework that ties emotional and instructional strategies to academic learning. Offered as a complementary model to SEL, cognitive-behavioral and related individual and group therapies can promote skill-building and coping that translates to better academic and behavioral outcomes for even the model vulnerable children (Ko et al., 2008).

School-based mental health services have gained prominence over the years, partly because of the growing need for such services, as well as an awareness that children's mental health directly impacts their ability to learn (Rones & Hoagwood, 2000). An overwhelming majority of children in need of mental health intervention receive services in school (70% to 80%), and this number continues to grow as federal and state guidelines mandate need-based programs. The "system of care" model described by Rones and Hoagwood (2000) emphasizes the importance of meeting the multiple needs of children who are severely impacted by emotional disorders by connecting agencies and systems – a theme very similar to that of the CBITS-integrated framework. It also focuses on providing services to children that are not "agency-specific" but "function-specific" (Stroul & Friedman, 1986); that is services are directed to children to address a particular need and are not bound to a model that assumes the same services fit all needs.

The Patient Protection and Affordable Care Act (ACA), the comprehensive health care reform signed into law in 2010, continues to emphasize the need for physical and mental health care in schools by authorizing funding to establish and expand school-based health centers. These are clinics that are located in or near school facilities through partnerships with community health providers. In this model, the community provider becomes part of the school community, and services for children are administered through the partnering organization. With the expansion of health care now underway under new federal policies, there is a strong likelihood that school-based health centers will become increasingly popular in schools that serve large percentages of children from high-poverty and disadvantaged backgrounds. To date, school-based mental health services have largely been comprised of screening and counseling services outside of the classroom, sometimes utilizing school-based health centers. However, toward the goal of integrating education and mental health in schools, experts in the field emphasize the importance of delivering services along a continuum by integrating SEL programs and providing ongoing support and professional development to teachers as they grapple with how to respond appropriately to the multiple needs of an increasingly diverse student body (Atkins, Hoagwood, Kutash, & Seidman, 2010).

Conclusion

The building blocks of resilience include supportive relationships and environmental contexts that are conducive to health and recovery. With a growing awareness of the impact of childhood adversities and trauma, experts on schools are looking at the teaching and learning of social emotional skills and competencies as a fundamental component of the core curriculum. In that children who have experienced adversities, such as abuse and neglect, are often provided fewer opportunities before they enter school to acquire requisite SEL skills, it is critically important that schools help fill this void so that all students are served equitably and in ways that maximize the learning for all who attend. Embedded in an integrated framework that provides the opportunity for children to receive targeted, function-specific interventions for mental health problems, SEL instruction can help equip children to succeed academically and to handle challenges they encounter over their lifetimes. Community schooling and other similar models (e.g. CBITS, TFC) focus on SEL in the context of a broader goal of serving children in need of mental health and physical health services – and of bringing families and community service providers closer to the school setting to help serve children more holistically. Emphasis within a community schools framework also extends to parents and other family members, who are viewed as potential collaborators and recipients of services at the same time. The benefit of comprehensive and integrated approaches to school-based services include allowing children access to care they need and to conveniently locate services in a central place known to families. Integrated services are a foundation for building resilience in vulnerable children impacted by family violence and other forms of adversity. Accumulating evidence shows that creating safe and welcoming school environments and providing children access to opportunities to learn a full array of skills for academic and life success is essential to all children and of paramount importance to those whose early lives are marked by hardship.

References

Atkins, M. S., Hoagwood, K. E., Kutash, K., & Seidman, E. (2010). Toward the integration of education and mental health in schools. *Administration and Policy in Mental Health and Mental Health Services Research, 37*(1–2), 40–47.

Brackett, M. A. & Rivers, S. E. (2014). Transforming students' lives through social and emotional learning. In R. Pekrun & L. Linnenbrink-Garcia (Eds.), *International Handbook of Emotions in Education* (pp. 368–388). London: Routledge.

Brackett, M. A., Rivers, S. E., Reyes, M. R., & Salovey, P. (2012). Enhancing academic performance and social and emotional competence with the RULER feeling words curriculum. *Learning and Individual Differences, 22*(2), 218–224.

Bradshaw, C. P., O'Brennan, L. M., & McNeely, C. A. (2008). Core competencies and the prevention of school failure and early school leaving. *New Directions for Child and Adolescent Development, 122*, 19–32.

Dryfoos, J. G. (1994). *Full service schools: A revolution in health and social services for children, youth, and families.* San Francisco, CA: Jossey-Bass.

Durlak, J. A., Weissberg, R. P., Dymnicki, A. B., Taylor, R. D., & Schellinger, K. B. (2011). The impact of enhancing students' social and emotional learning: A meta-analysis of school-based universal interventions. *Child Development, 82*(1), 405–432.

Frick, P. J., Cornell, A. H., Barry, C. T., Bodin, S. D., & Dane, H. E. (2003). Callous-unemotional traits and conduct problems in the prediction conduct problem severity, aggression, and self-report of delinquency. *Journal of Abnormal Child Psychology, 31*(4), 457–470.

Goncy, E. A., Sutherland, K. S., Farrell, A. D., Sullivan, T. N., & Doyl, S. T. (2015). Measuring teacher implementation in delivery of a bullying prevention program: The impact of instructional and procedural adherence and competence on student responsiveness. *Prevention Science, 16*(3), 440–450.

Herrenkohl, T. I. (2011). Resilience and protection from violence exposure in children: Implications for prevention and intervention programs with vulnerable populations. In T. I. Herrenkohl, E. Aisenberg, J. H. Williams, & J. M. Jenson (Eds.), *Violence in context: Current evidence on risk, protection, and prevention* (pp. 92–108). New York: Oxford University Press.

Herrenkohl, T. I., Chung, I. J., & Catalano, R. F. (2004). Review of research on predictors of youth violence and school-based and community-based prevention approaches. In P. Allen-Meares & M. W. Fraser (Eds.), *Intervention with children and adolescents: An interdisciplinary perspective* (pp. 449–476). Boston: Allyn & Bacon.

Klika, J. B., & Herrenkohl, T. I. (2013). A review of developmental research on resilience in maltreated children. *Trauma, Violence, and Abuse, 14*(3), 222–234.

Ko, S. J., Ford, J. D., Kassam-Adams, N., Berkowitz, S. J., Wilson, C., Wong, M., & Layne, C. M. (2008). Creating trauma-informed systems: Child welfare, education, first responders, health care, juvenile justice. *Professional Psychology: Research and Practice, 39*(4), 396–404.

Leadbeater, B. J., Schellenbach, C. J., Maton, K. I., & Dodgen, D. W. (2004). Research and policy for building strengths: Processes and contexts of individual, family, and community development. In K. I. Maton, C. J. Schellenbach, B. J. Leadbeater, & A. L. Solarz (Eds.), *Investing in children, youth, families, and communities: Strengths-based research and policy* (pp. 13–30). Washington, DC: American Psychological Association.

Luthar, S. (2006). Resilience in development: A synthesis of research across five decades. In D. Cicchetti & D. J. Cohen (Eds.), *Development and psychopathology: Risk, disorder, and adaptation* (pp. 740–795). New York: John Wiley.

Luthar, S., Cicchetti, D., & Becker, B. (2000). The construct of resilience: A critical evaluation and guidelines for future work. *Child Development, 71*(3), 543–562.

March, J. S., Amaya-Jackson, L., Murray, M. C., & Schulte, A. (1998). Cognitive-behavioral psychotherapy for children and adolescents with posttraumatic stress disorder after a single-incident stressor. *Journal of the American Academy of Child and Adolescent Psychiatry, 37*(6), 585–593.

Masten, A. S. (1994). Resilience in individual development: Successful adaptation despite risk and adversity. In M. C. Wang & E. W. Gordon (Eds.), *Educational resilience in inner city America: Challenges and prospects* (pp. 3–25). Hillsdale, NJ: Lawrence Erlbaum Associates, Inc.

Masten, A. S. (2001). Ordinary magic: Resilience processes in development. *American Psychologist, 56*(3), 227–238.

Mulloy, M. (2014). *Resilience-building schools for at-risk youth: Developing the social, emotional, and motivational foundations of academic success.* Kingston, NJ: Civic Research Institute.

NCTSN. (2012). Cognitive behavioural intervention for trauma in schools. Retrieved from www.nctsnet. org/sites/default/files/assets/pdfs/cbits_general.pdf

Rones, M., & Hoagwood, K. E. (2000). School-based mental health services: A research review. *Clinical Child and Family Psychology Review, 3*(4), 223–241.

Ruby, A., & Doolittle, E. (2010). *Efficacy of schoolwide programs to promote social and character development and reduce problem behavior in elementary school children.* Washington, DC: Institute of Education Sciences National Center for Education Research.

Stein, B. D., Jaycox, L. H., Kataoka, S. H., Wong, M., Tu, W., Elliott, M. N., & Fink, A. (2003). A mental health intervention for schoolchildren exposed to violence: A randomized control trial. *Journal of the American Medical Association, 290*(5), 603–611.

Stroul, B. A., & Friedman, R. M. (1986). *A system of care for severely emotionally disturbed children and youth.* CASSP Technical Assistance Center, Georgetown University Child Development Center, Washington, DC.

Trickett, P. K., Kurtz, D. A., & Pizzigati, K. (2004). Resilient outcomes in abused and neglected children: Bases for strengths-based intervention and prevention policies. In K. I. Maton, C. J. Schellenbach, B. J. Leadbeater, & A. L. Solarz (Eds.), *Investing in children, youth, families, and communities: Strengths-based research and policy* (pp. 73–95). Washington, DC: American Psychological Association.

US Department of Health and Human Services, Centers for Disease Control and Prevention. (2009). *School connectedness: Strategies for increasing protective factors among youth.* Retrieved from www.cdc.gov/healthyyouth/protective/connectedness.htm

Walker, H. M., & Shinn, M. R. (2002). Structuring school-based interventions to achieve integrated primary, secondary, and tertiary prevention goals for safe and effective schools. In M. R. Shinn, G. Stoner, & H. M.

Waker (Eds.), *Interventions for academic and behavior problems: Preventive and remedial approaches* (pp. 1–26). Silver Spring, MD: National Association of School Psychologists.

Warren, M. A. (2005). Communities and schools: A new view of urban education reform. *Harvard Educational Review, 75*(2), 133–139.

Webster-Stratton, C., Reid, M. J., & Stoolmiller, M. (2008). Preventing conduct problems and improving school readiness: Evaluation of the incredible years teacher and child training programs in high-risk schools. *Journal of Child Psychology and Psychiatry, 49*(5), 471–488.

Zins, J. E., & Elias, M. J. (2006). Social and emotional learning. In G. G. Bear & K. M. Minke (Eds.), *Children's needs III: Development, prevention, and intervention* (pp. 1–13). Bethesda, MD: National Association of School Psychologists.

29

Leader influences on resilience and adaptability in organizations

Paul T. Bartone

According to the renowned stress researcher Hans Selye, some amount of stress is a necessary condition of life. Even when fully at rest, our bodily systems are still working hard to maintain homeostasis. As Selye (1974) said famously, the only way to be completely free from stress is to be dead! And while life has never been without stress, it certainly appears that, as the pace of change has quickened in the modern era, the potential for stress has risen for many people. The need to adjust and adapt to changing circumstances has indeed grown substantially in today's world (Ilgen & Pulakos, 1999). New technologies, equipment, and systems appear at a fast pace, forcing changes in the way many jobs get accomplished (Thach & Woodman, 1994). Also, increasing globalization of operations for many organizations means that employees often must learn to function in unfamiliar cultures and languages (Molinsky, 2007). Given these increased demands, organizations are in need of employees who are highly resilient and able to adapt quickly to changing conditions. The present chapter explores the role of psychological hardiness in promoting resilience and adaptability and describes how leaders can foster these desirable qualities across the workforce.

Individual differences in responding to stress

Selye, despite his extensive attention to generalized patterns of responding to stress, also recognized that there are profound individual differences in how people respond to stressors. He observed that "the same stress which makes one person sick can be an invigorating experience for another" (Selye, 1978, p. xv). Much of the early human research in this area focused on the ill effects of various life stressors (e.g. Holmes & Rahe, 1967). More recently, attention has shifted to the study of resilient people, those who remain healthy and continue to perform well despite high levels of stress (Bonanno, 2004).

Recent years have seen a dramatic increase in the number of studies on "resilience," although there is little agreement as to what it means (Layne, Warren, Watson, & Shalev (2007). The term resilience has its roots in materials science, where it is defined as "the ability of a material to absorb and release energy, within the elastic range" (Gere & Goodno, 2009, p. 146).[1] Resilience was first applied to humans by developmental psychologists and psychiatrists, who used it to describe children who developed normally and adapted well despite having grown up in harsh environments that put them at higher risk for psychopathology and other poor outcomes (Garmezy, 1971; Garmezy, 1974; Rutter, 1979; Werner, Bierman, & French, 1971). Many stress researchers still new to this tradition and view resilience as basically the *absence of pathology* following stress exposure (Sroufe, 1997; Witmer & Culver, 2001).

In contrast to this view, many researchers see resilience as involving positive processes that are distinct from those associated with heightened vulnerability (Carver, 1998; Friborg, Hjemdal, Martinussen, & Rosenvinge, 2009; Werner & Smith, 2001). However, even among those focusing only on positive features, there is a wide diversity of views as to what factors constitute or contribute to resilience (Luthar, 2006). These range from individual attributes such as intellectual ability, self-control, flexibility, optimism, self-efficacy, spirituality, and confidence, to social factors such as support from family and friends, co-workers, and the broader socio-economic environment (Layne et al., 2007).

Resilience and adaptability

In a world of rapid change, resilience must also include the capacity to adjust and adapt in response to new circumstances. It is not enough to merely "bounce back" from stress into one's original state. In fact, some scholars see adaptability as the core feature of resilience. For example Folke et al. (2010) assert: "Resilience in this context is the capacity of a [system] to continually adapt and change yet remain within critical thresholds. Adaptability is part of resilience." Importantly too, adaptability involves the capacity "to learn, combine experience and knowledge, and adjust responses to external drivers and internal processes." While Folke et al. (2010) are addressing the resilience of social-ecological systems, the same is true for resilience at the individual level. Adaptability has been linked to resilience and performance of individuals (Burke, Pierce, & Salas, 2006); teams (Hackman, 2002); organizations (Weick & Sutcliffe, 2001; Zaccaro & Banks, 2004); and entire nations (Ben-Dor, 2004; Gaillard, 2007). Regardless, adaptability always has to do with the ability of a system to change or adjust in response to changing conditions (Mueller-Hanson, White, Dorsey, & Pulakos, 2005). A recent report by the Defense Science Board (2011) takes this even further, defining adaptability as "the ability and willingness to anticipate the need for change, to prepare for that change, and to implement changes in a timely and effective manner in response to the surrounding environment" (p. 3). This report also notes that in the new, rapidly changing global environment, the ability of organizations and personnel to adapt is essential to successful performance.

One of the most frequently studied variables contributing to stress resilience at the individual level is psychological hardiness (Eschleman, Bowling, & Alarcon, 2010). Hardiness is a constellation of psychological qualities found to characterize people who remain healthy and continue to perform well under a range of stressful conditions (Bartone, 1999; Bartone, Roland, Picano, & Williams, 2008; Kobasa, Maddi, & Kahn, 1982). The key facets of hardiness are commitment – an active engagement and involvement with the world, and a sense of meaning in life (versus alienation); control – a belief that through effort one can influence events and outcomes (versus powerlessness); and challenge – a receptiveness to variety and change in life (versus high need for security and predictability). Highly hardy persons typically regard experience as (1) overall interesting and worthwhile (commitment) and (2) something they can exert control over (control). When confronted with new or changing situations, they tend to see these as (3) challenging opportunities to learn and grow (challenge). Highly hardy persons also favor proactive, problem-solving coping strategies, as opposed to avoidant ones.

Since Kobasa's original (1979) report on hardiness and health in highly stressed executives, a substantial body of research has accumulated that generally confirms hardiness as a protective factor against the ill effects of stress on health and performance. Studies with diverse occupational groups have found that hardiness operates to moderate or buffer stress (e.g. Contrada, 1989; Kobasa et al., 1982; Maddi & Kobasa, 1984; Roth, Wiebe, Fillingim, & Shay, 1989; Wiebe, 1991). Hardiness was also found to be a moderator against the ill effects of combat exposure stress on Gulf War soldiers (Bartone, 1993; Bartone, 2000). Other groups where hardiness has been identified as a stress resilience resource include US Army casualty assistance workers (Bartone, Ursano, Wright, & Ingraham, 1989); peacekeeping soldiers (Bartone, 1996; Britt, Adler, & Bartone, 2001); Israeli soldiers in combat training (Florian, Mikulincer, & Taubman, 1995); Israeli officer candidates (Westman, 1990); former prisoners of war (Waysman, Schwarzwald, & Solomon, 2001); and Norwegian Navy cadets (Bartone, Johnsen, Eid, Brun, & Laberg, 2002). Studies have also found that military personnel who develop PTSD symptoms following exposure to combat stressors are significantly lower in hardiness, compared to those who don't get PTSD (Bartone, 1999; Escolas, Pitts, Safer, & Bartone, 2013). Moreover, there is evidence that highly hardy soldiers, not only adapt better during operational deployments, but also adjust more favorably in the months following their return home (Britt et al., 2001).

Relevant studies with military academy cadets found that hardiness predicts several important outcomes for these military officers in training. For example across multiple West Point classes, hardiness (commitment) predicts successful completion of a rigorous six-week Cadet Basic Training course (Bartone & Psotka, 2004). Hardiness-commitment also predicts retention throughout the four-year West Point experience and predicts successful graduation. Total hardiness and the hardiness facet of commitment were also found to predict military performance scores, which are the grades received by cadets for their performance of military and leadership tasks. Other studies found hardiness-commitment to be a stronger predictor of retention at West Point than the traditional weighted composite (Whole Candidate Score) of academic aptitude, leadership, and physical fitness indicators (Kelly, Matthews, & Bartone, 2005). In this same study, hardiness was second only to high school class rank in its relationship to military performance scores at the academy. A recent meta-analysis also found that hardiness is related to better health, as well as relevant performance outcomes (Eschleman et al., 2010).

Theoretical roots of hardiness

In order to better understand how leaders and organizations may influence hardiness, it is useful to delve a bit into some theoretical background. The hardiness concept derives theoretically from the work of existential philosophers and psychologists including Binswanger (1963), Frankl (1960), and Heidegger (1986), as discussed by Kobasa and Maddi (1977). It is a broad, generalized perspective that affects how one views oneself, others, work, and even the physical world (in existential terms, *umwelt*, the "around" or physical world; *mitwelt*, the "with" or social world; and *eigenwelt*, the world of the self). People high in hardiness see life as meaningful and worthwhile, even though it is sometimes painful and disappointing. The commitment facet of hardiness shares some features with Antonovsky's (1974) "sense of coherence," which also entails commitment and engagement with others and lends resistance to the ill effects of stress. Kobasa's understanding of commitment was also influenced by White's (1959) ideas on self-awareness and striving for competence. Hardiness-commitment thus includes a sense of internal balance and self-confidence, which aids the person in making realistic assessments of stressful and threatening situations.

The control facet of hardiness likewise derives from existential theory. According to Maddi, the core tendency in existential personality theory is the "striving for authentic being," which involves an honest and genuine acceptance of oneself and the world and a willingness to make choices and take responsibility for those choices (Maddi, 1989, pp. 128–130). The authentic person routinely chooses to engage with and act upon the world, rather than retreat into the safety of passive inaction. Highly hardy persons are authentic in this sense and see themselves as in control of their own destiny despite the reality of an uncertain and sometimes frightening future. The hardiness-control facet also shows some similarities to Rotter's concept of locus of control (Rotter, Seeman, & Liverant, 1962), and Lefcourt's (1973) on control beliefs. Kobasa's thinking on control was further influenced by multiple experimental studies showing that, when subjects are given control over aversive stimuli, the stress effects are substantially reduced, as compared to when the aversive stimuli are uncontrollable (Averill, 1973; Seligman, 1975).

The challenge hardiness element involves an appreciation for variety and change in the environment and a motivation to learn and grow by trying new things. The primary theoretical influences on challenge come from Fiske and Maddi's (1961) work on the importance of variety in experience, and Maddi's (1967) ideas on engagement versus alienation. Maddi (1967) used the term "ideal identity" to describe the person who lives a vigorous and proactive life, with an abiding sense of meaning and purpose, a belief in his own ability to influence things, and an appreciation for variety and change in experience. This is contrasted with the "existential neurotic," who shies away from change, seeking security and predictability in the environment. The influence of existential theorists is evident here as well, as the person high in hardiness is more courageous in choosing to look forward and take action in a world that is inherently unpredictable.

While it is often thought about as a personality variable, hardiness seems to be largely distinct from the "Big Five" personality dimensions of neuroticism, extraversion, openness, conscientiousness, and agreeableness (Costa & McCrae, 1992; Digman, 1990). For example in a study that examined hardiness alongside the Big Five dimensions, hardiness was a unique predictor of military cadet performance beyond the variance accounted for by the Big Five factors (Bartone, Eid, Johnsen, Laberg, & Snook, 2009). Also, it is important to remember that most psychological constructs are not fully trait-like or state-like but exist on a continuum between full trait and full state (Donnellan, Kenny, Trzesniewski, Lucas, & Conger, 2012; Hertzog & Nesselroade, 1987). So while hardiness is trait-like in that it is a relatively stable quality of individuals, it also shows state-like qualities and can increase or decrease depending upon social-environmental factors and training (Bartone & Hystad, 2010).

Theoretically, hardiness should also contribute to adaptability in several ways. Hardiness-commitment should help people to be more adaptable in novel and rapidly changing situations, since the high-commitment person tends to regard all experience as interesting and meaningful and also has a strong sense of self and confidence in his own abilities (Kobasa, 1979). People high in commitment are more actively engaged with the world, seeing their experience as generally meaningful and important. They are more interested in what's going on around them, more attentive, and thus more likely to perceive different aspects of situations, as well as to envision multiple possible response alternatives and adjust their behaviors accordingly. Hardiness-control should likewise lead to greater adaptability, since people high in control approach novel situations with the belief they can respond well and influence outcomes. Regardless of changing conditions, those with a strong sense of control tend to believe they can influence and manage events effectively. Studies have shown for example that hardiness increases the sense of self-efficacy which in turn can lead to more positive and healthy behaviors (Delahaija, Gaillard, & van Damb, 2010; Oman & Duncan, 1995). Finally, hardiness-challenge should also facilitate greater adaptability. By definition, challenge involves an abiding acceptance of change in life and a proclivity for variety. People high in challenge enjoy novelty and tend to see changing circumstances as an opportunity to learn. Thus, challenge should facilitate a person's adapting to changing conditions. Some confirmation for the influence of hardiness on adaptability comes from a longitudinal study of

US Army military academy cadets, which found that hardiness scores as freshman predicted later supervisor ratings of adaptability as junior officers (Bartone, Kelly & Matthews, 2013).

Leader influences on hardiness

How does hardiness operate to influence stress resilience? Although the underlying mechanisms are still not fully clear, a key feature of hardiness involves the meaning that people impute to events around them, as well as to their own actions. This involves the executive brain functions of memory, recognition, appraisal, and judgment. Again, highly hardy people tend to interpret their experiences as interesting and meaningful, amenable to control, and challenging, presenting opportunities to learn and grow. In organizations, this "meaning-making" process is something that can be influenced by leader actions and policies, as well as by peers.

Social identity theory suggests several possible avenues by which leaders may influence hardy or resilient thinking in groups. Social identity theory posits that social influence within groups occurs in large part due to self-categorization by individuals who see themselves as belonging to the group (Hogg, 1992; Turner, 1991). This identification with the group in turn makes the individual more susceptible to group norms of behaving and thinking. In many organizations the work is group-oriented and highly interdependent. The more interdependence among the workers, the more salient are the group categories for people, and the more likely that individuals will categorize themselves into their work groups (McGarty, 1999). Furthermore, categorization can also be imposed upon the worker by his/her superiors (Branscombe, Schmitt, & Harvey, 1999), providing another way that social identity with the group is increased.

Another important idea found in social identity theory is that group members tend to think and act similarly to those seen as prototypical within the group (Postmes, Haslam, & Swaab, 2005). To the extent leaders in organizations are admired and positively regarded, they would also come to represent the prototype that embodies the norms and values of the group. By the policies and priorities they establish, the directives they give, the advice and counsel they offer, and perhaps most importantly the example of their own actions, leaders may alter the manner in which their subordinates interpret and make sense of experiences. The narratives and stories told by more experienced members and leaders provide another avenue for influencing the thought and actions of individuals within the group (Weick & Roberts, 1993). Weick takes this even further, arguing that not only leaders but organizational policies and programs also exert powerful influence over how individuals within the organization "make sense of" or interpret their experiences, particularly work experiences (Weick, 1995; Weick & Roberts, 1993). There are many additional perspectives on how social processes can influence the creation of meaning by individuals. For example Janis (1982) used the term "groupthink" to describe how people in groups can come to premature closure on issues, with multiple individuals conforming to whatever is the dominant viewpoint in the group. In their classic work, Berger and Luckmann (1967) argue that "reality" or perceptions of individuals reflect "social constructions," an incorporation into the individual mind of social definitions of the world.

Data from multiple studies provide support for the notion that leaders high in hardiness can influence their subordinates to think and behave in more hardy or resilient ways. The idea that hardiness is linked to meaning making is supported by a study of US soldiers deployed to Bosnia (Britt et al., 2001), which found hardiness levels influenced perceptions that the deployment work was meaningful and was also associated with positive benefits. Several studies with West Point cadets have found that hardiness is associated with leader performance grades (Bartone, 1999; Bartone et al., 2009). Under the stressful environment of the West Point Military Academy, cadets high in hardiness perform more effectively as leaders, as indicated by external ratings of cadet peers and faculty supervisors. This is even more true for female cadets, where the correlation between hardiness and leader performance grades is stronger (Bartone & Snook, 2000). Leader performance ratings in part reflect how successful the leader's unit is in accomplishing group tasks, and these tasks are frequently highly stressful and conducted under time pressure. It appears then that highly hardy cadets are more effective leaders in part because they help the group to adapt and perform well under stressful conditions.

The positive influence of high-hardy leaders on their subordinates can also be understood as a form of contagion. Rajah and Arvey (2013) have discussed this as the "contagion of resilience" effect, which has also been identified in other leadership studies (Norman, Luthans, & Luthans, 2005). For example using an experimental design, Barsade (2002) showed that both positive and negative emotions and attitudes readily spread through working groups. A study done with Norwegian military cadets seems to support the notion that hardiness as displayed by leaders can be contagious. This study identified factors that help to increase cohesion in small units undergoing a stressful training exercise (Bartone et al., 2002). Results showed that hardiness and leadership influenced cohesion levels in a positive direction and that hardiness and leadership interacted to influence cohesion. This further suggests that what leaders do, and how they are perceived by their subordinates, can have a team-building or cohesion-enhancing effect on the unit. Subordinates appear to be modeling themselves after admired leaders, following the leader's example as to how to interpret and make sense of stressful events. In a study that looked specifically at leaders attempting to build hardiness in their subordinates, McNeese-Smith (1997) reported that nurse managers who actively encouraged hardiness qualities in their organizations had employees with higher job satisfaction, productivity, and organizational commitment and fewer stress-related problems. It thus appears that leaders can raise hardiness levels throughout their organizations through multiple avenues, both indirect (e.g. leading by example, positive contagion) and direct (e.g. training programs and policies to improve commitment, control and sense of challenge).

Relevant leadership theory

A number of leadership theories are also suggestive of pathways through which highly hardy leaders may exert positive influence on hardiness in their subordinates. Transformational leadership theory (Bass, 1998; Burns, 1978) for example indicates that "inspirational motivation" is necessary for stimulating extra effort and performance in work groups. According to Bass and Avolio (1994):

> [T]ransformational leaders behave in ways that motivate and inspire those around them by providing meaning and challenge to their followers' work. Team spirit is aroused. Enthusiasm and optimism are displayed. The leader gets followers involved in envisioning attractive future states. The leader clearly communicates expectations that followers want to meet and also demonstrates commitment to goals and the shared vision.
>
> *(p. 3)*

Thus, transformational leadership is believed to work in part through a process whereby leaders generate an increased sense of meaning, commitment, and challenge amongst their subordinates. Gal (1987) argues that transformational leaders exert their positive influence primarily by increasing commitment levels in their subordinates. In fact, some studies have found a direct positive relation between inspirational motivation and subordinate resilience and innovation (Elenkov, Judge, & Wright, 2005). The positive influence of transformational leaders appears then to be related to several important features of hardiness, including commitment and a strong sense of purpose or meaning.

The "path–goal" theory of leadership (House, 1971) also places heavy importance on leaders' building up commitment and motivation in their worker. This perspective focuses attention on how leaders influence the motivation of subordinates by identifying what are the important goals and then structuring situations so that subordinates experience personal rewards for attaining these goals (House, 1996). Leaders demonstrate *supportive, directive, participative,* or *achievement* leadership depending upon personal style and preference, as well as the demand requirements the situation (House & Mitchell, 1974). According to the theory, the achievement-oriented leader is able to tap into and even increase followers' motivation to overcome obstacles, and to apply this motivation in the pursuit of group goals. This is just how highly hardy individuals react to unexpected or highly stressful situations. They tend to interpret these situations as challenges and opportunities to learn and improve. At the opposite end of the continuum, the low-hardy, low-achievement person perceives changes more as threats or disruptions, things that should be avoided. Thus, the path-goal leadership theory suggests another pathway through which leaders who are high in hardiness (and achievement orientation) may influence the motivation, thinking, and behavior of subordinates in a positive direction.

A more recent perspective that builds on transformational leadership theory is known as "authentic leadership" (Avolio & Gardner, 2005). Authentic leaders are characterized by four principal qualities: (1) relational transparency, or honesty in relationships, including admitting mistakes; (2) internalized moral perspective, strives to do the right thing, including aligning actions with words; (3) balanced processing, being open to different perspectives and points of view; and (4) self-awareness, being aware of self and others, and how one's actions may impact on others. The authentic leader or person takes ownership over his own thoughts and actions and accepts responsibility for them. Authentic leaders are believed to exert influence in the workplace largely through positive role modeling (Avolio, Gardner, Walumbwa, Luthans, & May, 2004). This perspective is clearly related to existential ideas on authenticity; active engagement with the world, self, and others; and taking control and responsibility for one's own choices and actions (Maddi, 1989).

Recommendations for leaders: how to increase hardiness

Based on this discussion, several recommendations follow for steps that leaders can take to increase hardiness across their organizations. Perhaps most important, leaders should set a clear positive example, providing subordinates with a role model of the hardy approach to life and work, and how to cope with stressful experiences. Through their actions and reactions, leaders should demonstrate a strong sense of commitment, control, and challenge, responding to stressful circumstances with an attitude that says stress can be valuable and that stressful events always at least provide the opportunity to learn and grow. Subordinates observe their leaders closely and will tend to model themselves after the leader's example.

- Facilitate positive, group sense making of experience in how tasks and missions are planned, discussed, and executed and also in how mistakes, failures, and casualties are spoken about and interpreted. For example do we accept responsibility for mistakes and seek to learn from them, or do we blame others and avoid responsibility (and learning)? Leaders build resilience by setting high standards, while addressing shortfalls and failures as opportunities to learn and improve. While most of this "sense-making" influence occurs through normal day-to-day interactions and communications, it can also happen in the context of

361

more formal after-action reviews, or debriefings that focus attention on events as learning opportunities and create shared positive constructions of events and responses around events.

- Provide meaningful and challenging group tasks, while assuring that the work group has the needed resources to accomplish these tasks. When failures occur, look for what went wrong and seek to correct it, rather than punish or berate workers. What can be learned from the experience so that we do better next time? Capitalize on group success by providing recognition, awards, and opportunities to reflect on and magnify positive results, such as photographs, company newsletter stories, employee- or team-of-the-month awards, and so forth.
- Always communicate a high level of respect and commitment to subordinates and peers in the organization. This is done by means of respectful communications, as well as supportive actions and policies such as health promotion and personal/professional development opportunities. These help to foster a strong sense of commitment to the organization and its missions and goals.
- Build cohesion in teams and across the organization by providing opportunities for socializing and interacting both on the job and outside of work. At work, provide comfortable areas where workers can meet informally, such as lunch and break rooms. Sponsor offsite team activities such as sports competitions, community and charity benefit projects, and educational or professional development trips. These also build organizational cohesion and commitment.

Tables 29.1 to 29.3 present some further specific leader actions that can build hardiness commitment, control, and challenge, as well as actions that can diminish these hardiness tendencies. In considering these, it's important to remember that the hardiness facets overlap and interact with each other a great deal. Many leader actions and policies thus may influence more than one hardiness facet simultaneously.

Table 29.1 Leader actions to foster mental hardiness: commitment

How to build commitment	How to diminish commitment
✓ Support workers' attempts to give their own ideas; use their skills and talents to get tasks accomplished	✓ Do not accept feedback, input from subordinates
✓ Give recognition, awards, praise for accomplishments	✓ Criticize and denigrate worker initiative
✓ Plan teamwork-/cohesion-building activities	✓ Be self-absorbed and self-promoting
✓ Provide meaningful tasks where progress is visible	✓ Keep apart and take special privileges for yourself
✓ Support individual professional development (education, learning opportunities)	✓ Be unfair or stingy with rewards, benefits, recognition
✓ Be fair; do not show favoritism	✓ Avoid direct interactions with workers
✓ Be visible; spend time with workers	✓ Do not provide workers with information about the mission and goals of the organization, the purpose
✓ Share hardships with workers	✓ Show favoritism
✓ Provide information about what you are doing and why, purpose	✓ Show no interest in workers' individual aspirations

As the left side of Table 29.1 shows, hardy leaders build up commitment by taking steps to engage workers in the mission is significant ways, seeking their input and ideas. Worker initiative is welcomed and rewarded. Team- and cohesion-building activities also build enhanced commitment to the group and the shared values of the organization. Leaders who are fair and who do not take special privileges for themselves further inspire trust and a desire in workers to emulate them. When hardships occur, such as pay cuts or long hours to meet production deadlines, hardy leaders share those hardships evenly and do not exclude themselves. They are also visible and interact regularly with employees. Perhaps most important, they take the time and trouble to explain to workers what it is they are doing and why – what is our purpose? The more workers can understand the overall purpose and meaning behind their activities, the greater will be their sense of commitment. On the right side of Table 29.1 are listed some parallel actions that leaders should avoid, as they have the effect of diminishing worker commitment.

Leaders who wish to increase the sense of hardiness-control in their employees should see to it that the tasks assigned are within the capabilities and skill levels of those employees to perform. Tasks that are too easy can lead to boredom, while those that greatly exceed worker abilities can be overwhelming and anxiety-producing (Csikszentmihalyi, 1975). When work assignments match or slightly exceed a worker's abilities, he is likely to engage fully and realize success, enhancing the sense of control and mastery. Whether in training programs or production activities, it is best to follow a graduated schedule in which small, manageable tasks are presented first, followed by more demanding ones as skill and confidence develops. Research with security forces trainees has shown that this graduated approach, when coupled with supportive feedback from instructors, results in an increase in hardiness (Zach, Raviv, & Inbar, 2007). A contextual factor that is often overlooked involves resources. Workers should be provided the tools, supplies, and needed time to complete a job satisfactorily. No matter the worker's skills, if essential materials or time are unavailable, the job will not be done properly or to schedule. This can add to the worker's sense of powerlessness or inability to control outcomes. Related to this, the effective leader needs to make a realistic appraisal of what can be accomplished with the time, resources, and workforce available and set high but achievable standards of performance (see Table 29.2).

The challenge aspect of hardiness likewise can be encouraged across the organization by a number of leader actions and workplace policies. Number one is by leaders setting a good example to follow. The high-challenge person enjoys variety and sees change as a chance to learn and grow, rather than something to be feared and avoided. Leaders should demonstrate this approach in their own daily lives, especially at where they are most visible to employees – at

Table 29.2 Leader actions to foster mental hardiness: control

How to build control	How to diminish control
✓ Provide tasks that are challenging but within employees' capabilities to achieve	✓ Assign too many tasks for the time available
✓ Establish graduated training and production programs: crawl – walk – run	✓ Assign tasks that are too difficult for workers' skill levels
✓ Provide resources and time needed to accomplish goals	✓ Criticize and punish workers for failure
✓ Set achievable standards	✓ Do not listen to feedback
✓ Build on success; seek short-term wins to build on	✓ Do not provide needed resources

Paul T. Bartone

Table 29.3 Leader actions to foster mental hardiness: challenge

How to build challenge	How to diminish challenge
✓ Always emphasize value of change for learning	✓ Avoid change or surprise at all cost
✓ Incorporate surprises and variation into schedules	✓ Never take a risk
✓ Model enjoyment, fun in variety	✓ Restrict innovation and experimentation by requiring rules and permission for everything
✓ Be willing to change the plan to meet changing circumstances	✓ Never change the plan or schedule
✓ Treat failures as chance to learn	✓ Blame others for mistakes and failure
	✓ Denigrate others for failure

work. When confronted with some surprising event, even something negative, the highly hardy leader will show a calm demeanor and an interest in learning more and solving the problem if possible. He accepts responsibility for failures and avoids blaming others when things go wrong. Also, the highly hardy leader is willing to shift and change approaches in the face of changing conditions and is willing to experiment with new ideas. In addition to modeling these qualities, the leader also seeks to create a work environment that rewards and reinforces them across the workforce. This can be done for example via policies that permit flexible routines and schedule changes. Highly regimented schedules and inflexible systems tend to frustrate innovation and experimentation. While organizations differ in terms of the challenges and risks that must be managed, leaders should strive for a reasonable balance between standardization and flexibility (see Table 29.3). Even in high-risk organizations where the costs of failure can be very high, some flexibility in rules and routines can lead to increased resilience (Grote, Weichbrodt, Günter, Zala-Mezö, & Künzle, 2009).

Conclusion

Worker resilience has become a more important concern for leaders and organizations, in part because periods of rapid change and uncertainty can mean increased stress for workers and more stress-related problems. This has led many organizations to institute "quick-fix" training programs aimed at building individual "resiliency skills," most of which have met with limited success. As discussed by Cooper, Flint-Taylor, and Pearn (2013), this may be due to leaders failing to recognize and address contextual factors in the workplace that influence worker stress and resilience. This chapter has taken a close look at the concept of psychological hardiness, an individual trait as well as a state that contributes to stress resilience and adaptability across a range of circumstances and occupations. Understanding how the hardiness facets of commitment, control and challenge operate to make people more stress resilient, leaders can act to facilitate more positive and resilient thinking and behavior – increased hardiness – across the entire organization. Leaders exert positive influence on worker hardiness, adaptability and resilience by the examples they provide and by establishing policies that support high levels of engagement and commitment, personal control, and challenge perspectives in their employees.

Note

1 For an interesting account of the history of the resilience term, see A. McAsian, *The concept of resilience: Understanding its origins, meaning and utility*. Adelaide, Australia: Torrens Institute, 14 March 2010. Available at: http://torrensresilience.org/images/pdfs/resilience%20origins%20and%20utility.pdf.

References

Antonovsky, A. (1974). Conceptual and methodological problems in the study of resistance resources and stressful life events. In B. S. Dohrenwend & B. P. Dohrenwend (Eds.), *Stressful life events: Their nature and effects* (pp. 245–258). New York: Wiley.

Averill, J. R. (1973). Personal control over aversive stimuli and its relationship to stress. *Psychological Bulletin, 80*(4), 286–303.

Avolio, B. J., & Gardner, W. L. (2005). Authentic leadership development: Getting to the root of positive forms of leadership. *The Leadership Quarterly, 16*(3), 315–338.

Avolio, B. J., Gardner, W. L., Walumbwa, F. O., Luthans, F., & May, D. R. (2004). Unlocking the mask: A look at the process by which authentic leaders impact follower attitudes and behaviors. *The Leadership Quarterly, 15*(6), 801–823.

Barsade, S. G. (2002). The ripple effect: Emotional contagion and its Influence on group behavior. *Administrative Science Quarterly, 47*(4), 644–675.

Bartone, P. T. (1993, June). *Psychosocial predictors of soldier adjustment to combat stress.* Paper presented at the Third European Conference on Traumatic Stress, Bergen, Norway.

Bartone, P. T. (1996). *Stress and hardiness in US peacekeeping soldiers.* Paper presented at the Annual Convention of the American Psychological Association, Toronto, Ontario, Canada.

Bartone, P. T. (1999). Hardiness protects against war-related stress in army reserve forces. *Consulting Psychology Journal: Practice and Research, 51*(2), 72–82.

Bartone, P. T. (2000). Hardiness as a resiliency factor for United States forces in the Gulf War. In J. M. Violanti, D. Paton, & C. Dunning (Eds.), *Posttraumatic stress intervention: Challenges, issues, and perspectives* (pp. 115–133). Springfield, IL: C. Thomas.

Bartone, P. T., Eid, J., Johnsen, B. H., Laberg, J. C., & Snook, S. A. (2009). Big five personality factors, hardiness, and social judgment as predictors of leader performance. *Leadership & Organization Development Journal, 30*(6), 498–521.

Bartone, P. T., & Hystad, S. W. (2010). Increasing mental hardiness for stress resilience in operational settings. In P. T. Bartone, B. H. Johnsen, J. Eid, J. M. Violanti, & J. C. Laberg (Eds.), *Enhancing human performance in security operations: International and law enforcement perspective* (pp. 257–272). Springfield, IL: Charles C. Thomas.

Bartone, P. T., Johnsen, B. H., Eid, J., Brun, W., & Laberg, J. C. (2002). Factors influencing small-unit cohesion in Norwegian Navy officer cadets. *Military Psychology, 14*(1), 1–22.

Bartone, P. T., Kelly, D. R., & Matthews, M. D. (2013). Psychological hardiness predicts adaptability in military leaders: A prospective study. *International Journal of Selection & Assessment, 21*(2), 200–210.

Bartone, P. T., & Psotka, J. (2004, July). *Hardiness, transformational leadership and retention in a West Point officer cohort.* Presented at the Annual Convention of the American Psychological Association, Honolulu, Hawaii.

Bartone, P. T., Roland, R. R., Picano, J. J., & Williams, T. J. (2008). Psychological hardiness predicts success in US Army Special Forces candidates. *International Journal of Selection and Assessment, 16*(1), 78–81.

Bartone, P. T., & Snook, S. A. (2000, June). *Gender differences in predictors of leader performance over time.* Paper presented at the 12th Annual Convention of the American Psychological Society, Miami Beach, Florida.

Bartone, P. T., Ursano, R. J., Wright. K. M., & Ingraham, L. H. (1989). The impact of a military air disaster on the health of assistance workers: A prospective study. *Journal of Nervous and Mental Disease, 177*(6), 317–328.

Bass, B. M. (1998). *Transformational leadership: Industry, military, and educational impact.* Mahwah, NJ: Erlbaum Associates.

Bass, B. M., & Avolio, B. J. (1994). Introduction. In B. M. Bass & B. J. Avolio (Eds.), *Improving organizational effectiveness through transformational leadership* (pp. 1–9). Thousand Oaks, CA: Sage.

Ben-Dor, G. (2004). *The societal component of national resilience.* Israel: National Security Studies Center, Haifa University.

Berger, P. L., & Luckmann, T. (1967). *The social construction of reality.* Garden City NY: Doubleday.

Binswanger, L. (1963). *Being in the world: Selected papers of Ludwig Binswanger.* New York: Basic Books.

Branscombe, N. R., Schmitt, M. T., & Harvey, R. D. (1999). Perceiving pervasive discrimination among African Americans: Implications for group identification and well-being. *Journal of Personality and Social Psychology, 77*(1), 135–149.

Britt, T. W., Adler, A. B., & Bartone, P. T. (2001). Deriving benefits from stressful events: The role of engagement in meaningful work and hardiness. *Journal of Occupational Health Psychology, 6*(1), 53–63.

Bonanno, G. A. (2004). Loss, trauma and human resilience: Have we underestimated the human capacity to thrive after extremely aversive events? *American Psychologist, 59*(1), 20–28.

Burke, C. S., Pierce, L. G., & Salas, E. (2006). *Understanding adaptability: A prerequisite for effective performance within complex environments.* London: Emerald Group Publishing.

Burns, J. M. (1978). *Leadership.* New York: Harper & Row.

Carver, C. S. (1998). Resilience and thriving: Issues, models, and linkages. *Journal of Social Issues, 54*(2), 245–266.

Contrada, R. J. (1989). Type A behavior, personality hardiness, and cardiovascular responses to stress. *Journal of Personality and Social Psychology, 57*(5), 895–903.

Cooper, C., Flint-Taylor, J., & Pearn, M. (2013). *Building resilience for success.* New York: Palgrave Macmillan.

Costa, P. T., Jr., & McCrae, R. R. (1992). *The revised NEO Personality Inventory (NEO PI-R) and NEO Five-Factor Inventory (NEO-FFI) professional manual.* Odessa, FL: Psychological Assessment Resources, Inc.

Csikszentmihalyi, M. (1975). *Beyond boredom and anxiety.* San Francisco: Jossey-Bass.

Defense Science Board. (2011). *Enhancing adaptability of US Military Forces.* Washington, DC: Office of the Under Secretary of Defense for Acquisition, Technology, and Logistics. Retrieved from www.acq.osd.mil/dsb/reports/EnhancingAdaptabilityOfUSMilitaryForces.pdf

Delahaija, R., Gaillard, A. W. K., & van Damb, K. (2010). Hardiness and the response to stressful situations: Investigating mediating processes. *Personality and Individual Differences, 49*(5), 386–390.

Digman, J. M. (1990). Personality structure: Emergence of the five-factor model. *Annual Review of Psychology, 41*, 417–440.

Donnellan, M. B., Kenny, D. A., Trzesniewski, K. H., Lucas, R. E., & Conger, R. D. (2012). Using trait-state models to evaluate the longitudinal consistency of global self-esteem from adolescence to adulthood. *Journal of Research in Personality, 46*(6), 634–645.

Elenkov, D. S., Judge, W., & Wright, P. (2005). Strategic leadership and executive innovation influence: An international multi-cluster comparative study. *Strategic Management Journal, 26*(7), 665–682.

Eschleman, K. J., Bowling, N. A., & Alarcon, G. M. (2010). A meta-analytic examination of hardiness. *International Journal of Stress Management, 17*(4), 277–307.

Escolas, S. M., Pitts, B. L., Safer, M. A., & Bartone, P. T. (2013). The protective value of hardiness on military posttraumatic stress symptoms. *Military Psychology, 25*(2), 116–123.

Fiske, D. W., & Maddi, S. R. (Eds.). (1961). *Functions of varied experience.* Homewood, IL: Dorsey Press.

Florian, V., Mikulincer, M., & Taubman, O. (1995). Does hardiness contribute to mental health during a stressful real life situation? The role of appraisal and coping. *Journal of Personality and Social Psychology, 68*(4), 687–695.

Folke, C., Carpenter, S. R., Walker, B., Scheffer, M., Chapin, T., & Rockström, J. (2010). Resilience thinking: Integrating resilience, adaptability and transformability. *Ecology and Society, 15*(4), 20. [online] URL: www.ecologyandsociety.org/vol15/iss4/art20/

Frankl, V. (1960). *The doctor and the soul.* New York: Knopf.

Friborg, O., Hjemdal, O., Martinussen, M., & Rosenvinge, J. (2009). Empirical support for resilience as more than the counterpart and absence of vulnerability and symptoms of mental disorder. *Journal of Individual Differences, 30*(3), 138–151.

Gaillard, J. C. (2007). Resilience of traditional societies in facing natural hazards. *Disaster Prevention and Management: An International Journal, 16*(4), 522–544.

Gal, R. (1987). Military leadership for the 1990s: Commitment-derived leadership. In L. Atwater & R. Penn (Eds.), *Military leadership: Traditions and future trends* (pp. 53–59). Annapolis, MD: US Naval Academy.

Garmezy, N. (1971). Vulnerability research and the issue of primary prevention. *American Journal of Orthopsychiatry, 41*(1), 101–116.

Garmezy, N. (1974). The study of competence in children at risk for severe psychopathology. In E. J. Anthony & C. Koupernik (Eds.), *The child in his family: Vol. 3. Children at psychiatric risk* (pp. 77–97). New York: Wiley.

Gere, J. M., & Goodno, B. J. (2009). *Mechanics of materials* (7th ed.). Toronto: Cengage Learning.

Grote, G., Weichbrodt, J. C., Günter, H., Zala-Mezö, E., & Künzle, B. (2009). Coordination in high-risk organizations: The need for flexible routines. *Cognition, Technology & Work, 11*(1), 17–27.

Hackman, J. R. (2002). *Leading teams: Setting the stage for great performances.* Boston, MA: Harvard Business School Press.

Heidegger, M. (1986). *Being and time.* New York: Harper Collins Publishers.

Hertzog, C., & Nesselroade, J. R. (1987). Beyond autoregressive models: Some implications of the trait–state distinction for the structural modeling of developmental change. *Child Development, 58*(1), 93–109.

Hogg, M. A. (1992). *The social psychology of group cohesiveness: From attraction to social identity.* Hemel Hempstead, UK: Harvester Wheatsheaf.

Holmes, T. H., & Rahe, R. H. (1967). The social readjustment rating scale. *Journal of Psychosomatic Research, 11*(2), 213–218.

House, R. J. (1971). A path-goal theory of leader effectiveness. *Administrative Science Quarterly, 16,* 321–338.

House, R. J. (1996). Path-goal theory of leadership: Lessons, legacy, and a reformulated theory. *Leadership Quarterly, 7*(3), 323–352.

House, R. J., & Mitchell, T. R. (1974). Path-goal theory of leadership. *Journal of Contemporary Business, 3,* 81–97.

Ilgen, D. R., & Pulakos, E. D. (1999). Employee performance in today's organizations. In D. R. Ilgen & E. D. Pulakos (Eds.), *The changing nature of work performance: Implications for staffing, motivation and development* (pp. 1–20). San Francisco: Jossey-Bass.

Janis, I. (1982). *Groupthink* (2nd ed.). Boston: Houghton Mifflin.

Kelly, D. R., Matthews, M. D., & Bartone, P. T. (2005). *Hardiness predicts adaptation to a challenging military environment.* Paper presented at the International Applied Military Psychology Symposium, Washington, DC.

Kobasa, S. C. (1979). Stressful life events, personality and health: An inquiry into hardiness. *Journal of Personality and Social Psychology, 37*(1), 1–11.

Kobasa, S. C., & Maddi, S. R. (1977). Existential personality theory. In R. Corsini (Ed.), *Current personality theories* (pp. 243–276). Itasca, IL: Peacock.

Kobasa, S. C., Maddi, S. R., & Kahn, S. (1982). Hardiness and health: A prospective study. *Journal of Personality and Social Psychology, 42*(1), 168–177.

Layne, C. M., Warren, J. S., Watson, P. J., & Shalev, A. Y. (2007). Risk, vulnerability, resistance, and resilience: Toward an integrative conceptualization of posttraumatic adaptation. In M. J. Friedman, T. M. Keane, & P. A. Resick (Eds.), *Handbook of PTSD: Science and practice* (pp. 497–520). New York: Guilford.

Lefcourt, H. M. (1973). The function of the illusions of control and freedom. *American Psychologist, 28*(5), 417–425.

Luthar, S. S. (2006). Resilience in development: A synthesis of research across five decades. In D. J. Cohen & D. Cicchetti (Eds.), *Developmental psychopathology: Risk, disorder, and adaptation* (pp. 739–795). Hoboken, NJ: Wiley.

McGarty, C. (1999). *Categorization in social psychology.* London: Sage.

McNeese-Smith, D. K. (1997). The influence of manager behaviour on nurses' job satisfaction, productivity, and commitment. *Journal of Nursing Administration, 27*(9), 47–55.

Maddi, S. R. (1967). "The existential neurosis". *Journal of Abnormal Psychology, 72*(4), 311–325.

Maddi, S. R. (1989). *Personality theories: A comparative analysis.* Chicago, IL: Dorsey.

Maddi, S. R., & Kobasa, S. C. (1984). *The hardy executive.* Homewood, IL: Jones-Irwin.

Molinsky, A. (2007). Cross-cultural code-switching: The psychological challenges of adapting behavior in foreign cultural interactions. *Academy of Management Review, 32*(2), 622–640.

Mueller-Hanson, R. A., White, S., Dorsey, D. W., & Pulakos, E. D. (2005). *Training adaptable leaders: Lessons from research and practice* (ARI Research Report 1844). Arlington, VA: US Army Research Institute for the Behavioral and Social Sciences.

Norman, S. M., Luthans, B., & Luthans, K. (2005). The proposed contagion effect of hopeful leaders on the resiliency of employees and organizations. *Journal of Leadership and Organizational Studies, 12*(2), 55–64.

Oman, R. F., & Duncan, T. E. (1995). Women and exercise: An investigation of the roles of social support, self-efficacy, and hardiness. *Medicine, Exercise, Nutrition and Health, 4*(5), 306–315.

Postmes, T., Haslam, S. A., & Swaab, R. I. (2005). Social influence in small groups: An interactive model of social identity formation. *European Review of Social Psychology, 16*(1), 1–42.

Rajah, R., & Arvey, R. D. (2013). Helping group members develop resilience. In A. J. DuBrin (Ed.), *Handbook of research on crisis leadership in organizations* (pp. 149–176). Northampton, MA: Edward Elgar Publishing.

Roth, D. L., Wiebe, D. J., Fillingim, R. B., & Shay, K. A. (1989). Life events, fitness, hardiness, and health: A simultaneous analysis of proposed stress-resistance effects. *Journal of Personality and Social Psychology, 57*(1), 136–142.

Rotter, J. B., Seeman, M., & Liverant, S. (1962). Internal vs. external locus of control of reinforcement: A major variable in behavior theory. In N. F. Washburne (Ed.), *Decisions, values and groups* (pp. 473–516). London: Pergamon Press.

Rutter, M. (1979). "Protective factors in children's response to stress and disadvantage". In M. W. Kent & J. E. Rolf (Eds.), *Primary prevention of psychopathology: Vol. 3. Social competence in children* (pp. 49–74). Hanover, NH: University Press of New England.

Seligman, M. E. P. (1975). *Helplessness: On depression, development and death*. San Francisco: Freeman.

Selye, H. (1974). *Stress without distress*. Philadelphia, PA: J. B. Lippincott.

Selye, H. (1978). *The stress of life*. New York: McGraw-Hill.

Sroufe, L. A. (1997). Psychopathology as an outcome of development. *Development and Psychopathology, 9*(2), 251–268.

Thach, L., & Woodman, R. W. (1994). Organizational change and information technology: Managing on the edge of cyberspace. *Organizational Dynamics, 23*(1), 30–46.

Turner, J. C. (1991). *Social influence*. Milton Keynes, UK: Open University Press.

Waysman, M., Schwarzwald, J., & Solomon, Z. (2001). Hardiness: An examination of its relationship with positive and negative long term changes following trauma. *Journal of Traumatic Stress, 14*(3), 531–548.

Weick, K. E. (1995). *Sense making in organizations*. Thousand Oaks, CA: Sage.

Weick, K. E., & Roberts, K. H. (1993). Collective mind in organizations: Heedful interrelating on flight decks. *Administrative Science Quarterly, 38*(3), 357–381.

Weick, K. E., & Sutcliffe, K. M. (2001). *Managing the unexpected – Assuring high performance in an age of complexity*. San Francisco, CA, USA: Jossey-Bass.

Werner, E. E., Bierman, J. M., & French, F. E. (1971). *The children of Kauai*. Honolulu: University of Hawaii Press.

Werner, E. E., & Smith, R. S. (2001). *Journeys from childhood to midlife: Risk, resilience, and recovery*. Ithaca, NY: Cornell University Press.

Westman, M. (1990). The relationship between stress and performance: The moderating effect of hardiness. *Human Performance, 3*(3), 141–155.

White, R. W. (1959). Motivation reconsidered: The concept of competence. *Psychological Review, 66*(5), 297–333.

Wiebe, D. J. (1991). Hardiness and stress moderation: A test of proposed mechanisms. *Journal of Personality and Social Psychology, 60*(1), 89–99.

Witmer, T. A. P., & Culver, S. M. (2001). Trauma and resilience among Bosnian refugee families: A critical review of the literature. *Journal of Social Work Research, 2*(2), 173–187.

Zaccaro, S. J., & Banks, D. (2004). Leader visioning and adaptability: Bridging the gap between research and practice on developing the ability to manage change. *Human Resource Management, 43*(4), 367–380.

Zach, S., Raviv, S., & Inbar, R. (2007). The benefits of a graduated training program for security officers on physical performance in stressful situations. *International Journal of Stress Management, 14*(4), 350–369.

30

Promoting children's resilience by strengthening parenting practices in families under extreme stress

The Parent Management Training-Oregon model

Laura Supkoff Nerenberg and Abigail Gewirtz

Over the past sixty years, a strong body of empirical literature has emerged to facilitate an understanding of the correlates and predictors of children's resilience. We use the word 'resilience' to connote the capacity to function within the typical range (emotionally and behaviorally, in school, and in social settings) despite adverse life circumstances (Masten, 2001). What enables a child to survive and function competently despite living under conditions of extreme adversity? Several longitudinal studies have followed at-risk children over decades from childhood to adulthood in order to understand child and family factors that may be associated with resilience (Werner, 2013). The results of these studies indicate that there is a 'shortlist' of child and family factors that appear to be associated with resilience. Chief among the family factors is a child's access to an effective or competent parent or caregiver (Masten et al., 1999).

Parenting is generally seen as important for children's healthy development. Under high-risk conditions, parenting becomes even more crucial (Masten et al., 1999; Pettit, Bates, & Dodge, 1997), yet these same stressful conditions often threaten parenting. Family Stress Models document how stressors such as poverty, marital disruptions, and parental psychopathology increase parents' stress, in turn impairing their parenting capacities and increasing children's risk for emotional and behavioral problems (e.g. Conger et al., 2002). These models place parenting practices as *mediators* of the impact of stressful family contexts on children's adjustment. The detailed mechanisms through which impaired parenting detrimentally influences children's adjustment were proposed by Gerald Patterson (Patterson, 1982, 2005), whose Social Interaction Learning (SIL) model proposes that stressed parents engage in coercive interactions with their children that are reinforcing and eventually generalize across a child's social world. Coercive interactions are parent–child conflict bouts that are aversive, negatively reinforcing, and escalating. For example in a study of families with clinical levels of problems, conflict bouts occurred about once every sixteen minutes, and the observed relative rate of reinforcement was a significant predictor of out-of-home placement and police arrest two years later (Dishion & Patterson, 2006).

In efforts to reduce the risks to children's development conferred by coercive parent–child interactions, an intervention model was developed to reduce coercive parenting by teaching parents to implement effective, positive parenting practices. While coercive parenting contributes to behavioral disruptions in children and youth, positive parenting practices are protective for at-risk children; both positive and coercive parenting each predict unique variance in accounting for child outcome (Martinez & Forgatch, 2001). The five core effective parenting practices in the SIL model are teaching through encouragement, limit setting, monitoring and supervision, family problem solving, and positive involvement with children. The group of parenting interventions emerging from the SIL model is known as Parent Management Training-Oregon (PMTO). PMTO interventions – both treatment and prevention programs – have been tested in multiple clinical and prevention studies with diverse populations. In a foundational test of the SIL model, Forgatch developed and tested a PMTO group-based prevention program for divorcing and separating mothers (Forgatch & DeGarmo, 1999; Forgatch, Patterson, DeGarmo, & Beldavs, 2009). The program, Parenting Through Change (PTC), was tested in a randomized controlled trial with 238 mothers and their kindergarten to 3rd grade boys. At one year post-baseline, the program was associated with improvements in mothers' parenting, which in turn led to improvements in children's adaptive behavior, externalizing behavior, depression, and anxiety (Forgatch & DeGarmo, 1999). These improvements were sustained at three years post-baseline (DeGarmo, Patterson, & Forgatch, 2004; Forgatch, Beldavs, Patterson, & DeGarmo, 2008; Martinez & Forgatch, 2001). After *nine* years, the program demonstrated cascading improvements across the family system, evidenced in significant improvements to mothers' standard of living, as well as maintenance or improvements in children's adjustment across a variety of domains (Forgatch et al., 2009; Patterson, Forgatch, & DeGarmo, 2010).

A subsequent study, designed as a replication and extension of PTC is the Marriage and Parenting in Stepfamilies (MAPS) intervention targeting recently remarried families (Forgatch, DeGarmo, & Beldavs, 2005). Given the challenges in engaging this population, the program was administered with individual families, rather than in groups, with some involvement of children in addition to parents. Additionally, all families were offered a brief marital enhancement component (DeGarmo & Forgatch, 2007). As with PTC, MAPS results showed improvements in parenting practices, which mediated increases in child adjustment (Forgatch et al., 2005). Outcome data demonstrated that effects of the intervention extended beyond the impact on child behavior problems and included indirect effects on marital relationship processes through parenting practices (Bullard et al., 2010).

PMTO programs are offered as both prevention and treatment interventions in individual family and multifamily group modalities and in home, clinic, and community settings. The programs have been delivered and adapted for culture and context in the USA and Europe (Norway, Iceland, the Netherlands, and Denmark). For a comprehensive review of PMTO research, see Forgatch and Patterson (2010) and Forgatch, Patterson, and Gewirtz (2013).

While the PMTO model was originally developed for families facing a variety of normative stressors, until recently, less attention was paid to the most highly stressed families: those under threat from exposure to traumatic events including violence and its sequelae (dislocation, caregiving disruptions, etc.). Parenting practices are particularly susceptible to stress, and indeed, family exposure to traumatic events may be conceptualized as extreme examples of family stressors. We posit that parenting might especially suffer when parents are exposed to traumatic events and particularly when parents suffer from traumatic stress symptoms or post-traumatic stress disorder (PTSD) because of impairments in emotion regulation, and related challenges such as experiential avoidance that are inherent to PTSD (Brockman et al., 2016; Gewirtz & Davis, 2014).

In addition to posing threats to life and limb, traumatic events such as war and other types of violence engender chaos and disorganization, circumstances that themselves pose threats to parenting practices and children's adjustment (e.g. Patterson & Capaldi, 1991; Patterson & Dishion, 1988). Circumstances of war often mean that parents are preoccupied – seeking food and shelter for the family or fighting, for examples – with children left unmonitored, and potentially in danger, playing with unexploded landmines, being forced into combat, or exposed to other dangers (Gewirtz, Forgatch, & Wieling, 2008).

Earlier PMTO studies placed a heavier emphasis on the role of effective parenting practices in reducing or improving children's behavioral (i.e. externalizing) problems than on their emotional problems. However, an individual's (parent or child) response to traumatic circumstances often include anxiety and emotional distress (e.g. posttraumatic stress disorder). Little research has examined the role of effective parenting for children's emotional functioning in the aftermath of traumatic events (Gewirtz, DeGarmo, & Medhanie, 2011) and whether effective parenting interventions might improve children's emotional functioning in these circumstances (Sandler et al., 2003). Given these strong threats to children's development, teaching parents effective parenting practices may provide a strong buffer for children's adjustment in situations of extreme stress and trauma exposure (Gewirtz et al., 2008). For that reason, we have embarked on a research agenda to extend the PMTO model for families exposed to these kinds of stressors.

In this chapter, our focus is on extensions or adaptations of the PMTO model for the most highly stressed populations: those in which either parents or children are exposed to traumatic or extremely stressful events such as homelessness, war, family violence, and immigration due to economic or political instability. Common to all these stressors is a combination of external threats (e.g. violence) and family disruption or dislocation. Disruption or dislocation may occur as a result of violence, as, for example when an abused spouse flees the family home with her children. Conversely, violence may be a consequence of dislocation, as, for example when immigrants fleeing economic instability are violently preyed upon via human trafficking or when smuggled across borders. Thus, although we examine adaptations to PMTO for these populations separately, by category of stressor, in reality these stressors are often interconnected.

Adaptations of PMTO for highly stressed and traumatized families

Homelessness and supportive housing

Children and families experiencing homelessness and extreme poverty are at risk for a variety of negative psychosocial outcomes. These children have an increased likelihood of experiencing a broad range of risk factors including hunger, high family stress, low economic resources and social support, and exposure to domestic and neighborhood violence and may have parents who engage in substance abuse or have mental health problems (Bassuk, 1990; Bassuk, Weinreb,

Dawson, Perloff, & Buckner, 1997; Masten, Miliotis, Graham-Bermann, Ramirez, & Neemann, 1993). Disrupted family processes have also been associated with homelessness and housing instability, including less warmth and acceptance in parenting, less structured environments, and higher rates of child abuse (David, Gelberg, & Suchman, 2012; Gewirtz, Burkhart, Loehman, & Haukebo, 2014; Koblinsky, Morgan, & Anderson, 1997).

Given the pervasive risk factors that children may be exposed to within the context of homelessness and housing instability, coupled with possible impairments in parenting under these conditions, there have been efforts to utilize PMTO for this population via its delivery in supportive housing programs. Supportive housing (temporary or permanent housing with case management services) is an increasingly utilized solution for family homelessness and may serve as a platform for providing services to families that are often hard to reach (Gewirtz & August, 2008). PTC was integrated into an effectiveness trial of the Early Risers Skills for Success, a multicomponent prevention program conducted in a randomized controlled trial with sixteen supportive housing agencies (Gewirtz, 2007). Attendance and satisfaction were high and results demonstrated significant reductions in children's depression, improvements in parenting self-efficacy over time, and prediction of observed parenting practices by growth in self-efficacy (Gewirtz, DeGarmo, Lee, Morrell, & August, 2015; Perlman, Cowan, Gewirtz, Haskett, & Stokes, 2012).

PMTO offers a strengths-based approach that emphasizes the importance of building parent self-efficacy (Patterson, DeGarmo, & Forgatch, 2004; Patterson et al., 2010) and is implemented in a manner that considers the challenges regarding resources and buy-in of families and practitioners alike (Gewirtz, 2007). Many barriers remain regarding the use of parenting programs in shelter and housing settings, suggesting the continued importance of efforts to understand barriers to adoption and engagement (Perlman et al., 2012).

Immigration

Immigrant families often face a variety of contextual risks and stressors that may impact parenting practices and children's adjustment. These stressors may serve as the impetus for immigration, result from the move itself, or stem from adjustment to new living circumstances. Examples include poverty, difficulty finding work, threat of deportation, disconnection that can result from differing values and practices between parents and children, as well as the prejudice and marginalization that may be associated with minority group status (Baumann, Domenech Rodr guez, & Parra-Cardona, 2011; Domenech Rodr guez, Baumann, & Schwartz, 2011; Parra Cardona et al., 2009). Moreover, immigrant families often have less access to mental health services and supports, and there is often a lack of available culturally appropriate programming. Given these challenges, programs that support parenting are critical for promoting child and family well-being. One example of such programs is the adaptation and application of PMTO for Latino immigrants living in the United States.

Parra Cardona et al. (2009) engaged parents in order to address, not only the values and stressors of Latino immigrant parents, but also the many barriers to their participation in parenting groups, emphasizing the importance of understanding these topics in order to increase parents' perceptions of acceptability of programming and willingness to engage. Domenech Rodr guez et al. (2011) developed *Criando con Amor: Promoviendo Armon a y Superación* (CAPAS), an adaptation of PMTO for Spanish-speaking Latino parents, based on a theoretically driven cultural adaptation approach. Baumann et al. (2011) described the necessity of collaboration with community leaders and ethical considerations around decision-making processes when working with these under resourced and highly stressed families.

Parra Cardona et al. (2012) compared two culturally adapted versions of PMTO: CAPAS-Original, a translation of core components of original PMTO, and CAPAS-Enhanced, which included the addition of two culture-specific sessions based on themes raised by parents in focus groups conducted by Parra Cardona et al. (2009). Findings suggested that, though parents experienced high levels of satisfaction with both original and enhanced versions, they experienced significantly higher satisfaction in the enhanced version. Results, if replicated in a larger randomized control trial, highlight the importance of addressing the role of culture for engagement and satisfaction, which can be viewed as critical building blocks for successful program completion.

Parental deployment to war

The USA's involvement in two wars for over a decade has revealed psychosocial risks associated with a parent's deployment to war. Studies have demonstrated increased rates of psychosocial problems including distress, depression, anxiety, and conduct problems among children of deployed parents (Chandra, Martin, Hawkins, & Richardson, 2010; Flake, Davis, Johnson, & Middleton, 2009; Gewirtz, Erbes, Polusny, Forgatch, & DeGarmo, 2011). Deployment affects parents, too, both those who are sent to war, as well as those remaining behind (Gewirtz, Polusny, DeGarmo, Khaylis, & Erbes, 2010; Gibbs, Martin, Kupper, & Johnson, 2007; Samper, Taft, King, & King, 2004). Indeed, Flake et al. (2009) found parental stress to be the strongest predictor of child functioning during the period of deployment.

After Deployment: Adaptive Parenting Tools (ADAPT), a web-enhanced preventive intervention program based on PMTO principles, was developed to bolster parenting in military families in order to enhance children's adjustment postdeployment. This adaptation of the PMTO model is particularly appropriate given findings from a needs assessment with National Guard soldiers by Khaylis, Polusny, Erbes, Gewirtz, and Rath (2011) suggesting a greater preference for family-based interventions as compared to individual interventions. ADAPT was designed to address the needs of National Guard and Reserve military families in particular, given the increasing levels of deployment for these service members in recent years and their embeddedness in civilian communities with limited military support systems in place (Gewirtz, Pinna, Hanson, & Brockberg, 2014).

ADAPT included PMTO core components and modified the program using focus group and key informant interview data, as well as the empirical literature (Gewirtz et al., 2014). Adaptations addressed military culture and co-parenting after the separation of deployment. Adaptations particularly addressed the challenges to parenting associated with having spent time in a combat zone and combat stress symptoms, i.e. hypervigilance, reactivity, and experiential avoidance. Material focused on parents' emotion regulation and ability to respond to their children's emotions. Specific adaptations include mindfulness exercises and practice attending and responding to children's emotions using emotion coaching techniques. Web tools developed specifically for the ADAPT program were intended to increase access to content even if parents were not able to attend particular sessions.

Preliminary data suggest that ADAPT is both feasible and acceptable as a program for working with military families, and indicate benefits of the program at twelve months post-baseline on mothers' observed parenting and parenting self-efficacy as well as child outcomes (Gewirtz, DeGarmo, Zamir, & Forgatch, 2014; Gewirtz et al., 2014). Feasibility was measured by examination of weekly attendance, completion of practice assignments, and usage of online tools and acceptability by a feedback survey developed for PMTO interventions that was administered at the end of each ADAPT session.

Family exposure to war

Work in northern Uganda has sought to adapt PMTO for a population exposed to a lengthy war and the associated intergenerational transmission of violence, substance abuse, and harsh parenting (Wieling et al., 2015). Many of the parents in this region have experienced ongoing poverty, displacement, loss of family members, difficulty securing employment, responsibility for orphaned family members, worries about return of war, limited education (interrupted by war), and family violence and may have been exposed to abduction and murder.

Focus group data with parents informed the adaptation of the intervention. Due to constraints in regards to time and resources, only three of the five core PMTO components (positive reinforcement, setting limits, positive involvement) were included in the nine-session "Enhancing Family Connection" pilot, along with additional content on family and community legacies and understanding traumatic stress and related problems including substance abuse and domestic violence (Wieling et al., 2015). Other adaptations included translation, emphasis on visual presentation of concepts due to high illiteracy rates, and representation of time in a culturally understandable manner. Despite the many challenges associated with carrying out the initial pilot, preliminary findings suggested changes in positive parenting and decreases in aggressive parenting and family violence. Likewise, Wieling et al. (2015) reported that five-month follow-up interviews further suggesting the acceptability of the intervention.

Child maltreatment and family violence

Though few studies have directly measured the impact of family violence on parenting practices, there is reason to believe that literature regarding parenting in other stressful contexts would extend to this context. Indeed, Gewirtz et al. (2011) found that maternal parenting practices were associated with the trajectory of children's internalizing symptoms in over fourteen weeks following exposure to an incident of severe intimate partner violence. Following this, Gewirtz and Taylor (2009) piloted an adaptation of PTC with families who had been exposed to domestic violence and living in an emergency shelter. Initial findings suggested successful recruitment and retention, as well as high rates of participant satisfaction. Though these data are preliminary, and additional work will be needed to confirm the applicability and utility of PMTO-based programs within the context of domestic violence, this holds initial promise (Rains & Forgatch, 2012).

Efforts also have been made to integrate PMTO programming into statewide initiatives to address the needs of children exposed to family violence. The Kansas Intensive Permanency Project (KIPP), which represents a partnership between the University of Kansas School of Social Welfare, the Kansas Department of Children and Families, and four private providers of foster care in Kansas, selected PMTO as an intervention model to improve permanency for the highest-risk families with least likelihood for reunification (Akin et al., 2013; Bryson, Akin, Blase, McDonald, & Walker, 2014). Parental trauma was identified as a potential barrier for permanency, and developers subsequently collaborated with a PMTO researcher and implementer (second author) to add modifications addressing the needs of parents who have experienced trauma (Bryson et al., 2014). Other modifications included front-loading the intervention to move toward reunification, practicing parenting skills within the context of adult relationships due to limited contact with children during periods of out of home care, and facilitating the use of the opportunities for child contact during scheduled visits.

Many efforts were made to address challenges that arose regarding initial alliance with parents, particularly for parents who were experiencing strong negative emotions in response to the child welfare system, or those who had disengaged from the parenting role; the result was relatively high-parent participation in KIPP (Akin et al., 2013). Follow-up studies addressing the outcomes achieved by KIPP will be informative regarding the impact of PMTO on the process of reunification.

Conclusion

Across studies of development, parenting has been implicated as a key predictor of children's adjustment. Particularly important under conditions of stress, parenting practices can either buffer children or increase psychosocial risks to their development. Theory-driven efforts to improve parenting practices by teaching parents to implement effective, positive parenting practices have demonstrated efficacy and effectiveness in improving parenting practices, parent self-efficacy, and child functioning and show cascading effects over time. PMTO offers a powerful tool for changing parent and child trajectories supported by a strong research base of multiple clinical and prevention studies with diverse populations.

Given the utility of PMTO, coupled with the intense needs of families affected by traumatic and related stressors, it is critical that we engage in rigorous study of the adaptation and application of PMTO interventions for these families. Efforts described here to utilize and understand the impact of PMTO for families experiencing homelessness, immigration, exposure to war or parental deployment to war, child maltreatment, or family violence are promising steps towards addressing the needs of families under high stress. These adaptations described here represent initial efforts to address the feasibility and acceptability of adaptations alongside with effectiveness of adaptations, with an eye toward eventual widespread implementation.

The adaptations described here demonstrate good feasibility and acceptability, with some initial positive results regarding effectiveness. Given the extensive research base of PMTO, along with an established system for widespread implementation, we are optimistic that these adaptations will show positive outcomes as more data becomes available. Prioritizing how to engage families in programs has likely been critical to the success of the adaptations described here. Efforts undertaken by the research teams to engage community leaders and cultural liaisons, elicit parent input about contextual stressors and concerns, and carefully consider the constraints of the settings requires extensive investment of time and resources. However, such efforts have yielded knowledge about engagement that will continue to inform these and future efforts at adapting PMTO and other evidence-based parenting programs. Careful and continued efforts informed by work in the field of implementation science and cultural adaptation frameworks will create opportunities to understand the processes involved in expansion of the program.

Given the important role of parenting in buffering children in traumatic and highly stressful situations, promoting parenting practices that support children's development and adjustment to stress is a critical step towards investing in a positive future for our children. The science of promoting adaptive parenting practices has become significantly more sophisticated over the last few decades in regards to our knowledge about what works to positively impact parenting practices, and what maintains long lasting effects. Now, priorities must include focusing on the modifications, acceptability, uptake, and outcomes of effective programs, in order to reach increasingly diverse populations of parents and children.

References

Akin, B. A., Bryson, S. A., Testa, M. F., Blase, K. A., McDonald, T., & Melz, H. (2013). Usability testing, initial implementation, and formative evaluation of an evidence-based intervention: Lessons from a demonstration project to reduce long-term foster care. *Evaluation and Program Planning, 41,* 19–30.

Bassuk, E. L. (1990). Who are the homeless families? Characteristics of sheltered mothers and children. *Community Mental Health Journal, 26*(5), 425–434.

Bassuk, E. L., Weinreb, L. F., Dawson, R., Perloff, J. N., & Buckner, J. C. (1997). Determinants of behavior in homeless and low-income housed preschool children. *Pediatrics, 100*(1), 92–100.

Baumann, A., Domenech Rodriguez, M., & Parra-Cardona, J. R. (2011). Community-based applied research with Latino immigrant families: Informing practice and research according to ethical and social justice principles. *Family Process, 50*(2), 132–148.

Brockman, C., Snyder, J., Gewirtz, A., Gird, S. R., Quattlebaum, J., Schmidt, N., . . . DeGarmo, D. (2016). The relationship of military service members' deployment trauma exposure, PTSD symptoms and experiential avoidance to successful post-deployment family re-engagement. *Journal of Family Psychology, 30*(1), 52–62.

Bryson, S. A., Akin, B. A., Blase, K. A., McDonald, T., & Walker, S. (2014). Selecting an EBP to reduce long-term foster care: Lessons from a university–child welfare agency partnership. *Journal of Evidence-Based Social Work, 11*(1–2), 208–221.

Bullard, L., Wachlarowicz, M., DeLeeuw, J., Snyder, J., Low, S., Forgatch, M., & DeGarmo, D. (2010). Effects of the Oregon model of Parent Management Training (PMTO) on marital adjustment in new stepfamilies: A randomized trial. *Journal of Family Psychology, 24*(4), 485–496.

Chandra, A., Martin, L. T., Hawkins, S. A., & Richardson, A. (2010). The impact of parental deployment on child social and emotional functioning: Perspectives of school staff. *Journal of Adolescent Health, 46*(3), 218–223.

Conger, R. D., Wallace, L. E., Sun, Y., Simons, R. L., McLoyd, V. C., & Brody, G. H. (2002). Economic pressure in African American families: A replication and extension of the family stress model. *Developmental Psychology, 38*(2), 179–193.

David, D. H., Gelberg, L., & Suchman, N. E. (2012). Implications of homelessness for parenting young children: A preliminary review from a developmental attachment perspective. *Infant Mental Health Journal, 33*(1), 1–9.

DeGarmo, D. S., & Forgatch, M. S. (2007). Efficacy of parent training for stepfathers: From playful spectator and polite stranger to effective stepfathering. *Parenting, 7*(4), 331–355.

DeGarmo, D. S., Patterson, G. R., & Forgatch, M. S. (2004). How do outcomes in a specified parent training intervention maintain or wane over time? *Prevention Science, 5*(2), 73–89.

Dishion, T. J., & Patterson, G. R. (2006). The development and ecology of antisocial behavior. In D. Cicchetti & D. Cohen (Eds.), *Developmental psychopathology: Vol. 3. Risk, disorder, and adaptation* (Revised ed., pp. 503–541). New York: Wiley.

Domenech Rodriguez, M. M., Baumann, A. A., & Schwartz, A. L. (2011). Cultural adaptation of an evidence based intervention: From theory to practice in a Latino/a community context. *American Journal of Community Psychology, 47*(1–2), 170–186.

Flake, E. M., Davis, B. E., Johnson, P. L., & Middleton, L. S. (2009). The psychosocial effects of deployment on military children. *Journal of Developmental and Behavioral Pediatrics: JDBP, 30*(4), 271–278.

Forgatch, M. S., Beldavs, Z. G., Patterson, G. R., & DeGarmo, D. S. (2008). From coercion to positive parenting: Putting divorced mothers in charge of change. In M. Kerr, H. Stattin, & R. C. M. E. Engels (Eds.), *What can parents do?* (pp. 191–209). Chichester, UK: John Wiley & Sons, Ltd.

Forgatch, M. S., & DeGarmo, D. S. (1999). Parenting through change: An effective prevention program for single mothers. *Journal of Consulting and Clinical Psychology, 67*(5), 711–724.

Forgatch, M. S., DeGarmo, D. S., & Beldavs, Z. G. (2005). An efficacious theory-based intervention for stepfamilies. *Behavior Therapy, 36*(4), 357–365.

Forgatch, M. S., & Patterson, G. R. (2010). Parent management training – Oregon Model: An intervention for antisocial behavior in children and adolescents. In J. R. Weisz & A. E. Kazdin (Eds.), *Evidence-based psychotherapies for children and adolescents for children and adolescents* (2nd ed., pp. 180–199). New York: Guilford Press.

Forgatch, M. S., Patterson, G. R., DeGarmo, D. S., & Beldavs, Z. G. (2009). Testing the Oregon delinquency model with 9-year follow-up of the Oregon divorce study. *Development and Psychopathology, 21*(2), 637–660.

Forgatch, M. S., Patterson, G. R., & Gewirtz, A. H. (2013). Looking forward: The promise of widespread implementation of parent training programs. *Perspectives on Psychological Science, 8*(6), 682–694.

Gewirtz, A., Burkhart, K., Loehman, J., & Haukebo, B. (2014). Research on programs designed to support positive parenting. In M. E. Haskett, S. Perlman, & B. A. Cowan (Eds.), *Supporting families experiencing homelessness* (pp. 173–186). New York, NY: Springer New York.

Gewirtz, A., & Davis, L. (2014). Parenting practices and emotion regulation in National Guard and Reserve families: Early findings from the After Deployment Adaptive Parenting Tools/ADAPT study. In S. Mac-Dermid Wadsworth & D. S. Riggs (Eds.), *Military deployment and its consequences for families* (pp. 111–131). New York, NY: Springer New York.

Gewirtz, A., Forgatch, M., & Wieling, E. (2008). Parenting practices as potential mechanisms for child adjustment following mass trauma. *Journal of Marital and Family Therapy, 34*(2), 177–192.

Gewirtz, A., & Taylor, T. (2009). Participation of homeless and abused women in a parent training program: Science and practice converge in a battered women's shelter. In M. F. Hindsworth & T. B. Lang (Eds.), *Community participation and empowerment* (pp. 97–114). Hauppage, NY: Nova.

Gewirtz, A. H. (2007). Promoting children's mental health in family supportive housing: A community–university partnership for formerly homeless children and families. *The Journal of Primary Prevention, 28*(3–4), 359–374.

Gewirtz, A. H., & August, G. J. (2008). Incorporating multifaceted mental health prevention services in community sectors-of-care. *Clinical Child and Family Psychology Review, 11*(1–2), 1–11.

Gewirtz, A. H., DeGarmo, D. S., Lee, S., Morrell, N., & August, G. (2015). Two-year outcomes of the Early Risers prevention trial with formerly homeless families residing in supportive housing. *Journal of Family Psychology, 29*(2), 242–252.

Gewirtz, A. H., DeGarmo, D. S., & Medhanie, A. (2011). Effects of mother's parenting practices on child internalizing trajectories following partner violence. *Journal of Family Psychology, 25*(1), 29–38.

Gewirtz, A. H., DeGarmo, D. S., Zamir, O., & Forgatch, M. S. (2014, May). *Evaluation of After Deployment, Adaptive Parenting Tools: A web-enhanced parenting program for military families.* Washington, DC: Presented at the Society for Prevention Research.

Gewirtz, A. H., Erbes, C. R., Polusny, M. A., Forgatch, M. S., & DeGarmo, D. S. (2011). Helping military families through the deployment process: Strategies to support parenting. *Professional Psychology, Research and Practice, 42*(1), 56–62.

Gewirtz, A. H., Pinna, K. L. M., Hanson, S. K., & Brockberg, D. (2014). Promoting parenting to support reintegrating military families: After Deployment, Adaptive Parenting Tools. *Psychological Services, 11*(1), 31–40.

Gewirtz, A. H., Polusny, M. A., DeGarmo, D. S., Khaylis, A., & Erbes, C. R. (2010). Posttraumatic stress symptoms among National Guard soldiers deployed to Iraq: Associations with parenting behaviors and couple adjustment. *Journal of Consulting and Clinical Psychology, 78*(5), 599–610.

Gibbs, D. A., Martin, S. L., Kupper, L. L., & Johnson, R. E. (2007). Child maltreatment in enlisted soldiers' families during combat-related deployments. *JAMA, 298*(5), 528–535.

Khaylis, A., Polusny, M. A., Erbes, C. R., Gewirtz, A., & Rath, M. (2011). Posttraumatic stress, family adjustment, and treatment preferences among National Guard soldiers deployed to OEF/OIF. *Military Medicine, 176*(2), 126–131.

Koblinsky, S. A., Morgan, K. M., & Anderson, E. A. (1997). African-American homeless and low-income housed mothers: Comparison of parenting practices. *American Journal of Orthopsychiatry, 67*(1), 37–47.

Martinez, C. R., Jr., & Forgatch, M. S. (2001). Preventing problems with boys' noncompliance: Effects of a parent training intervention for divorcing mothers. *Journal of Consulting and Clinical Psychology, 69*(3), 416–428.

Masten, A. S. (2001). Ordinary magic. *American Psychologist, 56*(3), 227–238.

Masten, A. S., Hubbard, J. J., Gest, S. D., Tellegen, A., Garmezy, N., & Ramirez, M. (1999). Competence in the context of adversity: Pathways to resilience and maladaptation from childhood to late adolescence. *Development and Psychopathology, 11*(1), 143–169.

Masten, A. S., Miliotis, D., Graham-Bermann, S. A., Ramirez, M., & Neemann, J. (1993). Children in homeless families: Risks to mental health and development. *Journal of Consulting and Clinical Psychology, 61*(2), 335–343.

Parra Cardona, J. R., Domenech-Rodriguez, M., Forgatch, M., Sullivan, C., Bybee, D., Holtrop, K., . . . Bernal, G. (2012). Culturally adapting an evidence-based parenting intervention for Latino immigrants: The need to integrate fidelity and cultural relevance. *Family Process, 51*(1), 56–72.

Parra Cardona, J. R., Holtrop, K., Córdova, J. R., Escobar-Chew, A. R., Horsford, S., Tams, L., . . . Fitzgerald, Hiram E. (2009). "Queremos aprender": Latino immigrants' call to integrate cultural adaptation with best practice knowledge in a parenting intervention. *Family Process, 48*(2), 211–231.

Patterson, G. R. (1982). *Coercive family process* (Vol. 3). Eugene, OR: Castalia Publishing Company.

Patterson, G. R. (2005). The next generation of PMTO models. *The Behavior Therapist, 28*(2), 25–32.

Patterson, G. R., & Capaldi, D. (1991). Antisocial parents: Unskilled and vulnerable. In P. A. Cowan & M. Hetherington (Eds.), *Family transitions* (pp. 195–218). Hillsdale, NJ: Erlbaum.

Patterson, G. R., DeGarmo, D., & Forgatch, M. S. (2004). Systematic changes in families following prevention trials. *Journal of Abnormal Child Psychology, 32*(6), 621–633.

Patterson, G. R., & Dishion, T. J. (1988). Multilevel family process models: Traits, interactions, and relationships. In R. A. Hinde & J. Stevenson-Hinde (Eds.), *Relationships within families: Mutual influences* (pp. 283–310). Oxford: Clarendon Press.

Patterson, G. R., Forgatch, M. S., & DeGarmo, D. S. (2010). Cascading effects following intervention. *Development and Psychopathology, 22*(4), 949–970.

Perlman, S., Cowan, B., Gewirtz, A., Haskett, M., & Stokes, L. (2012). Promoting positive parenting in the context of homelessness. *American Journal of Orthopsychiatry, 82*(3), 402–412.

Pettit, G. S., Bates, J. E., & Dodge, K. A. (1997). Supportive parenting, ecological context, and children's adjustment: A seven-year longitudinal study. *Child Development, 68*(5), 908–923.

Rains, L. A., & Forgatch, M. S. (2012). Trauma-informed PMTO: An adaptation of the Oregon model of parent management training. *CW 360°: Trauma-Informed Child Welfare Practice, 24*, 24–25.

Samper, R. E., Taft, C. T., King, D. W., & King, L. A. (2004). Posttraumatic stress disorder symptoms and parenting satisfaction among a national sample of male Vietnam veterans. *Journal of Traumatic Stress, 17*(4), 311–315.

Sandler, I. N., Ayers, T. S., Wolchik, S. A., Tein, J. Y., Kwok, O. M., Haine, R. A., . . . Griffin, W. A. (2003). The family bereavement program: Efficacy evaluation of a theory-based prevention program for parentally bereaved children and adolescents. *Journal of Consulting and Clinical Psychology, 71*(3), 587–600.

Werner, E. E. (2013). What can we learn about resilience from large-scale longitudinal studies? In S. Goldstein & R. B. Brooks (Eds.), *Handbook of resilience in children* (2nd ed., pp. 87–102). New York: Springer.

Wieling, L., Mehus, C., Yyumbul, C., Möllerherm, J., Ertl, V., Laura A., . . . Catani, C. (2015). Preparing the field for feasibility testing of a parenting intervention for war-affected mothers in northern Uganda. *Family Process.* Ahead of publication. doi: 10.1111/famp.12189.

31

Family resilience

Positive psychology approach to healthy family functioning

Alena Slezackova and Irena Sobotkova

For decades, there has been a great deal of research interest in thorough understanding of the factors determining family functioning. Nowadays, many families are exposed to changing living conditions, increasing life demands, and persistent stresses. The concept of family resilience has become very important.

Family resilience is understood as a process that protects and recovers family functioning and involves positive transformation and growth. The family resilience framework is theoretically enshrined in the family systems approach. Knowledge about family resilience comes from family stress and coping research and also from the clinical work with families who are confronted with challenges. For decades, dysfunction and risk factors dominated the family resilience literature. Recently, new findings in the field of positive psychology have provided family resilience research with new knowledge and have revealed the factors behind well-functioning and flourishing families.

This chapter deals with positive factors and key processes of family resilience that contribute to optimal functioning of the family system and presents a research-informed overview of various approaches for understanding and strengthening family resilience. Practice applications, including strategies and interventions based on the positive psychology approach, are described. The application of principles following from resilience research in prevention and intervention strategies for promoting healthy family functioning through counselling and clinical interventions is also highlighted.

The development of the concept of family resilience

Resilience was initially studied at the level of an individual (Anthony & Cohler, 1987; Garmezy, 1976; Luthar, 2003; Masten, 2001; Rutter, 1987; Werner & Smith, 1982). However, it was found that, not only individuals, but entire families can sometimes cope with adverse situations more successfully than others. This inspired the emergence of family resilience research at the end of the twentieth century. Understanding of family resilience was enhanced through the synthesis of ecosystem and developmental approaches (Walsh, 2006). It became obvious that human development is embedded in the context of interconnected ecosystems (Bronfenbrenner, 1979, 1986) and that resilience varies over time and changing conditions.

Social scientists typically view the twenty-first century as a period in which increased demands are placed on families. In many countries, globalization, migration, and urbanization have resulted in an increased shift of population from rural to urban areas, precipitating change and requiring adaptation of the family system (Wissing, Potgieter, Guse, Khumalo, & Nel, 2014).

Most research on family resilience deals with family adaptation to stress. One of the first authors to address this issue was R. Hill, who studied the impact of World War II on the lives of American families (Hill, 1949). Subsequent researchers refined the concept of family resilience using information from extensive studies as well as clinical practice (Patterson, 2002a; Walsh, 2003). Many publications focused on family resilience in the context of grave illness or loss (e.g. McCubbin, Balling, Posin, Friedrich, & Bryne, 2002; McCubbin & Huang, 1989; McCubbin, Thompson, Thompson, & Futrell, 1999; Walsh & Anderson, 2014; Walsh & McGoldrick, 2004). Theories and models of family resilience were developed, together with measures capturing its various components (McCubbin, Thompson, & McCubbin, 1996). The importance of these studies lies especially (but not exclusively) in the fact that they provide a detailed analysis of protective and risk factors of family resilience. The concept of family resilience as a dynamic power was principally elaborated by J. Patterson (2002b).

A possible obstacle to a thorough understanding of family resilience is the discrepancy between the conceptualizations of family resiliency as a trait and family resilience as a process. Earlier research focused on individual characteristics associated with resiliency. Following this line, family resiliency is seen as the ability of a family to respond positively to an adverse event and become strengthened and more resourceful (Benzies & Mychasiuk, 2009; McCubbin, 1995; Simon, Murphy, & Smith, 2005). In contrast, the term family resilience refers to "coping and adaptational processes in the family as a functional unit" (Walsh, 2006, p. 15). Currently – in accordance with the systemic and developmental perspective – family resilience is more often defined as a process that protects the family under stress; helps to restore family functioning after crisis; and even allows the family to flourish, gain new competencies, and learn from the experience (DeHaan, Hawley, & Deal, 2013; Greeff, 2000; Karraker & Grochowski, 2006; Patterson, 2002b; Walsh, 2006, 2012).

Family resilience factors

As indicated earlier, researchers have arrived at the concept of family resilience as a process mainly through the investigation of protective and risk factors associated with family functioning. A complete understanding of family resilience requires the identification of all family resilience factors. McCubbin, McCubbin, Thompson, Han, and Allen (1997) proposed and empirically tested three types of factors that are generally accepted (e.g. Karraker & Grochowski, 2006): family protective factors, family recovery factors, and general resilience factors.

Family protective factors

Family protective factors include all competences, potentialities, and resources that help the family to withstand confrontations with challenges throughout the life cycle. Patterson (2002b, 2004) describes two types of protective factors as most important: family resilience resources and family coping strategies.

Family resilience resources represent all means – material and/or psychosocial – the family has to cope with a challenge. External resources of this kind include the socially supportive network, socioeconomic stability and cultural background of the family. Internal resources can either be found at a systemic level (cohesion, flexibility, shared spirituality, ordinary routines contributing to continuity and stability in family life, family traditions, clear communication, family hardiness, etc.) or an individual level (knowledge and skills of family members, mental and physical health, self-confidence, sense of humour, sense of meaningfulness, internal locus of control, etc.).

Internal family resilience resources were also described by authors studying healthy family functioning (see following). DeFrain and his colleagues (DeFrain & Asay, 2012; Olson & DeFrain, 2000; Stinnett & DeFrain, 1986) referred to internal family resilience resources as family strengths. They identified six family strengths in families across different cultures: commitment (loyalty, promoting each other's well-being); appreciation (expressing love, care for one another); positive communication; enjoyable time together; shared values and beliefs (including spirituality); and successful stress management. Family strengths can be considered as the foundation for growth and positive change in family functioning (Silberberg, 2001).

Family coping strategies include everything the family does to acquire and utilize resilience resources. They help to maintain family well-being and emotional stability of the family members. Family coping is one part of adjustment that represents the family's decisions and actions towards relieving stress (Bomar, 2004), such as seeking social or spiritual support, reframing a stressful situation, or taking an active approach to life challenges. Some coping strategies may be harmful (violence, aggression). Effective family coping means managing a stressful situation with no detrimental consequences for any family member (Boss, 2002). McCubbin et al. (1996) empirically identified several family coping strategies that are generally considered effective: strategies directed at the reduction of demands, the acquisition of additional resources, the ongoing management of tension, and the assessment of the situation and understanding its meaning to make it more manageable and acceptable.

Family recovery factors

These factors, in combination with family protective factors, play a key role in recovering family functioning after a crisis caused by severe hardships or disruptive life changes such as divorce, severe illness, untimely death, job loss, natural disaster, etc. These factors were studied especially in families with children with chronic conditions (Garwick, 2006; Karraker & Grochowski, 2006). A review of longitudinal findings revealed the following key family recovery factors (McCubbin et al., 1997):

- Family integration as the effort to keep the family together
- Family support from the community and friends
- Family recreation orientation
- Maintaining family life through organization and control
- Maintaining optimism and a sense of mastery

General resilience factors

These factors act protectively in adaptation to chronic stress, but also help in overcoming the crisis and restoring family functioning. On the basis of numerous studies, McCubbin et al. (1997) described ten general family resilience factors:

1 Family communication: transparent communication is essential for effective problem solving, communicating emotions, mutual support, etc.

2   Equality: especially gender equality.
3   Spirituality: helps to find meaning and purpose in difficult situations.
4   Flexibility: protects family stability in times of changes.
5   Truthfulness: for effective adaptation, the family needs sufficient amount of information.
6   Hope: successful adaptation requires realistic hope and positive outlook.
7   Family hardiness: commitment to values, ability to see difficulties as challenges, and a sense of control.
8   Family time and routines: customs and traditions (common meals, leisure activities, family celebrations, etc.) strengthen family continuity.
9   Social support: acts both as a protective and a recovery factor. Interactions with friends and relatives help the family to understand the meaning of the situation, identify effective coping strategies, and find courage to change.
10 Health: overall health and well-being of family members are key factors promoting resilience of the family system.

Interesting findings emerged from a meta-analysis by Benzies and Mychasiuk (2009) of more than forty studies on family resilience, which revealed twenty-four protective factors that foster resilience across three distinct but interactive levels: the individual, the family, and the community. The authors emphasize that these protective factors need to be always assessed in a context, as their functioning may be moderated or mediated by many influences. The individual protective factors that significantly contribute to family resilience include internal locus of control, emotion regulation, belief systems, self-efficacy, effective coping skills, high education and skills, health, temperament, and gender. The family protective factors that foster family resilience are family structure, intimate partner relationship stability, family cohesion, supportive parent–child interaction, stimulating environment, social support, family-of-origin influences, stable and adequate income, and adequate housing. Finally, community protective factors include involvement in the community, peer acceptance, supportive mentors, safe neighbourhoods, access to high-quality schools and child care, and access to high-quality health care.

Ayoub, Bartlett, and Swartz (2014) also stress the importance of positive community contexts that can promote resilience among families. External support systems that can assist in healthy family functioning include suitable education settings and parents' workplaces.

These protective factors offer a useful starting point for clinical interventions to support family resilience. Preventive interventions that help families develop strong protective factors were found to be more cost-effective than helping families already in crisis (Patterson, 2002b).

Key processes in family resilience

A crucial component of all conceptions of family resilience is adaptation. Chronologically, the classic theory of family resilience (McCubbin et al., 1996) distinguishes between "adjustment" and "adaptation". Adjustment is the immediate response of the family to stress, which draws particularly on protective factors. On the other hand, adaptation involves long-term processes activated in case of unsuccessful adjustment when the family finds itself in crisis. Thus, adaptation principally requires mobilization of family recovery factors (McCubbin et al., 1999).

Family resilience cannot be "measured" by ticking off a list of qualities, because, as Walsh (2003, 2006, 2012) points out, resilience is a complex process. Family resilience processes reflect how families balance strengths and resources (buffers) against challenges and demands. This balancing (family adjusting and adapting) is described by some authors as the process of family coping or achieving harmony (Karraker & Grochowski, 2006; Patterson, 2002b).

Walsh developed the Family Resilience Framework drawing on many years of research and clinical practice. She described key family resilience processes in three domains (Walsh, 2006): family belief system – making meaning of adversity, positive outlook, transcendence and spirituality; organizational patterns – flexibility, connectedness, and social and economic resources; and communication processes – clarity, open emotional expression, and collaborative problem solving.

In this condensed summarization of the model, some of the processes (positive outlook, flexibility, etc.) can be understood as qualities rather than processes. However, the author provides a detailed analysis of each concept separately within its nomological network (Walsh, 2006). For example connectedness incorporates mutual support, collaboration and commitment, respecting individual needs, differences and boundaries, seeking reconnection, reconciliation of wounded relationships, forgiving, and remembering. The word "processes" is therefore justifiable. On the other hand, it is obvious that these processes overlap partly with the list of protective, recovery or general resiliency factors. We therefore believe that the concepts need further specification both terminologically and semantically.

Positive psychology and resilience

Resilience is closely connected with other topics addressed by positive psychology, namely positive adaptation, effective coping in the face of adversity, and healthy functioning (Joseph, 2013; Joseph & Linley, 2008; Lemay & Ghazal, 2001; Masten, 2001; Seligman, 2011).

Positive psychology is the scientific study of optimal human functioning (Linley, Joseph, Harrington, & Wood, 2006), focusing on conditions and processes that contribute to the flourishing of people, groups, and institutions and understanding and facilitation of their positive developmental outcomes (Gable & Haidt, 2005; Seligman, 2011; Seligman & Csikszentmihalyi, 2000). Nowadays, positive psychology researchers pay increased attention to the role of family in promoting optimal development of the individual (Diener & Diener McGavran, 2008; Sirgy, 2012). Empirical studies show that family relationships along with other close interpersonal relationships are the key components of subjective happiness and meaningfulness in various cultural contexts (Delle Fave, Wissing, Brdar, Vella-Brodrick, & Freire, 2013; Diener & Seligman, 2002).

Healthy family functioning is in positive psychology represented especially by the term flourishing families. Flourishing can be understood as high levels of emotional, psychological, and social well-being, a combination of functioning effectively in life and feeling good about one's functioning (Keyes, 2002). Huppert and So (2011) identified ten features of flourishing combining hedonic and eudaimonic aspects of well-being: positive emotions, engagement, meaning, competence, emotional stability, resilience, optimism, vitality, self-esteem, and positive relationships. A similar perspective can be applied to evaluate flourishing in families. Hence, the study of flourishing families (healthy families, optimally functioning, etc.) is an important area of intersection between positive psychology and the psychology of resilience.

Healthy family functioning

Currently, family psychology places great emphasis on the research on healthy family functioning (Fisher, Giblin, & Regas, 1983; Greeff, 2000; Walsh, 2012). The shift from a deficit-centred to a strength-centred focus enables to see families as competent (Karraker & Grochowski, 2006). Ever more phenomena (homoparental families, single-parent families, etc.) are perceived as "normal" alternatives to traditional family structures and functioning (Walsh, 2012). The quality of family life does not depend so much on the family structure (e.g. two parents vs. one parent) as on what is going on within. Family functioning is determined mainly by family processes and relationships (Walsh, 2003, 2006). Healthy family functioning is also studied in connection with social, cultural, and other differences (Adams & Trost, 2005).

Compton and Hoffman (2012) point out that one of the first psychologists to address to issue of healthy family functioning was Alfred Adler (1930, with W. B. Wolfe; Adler, 1938), who argued that:

> Psychologically healthy families display four essential characteristics:
>
> 1   warmth and respect among family members,
> 2   democratic rather than authoritarian decision making,
> 3   emotional maturation and autonomy,
> 4   friendly and constructive relations with other families and the wider community.
>
> *(Compton & Hoffman, 2012, p. 118)*

Although there is still some terminological inconsistency in the area of family functioning today, the simple polarity "functional–non-functional" is no longer applicable. Instead, authors refer to healthy, well-functioning, harmonious, flourishing, or successful families. It is worth mentioning that healthy family is not problem-free family. All families face problems, but healthy families solve them efficiently.

Since 1980s, some authors (McCubbin et al., 1997; McCubbin et al., 1996; McCubbin, Thompson, Thompson, & Fromer, 1998; Olson et al., 1989) have conceptualized healthy family functioning through the process of family adaptation to stress. Healthy (or effective) family functioning is now generally understood as the ability of the family to cope with difficult or stressful life events and to adjust to change (Olson & Gorell, 2003; Ryan, Epstein, Keitner, Miller, & Bishop, 2005; Shapiro, 1983). Much research in this area regards families dealing with serious health issues (Edwards & Clarke, 2004; Pinsof & Lebow, 2005). Facing the burdens of a chronic illness or disability, the "healthiest" families are able to utilize their experience to improve their quality of life (Rolland, 2012). The family resilience framework draws together the findings of research aimed at identifying core elements of healthy family functioning (Walsh, 2006).

While family functioning is an extremely complex phenomenon, in generally involves three components: cohesion, adaptability (flexibility), and communication. Cohesion and adaptability are essential for organizing family resources to meet life changes (Walsh, 2006). At balanced (not extremely low or high) levels, both cohesion and adaptability are positively related to healthy family functioning (Olson, 2011). Communication is the most sensitive indicator of quality of family functioning and a key determinant of family atmosphere. Whereas direct and open communication acts as a protective factor, non-transparent, or impaired communication can amplify the impact of risks (Galvin, Braithwaite, & Bylund, 2015).

As each family is a unique system there is no single "correct" model of healthy family functioning. However, certain aspects of family life seem to be generally beneficial. Some authors describe them as positive family traits (Fisher et al., 1983; Greeff, 2000); others talk about family strengths (Stinnett & DeFrain, 1989). The most commonly reported characteristics of healthy families are cohesion in balance with personal autonomy, adaptability, coping with changes and loss, effective communication, collaborative problem solving, clear and flexible family structure, subjective satisfaction of members, partner sexual harmony, identical or compatible attitudes and values, compliance of leisure activities, and quality social support. Other cited factors include family pride, sense of humour, and fidelity as a conscious personal choice.

Becvar (2007) argues that flourishing families can be distinguished by specific dimensions that go far beyond the absence of pathology or dysfunction. Resilience, the capacity to respond effectively to crisis and to grow from the experience, is one of the most significant characteristics of such families. Other indicators include, for example respect of the maturation processes of each member, success in achieving personal goals, a healthy balance between openness and closeness, spending time together, enjoying each other and having fun together, and others. Baumrind (1991) pointed out that family flourishing is also significantly influenced by parenting styles. The healthiest parenting style, considered as most effective in building flourishing families, is the authoritative style, characterized by a high level of communication, high demands, high warmth and support, and reasonable rules.

Lopez (2009) mentions further characteristics of strong, happy families: predictable ways to deal with conflict that do not threaten the family, ritual formation, keeping traditions and ceremonies, availability of private space, but also making time and place to get together and share a quality time, etc.

While certain family characteristics, especially a loving marital relationship, clear rules and boundaries, negotiations among members in decision making, support for individuality, and warm parenting style are associated with family flourishing, social class or economic status do not necessarily play an important role (Wissing et al., 2014). Findings show that even very poor families can be resilient and flourishing although poverty adds extra stress and burden. The increasing body of research on optimally functioning and flourishing families that highlights healthy processes and communication patterns may be inspiring for practical interventions to strengthen family resilience (Rich, 2003).

Strategies and positive psychology interventions for building family resilience

Information on resilience factors and basic principles of healthy family functioning facilitates effective work with families in preventive programmes as well as therapy and counselling. Yates and Masten (2004, p. 530) state that "resilience research has the potential to inform and foster practical applications of positive psychology by highlighting how interventions may operate as protective processes in development".

There are currently many interventions and strategies to help families flourish through the facilitation of resilience (Becvar, 2007, 2013). Strategies for enhancing family resilience are based on the assumption that resilient responses to life challenges can be taught and learned (Black & Lobo, 2008).

Within the family resilience framework, family practitioners help the family members to improve their ability to communicate in a supportive and honest way, discuss problems together and share feelings (McCubbin & Huang, 1989). Black and Lobo (2008) point out the importance of family warmth despite financial problems, which may be serious in families experiencing chronic health conditions. Other typical recommendations for strengthening family resilience include forgiveness to avoid the emotional burdens, fostering of emotional closeness, adequate autonomy of family members, clearly formulated rules adopted by all members, deep commitment to family values, keeping up family traditions, and focusing on the present (DeFrain & Asay, 2012; Hawley, 2000; McCubbin et al., 1997; Simon, Murphy, & Smith, 2005; Walsh, 2006).

Focusing on strengths for promoting individual growth and optimal family functioning is fundamental also to the positive psychology approach. Positive psychology offers a whole range of tried-and-tested techniques and interventions (Linley & Joseph, 2004; Parks & Schueller,

2014), many of which can be used for promoting optimal functioning in families. However, as Rashid (2009) points out, positive interventions do not imply that other psychotherapies are negative. A central premise of positive interventions is that one cannot understand positives without comprehending negatives. The therapists encourage clients to identify and use their strengths to understand and cope with their weaknesses (Rashid, 2009). The treatment methods and intentional activities are aimed at cultivating positive feelings, positive behaviours, or positive cognitions, which enhance well-being (Seligman, Steen, Park, & Peterson, 2005). Out of the set of evidence-based strategies and interventions in positive psychotherapy, many can be used in couple and family therapy (Kauffman & Silberman, 2009).

Some of the positive psychological interventions (PPIs) are more thoroughly established than others and have an extensive empirical basis. Some of the most frequently used and verified PPIs include gratitude interventions, nurturing the capacity to savour, interventions for promoting forgiveness, empathy-related interventions, promoting meaning and purpose in life, and character strengths interventions. Emerging areas of interventions regard the constructs of creativity, flow, humour, patience, courage, and wisdom (Parks & Schueller, 2014).

A useful framework for working with children and families through promoting strengths and building capacity within individuals and the family system, rather than focusing on the resolutions of problems or remediation of deficiencies, is represented by Family-Centred Positive Psychology (FCPP; Sheridan, Warnes, Cowan, Schemm, & Clarke, 2004). The FCPP approach to family-based services is based on the premise that child and family well-being will be enhanced if all members participate in identifying their needs, establishing partnerships and social support, and developing new skills and competencies, rather than receiving services from professionals.

Family-centred positive psychology is rooted in the assumption that families have strengths and abilities, but systemic or environmental conditions may present difficulties in accessing, using and developing those strengths. Based on the principles of FCPP, family-centred services provide a framework for service delivery, which strives to create a context in which unique and relevant family dynamics can be empowered (Sheridan & Burt, 2009). Sheridan, Sjuts, and Coutts (2006, p. 151) suggest

> four operating principles to define family-centred approaches: 1) intervention efforts are based on families' needs; 2) existing strengths and capabilities of families are used to mobilize resources and promote abilities; 3) social networks are used as a source of support; and 4) specific forms of helping behaviours on the part of professionals promote acquisition of family competencies.

Conoley and Conoley (2009), who use a Positive Family Therapy (PFT) approach, provide a summary of therapeutic techniques that are consistent with a positive family system approach and specify which have evidence or best practice support. PFT combines positive psychology and system theory to derive an approach that builds upon the strengths of a family to enhance the growth of each individual member. The techniques are meant to clarify the family's values and goals and build upon their strengths as well as facilitate positive affect. The family moves toward each member's goal, so that the focus is on what the individuals want to happen instead of what they want stopped. Approach goals increase positive emotions as well as relationship satisfaction and closeness (Gable & Impett, 2012).

PFT (Conoley, Conoley, & Pontrelli, 2014) defines family strengths as helpful personal assets or qualities, which can include abilities (social skills, coping, creativity, humour, etc.); accomplishments (physical health, knowledge, job, income, and friendship); attitudes and emotions (love, hope, curiosity, and prosocial beliefs); and virtues (honesty, kindness, and courage). Focusing on strengths can lead to relationship enhancement, creating positive emotions, identifying goals and creating tools for their accomplishment, and modelling positive patterns of behaviour.

Specific PFT techniques include, for example capitalization (communicating good news and positive personal events to other family members, which can increase both individual and family well-being), success finding (uncovering a past goal's accomplishment), the miracle question (asking family members to visualize a miraculous disappearance of the existing problems and discussing what happens in the family system), identification of virtuous behaviour, expressing acknowledgement and gratitude, etc. (Conoley et al., 2014). Some of the PFT techniques draw on the Broaden and Build Theory of positive emotions (Cohn, Fredrickson, Brown, Mikels, & Conway, 2009; Fredrickson, 2001, 2008), which suggests that cultivating positive emotions can help build resilience to stressful events. Being able to generate positive emotions in the family through playing games and laughing together, doing physical activities, or enjoying quality-time any other way all contribute to family resilience. The aim of the family therapy using positive psychology approach based on evidence-based components is to reach optimal level of family functioning: "Successful PFT ends with everyone in the family feeling happier" (Conoley & Conoley, 2009, p. 26).

Positive psychology views the promotion of satisfaction in the family as a buffer against stress as well as an important factor of family resilience, which in turn produces many beneficial outcomes. As follows from a concept analysis of studies published on the topic of family resilience, there seem to be five basic consequences of family resilience: 1) acceptance of the situation, 2) changed life perspectives, 3) enhanced relationship qualities, 4) reinforced resilient properties, and 5) improved health-related outcomes (Oh & Chang, 2014).

All of this information suggests that happy individuals contribute to optimal family functioning, and vice versa. The mentioned practical interventions can be further developed to strengthen family resilience and help families to flourish.

Conclusion

Orientation in family resilience literature is sometimes difficult due to a considerable semantic overlap between various terms and concepts (e.g. healthy families and flourishing families, family strengths, and internal family resilience resources). We therefore find it necessary that further research continues to produce clearer definitions and operationalizations. Similarly, longitudinal studies would be helpful in shedding more light on family resilience processes and conditions of healthy family functioning. Finally, promoting closer dialogue and research collaboration between family practitioners and positive psychologists would also help the field to thrive.

Family resilience can be strengthen and nurtured – that is the main message of the present chapter. The first step of practical assistance is careful assessment of what the family needs and what are its resources. The most helpful approach in family-centred services is a strength-based approach. The concept of family resilience is universal because it takes into account the wide socio-cultural context of families and their changes in time. Strengthening family resilience leads both to the enhancement of family functioning and to a higher well-being of individual family members. People higher in well-being tend to form healthier, more resilient, and more successful families, which in turn serve as an important factor of optimal functioning of both the individual and the community.

References

Adams, B. N., & Trost, J. (2005). *Handbook of world families*. Thousand Oaks: SAGE Publications.
Adler, A. (1938). *Social interest: A challenge to mankind*. Oxford: Faber & Faber.

Adler, A., & Wolfe, W. B. (1930). *The pattern of life.* New York: Cosmopolitan Book Corporation.

Anthony, E. J., & Cohler, B. J. (1987). *The invulnerable child.* New York: Guilford.

Ayoub, C. C., Bartlett, J. D., & Swartz, M. I. (2014). Parenting and early intervention: The impact on children's social and emotional skill development. In S. H. Landry & C. L. Cooper (Eds.), *Wellbeing: A complete reference guide: Vol. I: Wellbeing in children and families* (pp. 179–200). Oxford: Wiley-Blackwell.

Baumrind, D. (1991). The influence of parenting style on adolescent competence and substance use. *Journal of Early Adolescence, 11*(1), 56–95.

Becvar, D. S. (2007). *Families that flourish: Facilitating resilience in clinical practice.* New York: W. W. Norton & Company.

Becvar, D. S. (2013). *Handbook of family resilience.* New York: Springer.

Benzies, K., & Mychasiuk, R. (2009). Fostering family resiliency: A review of the key protective factors. *Child and Family Social Work, 14*(1), 103–114.

Black, K., & Lobo, M. (2008). A conceptual review of family resilience factors. *Journal of Family Nursing, 14*(1), 33–55.

Bomar, P. J. (2004). *Promoting health in families: Applying family research and theory to nursing practice* (3rd ed.). Philadelphia: Saunders.

Boss, P. G. (2002). *Family stress management: A contextual approach* (2nd ed.). Thousand Oaks: SAGE Publications.

Bronfenbrenner, U. (1979). *The ecology of human development.* Cambridge: Harvard University Press.

Bronfenbrenner, U. (1986). Ecology of the family as a context for human development: Research perspectives. *Developmental Psychology, 22*(6), 723–742.

Cohn, M. A., Fredrickson, B. L., Brown, S. L., Mikels, J. A., & Conway, A. M. (2009). Happiness unpacked: Positive emotions increase life satisfaction by building resilience. *Emotion, 9*(3), 361–368.

Compton, W. C., & Hoffman, E. (2012). *Positive psychology: The science of happiness and flourishing.* Wadsworth: Cengage Learning.

Conoley, C. W., & Conoley, J. C. (2009). *Positive psychology and family therapy: Creative techniques and practical tools for guiding change and enhancing growth.* Hoboken: John Wiley & Sons.

Conoley, C. W., Conoley, J. C., & Pontrelli, M. E. (2014). Positive family therapy interventions. In A. C. Parks & S. M. Schueller (Eds.), *The Wiley-Blackwell handbook of positive psychological interventions* (pp. 233–245). Oxford: Wiley-Blackwell.

DeFrain, J., & Asay, S. M. (Eds.). (2012). *Strong families around the world: Strengths-based research and perspectives.* New York: Routledge.

DeHaan, L. G., Hawley, D. R., & Deal, J. E. (2013). Operationalizing family resilience as a process: Proposed methodological strategies. In D. S. Becvar (Ed.), *Handbook of family resilience* (pp. 17–29). New York: Springer.

Delle Fave, A., Wissing, M. P., Brdar, I., Vella-Brodrick, D., & Freire, T. (2013). Perceived meaning and goals in adulthood: Their roots and relation with happiness. In A. Waterman (Ed.), *The best within us: Positive psychology perspectives on eudaimonia* (pp. 227–247). Washington, DC: American Psychological Association.

Diener, M., & Diener McGavran, M. B. (2008). What makes people happy? A developmental approach to the literature on family relationships and well-being. In M. Eid & R. J. Larsen (Eds.), *The science of subjective well-being* (pp. 347–375). New York: Guilford Press.

Diener, E., & Seligman, M. E. P. (2002). Very happy people. *Psychological Science, 13*(4), 81–84.

Edwards, B., & Clarke, V. (2004). The psychological impact of a cancer diagnosis on families: The influence of family functioning and patients' illness characteristics on depression and anxiety. *Psycho-Oncology, 13*(8), 562–576.

Fisher, B. L., Giblin, P. R., & Regas, S. J. (1983). Healthy family functioning/goals of family therapy II: An assessment of what therapists say and do. *American Journal of Family Therapy, 11*(4), 41–54.

Fredrickson, B. L. (2001). The role of positive emotions in positive psychology: The broaden-and-build theory of positive emotions. *American Psychologist, 56*(3), 218–226.

Fredrickson, B. L. (2008). Promoting positive affect. In M. Eid & R. J. Larsen (Eds.), *The science of subjective well-being* (pp. 449–468). New York: Guilford Press.

Gable, S. L., & Haidt, J. (2005). What (and why) is positive psychology? *Review of General Psychology, 9*(2), 103–110.

Gable, S. L., & Impett, E. A. (2012). Approach and avoidance motives and close relationships. *Social and Personality Psychology Compass, 6*(1), 95–108.

Family resilience

Galvin, K. M., Braithwaite, D. O., & Bylund, C. L. (2015). *Family communication: Cohesion and change* (9th ed.). New York: Pearson.

Garmezy, N. (1976). *Vulnerable and invulnerable children: Theory, research, and intervention.* Washington: Journal Supplement Abstract Service of the American Psychological Association.

Garwick, A. (2006). Promoting resilience in families of children with chronic conditions. In M. W. Karraker & J. R. Grochowski (Eds.), *Families with futures: A survey of family studies for the 21st century* (p. 76). Mahwah: Lawrence Erlbaum Associates.

Greeff, A. P. (2000). Characteristics of families that function well. *Journal of Family Issues, 21*(8), 948–962.

Hawley, D. R. (2000). Clinical implications of family resilience. *The American Journal of Family Therapy, 28*(2), 101–116.

Hill, R. (1949). *Families under stress: Adjustment to the crises of war separation and reunion.* New York: Harper.

Huppert, F. A., & So, T. C. (2011). Flourishing across Europe: Application of a new conceptual framework for defining well-being. *Social Indicators Research, 10*(3), 837–861.

Joseph, S. (2013). *What doesn't kill us: The new psychology of posttraumatic growth.* New York: Basic Books.

Joseph, S., & Linley, P. A. (2008). *Trauma, recovery and growth: Positive psychological perspectives on posttraumatic stress.* Hoboken: John Wiley & Sons.

Karraker, M. W., & Grochowski, J. R. (2006). *Families with futures: A survey of family studies for the 21st century.* Mahwah: Lawrence Erlbaum Associates.

Kauffman, C., & Silberman, J. (2009). Finding and fostering the positive in relationships: Positive interventions in couples therapy. *Journal of Clinical Psychology: In Session, 65*(5), 520–531.

Keyes, C. L. M. (2002). The mental health continuum: From languishing to flourishing in life. *Journal of Health and Social Research, 43*(2), 207–222.

Lemay, R., & Ghazal, H. (2001). Resilience and positive psychology: Finding hope. *Child & Family, 5*(1), 10–21.

Linley, P. A., & Joseph, S. (2004). *Positive psychology in practice.* Hoboken: John Wiley & Sons.

Linley, P. A., Joseph, S., Harrington, S., & Wood, A. M. (2006). Positive psychology: Past, present, and (possible) future. *The Journal of Positive Psychology, 1*(1), 3–16.

Lopez, S. J. (2009). The future of positive psychology: Pursuing three big goals. In C. R. Snyder & S. Lopez (Eds.), *Oxford handbook of positive psychology* (pp. 689–694). New York: Oxford University Press.

Luthar, S. S. (2003). *Resilience and vulnerability: Adaptation in the context of childhood adversities.* Cambridge: Cambridge University Press.

Masten, A. S. (2001). Ordinary magic: Resilience processes in development. *American Psychologist, 56*(3), 227–238.

McCubbin, H. I. (1995). Resiliency in African American families: Military families in foreign environments. In H. I. McCubbin, E. A. Thompson, A. I. Thompson, & J. A. Futrell (Eds.), *Resiliency in ethnic minority families: African American families* (Vol. 2, pp. 67–98). Madison: University of Wisconsin Press.

McCubbin, H. I., McCubbin, M. A., Thompson, A. I., Han, S. V., & Allen, C. T. (1997). Families under stress: What makes them resilient. *Journal of Family and Consumer Sciences, 89*(3), 2–11.

McCubbin, H. I., Thompson, A. I., & McCubbin, M. A. (1996). *Family assessment: Resiliency, coping and adaptation – inventories for research and practice.* Madison: University of Wisconsin Publishers.

McCubbin, H. I., Thompson, E. A., Thompson, A. I., & Fromer, J. E. (1998). *Stress, coping and health in families: Sense of coherence and resiliency.* Thousand Oaks: SAGE Publications.

McCubbin, H. I., Thompson, E. A., Thompson, A. I., & Futrell, J. A. (1999). *The dynamics of resilient families.* Thousand Oaks: SAGE Publications.

McCubbin, M. A., Balling, K., Posin, P., Friedrich, S. H., & Bryne, B. (2002). Family resiliency in childhood cancer. *Family Relations, 51*(2), 103–111.

McCubbin, M. A., & Huang, S. T. (1989). Family strengths in the care of handicapped children: Targets for intervention. *Family Relations, 38*(4), 436–443.

Oh, S., & Chang, S. J. (2014). Concept analysis: Family resilience. *Open Journal of Nursing, 4*(13), 980–990.

Olson, D. H. (2011). FACES IV and the Circumplex model: Validation study. *Journal of Marital & Family Therapy, 3*(1), 64–80.

Olson, D. H., & DeFrain, J. (2000). *Marriage and the family: Diversity and strengths* (3rd ed.). Mountain View: Mayfield.

Olson, D. H., & Gorell, D. M. (2003). Circumplex model of marital and family systems. In F. Walsh (Ed.), *Normal family processes* (3rd ed., pp. 514–547). New York: Guilford Press.

Olson, D. H., McCubbin, H. I., Barnes, H. L., Larsen, A. S., Muxen, M. J., & Wilson, M. A. (1989). *Families: What makes them work* (2nd ed.). Los Angeles: SAGE Publications.

Parks, A. C., & Schueller, S. M. (2014). *The Wiley-Blackwell handbook of positive psychological interventions.* Oxford: Wiley-Blackwell.

Patterson, J. M. (2002a). Integrating family resilience and family stress theory. *Journal of Marriage and Family, 64*(2), 349–360.

Patterson, J. M. (2002b). Understanding family resilience. *Journal of Clinical Psychology, 58*(3), 233–246.

Patterson, J. M., Holm, K. E., & Gurney, J. G. (2004). The impact of childhood cancer on the family: A qualitative analysis of strains, resources, and coping behaviours. *Psycho-Oncology, 13*(6), 390–407.

Pinsof, W. M., & Lebow, J. L. (2005). *Family psychology: The art of the science.* New York: Oxford University Press.

Rashid, T. (2009). Positive interventions in clinical practice. *Journal of Clinical Psychology: In Session, 65*(5), 461–466.

Rich, G. J. (2003). The positive psychology of youth and adolescence. *Journal of Youth and Adolescence, 32*(1), 1–3.

Rolland, J. S. (2012). Mastering family challenges in serious illness and disability. In F. Walsh (Ed.), *Normal family processes: Growing diversity and complexity* (4th ed., pp. 452–482). New York: Guilford Press.

Rutter, M. (1987). Psychosocial resilience and protective mechanisms. *American Journal of Orthopsychiatry, 57*(3), 316–331.

Ryan, C., Epstein, N. B., Keitner, G., Miller, I. W., & Bishop, D. S. (2005). *Evaluating and treating families: The McMaster approach.* New York: Routledge.

Seligman, M. E. P. (2011). *Flourish: A visionary new understanding of happiness and well-being.* New York: Free Press.

Seligman, M. E. P., & Csikszentmihalyi, M. (2000). Positive psychology: An introduction. *American Psychologist, 55*(1), 5–15.

Seligman, M. E. P., Steen, T. A., Park, N., & Peterson, C. (2005). Positive psychology progress: Empirical validation of interventions. *American Psychologist, 60*(5), 410–421.

Shapiro, J. (1983). Family reactions and coping in response to the physically ill or handicapped child: A review. *Social Science and Medicine, 17*(14), 913–931.

Sheridan, S. M., & Burt, J. D. (2009). Family-centered positive psychology. In C. R. Snyder & S. J. Lopez (Eds.), *The Oxford handbook of positive psychology* (2nd ed., pp. 551–560). New York: Oxford University Press.

Sheridan, S. M., Sjuts, T. M., & Coutts, M. J. (2006). Understanding and promoting the development of resilience in families. In S. Goldstein & R. B. Brooks (Eds.), *Handbook of resilience in children* (pp. 143–160). New York: Springer.

Sheridan, S. M., Warnes, E. D., Cowan, R. J., Schemm, A. V., & Clarke, B. L. (2004). Family-centered positive psychology: Focusing on strengths to build student success. *Psychology in the Schools, 41*(1), 7–17.

Silberberg, S. (2001). Searching for family resilience. *Family Matters, 58,* 52–57.

Simon, J. B., Murphy, J. J., & Smith, S. M. (2005). Understanding and fostering family resilience. *The Family Journal: Counseling and Therapy for Couples and Families, 13*(4), 427–436.

Sirgy, M. J. (2012). *The psychology of quality of life: Hedonic well-being, life satisfaction, and eudaimonia.* Social Indicators Research Series, Vol. 50. New York: Springer.

Stinnett, N., & DeFrain, J. (1986). *Secrets of strong families.* New York: Berkley Books.

Stinnett, N., & DeFrain, J. (1989). The healthy family: Is it possible? In M. J. Fine (Ed.), *The second handbook on parent education: Contemporary perspectives* (pp. 53–73). San Diego: Academic Press.

Walsh, F. (2003). Family resilience: A framework for clinical practice. *Family Process, 42*(1), 1–18.

Walsh, F. (2006). *Strengthening family resilience* (2nd ed.). New York: Guilford Press.

Walsh, F. (Ed.). (2012). *Normal family processes: Growing diversity and complexity* (4th ed.). New York: Guilford Press.

Walsh, F., & Anderson, C. M. (2014). *Chronic disorders and the family.* London: Routledge.

Walsh, F., & McGoldrick, M. (2004). *Living beyond loss: Death in the family* (2nd ed.). New York: W. W. Norton & Company.

Werner, E. E., & Smith, R. S. (1982). *Vulnerable but invincible: A study of resilient children.* New York: McGraw-Hill.

Wissing, M., Potgieter, J., Guse, T., Khumalo, T., & Nel, L. (2014). *Towards flourishing: Contextualising positive psychology.* Pretoria: Van Schaik Publishers.

Yates, T. M., & Masten, A. S. (2004). Fostering the future: Resilience theory and the practice of positive psychology. In P. A. Linley & S. Joseph (Eds.), *Positive psychology in practice* (pp. 521–539). Hoboken: John Wiley & Sons.

32

Building resilient organizations

Introspection through the lens of psychological resiliency

Rabindra Kumar Pradhan

The very nature of change is changing, and for twenty-first century, every day new strategies are essential to flourish in the context of professional complexity. For organizations to move head on and face the challenges with positivity, they have to be able to welcome changes and be strategized to be changed by themselves. With today's knowledge and technical industries having short product lifecycles and braving a rapidly changing competition market, the ability to assess and engage itself becomes a key capability for survival and growth (Burnes, 2000). In this context, the business catastrophes with the wake of 9/11 has spread the idea of *organizational resilience* to address the requirements for managing uncertainty happening in economies around the globe, which is apparently intricate and increasingly interconnected (Hamel & Välikangas, 2003). Coutu (2002) has suggested that organizations require three key constituents for getting tagged as 'resilient': acceptance of reality, deeply held values that yield meaning, and the ability to improvise. Researchers have further acknowledged that forward planning, perception, and reaction to variations (Hollnagel, Woods, & Leveson, 2006); the ability to interpret events and manage complexities (Rerup, 2001); and the ability to correct errors immediately and learn from them (Weick & Sutcliff, 2001) are some of the pre-requisites for fostering organizational resilience. Therefore, such proven characteristics of resilience need to be assimilated into an organization's philosophy and culture, which will eventually ensure survival in times of hardship.

It is understood that a resilient organization gets 'toughened' to endure disorders of all kinds, and can become more competitive on a day-to-day basis. There are two important competencies that stand prima-facie in such occasions: one is the prudence and cognizance of present situation to prevent potentially emerging crises, and the other one is to turn crises into sources of tactical opportunity. However, many on-going projects of organization's sometimes utterly fail because the people involved with them are not equipped to deal with volumes of change the organization puts on them. This is predominantly happening because of lack of awareness happening with external environment, dearth of commitment among people to change, and reduced engagement of the workforce with their respective work profile, etc.

An organization with resilient people as well as resilient systems and processes can be more agile and productive as it can adapt to meet the changing needs of the market with confidence

(Reinmoeller & Van Baardwijk, 2005). Hence, resilience stands as a fundamental strategy to survive in today's turbulent global business world. It is also understood that individual and organizational resilience are closely related, and improving individual employees' psychological resilience will surely have a positive organizational impact. At the same time, many of the prevailing literatures have found to be outcome focused (Horne & Orr, 1988; Mallak, 1998), and there is likely to gain an understanding by being introspective about behavioral dimensions that may potentially allow the organization and its members to cultivate the ability for resilience. In this paper, we are going to identify and address the psychological aspects associated with organizations and how this capacity will enable an organization to allow human resources (HR) intervention programs more effective towards enhancing organizational resilience.

Contemporary HR challenges

Employees of organizations are becoming increasingly heterogeneous. As days go by, diversity is a resilient issue for the HR manager because of increasing number of young workers in the workforce, more women joining the work force, enhancement of mobility of workforce, and the fact that international experience is becoming a pre-requisite for career progression to many top-level managerial positions. Recent literature findings have supported the fact that the major challenge that has resulted from changing workforce demographic concerns like dual-career couples, couples where both partners are actively pursuing professional careers (Becker & Gerhart, 1996). However, the increasing number of dual-career professionals limits individual flexibility in accepting such assignments and may hinder organizational flexibility in acquiring and developing talent.

With the changes in workforce demographics, employee expectations and attitudes also have shifted. Traditional allurements such as job security, attractive remuneration, housing, and the like do not attract and motivate today's workforce (Haggerty & Wright, 2010). Employees demand empowerment and expect equality with the management. Previous notions on managerial authority are giving way to employee influence and involvement along with mechanisms for upward communication and due process.

At the organizational level, it is difficult to imagine circumstances that pose a greater challenge for human resource management (HRM) than reorganizations resulting from acquisitions, mergers, divestitures, or take-over threats. The reorganizations will have impact on organizational levels and employees (Schuler, 1992). Employees experience anxiety and uncertainty about their places in a new organization. The employees of both the 'taking over' as well as the 'taken over' companies will have anxious moments because of fear of loss of jobs; job changes, including new roles and assignments; transfers to new geographic locations; changes in remuneration and benefits; changes in career possibilities; changes in organizational power, status, and prestige; staff changes, including new peers and supervisors; and changes in corporate culture and loss of identity in the company.

In this era of uncertainty, only flexible and relentlessly dynamic HR policies can take appropriate actions and undergo transformation in response to unanticipated behavioral differences happening in a workplace events. It is said that in a market characterized by sudden jolts, a capacity for organizational resilience may be necessary for survival (Cynthia, Tammy, & Mark, 2011).

Organizational resilience: its construct and its attributes

Organization is defined as a "goal-directed, boundary-maintaining and socially constructed systems of human activity' (Aldrich & Ruef, 2006). However, ever-changing environmental conditions and discontinuities have amplified the likelihood of collapses within and between organizations (Burnard & Bhamra, 2011). During such uncertainties, resilience stands as a dynamic capability of organizational adaptableness for survival and sustenance (Wildavsky, 1988). Precisely, the concept denotes the ability to retain desirable organizational functions in the midst of external and internal pressure (Bunderson & Sutcliffe, 2002), the ability to rebound back from unpleasant happenings (Sutcliffe & Vogus, 2003), and most essentially the maintenance of positive adjustment under challenging conditions (Worline et al., 2004). An important perspective to resilience stresses an organizational system's capacity for learning, flexibility, and a keen inclination to reinvent itself (Christopher & Peck, 2004). This kind of attitude compels a system to have flexibility and agility so that environmental jolts are managed proactively (Woods, 2006). Resilience in its spirit is defined as the "ability and capacity to withstand systemic discontinuities and to adapt a new risk environment, based on actions such as diagnosing enterprise risks, implementing risk mitigation strategies and enduring increased risk and complexity" (Starr, Newfrock, & Dulurey, 2003).

Fiksel (2003) has identified four major characteristics that contribute to resilience including (1) *diversity* – the existence of multiple forms and behavior, (2) *efficiency* – performance with modest resource consumption, (3) *adaptability* – flexibility to change in response to new pressures, and (4) *cohesion* – existence of unifying relationships and linkages between system variables and elements. The construct of organizational resilience has some components in common with organizational features such as flexibility, agility, and adaptability. Flexibility is the ability to change on relatively short notice and at low cost (Ghemawat & Del Sol, 1998), while agility is the ability to develop and quickly apply dynamic, competitive moves (McCann, 2004), and adaptability is the ability to re-establish fit with the present environment (Chakravarthy, 1982). However, none of these said constructs can account for the overreaching comprehensiveness of organizational resilience as it comprehends distinctive features that make the term an inclusive and a wider construct in literature of management and behavioral science.

The available studies of organizational resilience include the behavioral approach, the sense-making approach, the self-renewal process approach, the risk management approach, and the systems approach. In the *behavioral approach*, a resilient organization demonstrates collective behavior and carries robust response capability for perceiving environmental changes quickly and implementing adaptive responses early (Horne & Orr, 1998). The *sense-making approach* conveys that the resilient organization is capable of making sense of disruptions and threats, i.e. sense-making actions precede cognition in crisis (Weick & Sutcliffe, 2001). The *self-renewal process approach* is important for an organization to establish early warning signals that would impede the self-renewal process (Välikangas, Hoegl, & Gibbert, 2009). In the *risk management approach*, a resilience paradigm oriented towards an organizational capacity to cope with uncertain, destructive, and collective events is underlined (Sheridan, 2008). In the *systems approach*, organizational resilience can be achieved by taking a broader view to cope with changes/crises by identifying potential factors of a viable organization (Ignatiadis & Nandhakumar, 2007).

Gibson and Tarrant (2010) have provided an understanding about the complexity and multidimensional nature of organizational resilience by examining several different conceptual models that demonstrates different and interrelated aspects of organizational resilience. Some of the models have established specific organizational attributes that can support an organization for dealing with ambiguity and hardship. One of them is the 'attributional model' of resilience developed by the Resilience Community of Interest (Resilience COI, 2009) has proposed the following key drivers for creating resilience:

1 *Organizational values* – establishing commitment, trust, and strong internal alignment and creating a common purpose

2   *Leadership* – establishing a clear strategic direction based upon understanding risk, empower-
    ing others to implement the strategic vision, and engendering trust

The 'values' and 'leadership' attributes creates an organizational culture and capability that is
aware of, and is sensitive to, internal and external change. This high level of change sensitivity
or acuity (understanding the past, monitoring the present, and foreshadowing the future) allows
indicators to be identified in the lead-up to dramatic change. This in turn facilitates closer integration of the disparate parts of the organization and through-chain interdependencies, enabling
them to better work cooperatively together to a common set of goals for unfolding disruptive
events. The operation of these various elements is enabled through open, adequate, and honest
communications, which provide an understanding on various emerging risks of the organization.
This awareness and communication enhance the organization's ability to learn from previous
disruptions and will provide a scope to better understand and adapt the newly emerging disruptions (Peche & Oakley, 2005).

    However, to explore how a model can relate to an individual organization's level of maturity
and the context it operates within it, a one-stop shop model has been recommended in the form
of the Herringbone model (Peche & Oakley, 2005). The model first identified that every organization owns a sizable range of competences to undertake a range of activities (collectively what
the organization 'does') that contributes inherently towards improved resilience. Additionally, the
organization displays a number of characteristics ('how' the organization operates), which affect
the effectiveness of the capabilities and activities to enhance the organization's resilience.

    While most of the capabilities, activities, and characteristics are critical to functioning in the
routine environment, it is the manner in which they can adapt to the non-routine environment
that will create resilience. It is pertinent to mention here that a few capabilities and activities are
specific for operations in the non-routine environment, such as business continuity and crisis and
emergency management. However, there are a few hidden characteristics some use to come into
their own towards creating a resilient state by helping all other aspects of the organization. Some
of these are critically important factors include:

1   *Acuity* – The ability to recognize precedence, what has occurred in the past; situational
    awareness, what is happening now; and foresight, what could happen in the future. Acuity
    provides the ability to take this information and identify early warning indicators of dra-
    matic change and provides an understanding of possible options for dealing with it.
2   *Ambiguity tolerance* – The ability to continue making decisions and taking action at times of
    high uncertainty.
3   *Creativity and agility* – Operating in novel ways to work around problems at a speed that
    matches volatility.
4   *Stress coping* – People, processes, and infrastructure continue to operate under increasing
    demands and uncertainty.
5   *Learnability* – The ability of the organization to use their own lessons and others' experiences
    to better manage the prevailing circumstances includes using lessons in real time as they
    emerge.

The relative contribution and importance to resilience of each of the capabilities, activities, and
characteristics will depend upon the nature of the changing circumstances being faced by the
organization. Organizational resilience is not just a momentary response to economic recession and severity measures; it is an important feature that most organizations require in order
to deal effectively with the challenges of usual market conditions injected by liberalization and

globalization, in which constantly changing competitive pressures and growing customer expectations are the standard.

Psychological resilience and its significance

Long hours and the constant pressure of meeting deadlines have been the hallmark of present-day organizational requirements, and there is a lot of pressure on people to perform. On the grounds of resilience, individuals and organizations are complementary to one another as employees take strength from the climate of the organization, and organizations derive tangible and intangible value from resilience in the form of coping and performing attitudes from its employees. Precisely, the organization's capacity for resilience is

> embedded in a set of individual level knowledge, skills, and abilities and organizational routines and processes by which a firm conceptually orients itself, acts decisively to move forward, and establishes a setting of diversity and adjustable integration that enables it to overcome the potentially debilitating consequences of a disruptive shock
> *(Lengnick-Hall & Beck, 2009)*

Therefore, an understanding of resilient individuals offers the beginning for outlining resilient organizations since actions and interactions among individual organizational members reinforces the emergence of a firm's collective capacity for resilience (Morgeson & Hofmann, 1999). In this connection, Charles Darwin has cited that, during adversity, "it is not the strongest species that survive, nor the most intelligent, but the most responsive to change can only thrive and prosper". A seminal study detailed by Maddi and Kobasa (1984) has found that resilience (as characterized by attitudes of 'commitment', 'control', and 'challenge') distinguished between those who flourished during the period and those who succumbed to stress-related illness and behavior (such as heart attacks, depression/anxiety disorders, and alcohol/drug abuse). The positive psychology movement has highlighted a shift in focus from what makes people psychologically ill to what keeps people psychologically healthy (Seligman & Csikszentmihalyi, 2000). Resilient individuals are surprisingly found to counterattack psychological agony in traumatic conditions because they remain optimistic, absorbed in their work, flexible, and pro-active. Therefore, solidification of psychological resilience (e.g. commitment, control, and challenge) is an important pre-requisite that moderates the feelings, thoughts, and behaviors of resilient individuals to the responses of change, which is essentially enabling them to survive develop and prosper effectively. Derek (2011), in his study on "Resilience and strengthening resilience in individuals", has proposed five factors that influence in building our personal resilience:

1   *Experiences:* The experiences we are gaining throughout our life contribute to our resilience, amongst which are professional challenges, education, and associated factors affecting our lives and other people's lives.
2   *Skills:* Skills in identifying purpose, planning, and organizing our lives at home and at work; our expertise in certain topics or hobbies that turn into a passion for the subject; our ability to resolve problems and challenges.
3   *Interaction:* Our ability to interact and communicate with others to survive and grow; our ability to engage with others, understanding that reciprocal support is essential to achieving our interests; our ability to act appropriately in different contexts; our understanding that we need to be an attractor for people and to engage with us effectively.

4   *Relationships:* Our understanding of who is important to us and how strong the relationship is; our ability to generate commitment and trust within relationships, using styles such as transaction, transformation, and adaptive techniques.

5   *Human capital:* The accumulated skills, knowledge, and experience acquired throughout life that equips us with our personal sense of worth, esteem, and confidence. Our capital is built from economic, cultural, political, romantic, and social factors around us.

There are several personal characteristics among individuals that serve for promoting one's capacity to be resilient. The key individual characteristics from several research and review articles (for e.g. Ong, Bergeman, & Boker, 2009; Richardson, 2002; Tugade & Fredrickson, 2004) are composed of attributes such as adaptive coping problem solving, emotional stability, and locus of control.

The aforesaid personal characteristics depict individual resilience as the ability to cope with extreme, stress-provoking events without experiencing signs or symptoms of personal stress. Mowbray (2012) stated two aspects of resilience: personal control and controlling the responses of others. He has stated that

> [E]ach of us has developed the skills and experience to build resilience in both of these aspects to a certain degree. Life events that we overcome without damage to ourselves influence our personal esteem in a positive way, and this raises our levels of resilience in the face of further adverse events.

It is suggested that personal control can best be achieved by linking personal values and beliefs to the personal activities of daily life. There is also, a direct link to the type of personality we are, and our innate ability to be flexible or rigid in the way we do everyday tasks. We are not always very good at personal control, and many people find that adopting techniques and approaches known to build personal resilience help to regain control over ourselves and the situation we are in. Controlling the responses of others is necessary for our own survival. We cannot exist without engaging with others. In a situation where we want to build our resilience, our interaction with others and the strength of important relationships stand out as the principal features of being resilient.

Therefore, it is inferred that psychological resilience typically goes beyond individual personality traits. It is a process that involves interaction between an individual, his or her past experiences, and current life context (Lepore & Revenson, 2006). Resilient people, through analyzing their past experiences and present context, choose not to become sufferers as they consciously rise to the occasion and reflect confidently with a solution-focused approach. Therefore, the key to psychological resilience is the ability to recognize one's own beliefs and harness the power of increased accuracy and flexibility of thinking to manage the emotional and behavioral consequences more effectively (Jackson & Watkin, 2004).

Towards building resilient organization

An average adult professional works with not only through his/her hands but also engages his/her heart (spirit) spending much of life-span, as much as a quarter or perhaps a third of his/her waking life at work. This gives employers unparalleled prospects to influence the well-being of their workers, including cultivating their resilience in an organizational setup. Warner and April (2012) in this connection has stated,

> [O]rganizations can significantly enhance the chances of success of a change initiative by ensuring that real hearts-and-minds change is created through emotional engagement,

intellectual alignment, coaxing the will of individuals through ensuring that the required new behaviors are trained, reinforced and cemented as processes that are part of the organizational culture.

Towers Watson study (2012) has recommended that employers should strive for "sustainable engagement through creating policies and practices that make it possible for employees to better manage their stress, to live more balanced lives, and to have more autonomy over when and where they get their work done". Nick Hayter, a senior consultant and regular blog writer on organizational resilience has stated that "an ideal scenario for fostering resilience is through providing employees with 'good work' – typified by a role that is stretching, purposeful and offers a clear line-of-sight between actions and outcomes". When employees are provided with a meaningful work assignment associated with a compelling organizational vision offering better future prospects, they will bring their *higher selves* to work, which will promote the culture of resiliency.

At the same time, organizations are complex social networks that have evolved, not just as a result of individual orientations and actions, but more so through interactions that professionals have among themselves and with the systems and processes (Lengnick-Hall, Beck, & Lengnick-Hall, 2011). Therefore, enhancing the resilience of an organization is a multi-level, collective task that emanates from the capabilities and behavior of core individuals within a well-designed organization. Hence, it is the prerogative of HR to choose the right set of people who have an attitude to align oneself to team and organizational needs. It is said that, when teams are well chosen and managed, high well-being and performance can be sustained even in difficult circumstances. Comcare (2014) stated that an Australian government agency has brought four factors that influence resilience at workplace and they are:

1   *Individuals:* A resilient individual is someone who usually maintains good mental health and productivity without being affected by stressful conditions or adversity. Skills in emotion regulation, awareness of when to ask for help, self-esteem, and confidence in individual ability and problem-focused coping skills are protective factors that may boost individual resilience. Stressful life events, a mismatch between skills and the job, prior mental ill health as well as chronic health problems and a low perception of one's own health are risk factors that may reduce individual resilience.
2   *Individual jobs:* A job that helps build resilience can only be created in a workplace that monitors risk and reduces this risk. Examples of protective factors that may improve individual job resilience include workplace engagement, role clarity with regular feedback and recognition, job satisfaction, and meaningful and flexible work. Meanwhile, risk factors that may reduce resilience at work include high demand, a lack of control over work, poor performance feedback, and job insecurity. Matching the job to the skills and abilities of a worker and providing appropriate training and support are very important for improving resilience.
3   *Teams:* A resilient team buffers its members against the adverse effects of stress and helps minimize known risk factors. Protective factors that can help to build resilience within a team include supportive managers, trust and respect between team members, the ability to make reasonable adjustments, as well as good communication. Resilient teams are based on mutual trust, social norms, participation, and social networks. Resilient teams are more likely to be productive and high-performing teams. However, conflict and breakdown in relationships, team stigma around mental health, and poor leadership and communication are risk factors that may reduce a team's resilience.

4   *Organizations:* Resilient organizations are characterized by strong leaders and by an ability to positively adapt to a changing environment. Protective factors that may build resilience at the organizational level include clear organizational goals and objectives, transparent and accessible senior management, and consultation and good support systems to take care of ill or injured workers. Conversely, risk factors that can reduce organizational resilience include lack of accountability, poorly managed organizational change, lack of action for a known problem, and lack of proper support of senior leaders for mental health.

Role of organizational leadership

In today's world, effective leaders have a tendency to subordinate their own egos and, instead, nurture leadership in others throughout the organization. Leveraging the power of leadership throughout the organization by the corporate leaders depends upon orienting subordinates towards performance beyond established standards and goals. It is to bring to the attention in today's organizations; flexibility, teamwork, trust, and information sharing are replacing rigid structures, competitive individualism, control, and secrecy. The best leaders have been found to have tendency of listening, motivating, and providing support to their people, and these are believed to be the core characteristics of professionals possessing an optimal amount of psychological resilience.

Though a complex concept, leadership is an ability to influence, motivate, and enable others to contribute to the effectiveness and success of the organizations of which they are members. Leaders use influence to motivate followers and arrange the work environment so that they do the job more effectively (House, Javidan, Hanger, & Dorfman, 2002; Javidan, Dorfman, Sully de Luque, & House, 2006). Present-day organizations have become less stable and predictable than before, and for that, bureaucratic rules have to be replaced by trust while defining expectations and relationships. Therefore, it would be absolutely correct if one is to say that effective management of business by the executives depends on trusting relationships with those whom they seek to lead. It is also correct that leadership is not restricted to the executive suite, but anyone in the organization may be a leader to address the uncertain upcoming times (Pearce & Conger, 2003). An executive at General Semiconductor, a global high-technology company says that his organization is quite serious when it talks about leadership even to a bench worker on the assembly line. Lots of people use to say, "Oh, I am not a leader", but when the organization points out that the essence of leadership is influence, they realize everyone has leadership qualities and responsibilities (Cole, 1999). Thus, the concept of leadership is present in the present-day world has to understand the factors of resilience than what we have believed for years. It is pertinent to say that conceptualization of leadership in today's organizational reality requires a paradigm shift in the minds of behavioral scientists, both academicians as well as practicing managers.

Conclusion

Building the ability for effective change management, an organization needs to engage a systemic approach wherein it can tap into people's natural competence to change by supporting change and building it as a basic part of organizational life (Buono & Kerber, 2010). In this connection, the psychological contract, or the unwritten agreement between employees and employers, is an important feature in defining the attitudes and associated behavior of people. It is said that the organization claims their people as their fundamental assets, then breaches of the psychological contract will have counterproductive implications for organizational resilience. For resilient individuals and organizations, an impediment is not seen as an end of the world – it should be recognized and experienced as a learning opportunity and a chance to do better next time. With respect to organizational resilience the message is clear – the *psychological contract between employer and employee counts*, and organizational investment for employees' capacity to be resilient is good for both employee and business. It is claimed that the psychological contract acts in the same way as Herzberg's hygiene factors. A robust contract will not necessarily guarantee superior employee engagement and performance, but violation of the contract will result in lower levels of commitment, higher levels of absenteeism and attrition, and poor performance (Sparrow, 1996).

Finally, the development of organizational resilience needs to be viewed as a deliberate and proactive management initiative for building organizational capability, something that all businesses should strive to do as a matter of course, rather than merely as a reaction to change. This kind of initiative requires a fundamental shift in thinking through enabling the HR policies to take care of employees' physical, mental, emotional, and spiritual needs, and thereby resilience will see the light of day.

References

Aldrich, H., & Ruef, M. (2006). *Organizational evolving* (2nd ed.). London: Sage.

Becker, B., & Gerhart, B. (1996). The impact of human resource management on organizational performance: Progress and prospects. *Academy of Management Journal, 39*(4), 779–801.

Bunderson, J. S., & Sutcliffe, K. M. (2002). Comparing alternative conceptualizations of functional diversity in management teams: Process and performance effects. *Academy of Management Journal, 45*(5), 875–893.

Buono, A. F., & Kerber, K. W. (2010). Intervention and organizational change: Building organizational change capacity. In Anthony F. Buono & David W. Jamieson (Eds.), *Consultation for organizational change* (pp. 81–112). Charlotte: Information Age Publishing.

Burnard, K., & Bhamra, R. (2011). Organisational resilience: Development of a conceptual framework for organizational responses. *International Journal of Production Research, 49*(18), 5581–5599.

Burnes, B. (2000). *Managing: An approach to organizational dynamics* (3rd ed.). Harlow: Prentice Hall.

Chakravarthy, B. S. (1982). Adaptation: A promising metaphor for strategic management. *Academy of Management Review, 7*(1), 35–44.

Christopher, M., & Peck, H. (2004). Building the resilient supply chain. *International Journal of Logistics Management, 15*(2), 1–14.

Cole, M. A. (1999). Become the leader followers want to follow. *Supervision, 60*(12), 9–10.

Comcare. (2014). *Four factors that influence resilience in the workplace*. Retrieved from www.comcare.gov.au/promoting/Creating_mentally_healthy_workplaces/building_a_resilient_workforce

Coutu, D. (2002). How resilience works. *Harvard Business Review, 80*(5), 46–55.

Cynthia, A., Tammy, E. B., & Mark, L. (2011). Developing a capacity for organizational resilience through strategic human resource management. *Human Resource Management Review, 21*(3), 243–255.

Derek, M. (2011). *Resilience and strengthening resilience in individuals*. Retrieved from www.mas.org.uk/uploads/articles/Resilience_and_strengthening_resilience_in_individuals.pdf

Fiksel, J. (2003). Designing resilient, sustainable systems. *Environmental Science and Technology, 37*(23), 5330–5339.

Gibson, E., & Tarrant, M. (2010). A conceptual model approach to organizational resilience. *The Australian Journal of Emergency Management, 25*(2), 6–12.

Ghemawat, P., & Del Sol, P. (1998). Commitment versus flexibility. *California Management Review, 40*(4), 26–42.

Haggerty, J. J., & Wright, P. M. (2010). Strong situations and firm performance: A proposed re-conceptualization of the role of the HR function. In A. Winkinson, N. Bacon, T. Redman, & S. A. Snell (Eds.), *The Sage handbook of human resource management* (pp. 100–114). Thousand Oaks, CA: Sage.

Hamel, G., & Välikangas, L. (2003). The quest for resilience. *Harvard Business Review, 81*(9), 52–63.

Hollnagel, E., Woods, D. D. & Leveson, N. C. (2006). *Resilience engineering: Concepts and precepts*. Aldershot, UK: Ashgate.

Horne, J. F. I., & Orr, J. E. (1998). Assessing behaviors that create resilient organizations. *Employee Relations Today, 24*(4), 29–39.

House, R. J., Javidan, M., Hanges, P., & Dorfman, P. (2002). Understanding cultures and implicit leadership theories across the globe: An introduction to Project GLOBE. *Journal of World Business, 37*(1), 3–10.

Ignatiadis, I., & Nandhakumar, J. (2007). The impact of enterprise systems on organizational resilience. *Journal of Information Technology, 22*(1), 36–43.

Jackson, R., & Watkin, C. (2004). The resilience inventory: Seven essential skills for overcoming life's obstacles and determining happiness. *Selection & Development Review, 20*(6), 13–17.

Javidan, M., Dorfman, P. W., Sully de Luque, M., & House, R. J. (2006). In the eye of the beholder: Cross cultural lessons in leadership from Project GLOBE. *Academy of Management Perspectives, 20*(1), 67–90.

Lengnick-Hall, C. A., & Beck, T. E. (2009). Resilience capacity and strategic agility: Prerequisites for thriving in a dynamic environment. In C. P. Nemeth, E. Hollnagel, & S. Dekker (Eds.), *Resilience engineering perspectives* (pp. 39–70). Aldershot, UK: Ashgate Publishing.

Lengnick-Hall, C. A., Beck, T. E., & Lengnick-Hall, M. L. (2011). Developing a capacity for organizational resilience through strategic human resource management. *Human Resource Management Review, 21*(3), 243–255.

Lepore, S. J., & Revenson, T. A. (2006). Relationships between posttraumatic growth and resilience: Recovery, resistance, and reconfiguration. In Lawrence G. Calhoun & Richard G. Tedeschi (Eds.), *Handbook of posttraumatic growth: Research and practice* (pp. 24–46). Mahwah, NJ: Lawrence Erlbaum Associates.

McCann, J. (2004). Organizational effectiveness: Changing concepts for changing environments. *Human Resource Planning, 27*(1), 42–50.

Maddi, S. R., & Kobasa, S. C. (1984). *The hardy executive: Health under stress.* Homewood, IL: Dow Jones-Irwin.

Mallak, L. A. (1998). Putting organizational resilience to work. *Industrial Management, 40*(6), 8–13.

Morgeson, F. P., & Hofmann, D. A. (1999). The structure and function of collective constructs: Implications for multilevel research and theory development. *Academy of Management Review, 24*(2), 249–265.

Mowbray, D. (2012). *The guide to personal resilience by Management Advisory Service Ltd.* Retrieved from www.mas.org.uk/management-advisory-service/managing-resilience/building-resilience.html

Ong, A. D., Bergeman, C. S., & Boker, S. M. (2009). Resilience comes of age: Defining features in later adulthood. *Journal of Personality, 77*(6), 1777–1804.

Pearce, C. L., & Conger, J. A. (2003). All those years ago: The historical underpinnings of shared leadership. In C. L. Pearce & J. A. Conger (Eds.), *Shared leadership: Reframing the hows and whys of leadership* (pp. 1–18). Thousand Oaks, CA: Sage Publications.

Peche, R. J., & Oakley, K. E. (2005). Hormesis: An evolutionary "predict and prepare" survival mechanism. *Leadership & Organization Development Journal, 26*(8), 673–687.

Reinmoeller, P., & Van Baardwijk, N. (2005). The link between diversity and resilience. *MIT Sloan Management Review, 46*(4), 61–65.

Rerup, C. (2001). Houston, we have a problem: Anticipation and improvisation as sources of organizational resilience. *Comportamento Organizacional E Gestão, 7*(1), 21–44.

Resilience COI. (2009). Report on the 2nd National Organizational Resilience Workshop, 1–4 December 2008. Published Sydney, February 2009.

Richardson, G. E. (2002). The meta-theory of resilience and resiliency. *Journal of Clinical Psychology, 58*(3), 307–321.

Schuler, R. S. (1992). Strategic human resource management: Linking people with the strategic needs of the business. *Organizational Dynamics, 21*(1), 18–32.

Seligman, M. E., & Csikszentmihalyi, M. (2000). Positive psychology: An introduction. *American Psychologist, 55*(1), 5–14.

Sheridan, T. B. (2008). Risk, human error, and system resilience: Fundamental ideas. *Human Factors, 50*(3), 418–426.

Sparrow, P. R. (1996). Careers and the psychological contract: Understanding the European context. *European Journal of Work and Organizational Psychology, 5*(4), 479–500.

Starr, R., Newfrock, J., & Dulurey, M. (2003). Enterprise resilience: Managing risk in the networked economy. *Strategy + Business, 30*, 1–10.

Sutcliffe, K. M., & Vogus, T. (2003). Organizing for resilience. In K. S. Cameron, J. E. Dutton, & R. E. Quinn (Eds.), *Positive organizational scholarship: Foundations of a new discipline* (pp. 94–110). San Francisco: Berrett-Koehler.

Towers Watson Staff. (2012). *Global workforce study: Towers Watson.* Retrieved from www.towerswatson.com/Insights/IC-Types/Survey-Research-Results/2012/07/2012Towers Watson-Global-Workforce-Study

Tugade, M. M., & Fredrickson, B. L. (2004). Resilient individuals use positive emotions to bounce back from negative emotional experiences. *Journal of Personality and Social Psychology, 86*(2), 320–333.

Välikangas, L., Hoegl, M., & Gibbert, M. (2009). Why learning from failure isn't easy (and what to do about it): Innovation trauma at Sun Microsystems. *European Management Journal, 2*(4), 225–233.

Warner, R., & April, K. (2012). Building personal resilience at work. *Effective Executive, 15*(4), 53–68.

Weick, K. E., & Sutcliffe, K. M. (2001). *Managing the unexpected: Assuring high performance in an age of complexity*. San Francisco: Jossey-Bass.

Wildavsky, A. (1988). *Searching for safety*. New Brunswick, NJ: Transaction Books.

Woods, D. D. (2006). Essential characteristics of resilience. In E. Hollnagel, D. Woods, & N. Leveson (Eds.), *Resilience engineering* (pp. 21–34). Burlington, VT: Ashgate.

Worline, M. C., Dutton, J. E., Frost, P. J., Janov, J., Lilius, J., & Maitlis, S. (2004). *Creating fertile soil: The organizing dynamics of resilience* (Working paper). Ann Arbor: University of Michigan School of Business.

33

Architects of our own survival

Can authorities empower individuals and communities by building resilience through self-reliance in the face of impending seasonal natural disasters?

Kathryn M. Gow and Francine M. Pritchard

While the disaster research focus has primarily been on recovering from natural disasters in communities and rebuilding, less effort has concentrated on preparedness for disasters up until the past few years. Of the investigations and research that have been undertaken around the world, and across the multiple kinds of natural disasters that world citizens in this century are being exposed to, the results are mixed with respect to preparedness of both individuals and communities. Undoubtedly, the variations are influenced by the regularities of a specific type of disaster such as floods in Bangladesh, bushfires in Australia, drought in Africa, cyclones and typhoons in Asian and Pacific islands, tornadoes in the USA, and earthquakes in Turkey and the Ring of Fire[1] in the Asia Pacific areas. It is imperative to ascertain the circumstances under which individual communities appear to be continuing to be ill prepared or well prepared for such events and which communities lack the requisite available resources (e.g. the aboriginal communities of Elcho Island, Milingimbi, Ramingining and Maningrida did not have sufficient resources when the cyclones hit). Recent events and preparedness scheduling in Australia are showcased to highlight what strategies worked under which conditions and locations in Queensland in the immediate hours and days following recent catastrophic disasters.

Preamble

Both authors have been involved, not only in researching and writing about the field of natural disasters, but also have been practically involved in mitigation, preparedness, intervention and postvention. They have lived in urban, peri-urban, semi-rural and city environments where cyclones, floods, severe drought, bushfires, severe storms, tornadoes and heat waves have impacted on the neighbourhoods in which they have lived and worked. The authors have observed major progress in educating Australian communities since the 2009 Victorian Bushfires and the 2011 SEQLD[2] floods to be prepared for natural disasters and to act appropriately.

Introduction

The chapter outlines the kinds of mega disasters that have increased in the twenty-first century and allegedly are now more frequent and more ferocious because of climate change factors (especially heat waves, droughts, wildfires and flooding due to sea level rise) (Gow, 2009). We then outline difficulties in the understanding of, and use of, the term resilience. Finally, we showcase what Australia achieved in the 2014/2015 disaster season in terms of building self-reliance for preparedness across a range of potential and actual catastrophic natural hazards.

At the time this chapter is being finalised for submission (March/April 2015), the world is being beset by mega disasters (man-made and natural), with the latter reminding us of the power of the four elements – Water, Fire, Air and Earth – that govern this planet. The crippling Californian four-year long drought[3] vies for news space with the worst flood[4] in eighty years in Chile, which had just endured a horrendous destructive forest fire[5] in March. Typhoons in Micronesia grab attention from the cyclone destruction of Vanuatu, while Australia draws breath before the next onslaught of bushfires, cyclones and floods. Four cyclones menaced Northern Australia with the innocent names of Marcia, Lam, Nathan and Olwyn. However, Marcia and Lam were not innocents as the just released documentary on 9 April 2015 on the SBS Television illustrated its violence in relation to its impact on remote aboriginal communities in the NT. When Lam struck the NT, Marcia wreaked havoc in QLD.

Mega disasters

A mega disaster is a major overpowering, widespread, highly destructive disaster that destroys people, livestock and animals; landscapes, habitats, farmlands and crops; natural resources including mining plants, waterways, communications, infrastructure (roads, bridges, water and sewerage, gas lines, power lines); and transport facilities and businesses and interrupts, if not destroys, communications, food supplies, fuel supplies, transport, electricity and gas and water supplies.

The number of people and animals killed or injured varies according to the total population and size of country and the density of population per hectare in urban, city, coastal or rural locations.

There are several different environments in which hazards impact on people, animals, vegetation, infrastructure, businesses and the environment. These all intersect at various points. The impact of a hazard will depend on the number of people (density) in the area impacted; the type and severity of the hazard; people's familiarity with the hazard; wealth status of the population; location (remote, coastal, rural, city, urban, peri-urban); age and health distribution. Education and experience in preparedness for dealing with natural disasters all affect their vulnerability and survivability.

For example, two natural disasters some decades apart irrevocably changed the lives and character of two cities – Cyclone Tracey, which annihilated Darwin (Australia) on Christmas day in 1974, and Hurricane Katrina, which destroyed the essence of New Orleans (USA) in 2005. The mapped size of Cyclone Pam before it struck Vanuatu and other islands in March 2015 could be compared with the size of Hurricane Katrina. Economically, in 2012, Hurricane Sandy led to the highest death rate and economic loss in USA history, whereas Cyclone Yasi in 2011(coupled with the tourism losses to Australia and QLD) was estimated to be a massive financial loss but without loss of life relating directly to the actual disaster.

The catastrophic 2011 Christchurch earthquake destroyed people, homes, history, architecture, security and economic prosperity; however, some hope remained, and determination has led to the rebuilding of the famous city, even though there have been further quakes disturbances since then. The Japanese earthquake in 2011 was so unspeakably diabolical that its multiple effects continue to this day and will continue for many years to come.

On Christmas Day in 1974, Cyclone Tracy literally wiped out the city of Darwin and was one of the worst natural catastrophes in Australian history. Almost all residential properties (about 40,000) were damaged or destroyed with over 61 people killed. The whole structure of the society and families was destroyed when people were simply airlifted to other cities in other states hundreds of miles away. The learnings from such mismanagement influenced decisions this season when Cyclone Nathan threatened the NT shores again. Some residents were airlifted from Wurruni island back to shore just in case, while others were left on islands when different cyclones came, in case there was a backlash against the authorities as had happened in 1974 after the forced evacuation of Darwin. The ND warnings to Australians now contain carefully worded cautions and warnings about staying put or leaving early.

So when talking about resilience and recovery, we need to keep in mind the ways of measuring loss: loss of lives; degree of destruction; ferocity of NDs in terms of fear impact on residents; and economic loss at individual, community, state and federal levels.

Factors involved in breakdown of community response

There are a number of factors involved in the breakdown of community recovery and reconstruction and impact on resilience. These include:

1   Lack of immediate financial and practical support for a number of reasons. Residents who had already suffered other disasters, world financial downturn, lack of insurance or non-payment or partial payment of insurance.
2   Age: those in their twenties (who had only seen the good times) witnessing one calamity after the other in the world and worried about their future, with peak oil, climate change, country riots and rebellions wars and famines and doomsday prophecies and a loss of trust in authority across the world. People over 65 who had retired and had not the strength or finances to rebuild.
3   Prior individual and community trauma leading to severe panic or trauma reactions, acute stress disorder (ASD) or post-traumatic stress disorder (PTSD) reactions or pervasive depression, sadness, grief, anger and loss of meaning and purpose in life.
4   Across many disasters, gender is a factor with women tending to be more affected in terms of distress than men (although this is not necessarily the case with drought populations, as then many more men suicided than women).
5   Widespread destruction of housing, businesses, infrastructure and transport
6   Forced evacuation leading to breakup of families and communities; subsequent isolation and separation.
7   Lack of support or interventions from individuals or communities and perceived betrayal and abandonment by local state and federal authorities and rescue organizations.

Multiple and compounding stresses and traumas weaken normal resilience. NDs can re-hook other unresolved or still fresh individual or community traumas.

There is also no doubt that compounding emotional triggers can exacerbate the shock and trauma of ND losses, when it occurs at a time that is full of anniversary dates that reactivate feelings of loss and sadness. For instance, while the cyclones, floods, severe storms and bushfires beset Australians over the 2014/2015 summer, the media reminded them of other anniversary events that killed or maimed or destroyed the homes of their countrymen: Cyclone Tracy forty years on, the Hobart Bridge Collapse (5 Jan 1975) forty years ago, the Newcastle Earthquake twenty-five years on (28 December 1989), the tenth anniversary of the Asian Boxing Day tsunami (26 December 1984), with months of reminders that the 25 April 2015 would see the hundred-year Gallipoli commemorations and 2015 the forty-year commemoration of the end of the Vietnam War in 1975.

We know that isolated communities in Northern Queensland are prepared for floods and it is generally women who undertake multiple tasks before "the wet season" to ensure that they have adequate provisions (up to four months in some locations), back-up power, and medical supplies, and that their school children have a place to stay in case of being isolated (see Cottrell, 2008). Cyclones, however, are far more unpredictable in terms of timing and ferocity than floods.

While some cyclones can be rated as catastrophic in terms of wind speed (rated as Category 5 if sustained wind speeds are above 200 km/hr and gusts above 279 km/hr; for hurricanes, wind speeds have to be rated above 252 km/hr)(Cyclone Yasi 2011 in QLD, Cyclone George 2007 in WA, Cyclone Ingrid 2005 in NT, Cyclone Joan 1975 in WA, Cyclone Mahina 1899 in Bathurst Bay, Cyclone Innisfail 1918 in QLD), they may not cause as much damage as others such as Cyclone Larry (2006) in Innisfail, QLD (Australia's most costliest cyclone), Typhoon Tip 1979 in Western Pacific, Super Typhoon 2013 Haiyan (strongest typhoon ever recorded at landfall), Hurricane Wilma 2005 in the Atlantic and Super Typhoon Maysak 2015 in Micronesia.

It is important to recognise that in 2005, multiple wind storms beset the same areas in the Atlantic and similarly the Pacific areas in 2015. When areas are targeted by multiple NDs within a few months of each other, it is extremely difficult for humans or vegetation or infrastructure to keep rebounding. Take for instance the NT communities affected by both Cyclone Lam and then a month later Cyclone Nathan. Thus, eco, personal, social and economic resilience are all affected within a short time frame. If cross-type NDs (drought, floods, bushfires, cyclones, heat waves, severe storms) are besetting a country or close neighbours, then the psychological traumatic impact starts to wear down people and those people, especially the younger age groups who have not been exposed to such disasters before, become anxious and elderly residents depressed and fearful.

Resilience and resourcefulness

Resourcefulness refers to the ability to access and employ internal and external resources to deal with the impact of the adverse or traumatic event (after being psychologically affected by it) and as such is linked with the concept of recovery in the literature on post-traumatic conditions (Celinski & Gow, 2005). This is an attribute that is rarely mentioned in the disaster literature.

Marek Celinksi (Celinski & Gow, 2005) maintains that resourcefulness is both a personality trait and a process that is goal oriented and rooted in a sense of mastery and self-efficacy; it is associated with confidence in the utilization of internal and external abilities, knowledge, emotions, skills and sources of support to achieve specific goals (manageability). In normal everyday life, we might call it know-how, native intelligence, a practical approach to life, being inventive and knowing how to source what you need and drawing on external and internal resources to achieve the goal of preparing for, and solving problems in reacting to, hazards as quickly and as effectively as possible within one's means and strengths. When you are not stressed, you might do that easily, but stress makes it harder as it interferes with a clear head and problem-solving approaches.

It is interesting that Marek Celinksi and Lyle Allen (in Celinski, Allen, & Gow, 2013) believe that resilience has priority over resourcefulness, because they consider that resilience guides our efforts at seeking resources; if a person is "not ready" for a certain action, then teaching specific skills or attempting to tap available resources may be futile. If we apply these statements to preparing for and reacting to impending natural disasters, the authors' experiences with community reactions seem to fit this concept, vis-à-vis the years of preparing people in bush land areas to prepare for the bushfire season ahead, only to find out that most residents only believe they are in danger when the fire is at the steps to their house (see Gow, Pritchard, & Chant, 2008). Mileti and Fitzpatrick (1992) had concluded also that, even if people perceive there is a risk, it does not necessarily mean that they will take appropriate action to protect themselves against the hazard.

Within the 2014/2015 disaster season, Queensland seemed to have achieved the success of purveying one universal message for all disasters to the general public, what Kolender and Bowman (2004, p. 6) term taking personal responsibility. They point out that within that one message there should be a subset of messages for each type of hazard; we noted that this occurred in many ways this disaster season and it was astounding how well the public reacted (see later section).

Kolender and Bowman (2004, p. 6) were wary of the apathy evident in populations about taking action in preparing for disasters. Again this disaster season gave ample evidence of this fact: obviously not all of the public cooperated with the warnings; some still tried to "face off" death by standing out on the beach while Cyclones Marcia and Lam came in, or went touring around the beach side roads as the cyclone was advancing and trees were flying through the air, or went board riding in the gigantic waves brought in by ocean surges along the famous beaches – risk takers all.

If we then move conceptually to Earvoline-Ramirez's idea that "the main antecedent to resilience is adversity" (2007, p. 78), we knew before this disaster season (by living through and examining many others) that, while it is true that some people become enabled (such as those men, whom we speak about in another page of this chapter, who purchased generators so that they would never be without electricity again), there were other flood victims four years later, who lost too much financially after the 2011 floods, who are still down on their knees – but praying for guidance has not helped. They have no closure, similar to, but obviously very different from, the families who are still searching for closure on the fate of their loved ones who disappeared in the Boxing Day Tsunami in 2004.

"Challenge, change, and disruption are all aspects of adversity which must be present before the process of resilience can occur" (Richardson, 2002, p. 78), and we have witnessed such a process in emergent leadership following natural disasters. By reference to Richardson, Neiger, Jensen, and Kumpfer's (1990) Resilience Model, Earvolino-Ramirez (2007, p. 78) noted that individuals, reacting to disruptive life events, make conscious or unconscious choices to restore their sense of inner integration. "It is the disruption that allows an individual to learn or tap into resilient qualities and achieve resilient reintegration" (Richardson, 2002, in Earvolino-Ramirez, 2007, p. 78). Others now talk about *bouncing forward* rather than being stuck at the *bounce back* stage, which fails to occur in many people who have been seriously affected by natural disasters. This concept of bouncing forward (Manyena, O'Brien, O'Keefe, & Rose, 2011) is relatively new and has been readily taken up by organisational leadership consultants (Allison-Napolitano,

2014), but it is not an easy one to comprehend; it requires the taking of a new path altogether as the old one cannot continue as planned.

Eco-resilience, personal resilience, social resilience and economic resilience

In terms of *personal resilience*, there are many different definitions, but they all agree that it is an inner strength, a characteristic of the person that is generally stable across time and situations, every after encounters with trauma.

Neil Adger (2000) defines *social resilience* as "the ability of groups or communities to cope with external stresses and disturbances as a result of social, political and environmental change" (p. 347). This is a very useful definition for our purposes for what was going on in Queensland at the time of the 2011 floods (see other section) and for the complicated nationwide reaction to the 2009 Victorian Bushfire holocaust.

Adger (2000) considers that generally *ecological resilience* is demonstrated in ecosystems by their ability "to maintain themselves in the face of disturbance" (p. 347). After the very long drought in Australia, when the floods came, in some places they led to better crops and the restoration of major waterways such as the Murray Darling System. In other areas, crops were badly damaged or destroyed and waterways severely affected by erosion, with altered water course flows and major deposits of sand and soil wash. In such long droughts or cycles of droughts, the economic and thereby the personal resilience of farmers and towns people are directly linked to ecological resilience, and if these ecological resources and stability are damaged, they will be adversely affected, such as in floods, bushfires and droughts.

Economic resilience is a critical term in disaster aftermaths, as failure to have adequate insurance or failure of the insurance companies to pay out honourably is known as a major knock to one's ability to regroup, to plan ahead and to feel hopeful about the future. The destruction of businesses takes away people's livelihoods with a flow on effect to loss of jobs for people in the area. The cost to governments and local councils can be draining, and when things are economically tight, one can almost understand a prime minister or his treasurer cutting back small payouts to disaster affected Australians from $1,000 to $700 – well, almost.

If we move our focus from developed countries to developing countries, Heather Mohay in our chapter on the breakdown of community resilience following natural disasters (Gow & Mohay, 2013) refers to the different recovery levels of residents in the Bangladesh floods, with the poorer people on the river flats not recovering due to lack of economic resources, while those higher up with better incomes or capital were less affected and could recover. Vietnam (still a developing country), which has been analysing the effects of climate change leading to increased flooding, has suffered great loss and damage from typhoons and seasonal flooding with resultant loss of life and buildings, and businesses have attempted to assess rising health risks under such conditions (Few, Pham Gia Tran, & Bui Thi Thuy Hong, 2004). Obviously for a post-war country, even though the economic development has been substantial following "DoiMoi"[6] after 1986, it cannot afford to put into place all the mitigation and reconstruction and health recovery responses needed yet. Thus, low socio-economic status is a large determinant of economic recovery, and this was true of many rural areas in Australia during the long drought, as well as in African countries.

Cuba, because of its geographical location, is susceptible to NDs of all kinds. However, while still at an economic disadvantage, their contribution to know-how in preparing for hurricanes and other NDs has been recognised by United Nations' officials (Bermejo, 2006), and they offer that know-how in the form of trained personnel to countries beset by NDs.

Breakdown in community resilience

In relation to the factors that will be seen to contribute to lack of resilience or a breakdown in individual and community resilience, these are many, but there are four that stand out as causing the greatest destruction of community resilience and perhaps, by default, individual resilience; these relate to temporary and permanent displacement of persons, total area and materials destroyed and infrastructure destruction, loss of life and injuries, and the history of the people and area destroyed.

Drawing on case study material in our books

"We know that some places turn into ghost towns like Darwin after Cyclone 'Tracey' in 1974 and New Orleans after Hurricane 'Katrina' in 2005; the damage is so extensive and so severe that the whole cohesiveness of the community is lost; buildings, fencing, trees, roads, bridges, subways, railways lines, pavements, shops, factories, industrial estates, schools, hospitals all are gone; infrastructure, water, electricity no longer function and the landscape is not recognisable as being the same well known place. Actual displacement of people appears to be a key factor when large numbers of residents are displaced locally or relocated away from their town or city" (Gow & Mohay, 2013, p. 259).

"The major difference is that drought spans a long time and erodes community resilience and undermines resourcefulness; most other natural disasters wreak havoc quickly and violently, such as earthquakes, floods, tsunamis, cyclones, hurricanes, avalanches and volcanic eruptions and wildfires. Thus, there is severity, immediate damage to the ecosystems, property and people, infrastructure, business, environment and animals, agricultural crops etcetera and an abrupt and dramatic shortage of transport, food and water in many instances (Gow & Mohay, 2013, p. 259).

"The psychological reactions and physical health issues are similar in certain ways and yet different in others. PTSD is far likelier to occur with non-drought effects, whereas severe depression and suicide is more likely to occur in long droughts. In the former, the individual's resourcefulness is first depleted and over time their resilience is drained. The mental health effects are different and the resources that people draw on are also different; in the great drought, across 1992 to 2007 in Australia, farmers and small town business owners kept plodding on, hoping that things would improve, convinced that the rain would come again and that all they had to do was to obtain a bigger bank loan to get them through to the next crop or the next sheep/cattle sale; but the rain did not come, year after year, after year (Gow & Mohay, 2013, p. 259).

"Marriages and families separated slowly at first and then the momentum built; small business owners including hotels and grocery stores (often the meeting hub of small communities) 'hung in there' for many years and then, bankrupt, closed their doors in grief and loss. Small towns died, school children were bussed (transported) to other towns or moved to larger towns or cities, banks foreclosed on the farmers and graziers and property prices slumped. And when the rains came again, the farmers were met with new challenges that they could not fight, coal mining companies took out mineral rights to their lands spreading coals dust for miles around, and later coal seam gas companies with no permission dug wells on their properties poisoning their water. When does one admit defeat and give up? When does resilience mean staying or leaving?" (Gow & Mohay, 2013, p. 259).

Preparedness and self-reliance

In interviewing residents in the Lockyer and Somerset and Ipswich regions, some of the men in the 2011 SEQLD floods were prepared with generators and diesel fuel, but most households did not own them even though many lived on acreage in rural areas. On questioning other community members three months after the 2011 flood, the authors found people buying generators even though the likelihood then of being without power in such circumstances (from three to eight days or more) was not high; the men clarified that they did not ever want to be placed in that situation of having no electricity ever again. Two years later, the severe 2013 floods arrived with widespread power outages vindicating the outlay of their hard earned money.

In the same year, the merging of the State Emergency Services (SES) and Rural Fire Brigade (RFB) in Queensland caused lots of problems as the "old guard" left and community commitments were scaled back because of large cuts in government funding. Little care was taken about disaster preparedness, with the new Queensland State Premier in 2010/2011 indicating that we did not need all of these services, and he decided to cut back on climate change, disaster and environmental outlays. One politician lost the respect of many people when he was quoted as saying that the fire brigade service men were overpaid. The very next month, there were lots of house and industrial fires and bushfires[7] across Australia, and then a short time later in Queensland, wildfires marched across the now dry landscapes, and these continued for many months.

Further north across the equator, Bangladesh was hit yet again by torrential floods and seemingly no amount of preparedness or warning or lessons from the past could save the people on the flats (see Gow & Mohay, 2013). In a 2014 meeting in South America, Pope Francis called on the world to consider the impact of climate change on the poor people, but journalists ignored the potential to conduct solid investigative journalism here to explain what he and others were specifically calling attention to. As in Bangladesh (floods) and the Philippines (hurricanes/cyclones), if people are poor they have no money or resources to prepare or make life better or the ability to move elsewhere to higher ground where flood waters and storm surges cannot destroy their lives.

Low economic status, however, is not the only reason for lack of disaster preparedness. The South East Queensland 2011 flood proved that even emergency service organisations could become complacent and governments nonchalant in their preparations following sixteen years of drought and a complete change in the weather pattern (this does not mean that they were not "pulling out all stops" to help drought stricken communities, but rather that all other natural disasters had simply faded from consciousness). Something marked had altered the people's reading of the skies and the pattern of weather.

To clarify the difference between being complacent and nonchalant about preparedness, but still being able to react with disaster intervention and recovery expertise, when the 1996 and 1999 floods occurred, these were handled well by the well-trained emergency services officers. What happened in the 2011 floods was that the emergency services officers were unable in some cases to get out of their own flooded areas or to get into the places that needed help; this was an extraordinary time of flooding with seventy-four out of seventy-five government areas coming under flood at some point in Queensland.

Now let us return to the historical political influences operating at that time. The previous Federal Government, under the leadership of Labour Prime Minister Kevin Rudd, had implemented and facilitated initiatives at home and abroad in relation to mitigating the effects of climate change. Unfortunately, the US financial crash and the economic downturn of certain European and Asian countries halted the emphasis on climate change as a threat to the future of the world's populations, and all attention reverted to surviving from day to day. The momentum that had been gained in Australia halted, and then the new incoming Federal Liberal government refused to acknowledge climate change effects for reasons the populace could only guess at, and the new Liberal Queensland State Premier closed down departments relating to the environment, fisheries, primary industries, climate change and related areas and opened up uranium, coal and gas mining along with changing the laws to protect trees from mass clearing, even though two decades previously the international "watch dogs" pointed out that QLD was clearing as many trees as Indonesia and the Amazon; that was why the strict tree clearing laws had been enacted. Overall, doors were closed with very loud bangs and stunned silence or non–dissent was the climate of the day. This was in spite of strong evidence (as far back as ten years previously) that the forecast for high and extreme fire danger was likely to increase by 4–25% by 2020 and 15–70% by 2050 (Hennessy et al., 2005).

Following the dramatic floods and destructive Category 5 Cyclone Yasi in 2011, that complacency was seen for what it was. But not before a period of real disaster trauma consequences was acknowledged finally and emotions settled so that the emergent leaders and the regular emergency services and a range of disaster experienced community agencies such as the Red Cross, Salvos, Volunteering QLD and volunteers from every walk in life stepped up. By this time, the Federal Government, fortunately still under Labour leadership, allocated large grants to state and local governments to implement disaster recovery programs, functions and services. By the end of 2011, a year that had witnessed massive disasters within Australia and with its neighbours, the lethargy was lifting, and those citizens who were committed to disaster preparedness, mitigation, reconstruction and recovery marched ahead with energy and vision. The memory of the fateful February 2009 Victorian Bushfires and the tiny Queensland town of Grantham being wiped out by an inland wall of water in 2011, captured live by TV cameras from helicopters and affected residents, was one that they would never forget. Across Australia, the programs were created, improved, trialled and perfected in many different ways.

As indicated in the section on resilience and resourcefulness, Queensland achieved success in purveying one universal message (as recommended by Kolender & Bowman, 2004) about getting ready and taking personal responsibility for one's life and property. Many strategies had been developed at all levels and across all types of organisations and regions. The warning systems by email and mobile text message were well received across the country and while occasionally misfiring, proved to be a much appreciated intervention. Television and radio warnings and updates were attention grabbing, and even city buses conveyed messages about disaster preparedness on the outside and inside of vehicles. Well-constructed websites full of disaster preparedness and recovery material were exceptional.[8]

It is interesting to note that the TV advertisement about being prepared for summer storms (Be Prepared!) appeared as scheduled on the same night as a major destructive hail storm hit segments of Brisbane and other areas (27 November 2014), leaving many thousands of vehicles to be repaired, along with houses being unroofed and trees smashing over power lines etcetera. It warned of being prepared, but no-one could have been prepared for large hail streaming sideways without warning. In Chinchilla, a mining town to the far west of Brisbane, the hail stones were as big as a woman's hand.

Australia experiences up to eleven cyclones per annum. In Queensland, many of the cyclones reduce in impact before they cross land, and if they are classified as a Category 5 off the coast line, by the time they cross land their power has generally fallen to a Category 3 or 2. In the past four years, Queensland was beset by three Category 5 cyclones, which did not abate as they crossed land; one was Cyclone Yasi which hit central Queensland in 2011 (a few months after the major 2011 flood that devastated SEQ, and the highly destructive earthquake (6.3) and ensuing aftershocks which crippled the beautiful town of Christchurch in New Zealand, followed swiftly by the terrifying destructive force of the dramatic earthquake in Japan and its ensuing tsunami and nuclear hazards). Before the 6 April, 2015, Northern Australia had encountered four severe cyclones within one month: Lam, Marcia, Nathan and Olwyn.

In the summer of 2014/2015, the most amazing plan for cyclone preparedness went into action.

Instilling self-reliance: mustering the Australian populace into disaster preparedness

Australians are used to the term mustering being used mostly in regard to large flocks of sheep, but it is also sometimes used to herd cattle across wide treks of isolated land. A review of what occurred in preparation before the 2015 cyclones approached the QLD areas of Brisbane and the Gold Coast is akin to a successful muster. The people had been trained well, over and over again, through every conceivable media and communication tool and educational process. Simple, short messages were conveyed to the population about being prepared and avoiding risk-taking behaviours. The authorities had spent millions of dollars over four years on education and preparedness publicity and programs, website and training. Over and over again, they reinforced the concept of self-reliance with messages such as follow.

Table 33.1 Targeting natural disaster preparedness with short direct commands

Direct message	Hazard
Get down low and go, go, go	House fires
Remember if it's flooded . . . forget it	Flash floods and tidal/riverine floods
Don't let your life go down the drain	Flash floods and storms
Clean out your gutters	Bushfires and storms
Tie down loose furniture and objects	Severe storm and cyclonic winds
If it's too late, stay and defend your houses	Bushfires
If it's too late, find the strongest room in the house and pad it out with mattresses etc.	Cyclones
You may lose power: get batteries for torches	Storms, cyclones, floods
Stock up for 3 days of tinned and dry food and water	Storms, cyclones, floods
Stay away from fallen power lines	Storms, cyclones, floods, bushfires
Listen to your local ABC radio for updates	Storms, cyclones, floods, bushfires

So, there is no way that the public or disaster review teams could say that the authorities had not done their homework or educated the public.

Generally, it all worked; the main lesson was: we can't stop nature from inflicting vast damage on our homes, infrastructure, businesses, animals and wildlife. All of these natural hazards are going to happen regardless of what we do; what we have done is to prevent the hazard from becoming any more severe a disaster than it could be.

However, as indicated earlier, you can't stop the risk takers. Over and over again, the TV news coverage showed individuals and small groups going out for the big hype and adrenalin rush, going up to the ocean edge only to get 'wacked' by a massive wave, driving around in coastal towns while trees were flying around and rooves and walls being blown off houses and electrical power poles and lines were strewn across the streets.

At the end of the preparation and warning stage, the authorities on TV warned residents, and the newly appointed Premier of the QLD state and the disaster management officials reinforced the severity of the situation by stating very firmly, "We have withdrawn our men from the danger of storms/cyclones/floods/bushfires"; that is we cannot risk their lives for people who continue to deny reality by putting themselves into danger. This had been reflected in Western Australia and South Australia: "Leave your homes while you can safely do so; there will come a time when it will be unsafe for you to do so and you will then have to stay and defend your property and yourselves" and "We cannot put our firefighters into such life-threatening situations". (In recent months, many fire-fighters had been injured or badly burned, and several died.)

Summary and conclusion

Our main question to be addressed in this chapter was: "Can disaster preparedness be inculcated into enough individuals, communities, and organisations to create self-sufficiency and self-reliance when communities are isolated in the immediate hours and days leading up to and following catastrophic disasters."

The answer is: yes, this can be achieved – with adamant wake up calls from unrelenting natural disasters hammering communities, firm purpose, rationale strategies, co-operation across intra-state and inter-government levels, education and marketing suited to the culture of the population, and the inherent resilience and resourcefulness within a developed country (in this case, Australia).

In addition, those who have been hit the hardest are a valuable psychological resource and have the practical knowledge of assisting in the immediate aftermath of horrific consequences. For example it was the survivors of the 2009 Victorian Bushfires who quietly became a major support system for the people in Grantham, Queensland, whose town was drowned in 2011. Australian emergency service teams moved from helping in South East QLD floods to their friends across the ocean when the Christchurch earthquake erupted. Their actions show support and "mateship" at the deepest level of human compassion and practical problem solving.

Similarly medical and emergency service teams from Darwin (this season was the fortieth anniversary of the annihilation of Darwin by Cyclone Tracy) were the first area to respond immediately to devastated Vanuatu in 2015. And, as if proving that kindness expands, Micronesia was then aided by the preparedness strategies set up for Vanuatu.

These examples (and there are many others) are proof that people across all races and countries can come together to give a helping hand in times of disaster and transfer survival skills and recovery strategies – in solidarity and friendship.

In the spirit of the ANZACS, we can teach more people to simply ask, "Are you all right, mate?" or "Do you need a hand?" – simple words with so much meaning. A simple acknowledgement that something is wrong, that trauma has been experienced and that we really do care.

Notes

1 http://en.wikipedia.org/wiki/ring_of_fire/.
2 Abbreviations used in this chapter: QLD – Queensland, SEQ – South East Queenland, ND – natural disaster; NT – Northern Territory; WA – Western Australia; SA – South Australia; NZ – New Zealand.
3 www.smh.com.au/world/cyclone-pam-dozens-feared-dead-in-vanuatu-20150314.
4 www.abc.net.au/2015-03-14/forest-fire-threatens-valparaiso/6319442.
5 www.skynews.c-stories/2015/04/05/death-toll-inchile floods-rises-to-25.html.
6 DoiMoi – opening up of the Vietnamese economy by negotiating external trade.
7 www.theguardian.com/australia-news/live/2015/jan06/bushfires-conditions-worsening-in-south-australia-and-wa-on-alert-live.
8 The Somerset region is home to two very large dams used mainly for water storage for Brisbane. Somerset Regional Council in Queensland was one of the severely flood affected regions to implement many initiatives involving training local volunteers, disaster preparedness and recovery websites full of useful

information, sign-on for email or mobile text warnings, area action committees for any future man-made or natural disasters and emphasising the role of new and existing disaster preparedness officers (www.somerset.qld.gov.au).

References

Adger, W. N. (2000). Social and ecological resilience: Are they related? *Progress in Human Geography, 24*(3), 347–364.

Allison-Napolitano, E. T. (2014). *Bounce forward: The extraordinary resilience of leadership.* California: Corwin Press.

Bermejo, P. M. (2006). Preparation and response in case of natural disasters: Cuban programs and experience. *Journal of Public Health Policy, 27*(1), 13–21.

Celinski, M. J., Allen, L. M., & Gow, K. M. (2013). Assessing resilience in the aftermath of mass trauma. In K. Gow & M. Celinski (Eds.), *Mass trauma: Impact and recovery issues* (pp. 77–92). New York: Nova Science Publishers.

Celinski, M. J., & Gow, K. M. (2005). Trauma clients: How understanding disintegration can help to reveal resourcefulness of the self. *Australian Journal of Clinical and Experimental Hypnosis, 33*(2), 195–217.

Cottrell, A. (2008). Quiet achievers: Women's resilience to a seasonal disaster. In K. Gow & D. Paton (Eds.), *The phoenix of natural disasters: Community resilience* (pp. 181–193). New York: Nova Science Publications.

Earvolino-Ramirez, M. (2007). Resilience: A concept analysis. *Nursing Forum, 42*(2), 73–82.

Few, R., Pham Gia Tran, P., & Bui Thi Thuy Hong. (2004). *Living with floods: Health risks and coping strategies of the urban poor in Vietnam.* Paper prepared by British Academy (Committee for South East Asian Studies), Hanoi.

Gow, K. (2009). Can we anticipate more heatwaves, wildfires, droughts and deluges? In K. Gow (Ed.), *Meltdown: Climate change, natural disasters & other catastrophes – fears and concerns of the future* (pp. 157–174). New York: Nova Science Publications.

Gow, K., & Mohay, H. (2013). When community resilience breaks down after natural disasters. In K. Gow & M. Celinski (Eds.), *Mass trauma: Impact and recovery issues.* New York: Nova Science Publishers.

Gow, K., Pritchard, F., & Chant, D. (2008). How close do you have to be to learn the lesson? Fire burns! *The Australasian Journal of Trauma and Disasters and Trauma Studies, 2.* Retrieved from http://trauma.massey.ac.nz/issues/2008–2/gow.htm

Hennessy, K., Lucas, C., Nicholls, N., Bathols, J., Suppiah, R., & Ricketts, J. (2005). *Climate change impacts on fire-weather in south-east Australia.* Canberra: CSIRO, Commonwealth of Australia.

Kolender, B., & Bowman, J. (2004). *San Diego regional fire prevention and emergency preparedness task force.* San Diego, CA: San Diego Fire-Rescue Department. Retrieved from www/sandiego.gov/fireandems/

Manyena, B., O'Brien, G., O'Keefe, P., & Rose, J. (2011). Disaster resilience: A bounce back or bounce forward ability? *Local Environment: The International Journal of Justice and Sustainability, 16*(5), 417–424.

Mileti, D. D., & Fitzpatrick, C. (1992). The causal sequence of risk communication in the Parkfield earthquake prediction experiment. *Risk Analysis, 12*(3), 393–400.

Richardson, G. E. (2002). The metatheory of resilience and resiliency. *Journal of Clinical Psychology, 58*(3), 307–321.

Richardson, G. E., Neiger, B., Jensen, S., & Kumpfer, K. (1990). The resiliency model. *Health Education, 21*, 33–39.

34

The concept of resilience in the context of counterterrorism

Mark Dechesne

Introduction

Resilience is increasingly considered a key ingredient to effectively manage terrorism. Fareed Zakaria (2008) has been among the first to make the point that is now recognized by many: "In some unspoken way, people have recognized that the best counterterrorism policy is resilience. Terrorism is unusual in that it is a military tactic defined by the response of the onlooker" (p. 16).

In order to fight terrorism, then, we need to invest in resilience; that is we need to invest in the capability of 'the onlookers' to withstand the destabilizing effect that acts of terrorism or the threat thereof may bring about. To illustrate, Barack Obama (2013) pondered in his exposition of the US Counterterrorism strategy that:

> Victory will be measured in parents taking their kids to school; immigrants coming to our shores; fans taking in a ballgame; a veteran starting a business; a bustling city street; a citizen shouting her concerns at a President. The quiet determination; that strength of character and bond of fellowship; that refutation of fear – that is both our sword and our shield.

The resilience angle has further been recognized by Public Safety Canada (2012) where building resilience has become a cornerstone of counterterrorism policy. Indeed, the very title of the strategy reads, "Building Resilience Against Terrorism". A passage of the strategy further states:

> Resilience is both a principle and an underlying theme of the Strategy. Building a resilient Canada involves fostering a society in which individuals and communities are able to withstand violent extremist ideologies and challenge those who espouse them. They support and participate in efforts that seek to protect Canada and Canadian interests from terrorist threats. A resilient Canada is one that is able to mitigate the impacts of a terrorist attack, ensuring a rapid return to ordinary life.

Given the central place that the notion of 'resilience against terrorism' has in contemporary counterterrorism policy, it is of pertinence to consider the meaning of the concept resilience in the context of counterterrorism.

Note that, in the citation of Public Safety Canada just provided, 'resilience' has two meanings. It refers to the ability to withstand violent extremist ideologies, *and* to mitigate the impacts of a terrorist attack. Moreover, building resilience pertains both to individuals and communities. In bringing up this variation in resilience, the question arises of what ties these forms of resilience together? And, are other forms of resilience relevant in the context of counterterrorism? Questions as these inevitably lead to more fundamental questions: what is actually meant by resilience in the context of counterterrorism? Is counterterrorism policy attending to all facets of resilience? And, if not, what can we do to increase specific facets of resilience?

Theoretical foundation

> Resilience's scientific value lies not in whether it can be easily captured and quantified but in whether it leads to novel hypotheses about the characteristics of – and relations between – stressors, various adaptive capacities, and wellness over time.
>
> (Norris, Stevens, Pfefferbaum, Wyche, & Pfefferbaum, 2008, p. 146)

Norris et al. (2008) have noted that resilience is a concept originally from physics used to describe "the capacity of a material or system to return to equilibrium after a displacement" (p. 127). In emergency management, it has become a metaphor to refer to the capacity of a community to return to 'life as usual' after being confronted with a disaster. Formally, Norris et al. (2008) define resilience in the context of emergency management as "a process linking a network of adaptive capacities (resources with dynamic attributes) to adaptation after a disturbance or adversity" (p. 127).

Terrorism is a complex and dynamic process (LaFree, Dugan, & Korte, 2009; McCauley & Moskalenko, 2011) that implicates disturbances and adversity at various levels. Hence, I propose that, in order to use the concept of resilience in the context of counterterrorism, one needs to take into account that terrorism is a complex, dynamic process involving multiple actors, and therefore, resilience in the context of terrorism takes on multiple forms. And indeed, if one adopts a singular angle to resilience, significant components of building a resilient society against terrorism may remain obscured.

The dynamics of terrorism

The point of departure of the present analysis is that terrorism, as we know it today, is a form of political violence, whereby a group or individual opposes current practices espoused by a government through the threat or actual use of violence. This violence may be targeted towards representatives of the government (e.g. government officials); symbols of the government (e.g. buildings but also non-governmental, high-profile public figures that support the government); or elements of the general populations that supports the government. The violence affects how the violent opposition is perceived by the general public and by (potential) supporters of the violent opposition within society. The government, in turn, is forced to respond, and how it does so affects perceptions of the government by supporting members of society, but also by opposing members and those supporting the violent opposition. The non-violent political opposition is also forced to make a stand and, thus, to choose sides with either the government or the violent opposition. In a globalized world, this dynamic occurs while an international community of state and non-state actors is observing and taking a stand towards the violent opposition and the government, while being held accountable by their respective constituencies.

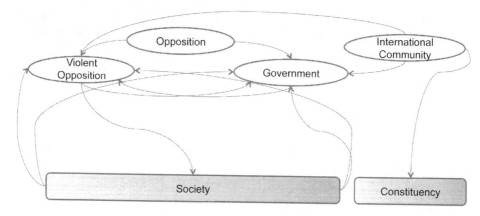

Figure 34.1   The dynamics of terrorism

Figure 34.1 provides a graphical depiction of the elements and relations involved in the process just described: note that society contains both supporters and opponents to the government. Supporters are depicted on the right, and opponents are depicted on the left of the "Society" box.

The many faces of resilience

Note that, in Figure 34.1, it is difficult to point to a single spot where 'resilience', as a singular construct, can be placed. Indeed, resilience can be put at different locations, with a different interpretation and set of implications at each location. First, one could consider the resilience of individuals directly under the threat of terrorism, e.g. threatened politicians or the victims of a terrorist attack. Here resilience is a *psychological capacity* to maintain equanimity in the presence of a real threat and the ability to bounce back after being exposed to terror-induced trauma. Second, one could also consider resilience in terms of the ability of a *society/community* to maintain cohesion under the threat of terrorism and to recover from terrorist attacks. Third, resilience may also be interpreted as the ability of potential supporters of the violent opposition to withstand the *ideology* of the violent opposition. Fourth, resilience may be the *political ability* of governing and opposing political parties to take a unified stance against violence while disagreeing over other, high-stakes issues. Finally, resilience may also pertain to ability of the government and country to maintain its *international reputation* while involved in counterterrorism efforts. Thus, in the context of terrorism/counterterrorism, resilience has many faces. It may refer to psychological resilience, community resilience, ideological resilience, political resilience, or international resilience. Figure 34.2 places these interpretations of resilience within the dynamic framework of terrorism.

The key point of the foregoing analysis is that the concept of resilience has many faces when considered in the context of (counter)terrorism. To the extent that building resilience is considered a core element of counterterrorism policy, it is critical to differentiate between the separate components of resilience. What do we know about the separate components?

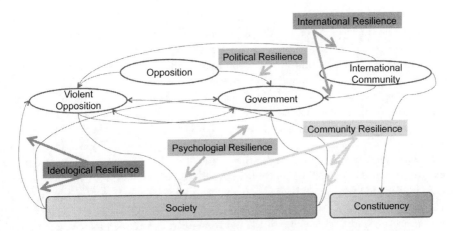

Figure 34.2 The place(s) of resilience in a dynamic framework of terrorism

Psychological resilience

There is ample research regarding the factors that foster the ability to maintain equanimity in the presence of a real threat and the ability to bounce back after being exposed to terror-induced trauma (see for example Dechesne, 2012, for a review). Some comes from experimental studies. Experiments inspired by terror management theory (e.g. Greenberg, Solomon, & Pyszczysnki, 1997; Pyszczynski, Solomon, & Greenberg, 2003), for instance, show that subtle reminders of death can lead to a variety of defensive responses, most notably a tendency for self-aggrandizement and a need to bolster one's worldview either by upholding those who share the same worldview or by derogating those who have different viewpoints. Experiments show that these responses are generally attenuated by two main factors: self-esteem, with the higher one's stable self-esteem, the lower the necessity to engage in psychological defense (e.g. Harmon-Jones et al., 1997), and a sense of meaning in life, with the greater sense of meaning, the lesser the apparent need to engage in psychological defense (e.g. Arndt, Greenberg, Solomon, Pyszczynski, & Simon, 1997). Perhaps relatedly or perhaps separately, there is also evidence that a firm belief in afterlife mitigates psychological defenses followed by death reminders (Dechesne et al., 2003). These experimental findings are of interest to describe in the context of resilience on terrorism, as there appears a marked similarity between the findings and the typical responses observed after terrorist attacks (see Pyszczynski et al., 2003, for details).

These experimental findings obtained from the mortality salience paradigm coincide, at least partially, with findings from real-life research based on the so-called cognitive adaptation theory (Taylor, 1983). Taylor and colleagues developed this theory on the basis of their research of breast cancer survivors. Counterintuitively, they found that illusory levels of self-enhancement, sense of control, and sense of meaning were correlated with more effective coping with breast cancer. In a classic follow-up review, Taylor and Brown (1988) demonstrated that, across a variety of health and performance domains, the effects of illusions about self-image, self-control, and meaning were indeed associated with adaptation, personal and social efficacy, and a positive outlook on life. Bolstering one's self-image, one's sense of control, and one's sense of meaning may thus contribute to psychological resilience.

Probably only limitedly aware of these findings, as they were reported in the psychological literature, a group of psychiatrists, all experts in the area of psychological adaptation and disaster management, once convened to name those elements for which evidence exists that they contribute to better adjustment in the face of disaster (Hobfoll et al., 2007). The psychiatrists identified safety, calmness, connected, self-efficacy, and hope as the key elements to adaptation. In one way or the other, the elements of connectedness, and in particular of self-efficacy and hope seems to be related to the elements of a positive self-image, self-control, and meaning, identified in the psychological literature. The elements of safety and calmness add a practical dimension. Clearly, even the strongest mind will need to establish a sense of safety and remain calm first, before adjusting mentally to the threats faced.

In a real-life investigation of the psychological factors involved in adaptive coping with, I together with colleagues from the Dutch Military Academy (Dechesne, Van den Berg, & Soeters, 2006) asked a group of Dutch soldiers either at rest in their European Headquarters or on site during a mission in Afghanistan about fear. In Afghanistan, fear levels were generally higher than at headquarters. This is no surprise, as the base in Afghanistan was frequently attacked by the Taliban. From a research perspective, one could argue that it therefore provided a good testing ground for resilience research. And, indeed, consistent with some of these findings, it was found that soldiers with a greater sense of self-efficacy, and a greater belief in the mission, were less likely to experience fear, and this was only found where the fear was tangible, at the mission site in Afghanistan.

Community resilience

The ability of a community to remain unaffected by terrorist attacks and, to the extent it is affected, to bounce back from the negative experience has received considerable attention in academic research and policy (see e.g. Norris et al., 2008; Galea et al., 2002, for reviews). Indeed, community resilience is probably the most commonly studied form of resilience, and by now, nations including the United States and Canada have an extensive repertoire of indicators and assessments to prevent major disasters from affecting communities in a lasting detrimental way. The events unfolding after Hurricane Katrina have particularly increased the awareness of the importance of community resilience assessment. And this has shown to be the case. When the massive storm Sandy hit the United States in 2012, the communal impact was significantly lower compared to Katrina, despite considerable havoc. At present, there is little attention concerning the difference between community resilience in the context of terrorism versus community resilience in the context of other disasters (but see Norris et al., 2008).

Research shows there are multiple factors that contribute negatively to community resilience. Community-level trauma as a result of continuous exposure to violence and disaster has been argued to negatively affect community resilience. It has been observed for example that, on a communal level, Palestinians typically show increased levels of PTSD, and it has been argued that this affects the community's ability to cope with the violence and wrongdoings in the Israeli-Palestinian conflict (Canetti et al., 2010; Post, 2010). Socio-economic status and ethnic minority status have also been observed to weaken community resilience. DiGrande et al. (2008) showed that low education levels, low income, and Hispanic ethnicity were predictors of reduced coping ability in the aftermath of the 9/11 World Trade Center attacks. Moreover, communal cohesion, family cohesion is particular, has been shown to positively contribute to effective coping. Henrich and Shahar (2008) have shown that close relationships with family and friends undermined the effects of rocket attack among a sample of Israeli middle school students. Silver et al. (2002) found marital separation a predictor of PTSD risk following the 9/11 attacks.

Ideological resilience

Ideological resilience refers to the ability of community to withstand extremist thought and to recover from extremist thought once it has become a significant part of the life of an individual or a community. Unlike psychological and communal resilience, there need not be a physical threat in order for ideological resilience to become relevant. Indeed, an assumption underlying the notion of ideological resilience is that a particular thought can also undermine the functioning of an individual or a community. Clearly, this is a controversial assumption. One cannot really tell whether a radical thought is really threatening for an individual or a community. In the context of terrorism and counterterrorism, the frequently heard saying "one man's terrorist is another man's freedom fighter" illustrates the difficulty of distinguishing the extreme from the sane and necessary. Of interest, Kruglanski et al. (2014) recently suggested that radicalism can be understood as a fixation on particular means to achieve a goal, a fixation that ironically reduces the chances that the goal is achieved. Thus, the commitment to violence as the only means to achieve a desired societal state, may ironically prevent the achievement the desired societal state. To underscore, the ETA, one of Europe's most active terrorist groups over the past decades, saw its number of supporters significantly increase after it disavowed its commitment to violence.

Both the prevention of the spreading of radical thoughts and the return to more moderate viewpoints after being exposed to radical thoughts have received considerable attention in the literature and in counterterrorism practice (see e.g. Dechesne, 2011). In the former case, the emphasis is on 'counterradicalization', in the latter case on 'deradicalization'. There seems to be general consensus that prevention is critical. In other words, the effectiveness of 'counterradicalization' is considered greater than the effectiveness of 'deradicalization', although most research attention has been devoted to the workings of deradicalization. Counterradicalization typically involves the mobilization of a particular community to identify and counteract on expressions of radicalism. This comes in the form of key leader engagement within a community to counteract on radical tendencies and to involve community workers, including physicians, teachers, and clergyman, to promote radicalization and to serve a liaisons to the government to avoid a splitting of particular elements from society at large.

Deradicalization aims for the reversal of extremist thoughts to more moderate points of view (see e.g. Horgan & Braddock, 2010). This reversal, although considered to be among the keys to an effective post-conflict recovery, turns out to be difficult to establish. A common understanding dictates that stopping radical behavior is much easier achieved than stopping radical thoughts. Especially early attempts to bring radical Islamists to more acceptable views have yielded disappointing results (see Rabasa, Pettyjohn, Ghez, & Boucek, 2011, for an extensive review). The dialogue initiative in Yemen, which focused on establishing religious dialogue between imprisoned extremists and moderate imams, failed to close the ideological divide. More extensive programs, such as in Saudi Arabia and most notably Singapore, that not only focus on ideological conceptions but also pay attention to the public, economic, and particularly the psychological components have reported greater successes. Yet, at present, in the absence of a clear understanding of the cognitive architecture of radical thoughts and the process of deradicalization, the results of deradicalization remain difficult to assess. Accordingly, it requires further theory development and research to effectively assess the level of ideological resilience.

Political resilience

Whereas psychological, community, and ideological resilience have received considerable research attention, few advances have been made to understand the factors contributing to political resilience or the breakdown of political resilience. This is quite remarkable. The ability of a political system to function effectively during an episode of terrorism may indeed be considered a key requirement for an effective response to terrorism. Oftentimes, it is assumed that terrorist attacks generally bring the general public together and also make politicians give up their differences and stand side by side against the perpetrators of terrorist attacks. This is for example conveyed in one of the most iconic images of the days after the World Trade Center and Pentagon Attacks, when members of the US Congress, indeed at that time already infamous for their divisions, were shown standing together on the stairs of Capitol Hill univocally singing "God Bless America".

It should be noted, however, that a key element to terrorist strategy is to show that a government and the larger political establishment is unequipped to deal with the terrorist perpetrators, that the system of governance will show its impotence and fall apart (e.g. Dechesne, 2012). And there are cases where governments were seriously put to the test by terrorist attacks. Independence movements in Israel and Algeria, often portrayed as terrorist by the ruling colonial powers, effectively used armed struggle as an instrument to drive a wedge within the colonial political establishment, eventually forcing the colonizers to withdraw. A very salient example of a failure of political resilience in the face of a terrorist attack can be found in Spain following the 3/11 Madrid Bombings of 2004, indeed the largest terrorist attack on Spanish soil (e.g. Levitt, 2014). It has created a rupture in the political landscape, especially because the attacks happened during election season. Eventually, the competing parties diverged in their interpretation of the attacks, with consequences up to this day. There are, for example multiple victim associations that are divided along political lines. Clearly, political division may constitute a hindrance for any country involved in counterterrorism campaigns, but at present, there is little known, academically, regarding the factors that contribute to political cohesion or factionalism in response to terrorist attacks.

International resilience

Even less attention has been paid to the factors that promote international resilience, i.e. the ability of a country to maintain its international reputation, while engaged in a counterterrorism campaign. Perhaps this lack of attention may be attributable to the labeling. International reputation and resilience are typically not considered under the same umbrella. International reputation may come from a country's respect for human rights or its ability to be a trusted partner in trade or simply its power on the international scene. Thus, at present, it may not be clear how reputation and resilience relate. Nonetheless, the Snowden scandal involving the publication of thousands of secret NSA documents show the extent to which damage to international reputation may undermine the ability of a country to engage in counterterrorism (Washington Post, 2013). As we are living in an increasingly globalized world, intelligence sharing between countries constitutes a key to any effective counterterrorism campaign. Having good standing with other countries will greatly facilitates this intelligence sharing. Therefore, despite its less-than-obvious linkage, consideration of resilience in the context of counterterrorism would benefit from inclusion of international relations.

Many faces of resilience but a shared basis in collective identity

An important outcome of the present reflection, then, is that resilience in the context of counterterrorism is not one 'thing'. Rather, it is a multi-fold strategy that involves building capacity to enable individuals, communities, ideologies, political systems, and nations vis-à-vis other nations to remain with equanimity when terror strikes and to bounce back after the damage is done.

Assuming the goal of building resilience in all its facets, the challenge thereby inevitably arises how to most effectively do so. One could create separate programs for each facet of resilience. Thus, building psychological resilience would require psychological resilience programs, building community resilience would require separate community resilience programs, etc. However, this approach overlooks the common basis of the separate forms of resilience. At least, in closing, I want to argue that, although there are separate forms of resilience against terrorism, these forms have an important common origin in a shared sense of identity. Building resilience in all its facets requires developing and maintaining a shared sense of identity, a perception of oneself as a people and the presentation of that identity to the outside world.

A shared sense of identity helps to bolster all aspects of resilience. A shared sense of identity will facilitate the individual's self-definition and serve a source of self-esteem for those who are part of the collective, features that have been shown in research to promote psychological resilience. A shared sense of identity as a people will strengthen community ties and thus promote community resilience. A shared sense of identity will also provide the individual within the community with values and ideas and thus with guidelines to differentiate between acceptable and extremist values and ideas, promoting ideological resilience. A shared sense of identity will also help politicians and public figures to engage in debate and to disagree while at the same time realizing that there is a common ground, enabling conditions for constructive dialogue, eliminating the necessity to resort to violence to advance political goals, and thus bolstering political resilience. Finally, having a shared identity clarifies one's position in the international sphere, thus enabling international resilience.

Characteristics of a balanced identity

Not all senses of shared identity will be equally equipped to bolster the forms of resilience outlined earlier. For instance, an identity based on absolutist ideas may considerably bolster self-definition and self-esteem and hence promote psychological resilience but, at the same time, may hamper non-violent political debate, and international dialogue, thereby undermining political and international resilience. What characteristics should the shared sense of identity have in order to optimally bolster all facets of resilience?

1 *Inclusiveness* seems to be a key feature. In order to bolster all forms of resilience, the shared sense of identity within a country should be truly shared among all constituents and cannot exclude particular groups.
2 *Plurality:* One of the implications of inclusiveness is that the sense of identity will be shared among different constituencies. Although all these constituencies endorse the same identity, this should not imply that all these constituencies will need to be the same. The shared sense of identity should recognize plurality among its adherents. "Out of many, one" so to speak.
3 *Tolerance:* In order for a plural sense of shared identity to function effectively, and to guarantee true inclusiveness, tolerance seems to be a third critical ingredient.
4 *Equity:* Tolerance, acceptance of the other, may not be enough. The shared identity should also be based on equity principles: adherence to the identity should come with rights, and contributions to strengthen the shared identity should come with rewards.
5 Finally, the principles associated with the shared identity should be *consequential*, in the sense that they are actively upheld by all members of the community, and violations of norms and values associated with the shared identity are dealt with.

Towards a counterterrorism strategy

How can the foregoing analysis be used to develop a comprehensive counterterrorism strategy? The key idea is that in order to deal with terrorist attacks, one needs to build resilience. Resilience in the context of terrorism comes in five different forms: psychological resilience, community resilience, ideological resilience, political resilience, and international resilience. While each type of resilience has its unique features, origins, and consequences, all types of resilience are considerably enhanced by bolstering a shared sense of identity. Not all shared senses of identity are equally equipped to bolster the separate elements of resilience, however. To build resilience against terrorism in all its facets, the optimal shared sense of identity should be inclusive, should recognize plurality, should be tolerant towards other conceptions, and should provide equity, and adherence to the identity should have consequences.

A program that seeks to build resilience against terrorism should thus explore opportunities for constructing common basis of identity for the community and seek ways to strengthen that identity. This common sense of identity, in turn, could serve as the foundation on which separate resilience program can be build.

References

Arndt, J., Greenberg, J., Solomon, S., Pyszczynski, T., & Simon, L. (1997). Suppression, accessibility of death-related thoughts, and cultural worldview defense: Exploring the psychodynamics of terror management. *Journal of Personality and Social Psychology, 73*(1), 5–18.

Canetti, D., Galea, S., Hall, B. J., Johnson, R. J., Palmieri, P. A., & Hobfoll, S. E. (2010). Exposure to prolonged socio-political conflict and the risk of PTSD and depression among Palestinians. *Psychiatry: Interpersonal and Biological Processes, 73*(3), 219–232.

Dechesne, M. (2011). Deradicalization: Not soft, but strategic. *Crime, Law and Social Change, 55*(4), 287–292.

Dechesne, M. (2012). The sociopsychological impact of terrorism: Key concepts, research, and theory. In U. Kumar & M. K. Mandal (Eds.), *Countering terrorism: Psychosocial strategies* (pp. 74–95). New Delhi: Sage Publications.

Dechesne, M., Van Den Berg, C. & Soeters, J. (2006). International collaboration under threat: A field study in Kabul. *Conflict Management and Peace Science, 24*(1), 25–36.

Dechesne, M., Pyszczynski, T., Arndt, J., Ransom, S., Sheldon, K. M., van Knippenberg, A., & Janssen, J. (2003). Literal and symbolic immortality: The effect of evidence of literal immortality on self-esteem striving in response to mortality salience. *Journal of Personality and Social Psychology, 84*(4), 722–737.

DiGrande, L., Perrin, M. A., Thorpe, L. E., Thaljl, L., Murphy, J., Wu, D., . . . & Brackbill, R. M. (2008). Posttraumatic stress symptoms, PTSD, and risk factors among lower Manhattan residents 2–3 years after the September 11: 2001 terrorist attacks. *Journal of Traumatic Stress, 21*(3), 264–273.

Galea, S., Ahern, J., Resnick, H., Kilpatrick, D., Bucuvalas, M., Gold, J., & Vlahov, D. (2002). Psychological sequelae of the September 11 terrorist attacks in New York City. *The New England Journal of Medicine, 346*(13), 982–987.

Greenberg, J., Solomon, S., & Pyszczynski, T. (1997). Terror management theory of self-esteem and social behavior: Empirical assessments and conceptual refinements. In M. P. Zanna (Ed.), *Advances in experimental social psychology* (Vol. 29, pp. 61–139). New York: Academic Press.

Harmon-Jones, E., Simon, L., Greenberg, J., Pyszczynski, T., Solomon, S., & McGregor, H. (1997). Terror management theory and self-esteem: Evidence that increased self-esteem reduced mortality salience effects. *Journal of Personality and Social Psychology, 72*(1), 24–36.

Henrich, C. C., & Shahar, G. (2008). Social support buffers the effect of terrorism on adolescent depression: Findings from Sderot, Israel. *Journal of American Academy of Child Adolescent Psychiatry, 47*(9), 1073–1076.

Hobfoll, S., Watson, P., Bell, C., Bryant, R., Brymer, M., Friedman, M., . . . Ursano, R. (2007). Five essential elements of immediate and mid-term mass trauma intervention: Empirical evidence. *Psychiatry, 70*(4), 283–315.

Horgan, J., & Braddock, K. (2010). Rehabilitating the terrorists?: Challenges in assessing the effectiveness of de-radicalization programs. *Terrorism and Political Violence, 22*(2), 267–291.

Kruglanski, A. W., Gelfand, M. J., Bélanger, J. J., Sheveland, A., Hetiarachchi, M., & Gunaratna, R. (2014). The psychology of radicalization and deradicalization: How significance quest impacts violent extremism. *Political Psychology, 35*(Suppl 1), 69–93.

LaFree, G., Dugan, L., & Korte, R. (2009). The impact of British counterterrorist strategies on political violence in Northern Ireland: Comparing deterrence and backlash models. *Criminology: An Interdisciplinary Journal, 47*(1), 17–45.

Levitt, J. (2014). *Analysis: On 10th anniversary of Madrid Al Qaeda 3–11 bombing, analysts apply lessons to fight terror in Israel.* The Algemeiner. Retrieved from www.algemeiner.com/2014/03/11/analysis-on-10th-anniversary-of-madrid-al-qaeda-3–11-bombing-analysts-apply-lessons-to-fight-terror-in-israel/

McCauley, C., & Moskalenko, S. (2011). *Friction: How radicalization happens to them and us.* New York, NY, US: Oxford University Press.

Norris, F. H., Stevens, S. P., Pfefferbaum, B., Wyche, K. F., & Pfefferbaum, R. L. (2008). Community resilience as a metaphor, theory, set of capacities, and strategy for disaster readiness. *American Journal of Community Psychology, 41*(1–2), 127–150.

Obama, B. (2013). *President Obama discusses US counter-terrorism strategy.* Retrieved from www.whitehouse.gov/the-press-office/2013/05/23/remarks-president-national-defense-university

Post, J. M. (2010). Commentary on 'Exposure to prolonged socio-political conflict and the risk of PTSD and depression among Palestinians': Bio-psychosocial foundations of contemporary terrorism. *Psychiatry: Interpersonal and Biological Processes, 73*(3), 244–247.

Public Safety Canada. (2012). *Building resilience against terrorism: Canada's counter-terrorism strategy.* Retrieved from www.publicsafety.gc.ca/prg/ns/2012-cts-eng.aspx

Pyszczynski, T., Solomon, S., & Greenberg, J. (2003). *In the wake of 9/11: The psychology of terror.* Washington, DC, US: American Psychological Association.

Rabasa, A., Pettyjohn, S., Ghez, J., & Boucek, C. (2011). *Deradicalizing Islamist extremists.* Washington, DC: RAND.

Silver, R. C., Holman, E. A., McIntosh, D. N., Poulin, M., & Gil-Rivas, V. (2002) Nationwide longitudinal study of psychological responses to September 11. *Journal of the American Medical Association, 288*(10), 1235–1244.

Taylor, S. E. (1983). Adjustment to threatening events: A theory of cognitive adaptation. *American Psychologist, 38*(11), 1161–1173.

Taylor, S. E., & Brown, J. (1988). Illusion and well-being: A social psychological perspective on mental health. *Psychological Bulletin, 103*(2), 193–210.

Washington Post. (2013). NSA secrets: Government spying in the internet age. Washington DC: Diversion Books.

Zakaria, F. (2008). *The Post-American world.* London: Allen Lane.

35

Diffusing portable radiation detectors among first responders

Device acceptance and implications for community resilience[1]

Brooke M. Fowler, Irina Illes, Brooke Fisher Liu,
Holly A. Roberts, Elizabeth L. Petrun
and Gary A. Ackerman

In the past decade, the US government has employed new national security technologies to meet rising security threats, technologies such as explosive, firearm, and chemical and biological weapons detectors (e.g. Hofer & Wetter, 2012, p. 278). Despite past tragedies such as the September 11 terrorist attacks and the important role police play in our society, there remains a gap in understanding how effective communication along with other motivators can enhance police technology adoption. In turn, effective technology adoption can enhance community safety and resilience (Anderson, Knutson, Giles, & Arroyo, 2002), though research on first responders' role in community resilience remains understudied (Wyche et al., 2011).

Due to the unique nature of police work and the structure of police departments, the adoption of new technologies can present challenges for police departments (Flanagin, 2002). While the public overwhelmingly expects emergency responders to use new technology, the reality is that police departments tend to be slow to incorporate new technology into their risk surveillance, prevention, and communication (American Red Cross, 2010; Heverin & Zach, 2010). New technology can greatly improve proactive policing (Dunlap, 2014; Flanagin, 2002). However, there remains a gap on *how* to actually use and incorporate these new technologies into departments and whether police use of specific new technologies increases community resilience versus yielding potential unintended consequences (e.g. negative media coverage and public responses to controversial security technology).

This chapter presents the current knowledge and gaps surrounding police as an example of first responders' technology adoption, with a particular emphasis on the diffusion of new security technologies. Then, the chapter reports perhaps the first field test where scientists from a US federal defense agency collaborated with communication scientists to test how police reacted to adopting portable radiation detectors (PRDs). We do so through an ethnographic field test during which we observed and interacted with fourteen police force members while they deployed the devices for the first time during a major public event.

Literature review

In this section, we first define PRDs and then introduce the theoretical foundation for our research: diffusion of innovation theory. We then move to an overview of police attitudes and behaviors surrounding these devices, followed by a synthesis of research on police technology adoption and the implications for community resilience.

Portable radiation detectors (PRDs) defined

Portable radiation detectors (PRDs) are instruments carried on the person that alert users to dangerous levels of radiation in their environment. The most modern version of PRDs – as discussed here – can inform authorities of radiation levels on a larger scale through collectively maintaining a constant yet fluid and dispersed network of detection when connected to a data system, such as through a carrier's cell phone. Consequently, these devices allow for comprehensive environmental coverage at an affordable price (Liu, Bunn, & Chandy, 2011). While much research focuses on the technical and implementation issues surrounding portable radiation detectors (e.g. Aloise, 2005; Vaseashta, Susmann, Braman, & Enaki, 2012), only two studies were found that focus on the adoption process itself among those at the front lines of community resilience: emergency responders, including police (Cameron, 2008; TECHBeat, 2012).

Diffusion of innovation theory overview

Diffusion of innovation is "the process by which an innovation is communicated through certain channels over time among the members of a social system" (Rogers, 2003, p. 35). The diffusion process includes (1) *knowledge* about an innovation's existence and how it works; (2) *persuasion*, which is when a favorable or unfavorable attitude is formed among potential adopters; (3) the *decision* on whether to adopt the innovation; (4) *implementation*, which is when adopters put an innovation into practice; and (5) *confirmation*, which is when adopters seek reinforcement regarding their decision to use the innovation (Rogers, 2003).

Innovations, such as PRDs, contain five attributes that can incentivize acceptance or create barriers to acceptance: relative advantage, compatibility, complexity, trialability, and observability (Chaudhuri, Aboulnasr, & Ligas, 2010; Rogers, 2003). Relative advantage reflects the benefits that an innovation may bring to a potential adopter compared to any other competing options. Compatibility refers to whether an innovation readily fits within a potential adopter's life, which includes being consistent with existing values, past experiences, and the adopter's needs. Complexity refers to a potential adopter's perception of how difficult it is to understand and/or use the innovation. Trialability refers to the ability to experiment with an innovation before making an adoption decision, and observability is the degree to which an innovation's results are visible to others. Finally, the time needed to adopt an innovation, clarity, and consistency of communication about an innovation, and social systems' perceptions and relative support of an innovation also impact an innovation's chances of diffusion within a particular group or community (Bratan, Stramer, & Greenhalgh, 2010; Rogers, 2003).

Police attitudes/behaviors surrounding PRDs

Of the two found studies that touch upon PRD adoption issues among first responders was the rollout of PRDs to the Suffolk County (NY) Police Department. This represented the introduction of radiological detectors to first responders in the suburbs. These responders possessed very

425

little prior knowledge of or experience with such devices. In this case, poor training and inadequate knowledge of the operation of PRDs resulted in adoption problems such as embarrassing false positives (Cameron, 2008).

A second case was the voluntary distribution of over 6,000 pager-size Polimaster PRDs to first responders in a pilot program in Illinois, beginning in 2010 (TECHBeat, 2012). Elements that were viewed as successful in this pilot were 1) the ability of the first responders to adjust the sensitivity of the detectors in order to account for different levels of expected background radiation, and 2) if high levels of radiation were detected, responders would be contacted by experts to verify the threat and provide assistance (i.e. reach back was provided).

In addition to these specific case reports, a number of sources discuss radiological detection or radiological/nuclear threats in general, from which some relevant inferences can be drawn. First, with respect to the potential barriers that might be experienced, a high rate of false positives might deter adoption (or at least proper usage) (Subgroup on Radon Epidemiology, 2009). Second, the implementation of new detection technologies can be hindered by the reluctance of institutions to reveal internal knowledge to other entities (Vaseashta et al., 2012). Cost and usability issues are also key – having a detector that is too expensive or that must be connected to a power source or computer to function will delay adoption (Record, 2012).

Police technology adoption

While limited literature is available specifically on police attitudes towards PRDs, there has been a clear shift in the role of police in society that may indicate a policing climate that is receptive to technology such as PRDs (Oliver, 2006). In the past, policing in the United States was primarily a reactive field; however, between the 1980s and 1990s, policing began to shift towards community policing and a proactive approach to crime prevention (Bratton, 2012; Oliver, 2006). Community policing has been defined in a variety of ways, but the core concepts are 1) a focus on the underlying problems that cause crime; 2) collaboration with community; 3) proactive and preventative action; 4) relationship building with local businesses, government, neighboring police agencies, and community members; and 5) rebuilding trust in police among citizens (Chappell & Gibson, 2009; Friedmann & Cannon, 2007; Maguire & Wells, 2002; Oliver, 2006).

After the September 11 terrorist attacks, a new approach to police work in the US began to take hold, known as homeland security policing (Chappell & Gibson, 2009; Friedmann & Cannon, 2007; Oliver, 2006). Homeland security policing focuses on 1) preventing terrorism, 2) collecting intelligence to aid in the prevention of terrorist attacks, 3) strengthening relationships between police and government agencies, and 4) preparing to respond to terrorist attacks (Chappell & Gibson, 2009; Friedmann & Cannon, 2007).

This shift occurred in part because of the increased fear of terrorism in the US (Oliver, 2006), which according to the Pew Research Center (2015) has remained a constant concern in the eyes of the public since September 11. After these attacks, the public began to expect the government to do more to prevent terrorism in the US (Oliver, 2006). Another reason for the shift is that the general consensus among researchers and practitioners was a new understanding of the crucial role police play in the prevention of terrorism in the US (Friedmann & Cannon, 2007), especially because of their scanning ability (Nunn, 2005). Police are in a good position to help prevent terrorism by being involved with and constantly collecting data on their communities (Nunn, 2005).

A better understanding of the perceived risk of radiation from intentional and unintentional sources may also facilitate PRD adoption among police. Alternatively, PRDs' association with radiation (even though detectors emit no radiation themselves) might present obstacles to adoption. If the perceived risk and stigmas of radiation are high enough, it may be possible that some police officers will associate this risk with the detectors themselves and thus perceive that using a device intended for detecting radiation carries high risk. Therefore, understanding how police officers perceive the risk of using PRDs may result in a better understanding of how to also encourage adoption of the technology. With respect to ameliorating such concerns, one study found that a higher perceived risk of using a device requires an increased emphasis on educating the user on the ease of use of that device in order to encourage adoption of the technology (Im, Kim, & Han, 2008). This study also found that, when encouraging the adoption of technology that is utilitarian in nature, the value of that technology to the user's job should be emphasized to encourage the use of the new technology (Im et al., 2008).

Police have a long history of adopting and creating new technologies to further their policing capabilities (Bratton, 2012; Flanagin, 2002). In a speech by William Bratton, the former chief executive of the Police Departments of Los Angeles, New York City, and Boston, he equated the adoption of technology in policing as "a [m]atter of [e]mbracing [c]hange" (2012, p. 22). "Policing is a profession that is all about change. If you're the kind of person who resists changes in how things are done, American policing is the wrong profession for you" (Bratton, 2012, p. 22). Despite this open attitude towards embracing new technology, police face organizational in addition to individual challenges when adopting new technology, especially budgets that may not allow for purchasing and supporting new technologies (Flanagin, 2002; Wexler, 2012). New technologies require training, and the cost and time of training officers on new technologies will have to be considered (Wexler, 2012). This means that new technologies will need to be able to demonstrate some level of return on investment (Gascón & Foglesong, 2010; Roberts, 2011) and produce measurable improvement (Bratton, 2012).

Method

The research team conducted an ethnographic field test of portable radiological/nuclear (RN) detectors. Ethnographic field research is ideal for in-depth exploration of how people perceive, understand, and attribute meaning in their everyday lives (Berg, 2009). By "being there" the researcher can come closer to "experiencing and understanding the 'insider's' point of view" (Hume & Mulcock, 2004, p. xi).

The observed field test involved distributing nine detectors to fourteen law enforcement officials who would monitor checkpoints for a July 4th, 2014, event in Washington, DC. Test detectors required a connection to a cell phone in order to function properly. The detectors connected to a cell phone in order to continuously transmit data to a central location for real-time analysis. Prior to the field test, officers attended a mandatory training on how to use and interact with the device, and a device support team was available throughout the field test to provide technical support. However, on the observation day, some detectors ended up delegated or handed off to other officers who did not receive training. Finally, during the field test, all officers also wore their standard PRDs, and the baseline defensive capability was not affected.

Field observations were conducted on July 4, 2014, to gain a realistic understanding of a densely populated and monitored event in the city. Police officers from various units assigned to monitor checkpoints and received the detectors in a small, green bag, designed to be worn on a belt. Each bag contained a detector and a cell phone.[2] Throughout the field test, an IT team was tasked with the technical operational success of the devices, checked battery charges, and addressed any technology-related concerns.

The research team consisted of four researchers, who split into teams of two, to observe user attitudes and behaviors regarding the detectors. Prior to the observations, the team compiled an analytic memo outlining the research purpose, objectives, protocols, and the following guiding field questions, derived from diffusion of innovation theory:

1   How do the officers physically handle the device?
2   How, if at all, do the officers discuss the device?
3   Is assistance/help requested with the detector? If so, what was requested and why?
4   What other factors, if any, appear to affect the extent to which the officers "adopt" the device during the field test?

The researchers were in the field for six hours and overlapped checkpoint coverage to document any changes in behaviors between research teams.

To analyze the data, the research team combined the researchers' field notes. They then used the coding techniques recommended by Corbin and Straus (2008): 1) using the study's primary research questions to guide coding, 2) identifying how content matches existing knowledge through theoretical comparison, 3) drawing on personal experience and knowledge while acknowledging potential biases and assumptions, 4) identifying findings that are similar and different from those already coded through constant comparison, 5) integrating the various meanings of words rather than taking meanings for granted, 6) waving *the red flag* to remind researchers not to take anything for granted, 7) looking at language to use the participants' exact words when possible for codes, 8) looking at expressed emotions and nonverbals to see how they match up with words, 9) thinking in terms of metaphors and similes to help explain findings, and 10) looking for the negative case or alternative explanations.

Results

In this section, findings from the ethnographic field test are organized by the five police check points in operation during the observed event. In the following section, the study's overall conclusions are presented, along with the implications for community resilience.

Check Point 1

At 10:00 a.m., the screening station[3] was lightly trafficked and well-staffed with ten to twelve officers consistently working. Researchers 1 and 2 introduced themselves to the officer in charge, who retrieved the device from its stationary position on a long picnic table near other officers. After retrieving it, the officer said, "It will make a noise or an alarm will go off, right?" – presumably justifying that, although the device was not being carried on his person, it nonetheless would be effective in alerting him to an issue. Researchers 1 and 2 instructed that it would not make a noise but would vibrate.[4] Seeming somewhat alarmed, the officer questioned, "*only* vibrate?" When confirmed, he looked for an area on his belt to secure the device, but there was none available. The officer threw up his hands as if to say "What am I supposed to do?" and ultimately placed it back on the table. While loading the phone back into its holster, the officer had some difficulty placing it in the bag with the device, as cords were taking up the space in the pocket intended for the phone portion. The officer could not zip up the device area and seemed mildly frustrated with the clumsiness. The device remained on the table except for a brief check-in from the technology team about an hour and a half later, after which it was returned to the table.

Device monitoring changed to another commanding officer once during observation. The second officer seemed as uninterested in the device as did the first. Additionally, people entering the event seemed not to notice the device, and researchers did not observe anyone questioning it.

Check Point 2

Upon arrival at 10 a.m., the screening station was crowded with a line of civilians down the block waiting to enter the event. After unsuccessfully scanning the area for an officer wearing the PRD, Researchers 3 and 4 approached an officer and asked about the device. The police officer pointed to his own vest, which showed that he had removed the detector and phone from the provided case and now had the detector on the right side and the phone on the left side. The screen of the phone faced the inside of the vest, and the officer shared that he had placed the detector in his vest so that he could see if it goes off. The officer stood in between the entrance and exit paths for the check point station giving him a wide range of coverage. Researchers 3 and 4 observed that the officer's arms were already bowed out because of the amount of items on his belt (gun on the right, walkie-talkie on the left, etc.). A few times the officer was called over to inspect certain bags. Even though the detector, chord, and phone were openly visible to the public, Researchers 3 and 4 did not observe any civilians inquiring about the device. The initial officer wore the device throughout the observation but ultimately ignored the device.

At 12:00 p.m., Researchers 1 and 2 moved to Check Point 2. At this time, the access point was moderately trafficked and was staffed with six officers. Upon arrival, one officer was wearing the device clipped on one end of his belt, allowing it to dangle. This officer mentioned that he was originally wearing the device parts in two pockets on his vest (one pocket housed the device, and the other, its attached mobile phone), but it became too heavy, and he needed to place it back in the provided holster.

The officer was with another commanding officer, and both officers commented on the device's size. One of these officers noted that he was able to clip the device on his belt because he did not have as much gear as other officers. The other officer showed that his belt was full and gave the example that the other officer carried a taser gun, whereas he did not. They also noted that larger officers have more room for holsters, as they have longer belts; smaller officers have less belt space available for holstering items.

The two commanding officers walked around Check Point 2; responded to minor issues as they arose (e.g. talking to people carrying items not permitted inside, helping file a report of a stolen bicycle); and occasionally sat in a police car to get off their feet and out of the heat. When taking breaks, the device-carrying officer took the device with him. He also carried his own additional personal radiation detector (PRD) on his belt. Both detectors stayed on the officer's person for the entire duration of observation.

The officer carrying the device being tested in this study mentioned several characteristics of the PRD that he would change. First, the color of any holster should correspond to the team's uniform colors. In his case, green contrasted with his team's primarily black uniforms. The officer explained that the color difference could cause the device to stand out and be more likely to be noticed and/or questioned by the public.[5] Further, both officers emphasized the long hours officers can often work, remarking that developers should keep in mind that the device could need to be worn and used by an individual for sixteen hours at an event such as the one we observed. Finally, like the former checkpoint, people entering the event seemed not to notice the device, and the researchers did not observe anyone questioning it.

Check Point 3

Researchers 1 and 2 entered Check Point 3 at about 2:30 p.m. and observed that the area was extremely crowded. The officer wearing the device was actively working the station and screening persons entering the event when researchers approached the station. However, observing this entrance was less fruitful than others as it did not provide a discreet location to monitor operations, and the officer wearing the device left shortly after the arrival of the researchers. He rested in his car while wearing the device for the remainder of the observation time. As such, people entering the event seemed not to notice the device, and the researchers did not observe anyone questioning it.

The station accommodated ten officers, including one K-9 unit.[6] The officers' blue uniforms also made the detector holster easy to spot. Officers who did not have the device seemed skeptical and somewhat on edge about the presence of the research team.

Check Point 4

At 12:30 p.m. Researchers 3 and 4 observed that check point four was moderately trafficked. The research team introduced themselves and noticed that the officer wearing the device had the pouch attached to his vest, but not through his belt loop as was intended. This ultimately placed the device in front of the officer rather than on his side. The officer wearing the PRD was directing foot traffic at the Check Point 4 exit. The officer shared that he had not heard anything and that "hopefully we won't find anything!"

Researchers 3 and 4 observed a conversation between the carrying officer and his colleague where he shared that he was concerned about the device being inaudible. The officer said to his partner, "I don't think I'd be able to hear anything." The two officers also appeared to discuss the screen functionality/sliding capabilities of the detector's phone counterpart. At one point, the officer with the device left his post to go to the bathroom. While he did not travel far, he did not pass the detector to the officer providing coverage at the check point exit. Aside from this temporary leave, the officer wearing the device remained at the check point exit and did not move around.

Researchers 3 and 4 observed that, aside from his conversation with his colleague, the carrying officer did not interact with the device. Furthermore, throughout the observation, there were no questions or comments from civilians regarding the device.

At 3:00 p.m., Researchers 1 and 2 visited Check Point 4. The officer wearing the device (the sergeant) attached it to his belt at his hip, similar to one of the officers from Check Point 2. Upon the arrival of the researchers, the sergeant had a few questions about the detector. The officer assumed the device would "make a sound" with "bells and whistles" upon detecting a problem, but he was uncertain about what to do if the PRD actively alerted him to a radiological or nuclear threat. He indicated his understanding was that he should do nothing because "the alarm will get sent back" and "they'll send people out to handle it." The officer did not know what he should look for on the screen or how to interpret it should the device emit a warning. He also was not sure whether the detector would vibrate at any time, and this could have influenced his decision to keep it attached to his belt instead of placing it on the table or off his person. Once again, people entering the event seemed not to notice the device, and the researchers did not observe anyone questioning it.

Check Point 5

At 2:45 p.m., Researchers 3 and 4 arrived at Check Point 5. The researchers could not identify who was wearing the PRD and approached the unit to locate the detector. Members of
the police unit, upon being asked to locate the PRD, could not confirm who was wearing the
detector. While the officers were searching for the device, one officer asked another, "Are you
wearing that thing that's gonna blow you up later?" After several minutes of questioning, the
PRD was found. The officer wore the PRD on his belt, or more specifically, on his back left hip
in the provided green pouch. He was also using the pouch to hold papers through one of the
exterior loops. The officer explained he was wearing the device because his commander's belt
was not big enough for the pouch to fit on it with all the other items they are required to wear.
The officer said the pouch was "cumbersome" and that he moved his walkie-talkie to make
room for it. The officer asked the researchers, "What's the range on this thing?" The officer
also suggested making the device so that it attached to the top of a police car. He believed this
would keep officers from having to add something else to their belts and also suggested hook-
ing the display of the car (in the dash) to the device so that police would not have to carry
and check a cell phone to view detector data. While the officer was very willing to discuss the
device, Researchers 3 and 4 did not see him interact with the detector during the course of the
observation, and no civilians shared any questions/concerns regarding the device during the
observation.

Discussion and conclusions

The direct observations cluster around three main themes: physical characteristics, technical features, and training and instructions. Before reviewing these themes, it is important to recall that
the officers studied here were also wearing their standard PRDs. Thus, the issues encountered
were with the new equipment and procedures they were helping to test, and baseline defensive
capability was not affected.

First, from the officers' perspective, the bulkiness, weight, size, and color detract from
device acceptance, and appear to be significant barriers to adoption, whereas perceived risk
from the devices does not. Officers commented on the minimal space available on their duty
belts for attaching items/devices and the discomfort associated with carrying large and/or
heavy items during long shifts (sometimes for sixteen hours). Device holster color could be
customizable to match various uniform colors to allow it to blend in with the area on which
it will be carried. Smaller, lighter devices that blend in with the officers' uniforms and fit
easily in provided holsters could enhance acceptance. Allowing for wireless detachment from
the device could also aid in reducing bulkiness. As currently designed, the relative advantage
and compatibility of the PRDs appear to inhibit adoption, which are two of the five key
attributes that affect whether an innovation is successfully adopted (Rogers, 2003). However,
device use did not appear to be affected by perceived risk, as has been found in prior studies
of technology adoption (Im et al., 2008).

Second, in terms of device technical features, all commanding officers that spoke with the
researchers, except for one who remembered being trained otherwise, exhibited the assumption
that the device would sound an audible alarm upon detecting a radiological or nuclear threat,
which is a common feature of some pager-sized PRDs (TECHBeat, 2012). Given this assumption, future iterations of the device should have an alarm with vibration as a default setting,
with options to choose one or the other as a customized setting. This finding again relates to
the compatibility of the PRD with officers' existing routines, and also speaks to the need to

provide PRDs that are as simple as possible. As diffusion of innovation theory states, the higher an innovation's complexity, the lower the likelihood it will be adopted (Rogers, 2003). Finally, this finding contradicts prior work that argued police are "all about change" (Bratton, 2012, p. 22). At least in this study, maintaining similar functionality across similar technologies (i.e. a PRD' alarm capacity) where appropriate and feasible can encourage proper device use and adoption.

Third, officers proved unaware of what to expect if the PRD indicated a significant threat. Further, in a few cases the PRD changed hands from an officer who received training to another who did not receive any training. Thus, the device should provide instructions and explanations so that any user could carry the detector. Such instructions could be attached to the device, such as on the back of the device. Instructions could include information on detection capabilities, circumference zones of detection surrounding the device, and troubleshooting. Guidance on interpreting and understanding readings and data visualization would also be helpful. All of these suggestions would improve the devices' compatibility and lower the device's complexity, as recommended by diffusion of innovation theory (Rogers, 2003). Reliable and accessible information is a hallmark of effective risk and crisis communication directed at the public (Palttala & Vos, 2011), which can be extended to risk information directed at first responders as studied here.

Additionally, explaining reasons for and how to deal with "false alarms," how the user should act upon receiving a warning, and when a user can expect backup and what that entails might help reduce potential feelings of anxiety. Prior research also pointed to the potential for false alarms as a potential barrier to adoption of PRDs among first responders (Cameron, 2008), and here we add to the list of potential obstacles the lack of the necessary knowledge to overcome these potential false alarms.

Further training suggestions include having all officers with access to the device attend formal training as opposed to training only those who are expected to carry the device. This approach makes all officers aware of what the device is, how it functions, and how to handle the device should a transfer be necessary. The field study clearly showed that observing others use the device while policing a large-scale public event was inadequate to encourage adoption. Instead, explicit training is needed, which is confirmed by prior diffusion of innovation research (e.g. Suther & Goodson, 2004).

From a community resilience perspective, the findings confirm prior research that found while the public overwhelmingly expects emergency responders to use new technology, the reality is that police departments tend to be slow to incorporate new technology into their risk surveillance, prevention, and communication (American Red Cross, 2010; Heverin & Zach, 2010). In this study, not a single member of the public passing through the police check points questioned the officers' use of the PRDs. Yet, the officers themselves questioned the utility and practicality of the devices, displaying reticence in adopting them as currently designed.

Furthermore, as noted in this chapter's introduction, there remain knowledge gaps on 1) the role of emergency managers in community resilience and 2) *how* first responders, including police, can incorporate new technologies into their routine behaviors to increase community resilience. Findings here reiterate the importance of providing training for all officers who may encounter a new technology, not just those currently charged with implementing the new technology, as recommended in prior research on police adoption of PRDs (Cameron, 2008). Findings here further highlight the importance of providing easily accessible ongoing technology support available in real time (i.e. instructions on the device) – a finding not mentioned in the nascent research on emergency managers' PRD adoption (Cameron, 2008; TECHBeat, 2012).

Future research should examine other first responders' reactions to adopting new technology that can increase community resilience if employed properly. Researchers have recognized first responders as unique workplace communities that impact community resilience (Wyche et al., 2011), but much more research is needed to understand the unique practices, policies, and behaviors of these communities separately and together before, during, and after disasters. Furthermore, researchers have theorized the importance of "pre-event functioning" adapted to the "pre-event environment" in models of community resilience (Norris, Stevens, Pfefferbaum, Wyche, & Pfefferbaum, 2008, p. 130); yet examinations of how workplace communities (and other communities) function pre-event remains understudied. Insights from this book chapter provide a starting point for understanding some pre-event functioning elements of police responders, including the importance of resilience initiatives – such as PRDs – integrating into regular routines, awareness of any pre-conceptions about resilience initiatives, ongoing and easily accessible information about new technology, and ongoing training.

Notes

1   *Disclaimer.* The views, opinions, and/or findings contained in this chapter are those of the author(s) and should not be interpreted as representing the official views or policies of the Department of Defense or the US Government. This research was funded by the Defense Advanced Research Projects Agency (DARPA) via the National Consortium for the Study of Terrorism and Responses to Terrorism (START). (Approved for Public Release, Distribution Unlimited.)
2   While test detectors required a connection to a phone in order to function properly, this may not be the case in the future as the PRD technology continues to evolve.
3   Before being allowed into the event, all civilians had to go through a screening station where bags and bikes were screened.
4   Alarms were purposefully turned off because of concerns about being discreet during the field test, but the system was monitored in real time at a command and control center.
5   Uniform and gear vary by county, state, and unit. Common colors of uniforms tend to be black, blue, or green.
6   K-9 units employ dogs in their operations.

References

Aloise, G. (2005). *Combating nuclear smuggling: Efforts to deploy radiation detection equipment in the United States and in other countries* (DHHS Publication No. GAO-05–840T). Washington, DC: United States Government Accountability Office.

American Red Cross. (2010). Web users increasingly rely on social media to seek help in a disaster. *American Red Cross disaster online newsroom.* Retrieved from http://newsroom.redcross.org/2010/08/09/press-release-web-users-increasingly-rely-on-social-media-to-seek-help-in-a-disaster

Anderson, M. C., Knutson, T., Giles, H., & Arroyo, M. (2002). Revoking our right to remain silent: Law enforcement communication in the 21st century. In H. Giles (Ed.), *Law enforcement, communication and community* (pp. 1–32). Philadelphia, PA: John Benjamins North America.

Berg, B. L. (2009). *Qualitative research methods for the social sciences* (7th ed.). Boston: Allyn & Bacon.

Bratan, T., Stramer, K., & Greenhalgh, T. (2010). 'Never heard of it'–Understanding the public's lack of awareness of a new electronic patient record. *Health Expectations, 13*(4), 379–391.

Bratton, W. (2012). William Bratton: Technology in policing is a matter of embracing change. In *Police Executive Research Forum: How are innovations in technology transforming policing?* (22–24). Retrieved from www.policeforum.org/assets/docs/Critical_Issues_Series/how%20are%20innovations%20in%20technology%20transforming%20policing%202012.pdf

Cameron, S. (2008). Securing the cities: Agencies working together to detect dangerous radiological materials. *The Police Chief, 75*(10), 142–156.

Chappell, A. T., & Gibson, S. A. (2009). Community policing and homeland security policing: Friend or foe? *Criminal Justice Policy Review, 20*(3), 326–343.

Chaudhuri, A., Aboulnasr, K., & Ligas, M. (2010). Emotional responses on initial exposure to a hedonic or utilitarian description of a radical innovation. *The Journal of Marketing Theory and Practice, 18*(4), 339–359.

Corbin, J., & Straus, A. (2008). *Basics of qualitative research: Techniques and procedures for developing grounded theory* (3rd ed.). Thousand Oaks, CA: Sage.

Dunlap, J. W. (2014). Communications and mass casualty events. In M. J. Fagel (Ed.), *Crisis management and emergency planning: Preparing for today's challenges* (pp. 141–154). Boca Raton, FL: Taylor & Francis Group.

Flanagin, A. J. (2002). The impact of contemporary communication and information technologies on police organizations. In H. Giles (Ed.), *Law enforcement, communication and community* (pp. 85–106). Philadelphia, PA: John Benjamins North America.

Friedmann, R. R., & Cannon, W. J. (2007). Homeland security and community policing: Competing or complementing public safety policies. *Journal of Homeland Security and Emergency Management, 4*(4), 1–20.

Gascón, G., & Foglesong, T. (2010). Making policing more affordable: Managing costs and measuring value in policing. In *New Perspectives in Policing* (pp. 1–19). Washington, DC: U.S. Department of Justice, National Institute of Justice. Retrieved from www.ncjrs.gov/pdffiles1/nij/231096.pdf

Heverin, T., & Zach, L. (2010). Twitter for city police department information sharing. *Proceedings of the American Society for Information Science and Technology, 47*(1), 1–7.

Hofer, F., & Wetter, O. E. (2012). Operational and human factors issues of new airport security technology–two case studies. *Journal of Transportation Security, 5*(4), 277–291.

Hume, L., & Mulcock, J. (2004). *Anthropologists in the field: Cases in participant observation.* New York: Columbia University Press.

Im, I., Kim, Y., & Han, H. (2008). The effects of perceive risk and technology type on users' acceptance of technologies. *Information & Management, 45*(1), 1–9.

Liu, A. H., Bunn, J. J., & Chandy, K. M. (2011). *Proceedings from information processing in sensor networks (IPSN) 10th international conference: Sensor networks for the detection and tracking of radiation and other threats in cities.* Chicago, IL: 10th International Conference on Information Processing in Censor Networks.

Maguire, E. R., & Wells, W. (2002). Community policing as communication reform. In H. Giles (Ed.), *Law enforcement, communication and community* (pp. 33–66). Philadelphia, PA: John Benjamins North America.

Norris, F. H., Stevens, S. P., Pfefferbaum, B., Wyche, K. F., & Pfefferbaum, R. L. (2008). Community resilience as a metaphor, theory, set of capacities, and strategy for disaster readiness. *American Journal of Community Psychology, 41*(1–2), 127–150.

Nunn, S. (2005). Preventing the next terrorist attack: The theory and practice of homeland security information systems. *Journal of Homeland Security and Emergency Management, 2*(3), 1–28.

Oliver, W. M. (2006). The fourth era of policing: Homeland security. *International Review of Law, Computers & Technology, 20*(1–2), 49–62.

Palttala, P., & Vos, M. (2011). Testing a methodology to improve organizational learning about crisis communication by public organizations. *Journal of Communication Management, 15*(4), 314–331.

Pew Research Center. (2015). *Terrorism worries little changes: Most give government good marks for reducing threat.* Retrieved from www.people-press.org/2015/01/12/terrorism-worries-little-changed-most-give-government-good-marks-for-reducing-threat/

Record, J. (2012). *Data logging radiation detector* (Honors Thesis). Retrieved from http://digitalcommons.library.umaine.edu/cgi/viewcontent.cgi?article=1075&context

Roberts, D. J. (2011). Technology's impact on law enforcement: Community interaction–technology talk. *The Police Chief, 78,* 78–82. Retrieved from www.policechiefmagazine.org/magazine/index.cfm?fuseaction=display_arch&article_id=2317&issue_id=22011

Rogers, E. M. (2003). *Diffusion of innovations* (5th ed.). New York, NY: Free Press.

Subgroup on Radon Epidemiology of the Advisory Group on Ionizing Radiation. (2009). *Radon and public health.* Retrieved from www.gov.uk/government/publications/radon-and-public-health

Suther, S. G., & Goodson, P. (2004). Texas physicians' perceptions of genomic medicine as an innovation. *Clinical Genetics, 65*(5), 368–377.

TECHBeat. (2012). Illinois distributes portable radiation detectors for first responders. *TECHBeat, 1,* 1–2. Retrieved from www.justnet.org/Interactive TechBeat/summer_2012/Radiationdetectors.pdf

Vaseashta, A., Susmann, P., Braman, E., & Enaki, N. (2012). Nuclear terrorism–dimensions, options, and perspectives in Moldova. In A. Vaseashta, E. Braman, & P. Susmann (Eds.), *Technological innovations in sensing and detection of chemical, biological, radiological, nuclear threats and ecological terrorism, NATO science for peace and security series A: Chemistry and biology* (pp. 101–114). Netherlands: Springer.

Wexler, C. (2012). How are innovations in technology transforming policing? *Police Executive Research Forum.* Retrieved from www.policeforum.org/assets/docs/Critical_Issues_Series/how%20are%20innovations%20in%20technology%20transforming%20policing%202012.pdf

Wyche, K. R., Pfefferbaum, R. L., Pfefferbaum, B., Norris, F. H., Wisnieski, D., & Younger, H. (2011). Exploring community resilience in workforce communities of first responders serving Katrina survivors. *American Journal of Orthopsychiatry, 81*(1), 18–30.

36

The use of resilience indicators to assist in the selection of personnel for employment in classified and covert environments

*Jeff Corkill, David J. Brooks, Julie Ann Pooley,
Lynne Cohen, Kira Harris,
Cath Ferguson and Craig Harms*

In the field of psychology, resilience is a phenomenon that has been subject to detailed examination. Resilience is understood as a multi-dimensional construct where individual attributes, family aspects and social environment all play a role in aiding individuals to deal with some form of adversity or vulnerability. Whilst there are many definitions of resilience based on theorists' different perspectives, most agree that resilience is represented by a minimum of two aspects; first that there is an adversity, and second that resilience is demonstrated by the individual dealing with the adversity in a way that demonstrates competence or adaptation to the environment and situation in a positive manner. However, contemporary approaches to resilience derive from a *strengths* perspective, where information sought from the individual results in an increase in options for interventions and improved life outcomes. This approach contributes a prophylactic benefit to the individual, organization or community. It is this perceived prophylactic benefit that has contributed to the systematic adoption of the concept of resilience into a diversity of domains outside of psychology.

Most notably this is evident in the national security discourse; however, it has also emerged as a phenomenon of discussion in the world of business and that of the environment sector. Resilience is referred to extensively in many elements of the literature about national security, critical infrastructure and the corporate security environment. The Australian Government's National Security Science and Innovation Strategy document clearly details the need to build a more prepared and resilient society (Department of the Prime Minister and Cabinet, 2009). The concept of resilience when considered within a security context has been difficult to define, due to the diversity and heterogeneous nature of security (Brooks, 2010). One approach may be through developing and supporting a resilient national security system maybe through the selection of resilient personnel.

Within the broadest context the national security domain consists of the various designated security agencies, law enforcement and border protection and significant components of the private security sector. Those employed in these domains are often bestowed rights not available to the wider community, provided access to information not available to the wider community and in many cases exposed to dangers those in the wider community would not expect to be exposed to. In order to select the right individuals to fill many of these roles a formal personnel vetting process is utilised to determine suitability. Some of the key criteria factored into selection include individual honesty, trustworthiness and loyalty. To determine suitability, the individual will be subjected psychological assessment, detailed background checking and a focused inter-view. Notwithstanding this rigorous process, significant breaches of trust, security and corruption still occur. The Edward Snowden case in the USA is a notable and recent example of a failure in the vetting process. The significance of the Snowden case, vetting and suitability failure has far greater consequences than just the compromise of secrets. Failure may manifest in poor team cohesion, skewing of management and leadership effort and associated post-employment health costs. Therefore, the imperative to enhance suitability assessment is not driven by security alone as there is also a significant potential financial benefit to be gained.

This chapter provides a rationale as to how and why the adoption of an instrument to measure resilience may make a significant contribution to improving or enhancing personnel security vetting and selection processes. The chapter begins with a brief examination of psychological resilience and the function of the lifespan resilience instrument. This is followed by a limited review of the security vetting processes as currently practiced in the national security environ-ment within Australia. Finally a discussion is presented of how a resilience measure may be exploited and incorporated by vetting agencies to better case manage those personnel operating in high-risk, high-security environments. Whilst this chapter is National Security-centric, it is nonetheless the assessment of the authors that the use of a resilience measure is important as an aid to effective selection and maintenance of personnel for employment across the wider security and law enforcement domain.

Psychological resilience

Over the lifespan, individuals may encounter challenging situations that place them at risk of negative psychological, social and physical consequences. Some of these individuals will respond negatively to these challenging situations and indulge in a range of negative behaviours, for example substance abuse or violence, whilst there will be others who effectively deal with these situations and go on to lead healthy and productive lives. Resilience has been defined in a variety of ways over the years. However, despite the vast range of definitions that are generally based in the researcher's interests and theoretical domain, to determine if someone is displaying a resilient profile two elements must co-occur: *adversity*, being a high-risk situation or threat, and *successful adaptation/competence* (Luthar, Cicchetti, & Becker, 2000; Masten, 2001; Schilling, 2008). Adver-sity is evaluated according to negative life circumstances, and adaptation is defined as successful performance on age-developmental tasks (Schilling, 2008). It is this aspect of threat exposure and successful adaptive behaviour that highlights to the security researcher a likely intersection of interest with those examining resilience in the psychology domain.

There is some debate within the psychological literature regarding whether resilience is a personality trait, being stable, fixed and measurable (Cicchetti & Rogosch, 2007; Flores, Cic-chetti, & Rogosch, 2005), whether it is a dynamic process that is contingent on context (Luthar et al., 2000; Rutter, 2007), whether there is a biological component (Cicchetti & Rogosch, 2007; Curtis & Cicchetti, 2007; Rutter, 2007), or whether it is a multi-dimensional construct, which also depends on one's cultural background (Ungar, 2004, 2005a; Ungar & Liebenberg, 2011).

The *Triarchic Framework* of resilience (Werner & Smith, 1982) was one of the first frameworks to include environmental factors, which suggested that protective and vulnerability processes need to be viewed on three levels, namely community influences, family influences and the individual. This framework therefore does not dismiss the role of the individual but rather proposes the need to consider additional aspects that may impact on the individual such as family and environment. This *Triarchic Framework* likely plays an important function when resilience is operationalised for prophylactic benefit in the security vetting environment.

Some researchers use the terms *resiliency* and *resilience* interchangeably. However, *resiliency* and *resilience* are two different constructs. Resiliency relates to a personality characteristic and resilience refers to a dynamic developmental process (Luthar et al., 2000). The use of these terms should be exercised with caution to avoid further confusion. For example *resiliency* refers to a personality trait and may lead to misconceptions that some people "do not have what it takes" (Luthar et al., 2000, p. 546) to overcome adversity. Luthar et al. (2000) indicated that there is a need for specificity in discussing resilient outcomes and that specific terminology such as *educational resilience, emotional resilience* and *behavioural resilience* should be used (see Luthar et al., 2000); as specific terminology reveals in what context an individual has displayed a *resilient profile*.

We argue that resilience is a dynamic process, contingent on context and culture, that it is a multi-dimensional construct that also depends upon the stage of lifespan development and may vary across the lifespan. Such belief has been developed over a number of years, during which the researchers have investigated resilience across a range of populations and contexts, have developed interventions to increase resilience and have seen the improvement of adaptive behaviour in a range of populations. A more recent definition proposed by Pooley and Cohen (2010) suggested that resilience is *the potential to exhibit resourcefulness by using available internal and external recourses in response to different contextual and developmental challenges*. Essentially, this definition adopts a broader understanding of the context of resilience and suggests the significant role played by the internal resources of the person and their access to external resources, while acknowledging the context and culture within which the person resides or works and recognises that resilience may change over the lifespan. The concept of *resources*, as proposed by the definition, is further discussed within the context of risk and protective factors. Furthermore this concept of resources is critical to the active case management of personnel operating in high-risk/high-security environments within the national security space.

Risk factors

The level of an individual's resilience can depend upon both internal and external resources. These resources may facilitate or inhibit positive adaptive behaviour. The resources that facilitate adaptive behaviour are generally referred to as protective factors; those that inhibit adaptive behaviour are termed risk factors. A number of protective and risk factors that either guard against or result in poor outcomes have been identified and unfavourable outcomes are usually defined as behavioural or emotional problems (Hawley & DeHaan, 1996). Protective factors can be considered 'buffers' between the 'person' and the 'stressful situation' (Hawley & DeHaan, 1996). Resilience research has demonstrated that individuals across all age groups have the ability to successfully negotiate challenges or adverse events despite many risk factors.

Risk factors include poverty, low socio-economic status, war, violence, sexual abuse, family dislocation, exposure to maltreatment or violence, loss of a parent, physical injury, mental illness, race or ethnicity, minority status, parental mental illness, parental relationship instability and community violence (Flores et al., 2005; Luthar et al., 2000; Martinez-Torteya, Bogat, von Eye, & Levendosky, 2009; Masten, 2001; Ungar, 2007). Many of these risk factors have been based on research into the resilience of children. In adults, many of these risk factors may affect behaviour; however, for adults there are additional risks of relationship problems, marital discord, substance abuse and domestic violence to name a few. *Buffers* between the person and the adverse circumstance provide the opportunity for mental health professionals to reduce the effect of negative events by focusing on a strength-based approach and develop interventions that increase protective factors (Anderson, 2008; Theron, 2008). Whilst factors such as poverty and low socioeconomic status are unlikely to apply in the national security domain many of the other identified risk factors are in fact likely to be amplified.

Protective factors

Protective factors can be classified into three main categories: those within the individual (psychological/dispositional attributes); family support/cohesion (and support from friends and peers); and external support (in terms of the environment/community systems) (Friborg, Hjemdal, Rosenvinge, & Martinussen, 2003; Hawley & DeHaan, 1996; Ribbens & McCarthy, 2006; Schilling, 2008) and coping processes.

The person (psychological dispositional attributes)

Dispositional attributes or internal factors attributed to the person may include self-esteem, coping skills, self-confidence, self-efficacy, internal locus of control, pro-social behaviour and empathy, optimism, positive self-image, intellectual functioning, self-regulation, intrinsic motivation, and pleasure in mastery (Cicchetti & Rogosch, 2007; Flores et al., 2005; Friborg et al., 2003; Luthar et al., 2000; Masten, 2001). In addition, with relation to dispositional attributes as protective factors, Curtis and Cicchetti (2007) mention the importance of positive emotion and emotion regulation. *Positive emotion* or self-esteem is found to be a protective factor strongly associated with resilience and improving coping. On the other hand, *emotion regulation* is a developmentally attained process and is characterised in diverse ways, including: emotional and stress reactivity, positive and negative emotionality and temperament.

Temperament and cognitive ability have been reported as protective factors in children (Martinez-Torteya et al., 2009). Children with *easy temperament*, such as a positive mood, low reactivity, high adaptability, approachability and regularity were found to demonstrate fewer behavioural problems than children with difficult temperaments. These children used effective coping strategies to deal with stress and regulated feelings of sadness and anger. In terms of cognitive ability, Martinez-Torteya et al. (2009) pointed out that well-developed verbal cognitive ability may facilitate verbal negotiation of conflict and can therefore lead to more suitable behavioural choices and better coping strategies.

Family support and cohesion

In terms of the second protective factor (family support/cohesion), positive or effective parenting, parental warmth and support are factors that predict positive adaptation in children when faced with adverse circumstances (Martinez-Torteya et al., 2009). Stable positive relationships are associated with resilience (Rutter, 2007). Other caregivers and adults that are not part of the immediate family are important to the resilience of high-risk adolescents (Ungar, 2004). Such relationships allowed the adolescent to believe in their ability to overcome adversity. Although much of this research has been conducted with children and adolescents, the knowledge is transferrable to adult populations.

External support: environment/community systems

The third protective factor is environment and community systems. The environment and community systems provide resources necessary for positive development (Ungar, 2005a, 2005b, 2007). Much of this international work has been conducted with children and adolescents; therefore, many of the community structures are based in this context. Systems have been identified as important external support factors, such as child welfare systems, mental health systems, correction systems, education systems, public health, political and legislative systems, spiritual communities and informal peer networks (Ungar, 2005a, 2005b). Again some of these systems are applicable for adult populations. For example for adults suffering from a diagnosed or undiagnosed mental illness, providing support to friends and families is important to developing the existing competencies and skills of an individual rather than focusing on the deficits (Cohen, Ferguson, Harms, Pooley & Tomlinson, 2011).

Coping process

Coping mechanisms are important to consider in terms of the resilience process (Rutter, 2007), and research is now investigating the issue of protective *processes*, that is what do individuals do in order to deal with the challenges they face? (Leipold & Greve, 2009; Rutter, 2007). Resilience results from *coping processes* that are influenced by situational and personal conditions (Leipold & Greve, 2009). The process involves an individual managing, in a positive manner, the challenging demands placed upon them. Therefore, resilience is the result of adaptive coping processes. In addition, an individual's competence in coping can be developed and learned (Leipold & Greve, 2009; Rutter, 2007), and resilience can be viewed as a "bridging concept between coping and development" (Leipold & Greve, 2009, p. 47) and needs to be explained in relation to coping and developmental theories.

Psychological resilience indicators

Currently, little attempt has been made to develop measures of resilience that can be applied across the lifespan. Scales that have been developed to measure resilience of the individual and the family do not fit with emerging ideas associated with resilience research. For example existing measures do not examine the relationship between the two types of resilience, individual and family. Nevertheless, current measures have been adapted by changing the items to measure resilience in adolescence (Hjemdal, Friborg, Stiles, Martinussen, & Rosenvinge, 2006) based on items developed to measure resilience in adults (Friborg et al., 2003).

Resilience scales

There are a large number of resilience measures, many of which are freely available to researchers and some that are subject to copyright. Resilience measures have generally assessed protective factors or resources that involve personal characteristics and coping styles (Connor & Davidson,

2003; Smith et al., 2008). These provide a useful summary of the types of resources that support positive adaptation. A range of measures have been designed to assess resilience in children (Prince-Embury, 2007); adolescents (*Resilience Scale for Adolescents [READ]*, Hjemdal et al., 2006); *Child and Youth Resilience Measure [CYRM]*, Ungar, 2008); and adults (Connor & Davidson, 2003; Friborg et al., 2003; Smith et al., 2008).

One of the shortest resilience scales contains only six questions and is unidimensional. The *Brief Resilience Scale (BRS)* (Smith et al., 2008) specifically assesses resilience as the ability to 'bounce back' or recover from stress and does not specify an age range, with initial testing conducted on undergraduate students and patients. As a brief one factor scale measuring within person aspects, the BRS will have its uses; however, it fails to capture the more extensive nature of resilience by failing to capture family and external resources aspects.

The *Connor-Davidson Resilience Scale (CD-RISC)* (Connor & Davidson, 2003) comprises of twenty-five items, which are rated on a five-point scale. The CD-RISC does not specify an age range and contains five factors of personal competence, high standards and tenacity; trust in one's instincts, tolerance of negative affect; positive acceptance of change and secure relationships; control; and spiritual influence. Although this measure claims to have five factors, all of these are internal to the individual and therefore does not encompass the extensive resilience literature that demonstrates the importance of family and external resources. Another resilience scale, developed by Wagnild and Young (1993), includes twenty-five questions that account for the two factors of personal competence and acceptance of self and life. This scale fails to account for the extended literature, as it includes only individual aspects.

The most recent and extensive scale to date is the *Resilience Scale for Adults (RSA)* (Friborg et al., 2003). The RSA is a thirty-seven-item self-report with five-point scale that measures protective resources that promote adult resilience. Five dimensions are outlined: personal competence, social competence, social support, family coherence and personal structure. It is important to note that the RSA covers all three categories of resilience mentioned in the literature, namely dispositional attributes, family cohesion/warmth and external support systems. This approach corresponds well to the overall categorisation of resilience as a multi-dimensional construct characterised by personal/dispositional attributed, family support and external support systems (Friborg et al., 2003; Ribbens & McCarthy, 2006; Schilling, 2008).

Resilience scales for vetting

Whilst these scales have their uses, none have been particularly designed to meet the needs of the security domain, specifically the security vetting function and the role of case managers in security aftercare. The researchers have developed a resilience measure that can be applied across the lifespan. It is anticipated that this scale will directly inform a specialised measure that is useful for both initial vetting on recruitment and as an ongoing tool to assess resilience in personnel.

From the literature, it is evident that resilience does not only depend on individual attributes, but also on the protective structures that operate around the individual, for example the family, the community and the environment. Models of resilience have adopted this view in terms of working with high-risk individuals. Importantly, one core principle by which resilience models or resilience program development operates is to *enhance resilience*. In order to achieve this, knowledge of protective factors needs to be reflected in the program development (Christiansen, Christiansen, & Howard, 1997).

The security environment

A core aspect of the national security environment is ensuring that its personnel are resilient in their character and ability. Vetting is the process used to determine an individual's suitability for access to classified information, environments and equipment. The positive vetting process is an intrusive and comprehensive process used for those individuals requiring access to information of the highest security classification. In addition to initial vetting, personnel with Top Secret Positive Vetting are subject to continuous review, assigned case managers and expected to keep their case managers advised of life changes that may influence their personal vulnerability. There are many similarities in the vetting and suitability assessment and subsequent management of security operatives who are employed in covert and undercover operations. The introduction of demonstrated resilience indicators will assist case managers to make better informed analysis of potential risk posed by personnel at times of change in circumstances or crisis.

Significance of resilience in the security context

Resilience is a vague but increasingly used term when considered within the context of security (Smith and Brooks, 2013). For example resilience is an undefined term when considered within the context of security. Nevertheless, resilience is a term that is used extensively in many Australian Government documents (Attorney-General's Department, 2009; Department of the Prime Minister and Cabinet, 2009) to define national security strategy, direction and policy. Furthermore, the National Security Resilience Policy Division (NSRPD) provides policy advice on emergency management, protective security, identity security, e-security, critical infrastructure protection and the security of chemicals (Attorney-General's Department, 2009).

Psychological resilience to stressors within military servicemen is believed to be increased by adaptive coping, personal control, hardiness and social support (Simmons & Yoder, 2013). It has been noted that military servicemen with high resilience are less prone to mental health issues and experience greater career and personal success; less resilient servicemen have increased risk of mental health issues such as post-traumatic stress disorder, anxiety, depression and substance abuse (Simmons & Yoder, 2013). Adaptive coping emphasises the ability to adapt to change and adverse situations. Personal control is the sense of control over one's fate and reduces fear. Preparation and adequate training before deployment positively influence this perception of control. Hardiness was described by Simmons and Yoder (2013) as personal characteristics of commitment and control in challenges. Finally, social support in the form of intra-unit support enhanced feelings of personal control and camaraderie, which increased resilience.

Psychometric testing has been a part of the Top Secret Positive Vetting process for more than ten years; however, the results into the value of psychometric testing as a predictor of potential for police officers to become corrupt suggested that the predictive value may be somewhat limited. Corruption was more likely to be influenced by environment, life stressors and disciplinary non-compliance (O'Connor-Boes, Chandler, & Timm, 1997). Girodo's (1991) study into drug corruption in undercover operations applied personality testing to 271 federal agents. The findings indicated that those with both high extraversion and high neuroticism produced the largest risk for corruption. Experience seeking and neuroticism appeared to be a poor combination as stress-induced behaviours mixed with disinhibition was correlated with disciplinary issues and drug abuse. From a vetting perspective, emotionality, impulsivity and disciplined self-image should be assessed. This appears to be consistent with Herbig's emerging evidence to suggest *significant life events* as being triggers for espionage (2008). Integrating this knowledge of the subject with an understanding of the degree of resilience they possess provides case managers with a context in which to situate a subjects likely response in the case of a significant life event.

The evidence does seem to suggest that the complexities of human behaviour, combined with the extensive variations in work environments and risk exposures, means optimal selection will not be perfect. Vetting and selection of personnel will be enhanced when a broader range of vetting and management tools are available to vetting and case management staff.

The use of psychological resilience markers as an aid to national security vetting and suitability assessment provides case managers with additional indicators for proactive intervention. These indicators will reduce the risks of possible compromise, corruption or espionage. The *Lifespan Resilience Scale* (Harms, Pooley, & Cohen, submitted) is suggested as a suitable tool that will assist vetting officers and case managers in ensuring national security through better risk management.

National security vetting

Personnel Security (PERSEC) is a process of both safeguarding the individual and ensuring that the individual is not a security risk. PERSEC should be developed in conjunction with an overall security policy and framework. Vetting is the most common form of PERSEC and consists of proving identity, background checking, referee checking and, in recent years, may include psychometric testing. Depending on the level of access to classified data, an individual will be assigned a level of aftercare. After vetting, personnel are subject to periodic security reviews with the frequency again determined by the level of access granted. Periodic review and the process of aftercare is recognition that individual circumstances change over time and with that, the individual's risk profile.

The security vetting process

Any decision about the suitability to access security classified information is based on the evaluation of an individual's character, attributes, background and actions (Attorney-General's Department, 2010). Therefore, the three objectives of personnel security are to verify one's identity, background and character (Defence Vetting Report, 2007).

As outlined in the Defence Vetting Report (2007), there are five levels of security clearance. These include restricted, confidential, secret, top secret (negative vetting), and top secret (positive vetting). Positive vetting involves an "intensive enquiry into the subject's life until suitability for clearance has been established beyond reasonable doubt" (Attorney-General's Department, 2010, p. 29). It is an intrusive process for individuals requiring access to information of the highest security classification i.e. Top Secret. Negative vetting, on the other hand, is less intrusive and aims to identify the individual's background and lifestyle likely to pose a security risk.

Vetting establishes the level of trust the organization has in an individual employee, determining the level of classified access that an individual employee may gain. Security clearances are granted on the basis of a need to know or access classified information. The vetting process has two primary aims:

1 Validating a person's identity: People have been known to present themselves as someone other than themselves. Therefore, the aim is to ensure that a person is who they say they are and that their background is as they claim.
2 Ensuring the integrity of the person and determining any personal security vulnerabilities: Their integrity is checked, which may include police checks, referee checks and perhaps a security assessment interview. The interview, which requires specialised skills, seeks to

confirm the suitability of the person for a security clearance by determining whether they have 'skeletons in their past'.

As outlined in the Protective Security Manual (Attorney-General's Department, 2010), the evaluation of suitability for clearance is based on *suitability indicators*: namely, maturity, responsibility, tolerance, honesty and loyalty. *Maturity* is evaluated by analysing a person's capacity for honest self-appraisal, personal life choices, hobbies, capacity to cope with stress, and the use of drugs and alcohol. *Responsibility* is evaluated by examining a person's history of financial responsibility and general personal history, including work information, educational background and security records. In addition, active involvement in community or charity organisations can indicate both maturity and responsibility.

Another suitability indicator is *tolerance*, which is evaluated by examining a person's appreciation of a 'broader perspective', for example an ability to accept other people's life choices or to respect those from other cultures or races. *Honesty* is evaluated by examining whether a person has a history of unlawful behaviour. Finally, *loyalty* is evaluated by examining a person's commitment to the democratic process with their primary loyalty to Australia.

The areas that are assessed in the vetting process include identity and background, drug use (including alcohol), sexual activities, financial responsibilities, overseas connections and travel, political extremism, influence of others, contact with foreign officials and diplomats, suspect associates, criminal activities, security record reliability, other personal issue and religion, that is involvement in extremist groups or cults (Defence Vetting Report, 2007). A person is not automatically entitled to clearance. The authorised officer must be satisfied that three criteria are met, namely that an individual is eligible, sufficient enquiries have been made for an adequate period of time and that within the Australian context the Australian Security Intelligence Service (ASIO) security assessment contains no information that the person presents a risk to national security (Attorney-General's Department, 2010).

The insider threat

The insider threat refers to the threat to the institution or organisation posed by disaffected employees or officers. It may be manifest as espionage in a national security context or corruption in a wider context. Factors linked to insider risk may be divided under stressors (personal, situational and life events), motivators and personality factors.

Stressors (personal, situational and life events)

In a report on insider threat, Shaw, Ruby, and Post (1998) from the Defense Personnel Security Research Center (PERSEREC) outlined that there are personal and situational stressors that may lead to insider risk. Such examples include:

- Embarrassment of being caught on video violating rules
- Feeling betrayed, rejected and criticized
- Conflict with co-workers and/or supervisors
- Illness or death in the family
- Personal medical problems
- Disappointments at work, for example professional frustrations, replaced, feeling exploited or loss of job
- Criminal and drug activities, for example alcoholism and substance abuse

- Family issues, for example marital problems and parents' separation)
- Financial stress

Shaw and colleagues mention that these types of stressors "can trigger an emotional reaction leading to impaired judgement and reckless or vindictive behaviour" (Shaw et al., 1998, p. 8), for example espionage, theft, fraud or sabotage. Likewise, Kramer and Heuer (2007) maintains that the decision to betray is triggered by a life event, whether in a person's personal or professional life that pushes stress beyond a person's breaking point. Kramer and Heuer suggest that *less emotionally stable* people may react to such situations by substance abuse, suicide or harming the organisation they work for. Herbig adds that triggers may include both positive and/or negative crises, for example divorce, death or starting a new relationship, that precedes an individuals' decision to commit espionage (2008, p. xi).

Motivation

Various authors (Gelles, 2005; Herbig, 2008; Shaw, Fisher, & Rose, 2009; Shaw et al., 1998) report that there are specific factors that can motivate a person to harm the organisation they work for. These motivators include money, disgruntlement, an expression of power to influence events, recognition, ego-satisfaction, conflicting loyalties, greed, anger, revenge, resolution of personal/professional problems, protection/advancement of career, challenging skills, impressing others, source of excitement and political reasons.

People will be tempted to commit a crime if they are unhappy, the crime is easy to commit, there is opportunity and the reward is sufficient (Smith, 1990). Motivation to commit a crime may increase if there is an intellectual challenge; to satisfy curiosity and to gain personal advantage, such as personal, financial, and competitive; and the motivation may be deeper than it appears (Gelles, 2005). Nevertheless, money is not only a motivation for what it can buy, but more for what it symbolises with power and success. As Herbig found, "since the 1990s, money has not been the primary motivator for espionage" (2008, p. xi). Individuals commit espionage to fulfil complex emotional needs (Gelles, 2005) or a combination of emotional and financial needs (Kramer & Heuer, 2007). Espionage cases that appear to be financially motivated are actually motivated by emotional needs, as money symbolises success, power, influence, a way to happiness and self-esteem.

Miller (2006) argues undercover recruits should have sufficient career experience to ensure a 'secure police identity'. Pogrebin and Poole's (1993) study into the effects of undercover policing found that the extended interaction with informants and targets can increase identification with criminals. They argue the identity forged during the undercover operation can be integrated into the officer's existing sense of self, which can have profound changes in their value system. The experiences of threat during the undercover period can increase bonding between the officer and criminals (Faupel & Watson, 1988). In addition, the undercover officer is purposefully developing personal relationships that they will eventually betray. With the dual identities and increased attachment to individuals, this betrayal can add to the stress (Miller, 2006).

Personality factors

Personality factors are important to consider in terms of prevention. General personality weaknesses include greed, impulsiveness, vindictiveness, alienation, paranoia and sensation seeking (Kramer & Heuer, 2007). Spies usually suffer from one or more personality disorders (Gelles, 2005) with the two most common being *antisocial personality disorder* and *narcissistic personality*. A person with *antisocial personality disorder* rejects rules, lacks feelings of guilt, is manipulative, is oriented toward immediate gratification and has no interest in learning from the past. He or she has little ability to form attachments or to develop a commitment to anyone or anything, therefore their ability to develop loyalty is compromised.

A person with a *narcissistic personality* has unwarranted feelings of importance or self-esteem, a sense of entitlement, lack of empathy for others; they are over-achievers, have a high self-image and a drive to be successful. Furthermore, they are unable to accept criticism or failure. Narcissists who feel undervalued by their organisations and/or supervisor may respond in rebellious or vindictive ways. Narcissism and psychopathic or sociopathic disorders have been associated with espionage (Shaw et al., 2009).

In addition to personality or character weaknesses, there are three factors that usually need to be present before a person commits a serious crime. These factors are personality or character weakness, a personal/financial/career crisis that puts a person with these weaknesses under stress and friends and co-workers who fail to recognise the signs of a serious problem and do not get involved (Gelles, 2005). These three factors indicate that factors related to espionage are multidimensional in nature and, similar to resilience, include personal attributes, a crisis or adversity and the involvement or lack of involvement of external resources.

Resilience as an aid to vetting and selection

It is proposed that the *Lifespan Resilience Scale* maybe a useful tool to assist staff responsible for security vetting and personnel selection in the wider security domain. Such a tool would assist case managers in clearance aftercare and allow proactive intervention.

Resilience as a vetting tool

The *Lifespan Resilience Scale* does not replace psychometric testing, background checking or other vetting tools; rather, it is an addition to the vetting toolbox. Nevertheless, there has been some concern over the efficacy of psychometric testing as a predicator towards future action. As O'Connor-Boes, Chandler and Timm stated, "predictive scales did very poorly during . . . cross-validation" (1997, p. iii). Therefore, the *Lifespan Resilience Scale* will provide an aid to case managers within the context of understanding how individuals' may respond to or cope with particular changes or triggers in their life or environment.

There is some evidence that suggests that vulnerability indicators such as illicit drug use, alcoholism and gambling are proving less relevant and trending downwards as causal factors in the current environment; however, there appears to be an increasing trend in significant life events triggering espionage. In addition, violators that had committed a breach of trust tended to have indicators that they were more maladjusted and irresponsible or were more immature (O'Connor-Boes et al., 1997, p. iv). Notwithstanding these factors, for the very small percentage of offenders who commit espionage after events such as divorce or workplace demotion, there are thousands more who encounter similar events or may be considered to be immature by work colleagues, but they do not commit an act of espionage (Herbig, 2008).

Individuals fall along a continuum of resilience, and determining where an individual sits on the continuum offers the vetting officer an insight into possible responses to a wide range of stressors. It is in this area the development of resilience markers have the greatest value. Being able to ascertain that individuals at x resilience are more likely to respond in a particular way for certain sorts of life events, case managers will be in a better position to assign indicators to monitor and determine thresholds at which active management intervention might be required. Moreover where it can be determined that an individual at *x* resilience manifesting *x* psychological profile is more likely to respond in a particular way in specific circumstances or in response to specific events, then an even more nuanced indicators and warning thresholds can be developed. Moreover, by determining resilience levels of individuals the real risk of vulnerable behaviours can be measured, allowing for better management of individuals who abuse alcohol and drugs. Aftercare then becomes tailored to the individual and adaptive to the circumstance. Furthermore it may be possible that by determining an individual is an *x* measure of resilience, a range of protective or coping measures may be introduced as a proactive and educative component of the aftercare process. More importantly, it may allow potential high-value recruits who, on a simple risk measure might be precluded from selection, to in fact be successfully engaged for the benefit of both the agency and individual.

Vetting intervention

Once a person breaches agency policy, they may feel incapable of reporting such a breach up, down or even sideways within the agency. Such stressors may lead a person to feel that they may lose their job, be rejected or criticized (Shaw et al., 1998). On the other hand, a person may feel resilient enough to self-manage the situation. In practice, it would not be uncommon for someone to be suspected of breaching trust to be reassigned to a non-trusted workplace or be stood down with or without pay. Research has suggested that one of the best predictors of violation has not been the pre-employment process, rather post-hired misconduct (O'Connor-Boes et al., 1997, p. v).

It is suggested that such self-management or "high" resilience is a greater concern, as many past breaches of national security has been by persons who are embedded within an agency and at a senior level. As Herbig indicates, "there has been a 'graying' of the American spy in the recent past" (2008, p. vii). Therefore, those that feel more in control and have greater authority within their organization may have a *higher* measure of resilience, whereas someone on the *low* or *normal* spectrum of the *Lifespan Resilience Scale* will be far more likely to display vulnerability indicators when stressed. Such a high measure of resilience may require greater aftercare, perhaps greater than those with low resilience, as this cohort may let the situation become dire until they are incapable of reporting their breaches. Intervention that acts as *external support* in providing the protective factor is important (Ungar, 2005a, 2005b). The clearance aftercare process could be equated to the protective factor, raising the efficacy of the clearance function in PERSEC.

Resilience as a protector

Resilience may be used as a protector, where markers aid national security vetting agencies. Such markers could develop a catalogue of life events and risk weighting in relation to resilience profiles. In addition a catalogue of psychometric profiles and risk weighting in relation to resilience profiles might be developed. Such understanding may resolve some vetting issues, be used as an aid for initial vetting and clearance aftercare and lead to improved vetting in the national security domain.

Resilience has been well research in the field of psychology; however, there is restricted research in the area of resilience markers or measurement scales? The transfer of the *Lifespan Resilience Scale* into the national security vetting domain will be a useful complementary tool.

Conclusions

Governments of all persuasions are fearful of international issues encroaching into their domestic environment, whilst increasing security capabilities and powers. Nevertheless, the danger of rouge insiders remains a significant threat. Security vetting has been the traditional tool employed, certainly at the national security level, to identify and detect the potential threat prior to and during employment, where identity, integrity and character are assessed. The level of clearance granted depends on the persons' need to access the security environment or information. The vetting process and maintaining clearance with aftercare is resource intensive, intrusive and has not always been successful. Nevertheless, such requirements are generally mandated by Governments for all departments and their personnel having exposure to the national security environment. The nature of what motivates an individual to commit an act of espionage or become corrupt has and continues to change, and there are many difficulties in dealing with the intelligent human insider threat.

The traditional process of security vetting is somewhat risk averse for clearly valid reasons, yet this has not prevented espionage and corruption from flourishing to various degrees. Moreover it is likely that many candidates with potentially exploitable capabilities have been rejected on security grounds. A tool or suite of tools that enables both more nuanced security selection and subsequent case management has potential to enhance the overall national security effort by allowing agencies to tap the human potential that has been in the past deemed too high risk to exploit.

From a psychological perspective, there are a number of factors that buffer people from stressors, such as risk or vulnerability, their ability to have some protective support and the person themselves. Resilience considers how a person may respond to such negative life situations or an adverse change in their environment, for example a marriage breakup, death or other trigger event. Within the context of this chapter, resilience is considered the potential to exhibit resourcefulness by using available internal and external recourses in response to different contextual and developmental challenges.

The chapter suggests the recently developed *Lifespan Resilience Scale* as an aid to national security, by providing government and non-government departments operating in the national security environment with an additional tool. Such a tool would assist case managers in clearance aftercare and allow proactive intervention. In addition, there is a need to develop resilience by working on such protective factors, understanding the resilience of the population and using resilience as a means to protect both the person and the agency.

References

Anderson, K. M. (2008). *Discovering how resilient capacities develop in the midst of surviving incest*. Canada: University of Toronto Press.

Attorney-General's Department. (2009). *National security resilience policy division*. Retrieved from www.ag.gov.au/www/agd/agd.nsf/Page/OrganisationalStructure_NationalSecurityResiliencePolicyDivision

Attorney-General's Department. (2010). *Protective security manual (PSM)*. Retrieved from www.ag.gov.au/www/agd/agd.nsf/Page/RWPE30AA68A4D5313EACA2571EE000AAF9F

Brooks, D. J. (2010). What is security: Definition through knowledge categorisation. *Security Journal, 23*, 225–239.

Christiansen, J., Christiansen, J. L., & Howard, M. (1997). Using protective factors to enhance resilience and school success for at-risk students. *Intervention in School and Clinic, 33*(2), 86–89.

Cicchetti, D., & Rogosch, F. A. (2007). Personality, adrenal steroid hormones, and resilience in maltreated children: A multilevel perspective. *Development and Psychopathology, 19*(3), 787–809.

Cohen, L., Ferguson, C., Harms, C., Pooley, J. A., & Tomlinson, S. (2011). Family systems and mental health issues: A resilience approach. *Journal of Social Work Practice: Psychotherapeutic Approaches in Health, Welfare and the Community, 25*(1), 109–125.

Connor, K. M., & Davidson, J. R. T. (2003). Development of a new resilience scale: The Connor-Davidson resilience scale (CD-RISC). *Depression and Anxiety, 18*(2), 76–82.

Curtis, W. J., & Cicchetti, D. (2007). Emotion and resilience: A multilevel investigation of hemispheric electroencephalogram asymmetry and emotion regulation in maltreated and nonmaltreated children. *Development and Psychopathology, 19*(3), 811–840.

Defence Vetting Report. (2007). *Defence vetting report: 22nd October 2007.* Canberra: Defence Teaming Centre Inc.

Department of the Prime Minister and Cabinet. (2009). *The national security science and innovation strategy.* Canberra: Author.

Faupel, C. E., & Watson, C. A. (1988). Undercover law enforcement stress: Some lessons from the analogy of academic field research. *The Justice Professional, 3*(2), 235–254.

Flores, E., Cicchetti, D., & Rogosch, F. A. (2005). Predictors of resilience in maltreated and nonmaltreated Latino children. *Developmental Psychology, 41*(2), 338–351.

Friborg, O., Hjemdal, O., Rosenvinge, J. H., & Martinussen, M. (2003). A new rating scale for adult resilience: What are the central protective resources behind healthy adjustment. *International Journal of Methods in Psychiatric Research, 12*(2), 65–76.

Gelles, M. (2005). Exploring the mind of the spy. *Employees' guide to security responsibilities: Treason, 101:* Texas A&M University Research Foundation.

Girodo, M. (1991). Drug corruption in undercover agents: Measuring risk. *Behavioral Sciences & the Law, 9*(3), 361–370.

Harms, C., Pooley, J. A., & Cohen, L. (Submitted). Measuring protective factors for psychological health: The development of a new measure of individual resilience (the Lifespan Individual Resilience Scale) and the relations between individual resilience, self-esteem, coping style, and life satisfaction. *Health Psychology Open.*

Hawley, D. R., & DeHaan, L. (1996). Toward a definition of family resilience: Integrating life-span and family perspectives. *Family Process, 35*(3), 283–298.

Herbig, K. L. (2008). Changes in espionage by Americans 1947–2007: Technical report 08–05. *Defense Personnel Security Research Centre.*

Hjemdal, O., Friborg, O., Stiles, T. C., Martinussen, M., & Rosenvinge, J. H. (2006). A new scale for adolescent resilience: Grasping the central protective resources behind healthy development. *Measurement and Evaluation in Counseling and Development, 39*(2), 84–96.

Kramer, L. A., & Heuer, R. J. (2007). America's increased vulnerability to insider espionage. *International Journal of Intelligence and CounterIntelligence, 20*(1), 50–64.

Leipold, B., & Greve, W. (2009). Resilience: A conceptual bridge between coping and development. *European Psychologist, 14*(1), 40–50.

Luthar, S. S., Cicchetti, D., & Becker, B. (2000). The construct of resilience: A critical evaluation and guidelines for future work. *Child Development, 71*(3), 543–562.

Martinez-Torteya, C., Bogat, G. A., von Eye, A., & Levendosky, A. A. (2009). Resilience among children exposed to domestic violence: The role of risk and protective factors. *Child Development, 80*(2), 562–577.

Masten, A. S. (2001). Ordinary magic: Resilience processes in development. *American Psychologist, 56*(3), 227–238.

Miller, L. (2006). Undercover policing: A psychological and operational guide. *Journal of Police and Criminal Psychology, 21*(2), 1–24.

O'Connor-Boes, J., Chandler, C. J., & Timm, H. W. (1997). *Police integrity: Use of personality measures to identify corruption-prone officers* (pp. 93). Monterey: PERSEREC.

Pogrebin, M. R., & Poole, E. D. (1993). Vice isn't nice: A look at the effects of working undercover. *Journal of Criminal Justice, 21*(4), 383–394.

Pooley, J. A., & Cohen, L. (2010). Resilience: A definition in context. *The Australian Community Psychologist, 22*(1), 30–37.

Prince-Embury, S. (2007). *Resiliency scales for children and adolescents: Profiles of personal strength.* San Antonio, TX: Harcourt Assessment, Inc.

Ribbens, A., & McCarthy, J. (2006). Resilience and bereaved children: Developing complex approaches. *Grief Matters, 9*(3), 58–61.

Rutter, M. (2007). Resilience, competence, and coping. *Child Abuse and Neglect, 31*(3), 205–209.

Schilling, T. A. (2008). An examination of resilience processes in context: The case of Tasha. *Urban Review, 40*(3), 296–316.

Shaw, E. D., Fisher, L. F., & Rose, A. E. (2009). *Insider risk evaluation and audit.* Monterey, CA: Defense Personnel Security Research Center.

Shaw, E., Ruby, K. G., & Post, J. M. (1998). The insider threat to information systems: The psychology of the dangerous insider. *Security Awareness Bulletin, 98*(2), 1–10.

Simmons, A., & Yoder, L. (2013). Military resilience: A concept analysis. *Nursing Forum, 48*(1), 17–25.

Smith, B. W., Dalen, J., Wiggins, K., Tooley, E., Christopher, P., & Bernard, J. (2008). The brief resilience scale: Assessing the ability to bounce back. *International Journal of Behavioural Medicine, 15*(3), 194–200.

Smith, C. L., & Brooks, D. J. (2013). *Security science: The theory and practice of security.* Waltham, MA: Elsevier.

Smith, M. R. (1990). Personnel security policies. *Computer Law & Security Report, 6*, 37–39.

Theron, L. (2008). *Resilience as a process: A group intervention program for adolescents with learning difficulties.* Canada: University of Toronto Press.

Ungar, M. (2004). The importance of parents and other caregivers to resilience of high-risk adolescents. *Family Process, 43*(1), 23–41.

Ungar, M. (2005a). Pathways to resilience among children in child welfare, corrections, mental health and educational settings: Navigation and negotiation. *Child & Youth Care Forum, 34*(6), 423–444.

Ungar, M. (2005b). Resilience among children in child welfare, corrections, mental health and educational settings: Recommendations for service. *Child & Youth Care Forum, 34*(6), 445–464.

Ungar, M. (2007). The beginnings of resilience: A view across cultures. *Education Canada, 47*(3), 28–32.

Ungar, M. (2008). Resilience across cultures. *British Journal of Social Work, 38*(2), 218–235.

Ungar, M., & Liebenberg, L. (2011). Assessing resilience across cultures using mixed methods: Construction of the child and youth resilience measure. *Journal of Mixed Methods Research, 5*(2), 126–149.

Wagnild, G. M., & Young, H. M. (1993). Development and psychometric evaluation of the resilience scale. *Journal of Nursing Measurement, 1*(2), 165–178.

Werner, E., & Smith, R. (1982). *Vulnerable but invincible: A study of resilient children.* New York: McGraw-Hill.

37

Psychological preparedness, combat performance and resilience

Rajbir Singh and Lokesh Gupta

Combat is cardinal to all military activities, and a positive outcome (combat success) is thus the desired goal. The present-day scenario has witnessed several events including changes in the political order from World War II onwards and up to very recent times, the end of the cold war, surges in technology, expanding economic ventures that have changed the need and role of militaries. Interventions far from the borders turn into cross-national conflicts, and even reorganization and restoration of political order, etc. are posing new challenges for combat preparedness in alien territories or in native borders, which tend to be quite often long term. Thus, a new orientation to applications of psychology in a military context that focuses upon the soldiers' traits and motivation is imperative.

The soldier is a basic and the important unit in military organizations. Without a soldier, a nation can never think about fighting. Among all the complicated machines used in combat, the most complicated are the men who operate the other machines, like tanks, planes and guns. What does them motivate or prepare the soldiers for combat?

Preparedness, a multi-faceted construct manifests at three levels: the cognitive level, the emotional level and the instrumental level (Mashiach & Dekel, 2012). The concept of psychological preparedness has been very well established in tackling problems in the area of health illness (Happell, Robins, & Gough, 2008; Houldin & Lewis, 2006; Hudson et al., 2013; King, Hartke, & Houle, 2010); disasters; and traumatic events (Basoglu et al., 1997; Broussard & Myers, 2010; Johnston et al., 2005; Mashiach & Dekel, 2012; Mishra, Suar, & Paton, 2011; Ronan, Johnston, Daly, & Fairly, 2001; Yermentayeva, Ayapbergenova, Issabaeva, & Asilova, 2013). It therefore is a construct suitable in the context of combat. The *cognitive level* here includes thinking about the combat before it happens and helps the soldiers to maintain their operational tempo at optimum level. All strengths combined help military personnel improve their cognitive level of preparedness. The *emotional level* implies the emotional aspects associated with the combat. Self-regulation is a key strength on the emotional level of preparedness, which helps a military personnel to control over their behaviour, feelings and thoughts to maintain their optimum level of operational tempo. The *instrumental level* focuses on the practicalities of the combat. Strengths like bravery, persistence and vitality make a military personnel prepared at instrumental level.

A model of psychological preparedness, combat performance and resilience: Empirical findings in various life contexts including military and extreme environments consolidate the view that a person (as soldier or commander) comes with several intrinsic, acquired and even temperamental dispositions. These are put as antecedent factors (individualistic) working at several levels in combination to determine combat preparedness. A tentative model is hereby presented around the key performance variable in the military context, that is combat performance and its outcome. In the traditional sense, it can be considered the dependent variable in military psychology and thus can be operationalized based on performance-based indicators. The net satisfying outcome of a combat (individual or/and unit level) is over-powering the opponent with least harm to self and maintain the pre-combat level preparedness for the future combat (immediate or remote). Naturally, such a performance shall be multi-dimensional and would pose a difficulty to circumscribe a composite of combat performance. Therefore, a construct so conceived is difficult to validate owing to difficulty in measuring/assessing war or war-like situations. Due to the seeming importance of combat, it therefore finds a central location in the model the duration and intensity of which is highly variable. There are two temporal sides to it – left, antecedent and right, outcome. In a way, combat preparedness is antecedent to the combat. The kind of combat is determined by two dimensions – intensity and duration – and is systemically related to the possible positive/negative outcome. High–intensity and long duration combat shall/may result into less satisfying outcomes despite desired individual characteristics and optimum preparedness for the first time. However, the proposed model is extendable and returns for restructuring the units, revisiting the comprehensiveness of preparedness and meeting the combat with resilience (reintegration) at the later stage.

Although high level of combat preparedness in all defence strategies is not necessarily to have combat but to achieve defence objectives by avoiding the combat. Therefore, the importance shifts from the event (of combat) to what is left of combat preparedness. It is not to have and display gestures and actions directly to convey the level of the preparedness to the opponent but rather to elicit a perceived state of preparedness to the level of opponent. It also deters the opponent from exercising the option of direct combat, and thus peace is achieved. It is perhaps another function of a high level of combat preparedness instead of a complacent approach in the absence of combat. There is a dynamic equilibrium between war and peace, which is exercised through a high level of combat preparedness. We value peace and preparedness of the armed forces at all levels in our lives and polity. Nonetheless, the composite outcome and human resources are proportionately related though mediated through combat preparedness.

Combat preparedness, here, implies usual military training and practice at the entry level, during service and especially pre-deployment including live exercises, etc. Each soldier or commander at various hierarchy levels undergoes all components of training mentioned earlier but at the individual level, and their preparedness varies a lot. Such individual differences are therefore critical to be appreciated by the unit commander before deployment so that the roles and placements are accordingly assigned. It is so important that the effectiveness of the preparations will be individualized and holistic at unit level. That is why the average unit's preparedness is material. Individually, preparedness is combined as interactive and additive at three serial levels: 1) cognitive, 2) emotional and 3) instrumental. It is, however, desirable to be fully prepared first at the cognitive level then at the emotional level leading to the instrumental level, but some would be more prepared at the cognitive level while others at an emotional level, and many, at the instrumental level, and few, at all levels. Why there would be more soldiers prepared better at the instrumental level is because training modules in general focus on instrumentality. Those who are well prepared at the emotional level may be either due to their temperament and experience or due to the emphasis and the recent inclusion of resource building at an emotional level including self-regulation in the training program among military officers. The acquisition of all the skills and development of resources through training and experience determines one's cognitive level of combat preparedness as well as the emotional and instrumental levels of combat preparedness as cognitions also determine one's understanding of emotion and action as well. The triad has omnipresence in all psychological constructs. This description leads to another question why do people in general and soldiers in particular would differ at different levels of combat preparedness. We, therefore, now go to the extreme left side of the model, which describes many traits and strengths. The model conceives them as antecedent, individualistic features leading to combat preparedness through various levels of psychological preparedness. Although there are yet more traits, our selection was based on rational-theoretical and/or empirical studies. Theoretically, *wisdom* has been linked to cognitive level. Similarly, regulation of emotion is linked to the emotional level of preparedness. On the other hand, bravery and courage relate to the instrumental level. It is to note that leadership is linked to overall combat preparedness. These traits may be expressed even thoroughly by a platoon/unit commander to determine combat preparedness at unit level. Though humanistic traits are ubiquitous, in military organizations these are implied implicitly at the unit level through leadership. Quite often, traits are emphasized at the time of selection in the military organization and further taken for granted.

Recent studies in various contexts, including military organizations, have amply demonstrated the power of individual strength, which can be inculcated, imbibed and grown through small training courses, graduated success models, savoring, resilience building etc. (Matthews, Eid, Kelly, Bailey, & Peterson, 2006; Peterson & Seligman, 2004). Combat preparedness as mentioned earlier is for several purposes, mainly pre-combat deployment to avoid an increase in the preparation period of combat by way of tactical deployment and strategies.

In the theatre of combat, a soldier acts with a lot of individual, social and physical resources. His own and his unit's overall preparedness is confronted by low, moderate and high risk/challenges (for example a low-intensity and high-duration combat is a moderate level of challenge whereas high-intensity and prolonged combat is categorized as high risk/challenge). Grossly speaking, either the combat shall be positively tackled with ease or may be with struggle. Might there be poor tackling, there shall be disruption leading to dysfunction (that is negative outcome). Whatever be the outcome, it entails and demands further processes where the combat experience reintegrates with the soldiers' characteristics especially resilience. A positive outcome in combat shall enhance a soldier's existing level of resilience, and therefore, he shall be well prepared for further combat. This usually happens when the combat event is less intense and of shorter duration. Whereas moderate challenges are likely to disrupt combat performance for some time, it will be temporary, and the soldier shall regain the optimum level of performance based on his preparedness. Such an outcome and experience shall also be integrated with the existing level of resilience greatly since the soldier has been able to regain and therefore shall be more efficacious. It could be possible that soldier fails to regain the optimum performance when the conflict is highly intense and prolonged; then the disruption shall be profound. The situation shall demand instituting more resources from the physical environment and resources from supply, including more men. If a soldier suffers injury yet is able to adapt in a post-combat situation, he is a more resilient soldier because he has been exposed to a grave situation. His cognition and overall preparedness shall be better in future because of resilience. Good training, desirable characteristics and overall preparedness do not always guarantee positive outcomes. As per the failure model of resilience, such soldiers shall experience psychological growth despite suffering permanent injury or trauma. The resources of such soldiers can therefore be fruitfully utilized in non-combat situation. After all, war is a war; the only safeguard is full preparedness (see Figure 37.1).

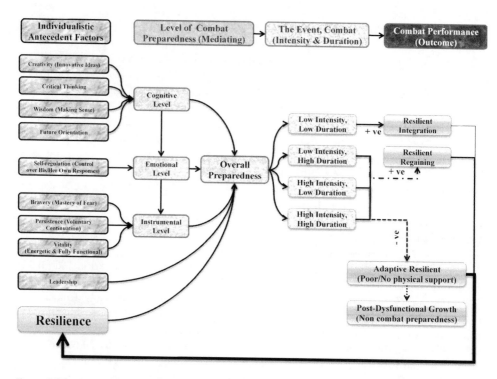

Figure 37.1 A model of psychological preparedness, combat performance and resilience
Source: Singh & Gupta, 2015.

Individual strengths for combat preparedness

A   Cognitive strengths

Cognitive strengths of an individual's like *creativity, critical thinking, wisdom and future orientation* effect cognitive level of psychological preparedness.

Creativity

"A creative man is motivated by the desire to achieve, not by the desire to beat others" (Ayn Rand, www.brainyquote.com). Creativity is best nurtured in an environment that provides many opportunities for intellectual, cultural and aesthetic stimulation; encourages the development of independent interests; flexibility; and supports free exploration that help in creativity growth.

   Significance in military contexts: A highly creative individual tends to work on several problems or projects simultaneously, frequently incubating ideas about while working on another and thereby permitting internal cross talk or cross-fertilization. A soldier/officer should be creative, through creativity, he solves an immediate practical problem, which is often seen as a sign of mental health and emotional well-being. One creative military personnel may inspire others to act creatively. A person can make a creative contribution to a particular domain with the help of mastery of the necessary knowledge and skills of the domain. In this way, creativity relates to love of learning and perspective.

Intervention strategies: Brainstorming technique enhances creativity within a group. People throw out ideas in a context that is explicitly uncritical, with the hope that other ideas will be stimulated, presumably good ones. Research findings on the effect of brainstorming are complex and do not allow simple conclusions about a best practice intervention embodying this strategy (Amabile, 1996; Paulus, 1999; Paulus & Nijstad, 2003; Rickards, 1999). An individual-level analogue of brainstorming entails deferring judgment about the quality of one's work at its initial stages (Parnes, 1963). The teaching of heuristics abstracted from the observation of creative people approaching their work can also work. Nickerson (1999) recommended enhancing creativity in persons through providing supportable beliefs about creativity; chiefly it takes years of training and effort to produce a work of genius.

Critical thinking

Analytical and synthetic minds employ such cognitive processes that browse through ideas and experiences very quickly, compare and weight them to productively solve problems.

Significance in military contexts: Critical thinking leads to good decisions and a coherent view of the world and also makes the examined life possible. Janis and Mann (1977) argued that a good thing is likely to happen when a decision is important, when the decision maker has time to make it and when it is possible that some outcome is acceptable. Tetlock (1986) shows that people think in a more actively open-minded way when they must make a judgment or decision involving values (goals) that are both strong and conflicting.

Intervention strategies: Critical thinking might be acquired like other values, partly from school, partly from home and partly from other media off acculturation. Studies indicate that education can reduce myside bias and change standards but, in many cases, does not do so. In military organization, a strength like critical thinking becomes very useful if a person has good judgment and thinks critically, which will be helpful in military operations/planning, etc.

Wisdom

An aggregate of experiences and the consolidated structure of learning to facilitate the quick understanding and abstraction.

Significance in military contexts: In military contexts, wisdom seems to be an important strength; if a soldier/officer has a strength of wisdom, he is able to make good judgments and use his wisdom for the well-being of himself and others. A wise military man may feel more confident, satisfied and psychologically and physically well and have psychological resources etc. Wisdom can be enhanced through deliberate intervention described earlier, which can suitably be adopted in various service courses time to time. Even enrollment in continuing education degree programs (education) also enhances wisdom.

Intervention strategies: Staudinger and Baltes (1996) showed experimentally that social collaboration – whether internally via a virtual inner dialogue or externally via discussion – facilitates reflection and later engagement. An intervention program for cultivating perspective is the Teaching for Wisdom program at Yale University (Sternberg, 1999, 2001) entails the following:

1   Classic works of literature and philosophy expose students to the "wisdom of the ages"
2   Discussion, projects and essays to draw out the lessons learned from reading
3   Encouragement for students to reflect on truth and values as they have meaning for one's self
4   Wisdom deployed for social ends (practical intelligence)
5   A Socratic method on the part of teachers to model perspective for students

For Baltes and Freund (2003) practical wisdom is described by their "select, optimize, and compensate" (SOC) model of effective life management. The model describes the role of wisdom in effective life management and optimal human functioning. *Selection* is the first step in life planning and is an integral part of personal development and well-being. *Optimization* refers to all the choices and actions that lead to successful goal achievement. The optimization element also includes the importance of repeated practice and effort in developing skills necessary for goal attainment. *Compensation* refers to developing alternative means for achieving and maintaining goals when previously effective means are blocked. Compensation strategies might involve finding new means and resources, activating unused resources, or relying on others for help and support.

Future orientation

"What you are is what you have been. What you'll be is what you do now" (Lord Buddha, www.achhikhabar.com). Hope seems more emotional than its cousins, and optimism, more purely exceptional. Future-mindedness and future orientation imply an articulate theory about what the individual needs to do to get from here to there (from the present to the desired future).

Significance in military contexts: The only well-documented downside of this strength is its link with what has been dubbed an optimistic bias in risk perception (Weinstein, 1989). Optimism is probably influenced by other characteristics of the individual plausibly based on genetic variation (attractiveness, intelligence, physical prowess, self-control, temperament and so on). Seligman, Steen, Park and Peterson (2005) speculated that singular events can be transformed, suddenly making someone more optimistic or pessimistic, but they also acknowledge that such a hypothesis is all but impossible to test. There is a risk of unrealistic optimism in a few.

Intervention strategies: Corsini (1984) recommends self-control strategies such as the relaxation response, meditation, biofeedback, autogenic training, progressive relaxation, systematic desensitization, hypnosis and behavioral self-management. McDermott and Hastings (2000) discussed school-based hope interventions that rely on the exposure of children to hopeful narratives: essays written by other children, children's books, and the like. This strategy is exciting not just because it increases hope but because it is cost-efficient and able to be deployed within an already existing institutional structure. Irving et al. (2004) tried a five-session pre-therapy motivational intervention targeting the components of hope agency and pathways. The pre-therapy intervention consisted of instruction in goal-setting and attainment. Initial levels of hope predicted good outcome, as did the change toward more hopeful ways of thinking.

B Emotional strengths

The emotional strength *self-regulation* effects the emotional level of psychological preparedness.

Self-regulation

"Conquer your passions and you conquer the word" (popular Hindu proverb). Lopez (2009) identified ten components of self-regulation: a) goals, b) plans, c) self-efficacy beliefs, d) standards of evaluation, e) goal-directed action, f) self-monitoring, g) feedback, h) self-evaluation, i) emotional reactions to these evaluations and j) self-correction.

Significance in military contexts: People with high self-control make better relationship partners and get along better with other people generally, sense of adjusting their behavior, report more satisfying relationships and better adjustment in their relationships (Finkel & Campbell, 2000; Vohs, Ciarocco, & Baumeister, 2003).

Effective self-regulation depends on multiple factors, and the failure of any of these can substantially impair self-control. Attention is crucial to the success of self-regulation, and indeed intentional processes often constitute the first step toward either success or failure at self-regulation. Reduced self-monitoring often precipitates factors in self-regulation because it is quite easy to lose track of one's status or quit regulating oneself when one cannot evaluate the distance between the current state the good state (e.g. Kirschenbaum, 1987). People who live only in the present moment are unlikely to exhibit good self-control, whereas future-mindedness will facilitate self-regulation. Conflicting or unclear standards undermine self-regulation (Emmons & King, 1988).

Intervention strategies: Throughout history we have counseled cultivating personal self-discipline as a way of building character and thereby strengthening the self for times of stress. It does suggest that it may be possible for parents, teachers, coaches and therapists to prescribe exercise that can build a young person's self-control. One promising route to increasing self-regulatory abilities involves cognitive strategies and behavioral interventions. Gollwitzer's (1993, 1999) implementation intentions theory considers the attainment of goals to be a function of action intentions – thoughts that enable people to cope with obstacles or initiate behaviors. The focus of implementation intentions is the way in which the person will achieve the goal, and intentions are often stated conditionally, such as when certain conditions are present, specific behaviors will be enacted. Empirical studies confirm the effectiveness of implementation intentions in helping people achieve goals. Gollwitzer (1993) proposed that implementation intentions render the response to be enacted more automatic and, thus, engaging in the response requires less effort and energy. If the actions become more automatic, then people will be less likely to experience self-regulation failure under demanding situations. Hence, one method of fostering effective self-regulation is to encourage people to create and maintain implementation intentions.

In the field of military psychology, the character strength of self-regulation is very important. Self-regulation can help military personnel to regulate their thoughts, emotions, impulses, performances and behaviors.

C Instrumental strengths

Instrumental strengths like *bravery, persistence and vitality of soldier* effect instrumental level of psychological preparedness.

Bravery (valor)

Bravery involves the mastery of fear rather than fearlessness. The military itself is interested in understanding the essence of bravery and the ways to reinforce it. Moran (1987) characterizes bravery as willpower overcoming fear and argues that soldiers displaying modest abilities make "good warfighter stuff".

Significance in military contexts: US studies dating from the end of the Korean War (Egbert et al., 1957) revealed individuals viewed as superior fighters (if not heroes) as more intelligent, socially and emotionally mature; more preferred by the peers; and displaying greater leadership potential. Accounts of combat episodes have shown superior combatants more frequently exposing themselves to gun fire, and to lead and encourage their fellow combatants (e. g. to advance towards the enemy's lines) or to support them (e.g. by fetching ammunition or assisting the wounded), displaying individual responsibility (e.g. being the last to leave the combat position) and preserving calmness in combat. Gal (1978) studied 283 Israeli soldiers decorated for bravery and found them in the top quarter on all psychological tests (superior intelligence, motivation, more stable personality). Combat skills, individual ability and responsibility should, therefore, be viewed as preconditions of bravery. Bravery is highly situational, it occurs in highly cohesive unit under a superior leader, in extraordinary situations, demanding strain and dedication (Filjak & Pavlina, 1998). Bravery and foolhardiness, which has fatal consequences, are two different things, however. Unreasonable exposure to danger is contained in military discipline, soldier preparedness and sensible leadership (Filjak & Pavlina, 1998).

Rachman (1990) found that, among groups of particularly brave soldiers, each was motivated to act primarily by the others. A valorous group of soldiers may help to knit the unit together, and the cohesive unit further supports bravery. There are several factors that may enable valor (Chaleff, 1996; Gross, 1994; Rogers, 1993; Shelp, 1984; Shepele et al., 1999; Way, 1995; Wilkes, 1981), such as contextual messages supporting courage, contextual support of pro-social behavior and an emphasis on truth telling, strong leadership, trust, clear expectations for behavior and community ties. Those who respond to challenges with a mastery orientation toward their own experience may be able to sustain brave activity easily than people without such a mastery orientation (cf. Dweck, 1986; Dweck & Leggett, 1988). Studies with military personnel suggest that social traits (e.g. sociability and a sense of belonging) contribute to the brave behavior (Gal, 1995). A group of combatants decorated for bravery or evaluated by peers as good fighters were more socially mature, more intelligent and more emotionally stable (Gal, 1995). In military contexts, bravery is an important virtue of a military personnel; without this virtue, it is impossible for personnel to sustain in military. They should be the masters of fear. An historical war of independence, the Indo-Pakistan Wars 1965, 1971 and 1999 are full with the stories of bravery of Indian soldiers (Singh, 2001).

Intervention strategies: Several popular psychology books attempt to teach bravery, but not built on a foundation of research, these books walk people through self-awareness exercises and share stories of bravery (e.g. Pearson, 1998; Williams & Paisner, 2001). Often these books and exercises involve showing people's triumphs over adversity and building a sense of common humanity through inspiring stories (e.g. Waldman & Dworkis, 2000). Robbins and CoVan's (1993) popular approach is based on physiological, habitual and attitudinal approach to cultivating bravery. Physiologically, people are encouraged to find a sense of courageousness within their body and use classical conditioning to associate some movement with the bodily sensation of power. Habitually, people are encouraged to become aware of their language and thought patterns and to break the ones that are especially limiting. Attitudinally, people are encouraged to engage in imagination and visualization exercises that help support valorous disposition and help them with emotion regulation. Toglen's practice (Chodron, 1991, 2001) is designed to use breathing techniques (Yogic-Pranayama). Finfgeld (1999) suggests that having a story values system, hope, optimism and self-confidence as the most important psychological factors that support bravery.

Persistence (perseverance, industriousness)

"Don't take a rest after your first victory because if you fail in second, more lips are waiting to say that your first victory was just luck" (a well-known quotation of A.P.J. Abdul Kalam, www.quotesthoughts.com. "Arise, awake and stop not till the goal is reached" (Swami Vivekanand, www.achhikhabar.com). In the past, persistence means persistence in effort; it now means persistence in engagement (Grimes, 2008).

Significance in military contexts: Military history presents almost endless examples of persistence, because hardly any 'general' was ever able to enjoy a long career without defeats, and setbacks, and the difference between the successful and unsuccessful ones often consisted of which one could learn from mistakes. Although persistence may be beneficial most of the time, persistence merely increases the total cost of effort, time and other resources that are expended fruitlessly. An archival study of airline and trucking industries showed patterns that parallel those of military history: initial success caused companies to persist with their strategies even as those become obsolete, and this persistence led to declines in performance (Audia, Locke, & Smith, 2000). In the military, for combat preparedness, strength of persistence seems to be important and significant. If military personnel possess persistence, they are well prepared and ready to face obstacles and difficulties with the necessary requirements.

Intervention strategies: Hickman, Stromme and Lippman (1998) exposed research subjects to high-effort training in the form of practicing with difficult and demanding tasks, and these people subsequently persisted longer than others at solving maze problems. Eisenberger, Kuhlaman and Cotterell (1992) found various benefits from effort training on persistence, and these benefits depended on individual differences. Persistence can be increased by teaching people to regard their initial failures as reflecting their own lacks of effort. Apparently, teaching people to blame failures on their own low effort encourages them to believe that outcomes are under their control and that they should keep going, preferably with an increase in effort.

Vitality (zest, enthusiasm, vigor, energy)

More a temperamental trait to be energetic, aroused and using bodily resources when the situation so demands.

Significance in military contexts: At a strictly psychological level, vitality is associated with experiences of autonomy, effectiveness and relatedness. Vitality not only appears to be a correlate of health and well-being but also may actually contribute to it.

Intervention strategies: Autonomy and relatedness or intimacy increased vitality (Reis, Sheldon, Gable, Roscoe, & Ryan, 2000). An intervention such as Outward Bound, ropes courses or other outdoor challenges explicitly claim to engender vitality, but so far there has been no specific empirical demonstration of this. For Myers et al. (1999), exercise also can yield increased vitality. Some programs that have fostered exercise in people's lives appear to increase energy and decrease depressive symptoms, provided that the activities are interesting or fun (Ryan & Frederick, 1997).

Leadership

Leadership is trait of an individual that can be helpful in building overall preparedness for combat.

Significance in military contexts: Sometime military officers behaved as "combat managers," but during the combat, the assigned role and the emerged role may be assumed by different soldiers. Platoon or units engaged in combat come up with good instances of situational leaders that organize resources afresh and think of on-the-spot, workable strategies. It has a special role in combat preparedness.

Intervention strategies: Strengths like creativity, kindness and persistence are other key army leader attributes (Matthews et al., 2006). Coalition forces, joint strikes, etc. are more common in the present.

In the military psychology of military personnel, leadership is one of the most important strengths of virtue at the time of combat preparedness. At the time of combat, if the military has an effective, visionary, helping, motivating, committed and self-confident leader, it helps the military to be well prepared for combat situations and lead to success. Leadership in military setups can be enhanced through interventions, which focus on dispositional quality of leadership and personal growth.

Resilience

Resilience is the ability to bounce back from adversity, positively adapt from adverse conditions and function well while facing unexpected harmful/adverse situation. Resilience is a hypothetical concept coupled with a situation. We can judge resilience in terms of the adaptive behavior of an individual with positive outcomes from risk/adversity.

Significance in military contexts: Nothing can be more salient a characteristic as resilience in a soldier because of the adverse nature of the combat and possible maladaptation/dysfunction. It may have serious consequences for the soldier and fellows in unit, like injury and loss of life, etc.

Intervention strategies: Training of military personnel make them prepared to face the adverse situations boldly and recover from their negative influences in better and adaptive ways (Singh & Gupta, 2015). It can be achieved by means of qualitatively enhancing and improving the protective factors around the soldiers, such as unit and family environment, social support system, welfare-oriented and trustworthy leadership and so on. As it has been seen, resilience is trainable, and impetus should be given to run dedicated programs for resilience building among soldiers. Empirical research concentrated on military population will make a long-lasting positive contribution towards making resilient future soldiers.

Conclusion

We all have different strengths/abilities/capacities or traits, for which some (including soldiers) are linked to performance in military context. Combat performance is a system variable and is centripetal, which is ensured through selecting men with desired traits/strengths. However, the optimal level of operational tempo is maintained and monitored through combat preparedness, which ought to be at the cognitive, emotional and instrumental levels all together, yet the varied intensity and duration of combat demands different levels of preparedness. Ultimately, combat performance shall depend upon host of variables in the form of socio-environmental resources, the combat preparedness of the opposing force and the resilient integration of the combat experience. The resilience integration depends upon the outcome of the combat and the experience during the combat. The real test of the preparedness is performance in the combat. Whatever be the outcome, the soldier shall attain growth even after dysfunction that can be utilized for future combat or other supportive roles.

References

Amabile, T. M. (1996). *Creativity in context*. Boulder, CO: Westview Press.

Audia, P. G., Locke, E. A., & Smith, K. G. (2000). The paradox of success: An archival and a laboratory study of strategic persistence following radical environmental change. *Academy of Management Journal, 43*(5), 837–853.

Baltes, P. B., & Freund, A. M. (2003). The intermarriage of wisdom and selective optimization with compensation: Two meta-heuristics guiding the conduct of life. In C. L. M. Keyes & J. Haidt (Eds.), *Flourishing: Positive psychology and the life well-lived* (pp. 248–273). Washington, DC: American Psychological Association.

Basoglu, M., Mineka, S., Paker, M., Aker, T., Livanou, M., & Gok, S. (1997). Psychological preparedness for trauma as a protective factor in survivors of torture. *Psychological Medicine, 27*(6), 1421–1433.

Broussard, L., & Myers, R. (2010). School nurse resilience: Experiences after multiple natural disasters. *Journal of School Nursing, 26*(3), 203–211.

Chaleff, I. (1996). Effective followership. *Executive Excellence, 13*(4), 16–18.

Chodron, P. (1991). *The wisdom of no escape and the path of loving-kindness.* Boston: Shambhala.

Chodron, P. (2001). *The places that scare us.* Boston: Shambhala.

Corsini, R. J. (1984). *Encyclopaedia of psychology-III.* USA: John Wiley & Sons, Inc.

Dweck, C. S. (1986). Motivational processes affecting learning. *American Psychologist, 41*(10), 1040–1048.

Dweck, C. S., & Leggett, E. L. (1988). A social-cognitive approach to motivation and personality. *Psychological Review, 95*(2), 256–273.

Egbert, R. L., Meeland, T., Cline, V. B., Forgy, E. W., Spickler, M. W., & Brown, C. (1957). *Fighter 1: An Analysis of Combat Fighters and Non-Fighters.* Washington, DC: George Washington University, Human Resources Research Office, Technical Report 44.

Eisenberger, R., Kuhlman, D. M., & Cotterell, N. (1992). Effects of social values, effort training, and goal structure on task persistence. *Journal of Research in Personality, 26*(3), 258–272.

Emmons, R. A., & King, L. A. (1988). Conflict among personal strivings: Immediate and long-term implication for psychological and physical well-being. *Journal of Personality and Social Psychology, 54*(6), 1040–1048.

Filjak, T., & Pavlina, . (1998). *Mi ljenja o juna tvu č asnika HV (Croatian Armed Forces Officers' Attitudes on Bravery).* Zagreb: Izvje će za potrebe Odjela za vojnu psihologiju MORH.

Finfgeld, D. (1999). Courage as a process of pushing beyond the struggle. *Qualitative Health Research, 9*(6), 803–814.

Finkel, E. J., & Campbell, W. K. (2000). Self-control and accommodation in close relationships: An interdependence analysis. *Journal of Personality and Social Psychology, 81*(2), 263–277.

Gal, R. (1978). *Characteristics of heroism.* Paper presented at the Second International Conference on Psychological Stress and Adjustment in Time of War and Peace, Jerusalem, Israel, June 19–23. In Kellett, A. (1984). *Combat motivation: The behavior of soldiers in battle.* Boston: Kluwer.

Gal, R. (1995). Personality and intelligence in the military. In D. H. Saklofske & M. Zeidner (Eds.), *International handbook of personality and intelligence* (pp. 727–735). New York: Plenum Press.

Gollwitzer, P. M. (1993). Goal achievement: The role of intentions. In W. Strobe & M. Hewstone (Eds.), *European review of social psychology* (Vol. 4, pp. 141–185). Chichester, England: Wiley.

Gollwitzer, P. M. (1999). Implementation intentions: Strong effects of simple plans. *American Psychologist, 54*(7), 493–503.

Grimes, G. A. (2008). Persistence as the 10th principle of war. *Small Wars Journal.*

Gross, M. (1994). Jewish rescue in Holland and France during the second world war: Moral cognition and collection action. *Social Forces, 73*(2), 463–496.

Happell, B., Robins, A., & Gough, K. (2008). Developing more positive attitudes towards mental health nursing in undergraduate students: Part 1 does more theory help? *Journal of Psychiatric and Mental Health Nursing, 15*(6), 439–446.

Hickman, K. L., Stromme, C., & Lippman, L. G. (1998). Learned industriousness: Replication in principle. *Journal of General Psychology, 125*(3), 213–217.

Houldin, A. D., & Lewis F. M. (2006). Salvaging their normal lives: A qualitative study of patients with recently diagnosed advanced colorectal cancer. *Oncology Nursing Forum, 33*(4), 719–725.

Hudson, P., Trauer, T., Kelly, B., O'Connor, M., Thomas, K., Summers, M., . . . White, V. (2013). Reducing the psychological distress of family caregivers of home-based palliative care patients: Short-term effects from a randomized controlled trial. *Psycho-Oncology, 22*(9), 1987–1993.

Irving, L. M., Snyder, C. R., Cheavens, J., Gravel, L., Hanke, J., Hilberg, P., & Nelson, N. (2004). The relationship between hope and optimism in the pre-treatment, beginning, and later phases of psychotherapy. *Journal of Psychotherapy Integration, 14*(4), 419–443.

Janis, I. L., & Mann, L. (1977). *Decision making: A psychological analysis of conflict, choice, and commitment.* New York: Free Press.

Johnston, D., Paton, D., Crawford, K., Ronan, B., Houghton, B., & Bürgelt, P. (2005). Measuring tsunami preparedness in coastal Washington, United States. *Natural Hazards, 35*(1), 173–184.

King, R., Hartke, R., & Houle, T. (2010). Patterns of relationships between background characteristics, coping, and stroke caregiver outcomes. *Topics in Stroke Rehabilitation, 17*(4), 308–317.

Kirschenbaum, D. S. (1987). Self-regulatory failure: A review with clinical implications. *Clinical Psychology Review, 7*(1), 77–104.

Lopez, S. J. (2009). *The encyclopedia of positive psychology.* New Jersey: Wiley-Blackwell.

McDermott, D., & Hastings, S. (2000). Children: Raising future hopes. In C. R. Snyder (Ed.), *Handbook of hope: Theory, measures, and applications* (pp. 185–199). San Diego, CA: Academic Press.

Mashiach, R. T., & Dekel, R. (2012). Preparedness, ideology and subsequent disasters: Examining a case of forced relocation. *Journal of Loss Trauma, 17*(1), 23–37.

Matthews, M. D., Eid, J., Kelly, D. R., Bailey, J. K. S., & Peterson, C. (2006). Character strengths and virtues of developing military leaders: An international comparison. *Military Psychology, 18*(Suppl.), S57–S68.

Mishra, S., Suar, D., & Paton, D. (2011). Self-esteem and sense of mastery influencing disaster preparedness behaviors. *Australasian Journal of Disaster and Trauma Studies.* Retrieved from http://trauma.massey.ac.nz/issues/2011–1/mishra.htm

Moran, L. (1987). *The anatomy of courage.* New York: Avery Publishing Group Inc.

Myers, A. M., Malott, O. W., Gray, E., Tudor-Locke, C., Ecclestone, N. A., Cousins, S. O., & Petrella, R. (1999). Measuring accumulated health-related benefits of exercise participation for older adults: The vitality plus scale. *Journal of Gerontology, 54*(9), 456–466.

Nickerson, R. S. (1999). Enhancing creativity. In R. J. Sternberg (Ed.), *Handbook of creativity* (pp. 392–430). New York: Cambridge University Press.

Parnes, S. J. (1963). The deferment of judgement principle: Clarification of the literature. *Psychological Reports, 12*(2), 521–522.

Paulus, P. B. (1999). Group creativity. In M. A. Runco & S. Pritzker (Eds.), *Encyclopedia of creativity* (Vol. 1, pp. 779–784). San Diego, CA: Academic Press.

Paulus, P. B., & Nijstad, B. A. (Eds.). (2003). *Group creativity.* New York: Oxford University Press.

Pearson, C. S. (1998). *The hero within: Six archetypes we live by.* San Francisco: Harper Collins.

Peterson, C., & Seligman, M. E. P. (2004). *Character strengths and virtues: A handbook and classification.* New York: Oxford University Press/Washington, DC: American Psychological Association.

Rachman, S. J. (1990). *Fear and courage* (2nd Ed.). New York: Freeman.

Reis, H. T., Sheldon, K. M., Gable, S. L., Roscoe, J., & Ryan, R. M. (2000). Daily well-being: The role of autonomy, competence, and relatedness. *Personality and Social Psychology Bulletin, 26*(4), 419–435.

Rickards, T. (1999). Brainstorming. In M. A. Runco & S. Pritzler (Eds.), *Encyclopedia of creativity* (Vol. 1, pp. 219–227). San Diego, CA: Academic Press.

Robbins, A., & CoVan, F. L. (1993). *Awaken the giant within: How to take immediate control of your mental, emotional, physical, and financial destiny.* New York: Simon & Schuster.

Rogers, A. (1993). Voice, play, and a practice of ordinary courage in girls' and women's lives. *Harvard Educational Review, 63*(3), 265–295.

Ronan, K. R., Johnston, D. M., Daly, M., & Fairley, R. (2001). School children's risk perception and preparedness: A hazard education survey. *The Australasian Journal of Disaster and Trauma Studies.* Retrieved from www.massey.ac.nz/Etrauma/issues/-2001-1/ronan.htm.

Ryan, R. M., & Frederick, C. (1997). On energy, personality, and health: Subjective vitality as a dynamic reflection of well-being. *Journal of Personality, 65*(3), 529–565.

Seligman, M. E. P., Steen, T. A., Park, N., & Peterson, C. (2005). Positive psychology: Empirical validations of interventions. *American Psychologist, 60*(5), 410–421.

Shelp, E. E. (1984). Courage: A neglected virtue in the patient-physician relationship. *Social Science and Medicine, 18*(4), 351–360.

Shepela, S. T., Cook, J., Horlitz, E., Leal, R., Luciano, S., Lutfy, E., . . . Worden, E. (1999). Courageous resistance: A special case of altruism. *Theory and Psychology, 9*(6), 787–805.

Singh, J. (2001). *With honour & glory: Wars fought by India 1947–1999 .* New Delhi: Lancer.

Singh, R., & Gupta, L. (2015). Resilience: Relevance to military context. In U. Kumar, Archana & Vijay Parkash (Eds.), *Positive psychology: Applications in work, health and well-being* (pp. 148–162). New Delhi: Pearson Education.

Staudinger, U. M., & Baltes, P. B. (1996). Interactive minds: A facilitative setting for wisdom-related performance? *Journal of Personality and Social Psychology, 71*(4), 746–762.

Sternberg, R. J. (1999). School should nurture wisdom. In B. Z. Presseisen (Ed.), *Teaching for intelligence* (pp. 55–82). Arlington Heights, IL: Skylight Training and Publishing.

Sternberg, R. J. (2001). Why schools should teach for wisdom: The balance theory of wisdom in educational settings. *Educational Psychologist, 36*(4), 227–245.

Tetlock, P. E. (1986). A value pluralism model of ideological reasoning. *Journal of Personality and Social Psychology, 50*(4), 819–827.

Vohs, K. D., Ciarocco, N., & Baumeister, R. R. (2003). *Interpersonal functioning requires self-regulatory resources.* Unpublished manuscript, University of Utah, Salt Lake City.

Waldman, J., & Dworkis, J. L. (2000). *The courage to give: Inspiring stories of people who triumphed over tragedy to make a difference in the world.* Berkeley, CA: Conari Press.

Way, N. (1995). "Can't you see the courage, the strength that I have?": Listening to urban adolescent girls speak about relationships. *Psychology of Women Quarterly, 19*(1), 107–128.

Weinstein, N. D. (1989). Optimistic biases about personal risks. *Science, 246*(4935), 1232–1233.

Wilkes, J. (1981). *The gift of courage.* Philadelphia: Westminster Press.

Williams, M., & Paisner, D. (2001). *A dozen ways to Sunday: Stories of hope and courage.* Carlsbad, CA: Hay House.

Yermentayeva, A. R., Ayapbergenova, A. Z., Issabaeva, Z. M., & Asilova, R. O. (2013). Testing of psychological preparedness of master's studies undergraduates for pedagogical communication. *World Applied Sciences Journal, 26*(6), 719–723.

Index

Note: Page numbers in italics indicate figures, tables, or charts.